CURRENT NEPHROLOGY
Volume 7

CURRENT NEPHROLOGY

Volume 7

Edited by

Harvey C. Gonick, M.D.
Adjunct Professor of Medicine
University of California, Los Angeles
School of Medicine
Clinical Chief, Division of Nephrology
Cedars-Sinai Medical Center
Los Angeles, California

Distributed by
YEAR BOOK MEDICAL PUBLISHERS • INC.
35 EAST WACKER DRIVE, CHICAGO

Managing Editor, Serial Books: Megan E. Thomas
Cover design: Wanda Lubelska

Copyright © 1984 by John Wiley & Sons, Inc.

All rights reserved. Published simultaneously in Canada.

Reproduction or translation of any part of this
work beyond that permitted by Sections 107 or 108
of the 1976 United States Copyright Act without the
permission of the copyright owner is unlawful. Requests
for permission or further information should be addressed
to the Permissions Department, John Wiley & Sons, Inc.

ISBN 0-471-88992-X
ISSN 0148-4265

Printed in the United States of America

10 9 8 7 6 5 4 3 2 1

Contributors

Jose A. L. Arruda, M.D.
Professor of Medicine
Chief, Division of Nephrology
University of Arkansas for Medical Sciences
Little Rock, Arkansas

John A. Bertolatus, M.D.
Associate in Internal Medicine
Division of Nephrology
University of Iowa Hospitals and Clinics
Iowa City, Iowa

Nachman Brautbar, M.D.
Professor of Medicine
Division of Nephrology
University of Southern California
School of Medicine
Los Angeles, California

Vito M. Campese, M.D.
Professor of Medicine
Division of Nephrology
University of Southern California
School of Medicine
Los Angeles, California

Matthew E. Conolly, M.D.
Associate Professor of Medicine and Pharmacology
University of California, Los Angeles
School of Medicine
Los Angeles, California

Ralph E. Cutler, M.D.
Chief, Clinical Pharmacology Section
Loma Linda University Medical Center
Associate Chief, Nephrology Section
Jerry L. Pettis Veterans Administration Hospital
Loma Linda, California

Gary M. Davis, M.D.
Fellow in Nephrology
Loma Linda University Medical Center
Loma Linda, California

Eben I. Feinstein, M.D.
Assistant Professor of Medicine
Division of Nephrology
University of Southern California
School of Medicine
Los Angeles, California

Marshal P. Fichman, M.D.
Clinical Professor of Medicine
University of Southern California
School of Medicine
Medical Director, Dialysis Unit
Cedars-Sinai Medical Center
Los Angeles, California

William J. Flanigan, M.D.
Professor of Medicine
Director of Transplantation
University of Arkansas for Medical Science
Little Rock, Arkansas

Steven C. Forland, Pharm.D.
Assistant Professor of Pharmacology
Loma Linda University Medical Center
Loma Linda, California

Robert Gold, M.D.
Instructor in Medicine
Division of Nephrology
Fellow, National Kidney Foundation
University of Arkansas for Medical Sciences
Little Rock, Arkansas

Michael Golub, M.D.
Assistant Professor of Medicine
University of California, Los Angeles
School of Medicine
Los Angeles, California
Assistant Chief, Division of Hypertension
Sepulveda Veterans Administration Medical Center
Sepulveda, California

Helen Gruber, M.D.
Professor of Medicine
Division of Nephrology
University of Southern California
School of Medicine
Los Angeles, California

Lawrence G. Hunsicker, M.D.
Associate Professor of Internal Medicine
Division of Nephrology
University of Iowa Hospitals and Clinics
Iowa City, Iowa

Joel D. Kopple, M.D.
Professor of Medicine and Public Health
University of California, Los Angeles
School of Medicine
Los Angeles, California

David B. N. Lee, M.D.
Associate Professor of Medicine
Chief, Division of Nephrology
Sepulveda Veterans Administration Medical Center
Sepulveda, California

Robert T. Misson, M.D.
Fellow in Nephrology
Loma Linda University Medical Center
Loma Linda, California

John Z. Montgomerie, M.D.
Professor of Medicine
University of Southern California
School of Medicine

Los Angeles, California
Chief, Infectious Disease Division
Rancho Los Amigos Hospital
Downey, California

Karl D. Nolph, M.D.
Professor of Medicine
University of Missouri Health Sciences Center
Director, Division of Nephrology
Harry S. Truman Memorial Veterans Administration Hospital
Columbia, Missouri

Gerhard Opelz, M.D.
Professor of Surgery
Director, Transplantation Immunology
University of Heidelberg
Heidelberg, West Germany

Shiva Rastogi, M.D.
Assistant Professor of Medicine
Division of Nephrology
University of Arkansas for Medical Sciences
Little Rock, Arkansas

Ronald Skowsky, M.D.
Associate Professor of Medicine
California College of Medicine
University of California at Irvine
Irvine, California
Chief, Endocrinology and Metabolism
Veterans Administration Medical Center
Long Beach, California

James Sowers, M.D.
Associate Professor of Medicine
University of California, Los Angeles
School of Medicine
Los Angeles, California
Assistant Chief
Division of Endocrinology and Metabolism
Sepulveda Veterans Administration Medical Center
Sepulveda, California

John C. Van Stone
Associate Professor of Medicine
University of Missouri School of Medicine
Columbia, Missouri

Richard Wheeler, M.D.
Instructor in Nephrology
University of Arkansas for Medical Sciences
Little Rock, Arkansas

Marsha Wolfson, M.D.
Associate Professor of Medicine
Oregon Health Sciences University
Portland, Oregon

Preface

He possesses two out of the three qualities necessary for the ideal detective. He has the power of observation and that of deduction. He is only wanting in knowledge, and that may come in time.

Sir Arthur Conan Doyle, *The Science of Deduction*

Arthur Conan Doyle was a physician before he became better known as the creator of that most astute fictional character, Sherlock Holmes. Conan Doyle must have extrapolated from his own earlier experience that, although observation and deduction are essential skills, the accumulation of knowledge is a never-ending but requisite task for the successful practitioner, whether physician or detective. As with past editions of *Current Nephrology*, the editor and authors of this volume hope that we have lightened this burden for our colleagues.

Harvey C. Gonick

Preface to Volume 1

For education the lesson is clear: its prime objective must be to increase the individual's "cope-ability"—the speed and economy with which he can adapt to continual change.

Alvin Toffler, *Future Shock*

Nephrology has indeed come of age as a subspecialty of internal medicine. Not only are there several excellent textbooks and journals in this field, but also symposia addressed to specific areas within nephrology appear each year. Why then yet another treatise? Nephrology is still a rapidly evolving field in which the busy clinician may easily fall behind if he does not have ready access to new information. This problem is of course not unique to nephrology, but is equally pertinent to all fields in which the rate of explosion of knowledge exceeds the capacity of the postgraduate to assimilate recent data and apply it in his daily work.

In addressing ourselves to this issue, we sought to provide a partial solution by creating an annual volume in which the literature within the disciplines of nephrology published within the preceding year was reviewed by an authority in each area, and placed in the perspective of existing knowledge. After much deliberation, certain ground rules were established. Each contributor agreed to survey all of the English language literature within the assigned year (October 1, 1975 to September 30, 1976), and to orient his presentation toward the clinician. Thus clinical studies were to be emphasized over animal experimentation, and animal studies were to be discussed in the context of the relevant clinical problem. The contributors had complete freedom to express their own views of the validity and significance of these articles. To the extent possible, the style was to be informal and informative. Each chapter was to begin with an introduction reviewing the state-of-the-art in that discipline prior to the year's articles. The individual chapters were to be illustrated by figures and tables reprinted from selected key articles, and on occasion, by original material from the contributors.

I believe that we have come close to satisfying these objectives. As this was the first volume, flexibility was allowed in the assigned year in order that important articles appearing a few months before or after the review dates could be included. Also, earlier pertinent references have been included to provide a background for discussion. It proved somewhat difficult to limit the basic researchers in our group in their discussion of critical animal experiments. In certain chapters it was possible to review every article published within the review period, but in others, because of the extensive amount of material, it was necessary to delete articles which in the opinion of the contributor did not add significantly to the knowledge in the field. Thus, this review cannot be considered to be exhaustive in scope. There is also considerable variability in chapter lengths, reflecting, in part, the degree of current interest, and therefore, investigation in each discipline.

The contributors and I consider that we have benefited from this intensive review of articles related to our special fields of interest. We hope that we have presented the information to you, the reader, in a manner that is easily assimilated. The proximity of the contributors has made it possible for us to coordinate our efforts and interact more closely than is usually the case in multiauthored publications, and we think that the publication has benefited from these continued discussions. We apologize to those authors whose contributions we may have deliberately or inadvertently deleted, and extend our appreciation to those authors and publishers who have graciously permitted the use of their data and figures.

To Dr. Charles Kleeman, Professor of Medicine and Chief of Nephrology at U.C.L.A. Medical Center, we extend our deepest appreciation for his leadership and guidance. Many of us had Dr. Kleeman as our mentor and have greatly benefited from his stimulating and innovative approaches to new problems.

Harvey C. Gonick

Contents

1 **Peritoneal Dialysis** 1
  Karl D. Nolph

2 **Hemodialysis** 57
  John C. Van Stone

3 **Clinical Transplantation** 107
  William J. Flanigan and Gerhard Opelz

4 **Pharmacology of Drugs in Renal Failure** 131
  Ralph E. Cutler, Steven C. Forland, Gary M. Davis, and Robert T. Misson

5 **Parenteral Nutrition in the Treatment of Acute Renal Failure** 175
  Eben I. Feinstein, Marsha Wolfson, and Joel D. Kopple

6 **Glomerulonephritis and Nephrotic Syndrome** 197
  John A. Bertolatus and Lawrence G. Hunsicker

7 **Urinary Tract Infections** 251
  John Z. Montgomerie

8 **Hypertension** 267
  Vito M. Campese, James Sowers, Michael Golub, and Matthew Conolly

9 **Acid-Base Metabolism** 299
  Jose A. L. Arruda, Robert Gold, Richard Wheeler, and Shiva Rastogi

10 **Disorders of Calcium, Phosphorus, and Magnesium** 371
  Nachman Brautbar, Helen Gruber, and David B. N. Lee

11 **Physiology and Disorders of Water Metabolism** 489
  Ronald Skowsky and Marshal P. Fichman

Index 555

CURRENT NEPHROLOGY
Volume 7

CHAPTER 1

Peritoneal Dialysis

Karl D. Nolph

With few exceptions, the papers reviewed herein cover the period from September 1981 through September 1982. By the fall of 1982 there were over 16,000 patients on continuous ambulatory peritoneal dialysis (CAPD) worldwide and over 7,000 CAPD patients in the United States. In some countries, patients on CAPD represented more than 20% of the dialysis population (Canada, the United Kingdom, Australia, New Zealand, and South Africa). In Scandinavia, 15% of the patients were on CAPD. In the United States, the CAPD population represented 11% of the dialysis population. Intermittent peritoneal dialysis (IPD) continues to be used as a chronic form of therapy in some centers although it is used mainly for acute or transient problems in most centers. There is growing interest in continuous cycling peritoneal dialysis (CCPD). All of these activities have resulted in a continuing rapid expansion of the peritoneal dialysis literature.

ANATOMY, PHYSIOLOGY, AND PERITONEAL TRANSPORT

Peritoneal Ultrafiltration

A hypothesis has been published to explain many of the characteristics of osmotically induced peritoneal ultrafiltration (1). This hypothesis relies on morphologic and functional evidence that suggests that proximal capillaries are less permeable than venules. High concentrations of glucose in the peritoneal interstitium should exert more effective osmotic pressure across the proximal capillary wall. The proximal capillary is the site of higher hydraulic pressure. Thus, the bulk of peritoneal ultrafiltration could occur across a less permeable portion of the microcirculation.

A review of this hypothesis mentions our state of ignorance regarding the distribution of glucose concentrations from the peritoneal cavity to the interstitium to the capillary blood (1). It is not known whether there are significant glucose concentration gradients across both capillary walls and mesothelium or whether mesothelium is so permeable that interstitial glucose concentrations quickly approach those of dialysis solution. Much of the interest in peritoneal anatomy and its influence on peritoneal transport in the past year has focused on the role of the mesothelium. In our previous reviews we focused on in vitro and in vivo studies suggesting that mesothelium is very permeable and offers little resistance to passive solute transport during peritoneal dialysis. There is some debate as to whether relatively wide mesothelial intercellular gaps are true representations of in vivo conditions or are merely artifacts.

It is well known that during peritonitis, glucose absorption increases and ultrafiltration decreases. Protein losses increase. All of these findings suggest increased peritoneal permeability during peritonitis. The loss of ultrafiltration represents the effects of rapid glucose absorption and loss of the osmotic gradient for ultrafiltration. In a study this year by Rubin and colleagues (2) these changes in patients caused by peritonitis were nicely demonstrated. Peritoneal transport characteristics return toward normal following resolution of the infection.

In our previous reviews we have emphasized the importance of the peritoneal microcirculation to peritoneal transport. The changes with peritonitis could thus represent vasodilatory effects of inflammation, perhaps secondary to the endogenous release of vasodilatory substances, such as histamine, bradykinin, and prostaglandins. Several recent studies, however, suggest that changes in mesothelium could also contribute to these transport alterations (3). Peritoneal biopsies obtained from 15 cadavers and from 13 patients on CAPD suggested that loss of ultrafiltration was associated with higher permeability and rapid glucose absorption secondary to patchy or total destruction of the mesothelium in certain areas of the peritoneum. The endothelium of capillaries was normal but the distance separating capillaries from the peritoneal cavity seemed to be diminished adjacent to areas of mesothelial denudation.

Even more recent studies in rats show rapid glucose absorption and loss of ultrafiltration with peritonitis or mesothelial drying (4). Protein losses in dialysate also increased (Figs. 1–3). With either peritonitis or mesothelial drying, morphologic studies showed loss of mesothelial villae and widening of mesothelial intercellular gaps. With peritonitis, there were deeper peritoneal changes, including interstitial inflammation and vasodilatation. Round cells could also be seen moving through the widened mesothelial or intercellular gaps in peritonitis (Fig. 4). These studies are interesting in that similar mesothelial alterations were associated with the same alterations in transport, even though with drying, the deeper peritoneum and the microcirculation seemed unchanged (4). Thus, these recent

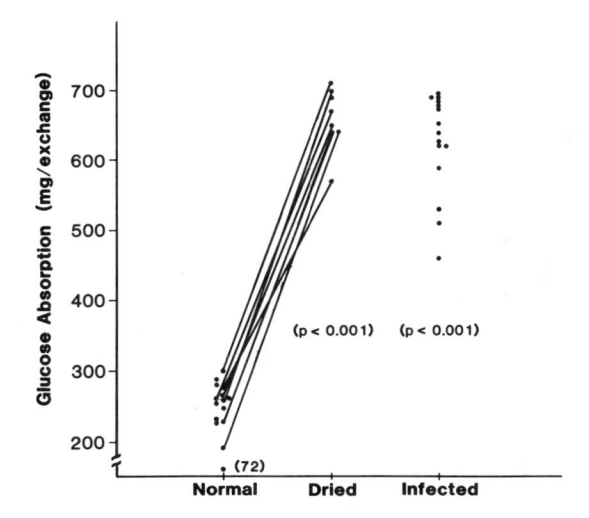

Figure 1. Glucose absorptions from peritoneal dialysis exchanges in rats. The solution contained 4.25% dextrose. Instillation volume was 22 ml. Total cycle time was 2 hours. Following control exchanges (normal) rats underwent laparotomy and gentle drying of the mesentery for 10–20 minutes. Following closure, transport studies were repeated after 10 hours. Transport studies were also performed in another group of rats during acute peritonitis which developed following catheter implantation. Absorption postdrying and with infection is compared to normal values by paired and nonpaired t analysis. (Verger C et al: Acute changes in peritoneal morphology and transport properties with infectious peritonitis and mechanical injury. *Kidney Int* [in press]. Reprinted with permission.)

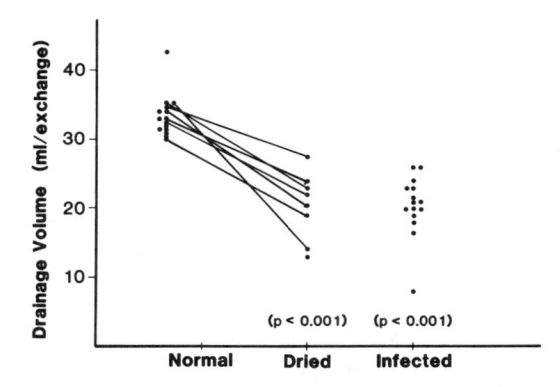

Figure 2. Drainage volumes for the same studies as in Fig. 1. (Verger C et al: Acute changes in peritoneal morphology and transport properties with infectious peritonitis and mechanical injury. *Kidney Int* [in press]. Reprinted with permission.)

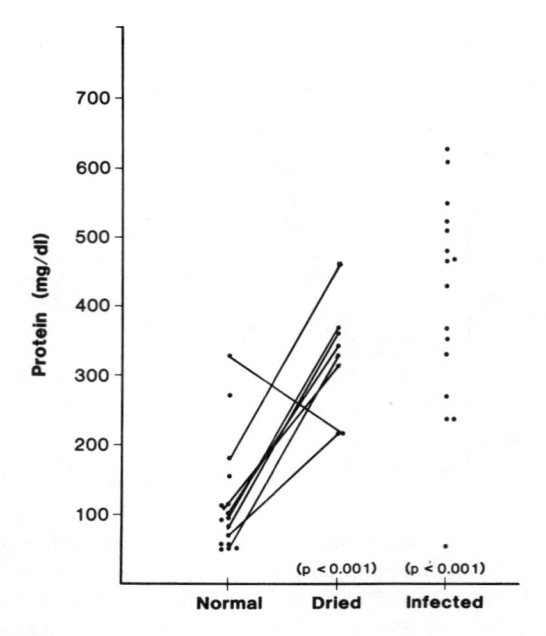

Figure 3. Dialysate protein concentrations from the same studies as in Fig. 1. (Verger C et al: Acute changes in peritoneal morphology and transport properties with infectious peritonitis and mechanical injury. *Kidney Int* [in press]. Reprinted with permission.)

findings suggest that the mesothelium may be an important resistant site and changes therein may in part explain transport changes that occur with peritoneal injury.

One study reported ultrastructural analyses of the peritoneum of normal rats, mice, and humans, uremic patients, and patients on CAPD (5). The ultrastructural features of mesothelium and subadjacent tissues in normal man, animals, and uremic patients, were very similar. Patients on CAPD showed some areas of cellular degeneration and edema in the mesothelium. The cause of these alterations, or their importance, is unknown.

Additional work with a variety of polyanions as osmotic agents in a simulated in vitro model of peritoneal dialysis was reported (6). These studies, like previous ones, show that sodium salts of large polyanions can exert osmotic pressure in situations simulating peritoneal dialysis. Since animal studies of toxicology are just beginning in this area, it will be some time before clinical studies can be initiated.

In 16 patients, the net sieving coefficients for sodium, potassium, urea, creatinine, and inulin were measured during 2.066 liter, 4.25% dextrose exchanges with 10 minute inflow, 20 minute drainage, and dwell time of 10, 20, or 30 minutes (7). Dialysis solution concentrations at instillation were set to eliminate initial concentration gradients for net diffusion.

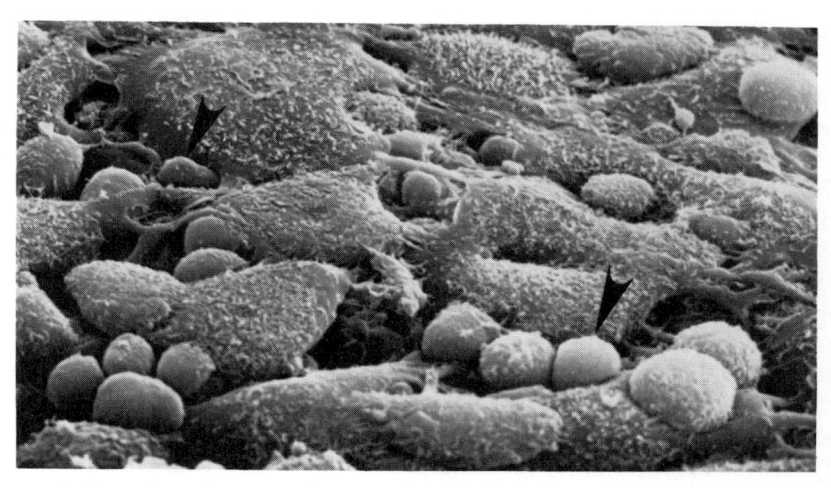

Figure 4. Scanning electron micrograph of infected rat mesentery. Round forms appear to be moving through widened intercellular spaces (arrows). There is loss of mesothelial surface villae. ×1,500 (Verger C et al: Acute changes in peritoneal morphology and transport properties with infectious peritonitis and mechanical injury. *Kidney Int* [in press]. Reprinted with permission.)

Mean net sieving coefficients with 30 minute dwells are shown in Table 1. Variations in dwell time in the range mentioned did not result in significant changes. The authors contend that the low net sieving coefficients support the concept that a portion of the ultrafiltrate might follow a transcellular route to the peritoneal cavity. They suggest that "water movement could be in part through extracellular pathways with low resistance" and "in part through transcellular routes with high resistance to solute movement." They call this the "two pipe" model. High resistance routes through extracellular channels could also explain their data.

Augmentation of Peritoneal Clearances

Arachidonic acid has been shown to increase peritoneal clearances, perhaps due to increased synthesis of vasodilatory prostaglandins (8).

Table 1. Net Sieving Coefficients (Peritoneal) (Mean ± SEM)

Solute	Sieving Coefficient	n
Sodium	0.56 ± .04	14
Potassium	0.40 ± .04	11
Urea	0.63 ± .06	10
Creatinine	0.57 ± .09	8
Inulin	0.41 ± .08	6

SOURCE: Rubin J et al: *ASAIO* 5:9–15, 1982. Reprinted with permission.

Docusate sodium increases peritoneal clearances in rabbits. Clearance increases for urea and creatinine range from 74% to 244%. Mechanisms for the effects of this substance on clearances are unknown (9).

In seven uremic patients on CAPD, it was shown that combining nitroprusside (4.5 mg/liter), hypertonic exchanges (4.25 g/dl), warming dialysate to 42°C, and dialysate flow rates of 3.4 liters/hr increased peritoneal urea clearances to values ranging from 30.3 to 42.2 ml/min/1.73 m^2, with a mean value of 35.6 (10). Most reported peak values of urea clearance in humans undergoing peritoneal dialysis are in this same range. The synergistic effects of these maneuvers optimize vasodilatation, blood flow, and dialysate flow, as well as convective transport. Limitations probably reflect stagnant fluid films, membrane resistances, and a limited number of capillaries involved in exchange.

Studies in an in vitro model demonstrated that conventional peritoneal dialysis is probably limited by stagnant fluid films within the peritoneal cavity and that the disruption of these films can augment clearances (11). The studies consisted of in vitro simulations of peritoneal dialysis with and without vigorous mixing of the dialysate compartment. The studies also included peritoneal clearance measurements in quiescent rats and in rats undergoing external massage of the abdomen every 10 seconds. Clearances were augmented in both in vitro and in vivo studies, presumably by better mixing within the peritoneal cavity. The application of these studies to clinical dialysis is unknown since there are obvious limitations to the amount of mixing that can be tolerated.

New studies have identified the vasodilatory components of commercially available peritoneal dialysis solutions (12). Microscopic observations of blood vessels in anesthetized rats were carried out with in vivo television microscopy. Small arterial diameters were quantitated. Hyperosmolality produced submaximal dilatation. Dextrose, sucrose, or sodium chloride could be used to create a hyperosmolar solution. The rate of dilatation differed depending on the substance used to increase osmolality. Near isotonic solutions with acetate (74 mmol) or lactate (45 mmol) produced slow submaximal dilatation. Hyperosmolar solutions containing acetate or lactate at the same concentrations as above produced rapid maximal dilatation of these vessels. Thus, the dilatory effects of commercial solutions appear to be due to the combinations of high osmolality and the buffer anions acetate or lactate.

The effect of protamine, a polycationic protein, on mesothelial permeability and ultrastructure was evaluated in a rat model of peritoneal dialysis (13). Following intraperitoneal instillation of protamine sulfate in varying concentrations, peritoneal permeability to urea and inulin were measured. Effects on the ultrastructure of the omentum were also assessed. In animals receiving 5–30 µg/ml of protamine, decreases in permeability to inulin were seen without significant alterations in permeability to urea. At protamine concentrations of 30–75 µg/ml, the peritoneal permeability to urea increased by 50% and to inulin by 20%. At these same concentrations, mesothelial cells showed a loss of microvillae and minor changes in submembranous cytoplasmic microfilaments, but the intramembranous structure of occluding junctions showed no significant changes. When protamine sulfate was instilled at concentrations of 100 µg/ml, there was an irreversible doubling of permeability to inulin without a comparable effect on permeability to urea. Disruptions of occluding cell junctions were seen in focal areas. The authors suggest that inulin diffuses primarily paracellularly, whereas urea moves mainly through the transcellular pathways; protamine could affect both pathways, depending on the intraperitoneal concentration used. They further suggest that permeability changes induced by protamine may be mediated through the cytoskeleton of the mesothelial cell.

Assessment of Peritoneal Transport

Lactate in commercial solutions is present in racemic configuration (14). The peritoneal uptakes of L(+) and D(−) lactate from the peritoneal cavity during peritoneal dialyses with short cycle exchanges and long cycle exchanges were compared. L(+) lactate was absorbed more rapidly from the peritoneal cavity, suggesting that the passive movement of lactate across the peritoneal membrane is relatively stereospecific. Since patients have been maintained on racemic lactate solutions, it seems apparent that both isomers must be absorbed and metabolized, even if at somewhat different rates.

Peritoneal dialysis is used to treat some very severe cases of psoriasis. Although controlled studies have yet to be published, many patients appear to receive some benefit from this treatment. Solute equilibration studies were performed in patients with psoriasis and normal renal function and compared to similar studies in patients with renal failure undergoing peritoneal dialysis (15). Calcium, phosphorus, uric acid, and protein equilibration rates were faster in uremics. Mechanisms for such differences are unknown, but they raise questions as to possible effects of uremia on the permeability of biologic membranes.

Transport kinetics were assessed for multiple substances (16–18). A positive net transfer of calcium from dialysis fluid to blood was demonstrated in several groups of patients undergoing intermittent peritoneal dialysis (17). Peritoneal clearances of theophylline were found to average 11.67 ml/min (18). The average theophylline to creatinine clearance ratio was 0.85.

Peritoneal dialysis kinetic studies were reported in six puppies and five adult dogs (19). Peritoneal dialysance values and permeability indices were examined for multiple solutes. Dialysances of inulin and urea per kilogram of body weight and permeability indices were higher in the young dogs. The data are compatible with the young having an increased peritoneal

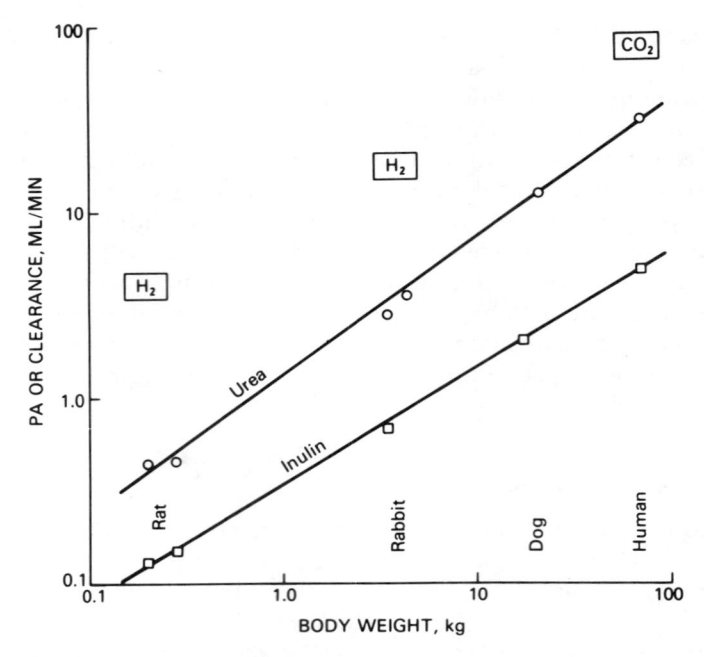

Figure 5. Mass transfer coefficient or clearance for urea and inulin in several species. Urea: rat, rabbit, dog, human. Inulin: rat, rabbit, dog, human. For reference, dissolved gas clearance is shown for hydrogen in the rat and in the rabbit, and for carbon dioxide in humans. (Dedrick RL et al: Is the peritoneum a membrane? *ASAIO* 5: 1–8, 1982. Reprinted with permission.)

membrane permeability and/or increased functional peritoneal surface area relative to body weight. The increases in solute movement were independent of dialysis mechanics and were thought to reflect age-related differences in the intrinsic characteristics of the peritoneal membrane.

An experimental model for studies of continuous peritoneal dialysis in uremic rabbits was described (20). Partial nephrectomy of one kidney and partial (five-sixths) destruction of the cortex of the remaining kidney by electrocauterization provided a simple and reproducible model. CAPD resulted in adequate control of uremia in the animals, but decreases in total plasma proteins and weight were noted. The model is felt suitable for studies of the metabolic complications of CAPD. Peritoneal transport studies could also be carried out in this model.

The movement of solutes between the peritoneal cavity and blood has been described theoretically as a process spatially distributed in tissues (21). Predictions of peritoneal permeabilities from microcirculatory observations and intratissue diffusivity were consistent with reported transport parameters as a function of solute molecular weight and body weight. Effective peritoneal area should exhibit a two-thirds power dependence on body weight. Figure 5 shows a summary of multiple measurements of mass transfer coefficients or clearances of urea and inulin related to body weight. Overall values are proportional to (body weight)$^{0.68}$, an exponent near the predicted 0.66.

CONTINUOUS AMBULATORY PERITONEAL DIALYSIS (CAPD)

Much of the peritoneal dialysis literature represents reports from many centers summarizing their experiences with CAPD (22–70). Most of these focus on speculations as to the eventual place of CAPD in end-stage renal disease therapy, dropout rates, experiences in patients with diabetes mellitus, and a variety of clinical observations. One report notes that CAPD now allows home dialysis as an option for many more patients with end-stage renal disease (29).

In this section I focus on studies that relate to the National CAPD Registry, patient survival, patient dropout, comparisons with other forms of dialysis therapy, nutritional and metabolic aspects of CAPD, modifications in CAPD technique, kidney transplantation in patients on CAPD, experiences with CAPD in patients with diabetes mellitus, and other observations relative to transport and problems that may be primarily a manifestation of CAPD. Peritonitis and a variety of complications not unique to CAPD but described under CAPD in the peritoneal dialysis literature are reviewed in separate sections.

National CAPD Registry, Patient Survival, Technique Survival, and Comparisons with Other Forms of Therapy

The National Institutes of Health have sponsored a National Registry for patients on continuous ambulatory peritoneal dialysis. As of November, 1982, there were over 5,000 patients in the National Registry, representing a high fraction of the over 7,000 patients on CAPD in the country at that time. The CAPD Registry is voluntary. Follow-up data on registered patients is in the early stages of collection and results on the national level are preliminary and not yet published. However, during 1981, 14 centers participated in a pilot phase collection of follow-up data. These centers were selected on the basis of experience and the size of their CAPD programs to test the feasibility of the Registry format. The results of this pilot study may not be indicative of more widespread experience. Patients at those centers who began CAPD during 1981, or who were on CAPD at the beginning of 1981, were followed. Data from 567 patients monitored for 320 patients years were analyzed (71). The average time on CAPD therapy was 14 ± 9 (SD) months with a range of 0.4–55 months. Experiences prior to CAPD included 37.9% on hemodialysis, 36.3% on no dialysis therapy, 22.2% on intermittent peritoneal dialysis (IPD), and

Table 2. Annualized Rates for Selected Outcome Measures (Pilot Study)

Measure	All Patients	Nondeath Dropouts
Patients	567	95
Patient-years	320	40
Peritonitis[a]	1.98	4.16
Exit or tunnel infections[a]	0.72	1.00
Catheter replacements[a]	0.40	0.70
Hospital admissions[a]	2.52	4.79
Hospital days[a] (any reason)	25.9	52.3

SOURCE: Nolph KD et al: *Kidney Int* 23:3–8, 1983. Reprinted with permission.

[a] Per patient-year.

3.5% had a failed kidney transplant. Nearly 25% of the pilot study patients were diabetic.

Annualized rates for selected outcome measures are shown in Table 2 for the entire population. Table 3 shows the distribution of days hospitalized by four specified categories as a percentage of total hospital days in all patients.

Table 4 shows life-table analyses of important outcome measures in the pilot study. These early projections show cumulative patient survival on CAPD of 89.5% of 1 year; cumulative percent of patients remaining on CAPD at one year is 59.5%. Dropout here includes death and all reasons for leaving CAPD. Although the numbers are preliminary, they are compatible with dropout rates seen in Australia and Europe. Thirty-eight percent of patients remained on CAPD without peritonitis at the end of the first year. Much higher percentages escape exit and tunnel infections. The cumulative percentage escaping hospitalization during the first year is only 19.7%. There are many reasons for dropout and hospitalization in this population; not all are related to problems with CAPD. No fair comparisons can be made with other forms of dialysis therapy at the

Table 3. Distribution of Days Hospitalized (% of 6540 days) (Pilot Study)

Dialysis related complications	48.1
Cardiovascular problems	10.5
Other medical problems	32.9
Training	8.5

SOURCE: Nolph KD et al: *Kidney Int* 23:3–8, 1983. Reprinted with permission.

Table 4. Life Table Analyses (Pilot Study)[a]

Months on CAPD	Patients at Risk[b]	Remained Alive on CAPD	Still on CAPD	No Peritonitis	No Exit/Tunnel Infections	No Catheter Replacement	Not Hospitalized
3	184–194	92.1	92.1	70.7	79.6	87.6	55.2
6	68–122	92.8	78.5	49.4	69.9	84.0	39.6
9	28–60	89.5	68.0	41.1	64.5	72.0	24.1
12	6–16	89.5	59.5	30.8	64.5	66.0	19.7

SOURCE: Nolph KD et al: *Kidney Int* 23:3–8, 1983. Reprinted with permission.
[a] Numbers for outcomes represent cumulative percentages of patients at risk.
[b] Numbers differ for each column; the range is given.

Table 5. Last Reported Status (% of 567 Patients) (Pilot Study)

Still on CAPD	76.1
Hemodialysis	10.4
Dead	7.1
Kidney transplant	3.0
IPD	2.1
Return of renal function	0.9
Stopped dialysis	0.4
Unknown	0.2

SOURCE: Nolph KD et al: *Kidney Int* 23:3–8, 1983. Reprinted with permission.

present time. Randomized perspective comparisons in similar populations (matched for age, cardiovascular disease, and diabetes) are not available.

Table 5 shows the last reported status as a percentage of the 567 patients. These represent absolute percentages rather than actuarial analyses.

Table 6 shows reasons for leaving CAPD other than death, transplant, or return of renal function. These numbers represent percentages of 69 patients in the pilot study who left CAPD for reasons other than those indicated above. The most frequent reason for leaving CAPD was related to medical problems not considered a complication of CAPD per se but that interfered with the patient's ability to carry out the technique. Stroke, progressive debilitation with malignancy, visual difficulties associated with diabetes mellitus, and crippling arthritis are examples. Recurrent peritonitis and technique problems account for the second largest category of dropouts.

Table 7 shows the percentage of pilot study patients followed during 1981 who fell into specific categories of rehabilitation or complications. As a simple index of mobility, 86.2% were able to go outside their home

Table 6. Reasons for Leaving CAPD other than Death, Transplant, or Return of Renal Function (% of 69 Patients) (Pilot Study)

Medical problems not CAPD-related	34.8
Recurring peritonitis or technique problems	24.6
Socioeconomic and patient preference	20.3
Poor control of chemistries or fluid	14.5
Other or unknown	5.8

SOURCE: Nolph KD et al: *Kidney Int* 23:3–8, 1983. Reprinted with permission.

Table 7. Frequency Distributions for Selected Outcomes (% of 567 Patients) (Pilot Study)

Outcome	Percentage
Rehabilitation	
Able to go out alone	86.2
Works more than 10 hr/wk	54.6
No hospital admission	36.2
Complications	
No catheter replacement	82.2
No exit or tunnel infection	75.3
No peritonitis	48.5

SOURCE: Nolph KD et al: *Kidney Int* 23:3–8, 1983. Reprinted with permission.

without aid; 54.6% were able to perform some kind of work beyond self-care and hygiene.

In many areas of the world, CAPD programs begin with problem patients. Frequently CAPD is offered as an alternative to death. Often there is little else to offer. These facts must be taken into account when evaluating this data. Advanced technologies may improve outcomes. Changes in patient selection may have impact. These pilot results must be considered preliminary. Results may differ with larger numbers on a national scale and with changes in CAPD techniques and patient selection.

Numerous papers have dealt with patient survival and technique survival on CAPD (71–74). In our own program at the University of Missouri we have observed patient survival rates and technique survival rates by actuarial analyses that are not significantly different for CAPD, home hemodialysis, center hemodialysis, and cadaveric transplantation (Figs. 6 and 7) (73). These were multiple biased, nonrandomized, uncontrolled studies. Outcomes may be affected more by population differences than by the form of end-stage renal disease therapy. Recent studies in Canada suggest that age, diabetes, and cardiac status may have a greater impact on patient survival in end-stage renal disease therapy than the choice of therapy (76). Studies of center hemodialysis and home hemodialysis usually only report patient survival and do not give technique survival. A recent report from the state of Michigan showed two year patient survivals on center hemodialysis at 54% (77). Since the age of the dialysis population has increased and as the number of patients with debilitating disease increases, decreases in patient survival and technique success are anticipated. There is no good evidence to suggest that CAPD is better or worse than hemodialysis in regards to these outcomes; only prospective randomized comparisons to correct for population differences would ever allow for legitimate comparisons.

Several reports dealt with comparisons of costs for CAPD and various forms of hemodialysis therapy (74,75). Successful outpatient therapies

14 CURRENT NEPHROLOGY

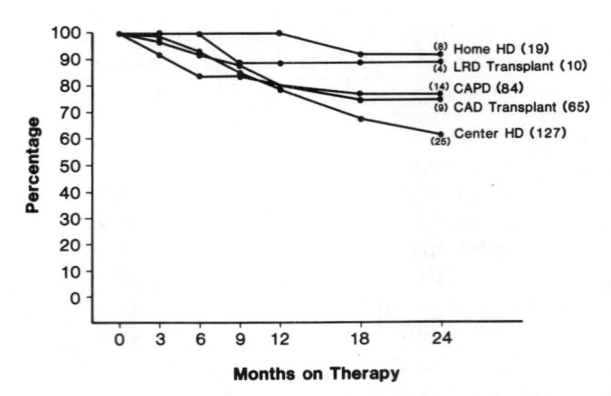

Figure 6. Actuarial patient survivals at the University of Missouri from 1977 to 1981 for patients placed on different end-stage renal disease therapies. Larger numbers in parentheses represent patients starting that mode of therapy; smaller numbers in parentheses indicate patients at risk after 2 years. Survivals were not significantly different. HD, hemodialysis; LRD, living related donor; CAPD, continuous ambulatory peritoneal dialysis; CAD, cadaveric. (Prowant B et al: Actuarial analysis of patient survival and dropout with various end-stage renal disease therapies. *Am J Kid Dis* [in press]. Reprinted with permission.)

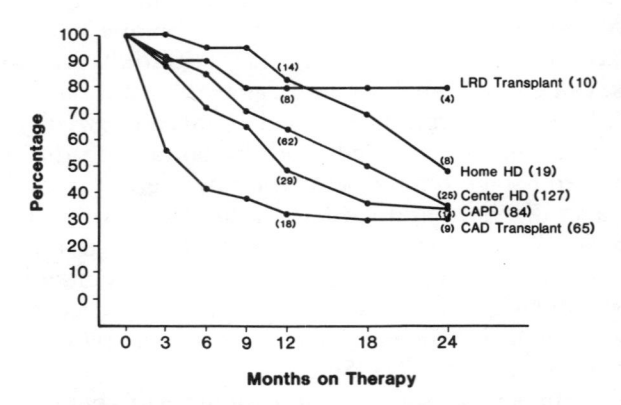

Figure 7. Actuarial survivals of dialysis technique and transplant grafts at the University of Missouri from 1977 to 1981. Death or cessation of therapy for any reason would count as a dropout. Numbers in parentheses are as in Fig. 6. Results with living related donor transplant are significantly better than with other forms of therapy. Results with other therapies were not significantly different. Living related transplant recipients were younger and matches were excellent. (Prowant B et al: Actuarial analysis of patient survival and dropout with various end-stage renal disease therapies. *Am J Kid Dis* [in press]. Reprinted with permission.)

using home hemodialysis or CAPD, probably cost from $15–18,000 annually. Center hemodialysis probably costs $25–30,000 annually. Differences in hospitalization rates and dropout rates could certainly contribute to additional costs, but legitimate comparisons of hospitalization rates independent of population biases are not available.

CAPD and Nutrition

Nutrition was the focus of many publications during this period (78–90).

A comprehensive evaluation of protein losses in 30 patients undergoing maintenance IPD, 12 patients undergoing acute IPD, and eight patients undergoing CAPD was published. Weekly losses of protein based on the usual treatments per week was similar with the three modes of peritoneal dialysis. With CAPD, 8.8 ± 1.7 (SD) grams of protein were removed per 24 hours on the average (79). In 19 CAPD patients, mean nitrogen balance was positive (mean was 3.14 g of nitrogen per day) after 2–4 months on CAPD, and was correlated with protein and energy intake as well as with an increase in body weight. Plasma free amino acid concentrations were normal but the tyrosine/phenylalanine ratio was decreased compared to ratios in healthy subjects. Glucose tolerance did not deteriorate. Serum concentrations of triglyceride and cholesterol were increased due to a rise of very low density lipoprotein (VLDL)-triglyceride and VLDL-cholesterol (80).

In one study, seven patients underwent balance studies on an outpatient basis. Estimation of total nitrogen balance was slightly positive while nutrition-related serum proteins remained comparable to those in other dialysis patients (81).

Net urea generation (urea nitrogen appearance) and losses of various nitrogenous constituents were measured during 12 metabolic studies in patients on CAPD (82). Patients ingested diets containing either 1 or 1.4 g of protein per kilogram of body weight per day. There was a reduction in the fraction of nitrogen appearing as urea, which was largely accounted for by losses of protein and free amino acids in dialysate. These latter constituents accounted for 11.5% and 4.4% of the total nitrogen output.

In another study, balance studies for nitrogen, potassium, magnesium, phosphorus, and calcium were carried out in eight men undergoing CAPD. Patients ingested either 0.98 or 1.44 g of primarily high biologic value protein per kilogram of body weight per day (83). Mean nitrogen balance was neutral with the lower protein diet (+0.35 ± 0.83 SEM g/day) and strongly positive with the higher protein diet (+2.94 ± 0.54 g/day). With the higher protein diet, balances of potassium, magnesium, and phosphorus were also strikingly positive. There was an increase in body weight in all patients and a rise in mid-arm muscle circumference in most. The authors recommend a 1.1 g/k/day protein intake for CAPD patients. Potassium balance correlated directly with nitrogen balance. High fecal potassium losses (19 ± 1.2 mEq/day) in all patients probably helped maintain normal serum potassium concentration. Mean serum magnesium concentration was increased (3.1 ± 0.1 mg/dl) and magnesium balances were positive, suggesting that dialysate magnesium is excessive. There was a net gain of calcium from dialysate that averaged 84 ± 18 mg/day and correlated inversely with serum calcium.

Free amino acid losses in the dialysate during a 24 hour period were measured in 14 studies in nine stable men on CAPD (86). Total amino acid losses were 3.4 ± 1.2 (SD) g/24 hr and represented 3.9 ± 1.9% of total nitrogen output. The sum of plasma essential, nonessential, and total amino acid concentrations was normal, although some specific amino acids had elevated or reduced concentrations. The authors conclude that during CAPD, postabsorptive plasma amino acids are generally well maintained. Daily losses of free amino acids during CAPD are small and easily replaced by food intake.

Six nondiabetic CAPD patients were infused over 6 hours with 2 liters of dialysis solution containing 2 g/dl of a mixture of essentials and nonessential amino acids (87). The osmolality of the solution and the amount of ultrafiltration induced was similar to that of a 4.25 g/dl dextrose solution. Thus, the amino acid solution appeared to exert an efficient osmotic effect. By the end of six hours, 80–90% of the amino acids had been absorbed. One hour after infusion, plasma amino acid levels increased threefold and subsequently decreased to the initial value by the sixth hour. The authors recommend further work to determine whether long-term administration of amino acids by this route will improve nutritional status of these patients and prevent side effects of daily absorption of large amounts of glucose.

Fasting plasma amino acid levels and 24 hour plasma amino acid losses in dialysate were measured in six nondiabetic females and six diabetic males on CAPD (88). Comparisons of plasma amino acid levels with six matched controls showed that CAPD did not restore the plasma amino acid levels of these patients to normal, and that the abnormalities in the nondiabetics were more marked than in the diabetics. Daily amino acid losses relative to protein intake were small, averaging 2.25 g/day. Losses were similar for nondiabetics and diabetics. The authors concluded that the losses of amino acids in the dialysate did not account for the abnormal plasma patterns. The latter may relate more to dietary habits.

Plasma lipid and lipoprotein cholesterol concentrations were reported in 13 normal lipidemic and eight hyperlipidemic patients undergoing CAPD (89). After 3–6 months of CAPD, a significant elevation of high-density lipoprotein (HDL) cholesterol occurred in the normal lipidemic group. The HDL cholesterol rose from a decreased level to within the normal range using a normal Toronto reference population. In the hyperlipidemic group there was a trend toward a higher plasma triglyceride (mainly VLDL-triglyceride), but this did not reach significance.

Serial dietary, biochemical, total body nitrogen and potassium, anthropometric, and immunologic assessments were performed on 13 patients during the first year on CAPD (90). In these patients there was a tendency for dietary protein and caloric intakes to decline. The decline was associated with a fall in total body nitrogen without significant changes in muscle mass or total body fat as assessed anthropometrically. There was an actual increase in body weight and an increase in total body potassium. The discrepancy in changes in total body nitrogen and potassium suggests that total body potassium may not be a good index of lean body mass in these patients. The authors concluded that CAPD patients may be in a long-term negative nitrogen balance if their protein intake is inadequate and if they do not receive nutritional support during intercurrent illnesses such as peritonitis.

Innovations in Technique

Many studies have described assessment of equilibrium kinetics with standard approaches to CAPD (usually four 2 liter exchanges per day) or with new innovations (91–102). Studies in Poland have shown the advantages of using increased exchange volumes when possible (91–94). Publications to date by this group have emphasized the use of 2.5 liter exchanges. I am also aware of preliminary work by some of this group with 3 liter exchanges. Increased volumes allow equal or greater amounts of solute clearance with reduced number of exchanges.

One paper described a new closed system with two bags connected to the permanent Tenckhoff catheter (96). Two clamps alternately allow outflow and inflow of peritoneal dialysate. When the exchange maneuver is completed, the patient frees the whole system from the needle and discards it. Results in 24 patients treated with this technique suggest a low incidence of peritonitis (one episode every 22.5 patient months).

Studies were also reported with CAPD plus hemoperfusion once a week (97), 6 liter daily CAPD (98,100), and other schemes to allow reduction in daily bag exchanges (101).

Transplantation in CAPD

A published survey of CAPD centers suggests that the incidence of transplantation in CAPD patients is relatively low compared to that in hemodialysis patients (103). Reasons for this are not explained entirely by age differences in the population nor by the incidence of debilitating diseases. Most centers have little or no reservations about transplanting patients maintained on CAPD or even using CAPD for postoperative dialysis (103–105). In one report over a 2-year period, 15 patients on CAPD and 65 patients treated predominantly by hemodialysis received first grafts (105). There was no difference in graft survival in the two groups. In the CAPD patients there were no postoperative episodes of peritonitis apart from one patient who had peritonitis at the time of transplantation. No technical difficulties were encouraged at the time of grafting. CAPD was not considered a contraindication to transplantation.

Diabetes Mellitus in CAPD

There continues to be interest in the use of CAPD and/or intraperitoneal insulin for the diabetic patient (105–135). One report in a small series of patients suggests improved survival of diabetic patients on CAPD as compared to other forms of dialysis therapy (107). In addition, an entire symposium on diabetes mellitus in CAPD was published in the *Peritoneal Dialysis Bulletin*, representing the proceedings of a workshop held in Toronto in February 1982 (108–122). The highlights of these proceedings are summarized below.

One report described experiences with 20 diabetics with end-stage renal disease who had never previously received dialysis treatment (108). They were treated with CAPD for periods of 2–36 months (mean 14.5 months). Intraperitoneal insulin achieved good control of blood sugar. Hemoglobin and albumin levels increased significantly. There was a significant increase in serum triglycerides. Blood pressure became normal without medication in all but one of the patients. Retinopathy, neuropathy, and osteodystrophy remained stable. Peritonitis developed once in every 20.6 patient months, a rate similar to that in nondiabetics. Calculated patient survival was 92% at 1 year, and the rate of continuation of CAPD was 87% at 1 year.

Experiences were reported with 64 diabetics treated with CAPD by a collaborative dialysis group in Toronto (109). Results in these diabetics were compared with results in 345 nondiabetics undergoing CAPD over the same period. The mean age of the diabetics was 46.7 and of the nondiabetics 51.4 years. One year and 2 year survival rates were not significantly different between the two groups (93% and 82% for the nondiabetics; 90% and 72% for the diabetics). Diabetics were transplanted at a higher rate than nondiabetics (20% versus 9%). Overall technique success rate, rates of transfer to alternative dialysis modalities, and the incidence of peritonitis were similar in the two groups.

IPD was used to treat 16 patients with end-stage renal disease and diabetes (110). One year patient survival was 48%. Blood pressure, serum potassium, and fluid and blood sugar control were considered poor compared to results with CAPD.

Many papers in this symposium dealt with the importance of good blood glucose control and experiences with intraperitoneal insulin administration in CAPD (112–114). Very helpful protocols for insulin administration in diabetics on CAPD were included (Tables 8 and 9).

Additional papers dealt with psychosocial and sexual aspect of diabetics on chronic peritoneal dialysis (115), psychiatric aspect of diabetics on

Table 8. Protocols of Insulin Administration in Diabetics on CAPD in Four Toronto Hospitals

	TWH	TGH	SMC	WH
Insulin administration	Intraperitoneal	Intraperitoneal plus subcutaneous	Intraperitoneal	Intraperitoneal
Inital dose per bag	$\frac{1}{4}$ previous daily requirement	Arbitrary—reflects previous requirements	$\frac{2}{3}$ original daily requirement	Arbitrary—reflects previous requirement
Nighttime	Reduced 30–50%	Reduced 50–90%	Unchanged	Reduced 50–60%
Insulin units per glucose concentration				
0.5 g%	$\frac{1}{4}$ previous + 0	0–12(6)[a]	0	0
1.5 g%	$\frac{1}{4}$ previous + 1	2–35(12)[a]	12–24(17)[a]	0–20(7)[a]
2.5 g%	$\frac{1}{4}$ previous + 2	3–24(13)[a]	20–32(26)[a]	not used
4.25 g%	$\frac{1}{4}$ previous + 3	4–38(16)[a]	20–40(26)[a]	15–35(25)[a]
Subcutaneous	not used	0–45(18)[a]	not used	0–100(30)[a]
Daily range	70–200(—)	9–123(62)[a]	56–108(58)[a]	30–210(87)[a]
Number of CAPD exchanges per day	Four	Three/four	Three/four	Three/four
Diet				
Calories kcal/kg body weight	20–25	20	20–25	20–25
Protein g/kg body weight	1.2–1.5	1.2	1.2–2	1.2–2

SOURCE: Roscoe JM: *Perit Dailys Bull* 2:S27–S29, 1982. Reprinted with permission.
[a] Average insulin requirements.

Table 9. Protocols of Insulin Administration in Diabetics on CAPD in Pitie-Salpetriere (France) and Iowa Lutheran (USA) Hospitals

Protocol	Pitie-Salpetriere	Iowa Lutheran
Insulin administration	Intraperitoneal	Intraperitoneal
Initial dose per bag	Arbitrary—reflects previous requirement	Total previous daily requirement
Nighttime	Unspecified	0.3 of 1.5% dose; 0.5 of 2.5% dose or 4.25% dose
Glucose concentration (g/dl)	Insulin units	Time of day
0.5	0	0600 20–100(53)
1.5	4-30(18)	1400 12–90(43)
2.5	Unspecified	2200 10–70(33)
4.25	10–45(30)	
Subcutaneous	Not used	Not used
Daily range	36–96(68)	42–260(129)
No. of CAPD exchanges per day	Three/four	Three
Diet:		
Calories kcal/kg body weight	Not specified	Not specified
Protein g/kg body weight	Not specified	Not specified

SOURCE: Roscoe JM: *Perit Dialys Bull* 2:S27–S29, 1982. Reprinted with permission.

CAPD (116), training of the diabetic patient on CAPD (117), evolution of retinopathy in diabetics on CAPD (118), care of the diabetic foot (120), nutritional considerations in diabetic patients on CAPD (121), and electrophysiologic studies in peripheral nerves of diabetics undergoing CAPD (122). Some of the highlights of these papers include observations that six of 17 patients were sexually active (115). In 17 patients, sexual activities were minimal for periods ranging from 2 months to 10 years. Special tools may need to be designed for visually handicapped patients (117). Visual acuity remained unchanged in 13 of 16 eyes in eight patients on CAPD (118). In three eyes, visual acuity deteriorated. Many diabetics have the anorexia, nausea, vomiting syndrome on CAPD (121). In some patients this may reflect gastroparesis as a result of autonomic neuropathy. In others this may reflect primarily constipation, lack of physical activity, or side effects of medications. In 12 diabetics maintained on CAPD for 1 year or more there was no evidence of progression of neuropathy by serial electrophysiologic studies (122). There were numerous other publications in addition to those from the special symposium relating to CAPD and diabetes mellitus (124–135). Many of these focused on intraperitoneal insulin administration (125–127,130,133–134). In five diabetics on CAPD, intraperitoneal insulin achieved satisfactory control of blood glucose, and the rate of peritonitis was not increased. However, regardless of whether blood glucose was well controlled or not, hemoglobin A1, as well as triglyceride values, rose in diabetics on CAPD (130). There continue to be successful reports of CAPD in blind diabetic patients (132,134,135).

Additional Observations

There has been interest in the long-term effects of peritoneal dialysis using CAPD on membrane permeability characteristics. Histologic and functional characteristics of the peritoneal membrane in a diabetic patient after 34 months of CAPD were reported (136). Even though this patient had frequent episodes of peritonitis over nearly 3 years, the morphology of the peritoneum at autopsy (following a massive myocardial infarction) was essentially normal other than the typical capillary basement membrane changes of diabetes. Transport appeared to remain stable in the peritoneum over the 3 year period. Membrane permeability changes were monitored in patients undergoing CAPD for 1 or more years. In most patients, transport remains quite stable even with frequent peritonitis (137).

Observations were made retrospectively and prospectively over 1 year in nine patients undergoing CAPD (138). Within 5 months, hematocrit increased to normal in four of nine patients; five others remained anemic. There was no significant difference in serum creatinine levels. The serum erythropoietin level in the four patients who responded was greater than in those who did not respond. The authors suggest that CAPD can normalize the hematocrit in patients with end-stage renal disease who were anemic on other modalities with little or no change in serum creatinine provided the remnant kidneys are capable of producing sufficient erythropoietin. Parathyroid hormone levels were higher in patients who responded than in those who did not.

Other studies have documented increases in red cell mass and hematocrit in patients on CAPD (139). In another study, in 11 uremic patients mean bleeding time improved on CAPD and became normal in six of seven patients who had had a prolonged bleeding time prior to CAPD (140). There was a concomitant improvement in platelet aggregation and mean platelet count increased. The result suggested that CAPD treatment improved uremic bleeding tendencies even in patients previously on hemodialysis treatment.

Serum carnitine and serum triglycerides were measured in 45 patients on CAPD and in 14 controls (141). There were no significant differences between mean carnitine levels in the two groups. Furthermore, there was no correlation between serum carnitine and serum triglycerides. The authors felt that these data cast doubt on a proposed role for carnitine in the development of hypertriglyceridemia in patients on CAPD and on the need for carnitine supplementation in these patients.

The mean peritoneal clearance of digoxin was reported to be 3.6 ± 0.4 SEM ml/min during CAPD (142). Patients lost 3.7–13.3% of their daily oral digoxin into the dialysate. The mean ratio of dialysate to serum digoxin concentration in long-dwell exchanges was 0.59.

A special program for the prevention and treatment of back pain in patients undergoing continuous ambulatory peritoneal dialysis was presented (143). Back supports, exercise, and other aspects of this special program were explained (123).

Aluminum mass transfer studies were reported in three CAPD patients (143). The results suggested that dialysate aluminum concentrations in commercially available solutions are low. Aluminum appears to be removed from CAPD patients in proportion to plasma aluminum concentrations.

The disposition of cimetidine was studied following a single intravenous dose of 300 mg over 10 minutes in six male patients with end-stage renal disease on CAPD (145). Cimetidine disappearance from plasma was biphasic with a half-life varying from 6.1 to 7.4 hours. Peritoneal clearance ranged from 1.9 to 4.0 ml/min. The total amount of cimetidine removed in the dialysate varied from 3.1 to 8.3 mg representing 1.2–2.7% of the dose administered over 24 hours. The authors concluded that very little cimetidine is removed by CAPD. A dose of 200 mg of cimetidine every 12 hours was recommended.

The clearance of quinidine was evaluated in a patient on CAPD (146). Peritoneal clearance of quinidine was 0.793 ml/min, representing only 0.61% of the total body clearance of the drug. Elimination half-life was 5.44 hours. The authors suggested, based on their results, that adjusting the dosage of quinidine did not appear necessary for patients on CAPD.

Effects of CAPD on parathyroid hormone and mineral metabolism were evaluated in 10 patients (147). It was found that CAPD removes significant amounts of parathyroid hormone. Normal 25-hydroxy vitamin D and vitamin D binding protein levels are maintained with CAPD despite large protein losses. Substantial amounts of phosphorus are removed with CAPD but not to an extent that precludes use of phosphorus binders. Dialysate containing lower magnesium and possibly higher calcium concentrations should be made available to improve mineral homeostasis.

PERITONITIS

The pilot study of the national CAPD Registry shows a frequency of peritonitis near two episodes per patient year (71). Peritonitis occurs at a much lower incidence in intermittent peritoneal dialysis. During the past year there were many descriptions of experiences with peritonitis in general and reviews of approaches to peritonitis (148–167).

A symposium on peritonitis in patients on CAPD was held in Toronto in February 1981 and published as a supplement to the *Peritoneal Dialysis Bulletin* in September 1981 (156–159). I will mention some of the highlights of these proceedings.

Patients who remain free of peritonitis for one year are unlikely to develop recurrent peritonitis (156). It has been recommended that patients who have three or more episodes of peritonitis within the first year should be withdrawn from the CAPD program (156). Another mode of dialysis may be appropriate for such patients.

The incidence of peritonitis at different institutions in Toronto over a 3 year period was reviewed (157). The overall incidence of peritonitis in nondiabetics was one every 10.5 patient months and in diabetics, one episode every 9.6 patient months.

The treatment of peritonitis was reviewed (159). The therapy recommended included a short lavage with three in-and-out exchanges to remove inflammatory products that may contribute to pain; loading doses of antibiotics; the addition of heparin to dialysis solutions; intraperitoneal antibiotics with continued CAPD; discontinuation of all drugs containing aluminum hydroxide to avoid aggravation of constipation (so common in patients with peritonitis); and increased protein intake because of the increased losses of protein during peritonitis. Catheter removal was recommended if peritonitis persisted for more than 4–5 days despite the use of appropriate antibiotics, in the presence of fungal peritonitis, for severe skin exit infection, for tuberculous peritonitis, and in patients with suspected fecal peritonitis. I would agree with the trend toward earlier catheter removal in refractory cases. In my experience, there may be occult tunnel infection or there may be organisms harbored in tissues within or coating the catheter and inhibiting resolution of the infection (161). Most of these approaches to peritonitis have been reviewed in detail previously.

In Toronto, the median time to the first infection in CAPD is about 260 days. The median time between the first and second infection is approximately 300 days (162). Patients who entered programs later tended to experience lower infection rates. The increased risk of failure on the CAPD program for patients who have at least one infection in the first 90–150 days is greater than threefold.

Vas has reviewed the overall trends in peritonitis during CAPD (160). In programs of long duration the trend has been for infection rates to decrease as the programs mature (161). The value of the dialysate cell count in the diagnosis of peritonitis continues to be emphasized (165). Connection techniques may influence infection rates (163). Infectious peritonitis was studied in 164 patients with renal failure, receiving 24,282 intermittent peritoneal dialysis treatments over a 5 year period (164). The overall incidence of peritonitis was 0.66 episodes per 100 dialyses. Infectious peritonitis was the most common complication among outpatients and was the major cause of dropout. Thirty-nine percent of the patients transferred to hemodialysis. The most common microorganisms were *Staphylococcus aureus* and micrococci, accounting for 50% of the cases; 46% of the cases caused by *Staphylococcus aureus* were preceded by wound or catheter tunnel infections.

Life-table analysis considering the first episode of peritonitis as an end event has been recommended by some investigators as the simplest method of expressing the probability of developing peritonitis (166). Comparison of two subpopulations of dialysis patients for the performance of two units can be done by comparing the two peritonitis probability curves calculated from respective data. Regression analysis between the probability to develop peritonitis within a specific interval on CAPD and calendar time of entrance into the program is a simple way to assess changes in the performance of the dialysis program over time.

Nonbacterial Peritonitis

Steiner has reported clinical observations on the pathogenesis of peritoneal dialysate eosinophilia (168). In all of his three cases, eosinophilia in dialysate was asymptomatic and the process resolved spontaneously after 2–7 weeks. IgE levels in dialysate were not elevated. It did not seem that IgE, a potent eosinophilotactic agent, was involved in the development of the disorder.

Three other cases of sterile peritonitis in CAPD patients were described where the predominant white cell type in the peritoneal dialysis fluid was the eosinophil (168). Bacterial and fungal organisms were not isolated on repeated cultures of the dialysis fluid. All patients had a benign course. Eosinophilic response occurred very soon after starting CAPD. All patients were asymptomatic and did not require antibiotic therapy.

We have reported a case of asymptomatic peritonitis and dialysate showing predominantly eosinophils (170). In our patient, the process also began shortly after commencement of CAPD and resolved spontaneously after 3 weeks.

A 43-year-old patient developed acute abdominal symptoms 7 days after completion of an intermittent peritoneal dialysis treatment (171). The peritonitis was attributed to starch powder and resolution occurred rapidly after removal of the powder. Starch peritonitis after peritoneal dialysis can be obviated by careful washing of gloves.

In 10 patients undergoing maintenance peritoneal dialysis, large numbers of eosinophils were found in the peritoneal fluid (172). Several patients complained of episodic abdominal pain, but there was no correlation between symptoms and the number of peritoneal fluid eosinophils. Cultures were negative as were the results of tests for endotoxin in dialysate. Eosinophil counts were elevated soon after catheter insertion.

Table 10. Unusual Organisms Causing Peritonitis (1981–1982)

Organism	Reference
Vibrio alginolyticus	173
Mycobacterium chelonei-like	174
Mycobacterium tuberculosis	175
Pseudomonas cepacia	176
Fusarium species	177

In some patients, peritoneal fluid eosinophil count spontaneously returned to normal despite continued peritoneal dialysis.

Unusual Organisms

There were several reports of peritonitis due to unusual organisms (Table 10) (173–177). These infecting agents included *Vibrio alginolyticus* (173), *Mycobacterium chelonei*-like organisms (174), tuberculosis (175), *Pseudomonas cepacia* (176), and *Fusarium* species (177). An epidemic of HB_sAg-positive hepatitis involving six patients and four staff members was described; the source was identified as a chronic in-center peritoneal dialysis patient in whom both serum and peritoneal fluid were persistently HB_sAg-positive (178). The authors concluded that peritoneal dialysis of HB_sAg-positive individuals represent a significant risk for the transmission of HB_sAg and clinical hepatitis.

Factors Predisposing to Peritonitis

Thirty patients undergoing long-term home-based peritoneal dialysis were monitored for 13 months for carriage of *Staphylococcus aureus* in the nares and for the development of infectious complications (179). With regard to *Staphylococcus aureus* carriage, there were three groups: chronic carriers, intermittent carriers, and noncarriers. Twenty-five episodes of peritonitis and twenty episodes of catheter exit site infections occurred during 268 patient months of observation. *Staphylococcus aureus* accounted for eight episodes of peritonitis and for 12 episodes of exit site infection. Chronic and intermittent carriers of *Staphylococcus aureus* were found to be at higher risk of developing infection than noncarriers.

In patients on continuous ambulatory peritoneal dialysis, peritonitis was shown to be associated with vaginal leakage of dialysis fluid (180).

Prevention and Therapy

Commercial peritoneal dialysis solutions were shown to suppress the activity of peripheral blood leukocytes as measured by chemiluminescence, phagocytosis, and bacterial killing (181). Suppression was found to be related to the low pH and high osmolality of the fluid. The pH increased to noninhibitory levels in vivo within 30 minutes, while osmolality changes were less rapid and remained at inhibitory levels for fluids of higher dextrose concentration (4.25%). Urea at concentrations normally found in dialysate and heparin at concentrations routinely added to fluid inhibited only chemiluminescence. Creatinine and insulin were not inhibitory. High fluid volume also resulted in decreased efficiency of bacterial killing. These studies suggest that peritonitis may be better treated with long-dwell exchanges rather than with rapid lavage.

Regular twice daily cultivation of dialysate drainage in a tube of nutrient medium was undertaken to see if latent peritoneal infection could be detected before symptoms appeared (182). Clinical peritonitis could then be prevented by early antibiotic therapy. The authors felt that the screening technique was helpful and contributed to a reduction of the incidence of peritonitis in their program from 5.6 to 0.5 episodes per patient year.

Oral doses of flucytosine and intravenous doses of miconazole appeared effective in eradicating a case of *Candida parapsilosis* peritonitis in a patient on CAPD (183). CAPD interruption was not necessary, and the authors measured acceptable flucytosine levels in serum and dialysate. Removal of the dialysis catheter was not necessary. These observations need further evaluation since most centers have found fungal peritonitis very refractory to therapy without catheter removal.

The current principles of the treatment of acute peritonitis were reviewed (184). Peritoneal sclerosis has been reported in patients on chronic intermittent peritoneal dialysis. Experiences with peritoneal sclerosis and concerns for patients on chronic peritoneal dialysis were reviewed by Schmidt and Blumenkrantz (185).

Two papers assessed changes in solute transport in ultrafiltration with peritonitis in CAPD patients with results confirming those mentioned in the section on physiology (186,187). Peritonitis was associated with decreased dialysate fluid volume, increased absorption of glucose, increased clearances of urea and creatinine, and increased protein losses. Following therapy these changes appeared reversible in days to weeks.

Pharmacokinetics

Transperitoneal movements of antibiotics and antibiotic stabilities in dialysis solution were frequently assessed (186–197). Some of the highlights of these studies will be mentioned (Table 11).

Stabilities of cephaphirin, gentamicin, penicillin G, nafcillin, ticarcillin, and vancomycin were tested in peritoneal dialysate at 25°C for 24 hours (190). All of the agents were stable except penicillin G, which lost 25% of its activity over 24 hours. Once daily preparation of drug dialysate solution

Table 11. Antibiotic Studies (1981–1982)

Antibiotic	Types of Study	Reference
Cephaphirin	Stability[a]	190, 198
Gentamicin	Stability	190, 198, 199
	Kinetics	190
Penicillin G	Stability	190
Nafcillin	Stability	190
Ticarcillin	Stability	190
Vancomycin	Stability	190, 199
Trimethoprim-sulfamethoxazole	Kinetics	192
Cefuroxime	Kinetics	195
Tobramycin	Stability	198
Amikacin	Stability	198
Sisomicin	Stability	199
Neitilmicin	Stability	199

[a] Activity in peritoneal dialysis solution.

was considered feasible for the treatment of peritonitis in patients on CAPD.

Gentamicin kinetics were determined after intravenous or intraperitoneal injection in five patients undergoing CAPD (191). After intraperitoneal instillation of 1 mg/kg in the CAPD fluid and during a 6 hour dwell exchange, the antibiotic appeared in the serum within 15 minutes in four or five patients studied. Peak serum concentrations ranged between 1.6 and 7.2 mg/liter and the time required to reach peak concentration was 3.8 hours. Peritoneal gentamicin clearance was 13 ml/min. Percent extraction from peritoneal dialysis fluid within the 6 hour fluid exchange ranged from 65% to 100% with a mean of 86.8%. When the same dose of gentamicin was injected intravenously, no gentamicin could be detected in the peritoneal fluid in three of five patients, and only small amounts of drug were present for brief periods in the remaining two. In two patients with acute peritonitis treated with intraperitoneal gentamicin, peak serum concentrations were found to range between 3.5 and 4.5 mg/liter. The authors concluded that gentamicin is rapidly absorbed from the peritoneal fluid into the blood compartment, but net removal rates are low. Thus, CAPD has little impact on the elimination characteristics of intravenous gentamicin, and intraperitoneal instillation allows rapid absorption to reach therapeutic serum concentrations. Other reports support these findings (197).

The pharmacokinetics of the fixed combination of trimethoprim-sulfamethoxazole (TMP-SMZ), including peritoneal transfer, were studied in patients on CAPD and on intermittent peritoneal dialysis (192). Peritoneal dialysance of both TMP and SMZ after oral administration was very low. In contrast, absorption after intraperitoneal administration was high and was increased during peritonitis. In patients with peritonitis, intraperitoneal administration of TMP-SMZ resulted in immediate high local concentrations and serum concentrations of both drugs in therapeutic ranges within 6–12 hours.

Four patients received 1 g vancomycin in 2 liters of dialysate during 6 hour cycles (194). Fifty-four percent of the amount introduced into the peritoneal cavity was absorbed systemically during a 6 hour cycle. Peak serum concentrations averaged 23.7 µg/ml.

Eight patients on chronic intermittent peritoneal dialysis were administered 1 g of cefuroxime as an intravenous bolus 1 hour before the start of dialysis (195). Mean plasma levels fell from 80 µg/ml at 1 hour to 40 µg/ml at 6–8 hours. In peritoneal fluid, levels reach 16.7 µg/ml at 1 hour and 7.55 µg/ml at 6 hours. Seven patients received cefuroxime added to dialysis solution at a dose of 2.5 g/10 liters. After 6 hours of peritoneal dialysis, plasma levels of 60 µg/ml were reached. The results demonstrate that this antibiotic administered intravenously easily diffuses from blood to peritoneal fluid. Antibiotic added to peritoneal dialysis solution is readily absorbed. Either route of administration was considered adequate to treat peritoneal infections associated with peritoneal dialysis.

Preliminary studies with epsilon aminocaproic acid, an antifibrinolytic agent, were carried out in two patients undergoing peritoneal dialysis (196). Total body clearance of epsilon aminocaproic acid was 25% of clearance in patients with normal renal function. Dialysis clearance accounted for 58% of total body clearance. Alternative routes of elimination must also exist. The authors suggest that patients undergoing peritoneal dialysis should receive 25% of the usual dose.

Antibacterial activities of seven cephalosporins, gentamicin, tobramycin, and amikacin in commercially available peritoneal dialysis solutions were assessed (198). There were no physical incompatibilities between any of the antibiotics and the solution. None of the cephalosporins was bactericidal in the solution whereas bactericidal concentrations of aminoglycosides in solution approximated those of aminoglycosides in serum. The authors concluded that cephalosporins may not be ideal agents for intraperitoneal therapy when they are administered in solution. These findings may explain the slow response to intraperitoneal cephalosporins in some patients, whereas in vitro sensitivities would predict prompt resolution of the infection. In such patients cure often follows addition or substitution of aminoglycosides. These studies warrant further investigations.

Another report noted that vancomycin, gentamicin, sisomicin, and neitilmicin are sufficiently stable in peritoneal dialysis solution so that the drugs can be added to dialysis concentrate when peritoneal administration of the antibiotic is indicated in patients undergoing chronic intermittent peritoneal dialysis (199). Tobramycin was found to be a more labile aminoglycoside and the authors suggest that if tobramycin is administered intraperitoneally in dialysis concentrate, it should be used promptly after reconstitution.

Miscellaneous

One report described a patient on continuous ambulatory peritoneal dialysis who developed multiple hepatic abscesses (200).

OTHER COMPLICATIONS (Table 12)

Bowel and Hernias

A spontaneous colonic perforation during chronic intermittent peritoneal dialysis was reported (201). The relationship to peritoneal dialysis is not clear.

Hernias and complications related thereto continue to be frequently reported in peritoneal dialysis patients (202–209). Abdominal hernias were found in 12 of 51 patients trained for CAPD (203). Five of these patients were noted to have abdominal hernias before the start of continuous ambulatory peritoneal dialysis. Four of the patients had incarcerations. The authors suggest that a careful search for the presence of hernias be performed prior to peritoneal dialysis. Continued monitoring for hernias is essential and, if found, elective repair should be performed. Other reports include a Richter's hernia (204), clostridial myonecrosis originating from an obturator hernia (205), hydrocele (206), and a hernia of Morgagni (207).

In a larger series of 192 patients, 22 patients developed 31 abdominal hernias (208). Fifteen of these were incisional and developed at the site of catheter implantation; five of these became incarcerated and produced complete or partial intestinal obstruction. More than half of the hernias developed during the first year of CAPD. All but six of the hernias were repaired surgically. Most of the patients returned to CAPD after temporary intermittent peritoneal dialysis or hemodialysis. Factors predisposing to hernia seem to be increases in intraabdominal pressure during CAPD combined with weak abdominal walls. The authors suggest that incisional hernias at the site of catheter insertion might be reduced by using a paramedial incision through the rectus muscle.

Two cases of acute small bowel obstruction complicating CAPD were presented (209). In both, bowel herniation occurred through the peritoneal opening around the dialysis catheter. Both patients had sudden onset of obstructive symptoms relieved by surgery. One patient returned to CAPD with no further problems. The other patient transferred to chronic in-center hemodialysis.

A 63-year-old patient on CAPD developed severe colitis extending from the upper part of the rectum to the splenic flexure associated with abdominal pain and rectal bleeding. The episode was associated with hypotension (210). The authors argued that the etiology of the colitis was

Table 12. Other Complications (1981–1982)

Complication	Reference
Richter's hernia	204
Obturator hernia	205
Hydrocele	206
Hernia of Morgagni	207
Incisional hernias	208, 209
Ischemic colitis	210
Hydrothorax	211–214
Hyperlipidemia	221–223
Acute aluminum intoxication	227
Peripheral ischemia	228
Low serum folate	229
Hepatitis B antigen positivity	230

ischemia. With correction of body weight and blood pressure, the colitis improved rapidly.

Pulmonary Complications

Four patients with massive hydrothorax were reported (211–214).

A patient developed a right pleural effusion soon after starting CAPD (211). Macroaggregated albumin was labeled with ^{99m}Tc administered intraperitoneally followed by 2 liters of dialysate. Transdiaphragmatic leakage was clearly demonstrated and confirmed by high count rates of pleural fluid and a negligible blood count. This method can safely be used to demonstrate transdiaphragmatic fluid leakage in peritoneal dialysis patients.

A 51-year-old woman presented with a massive right-sided hydrothorax after 84 days on CAPD (212). The presence of dialysate in the right pleural cavity was demonstrated by the recovery of fluid of intraperitoneal methylene blue injected in the peritoneal space. Talcage of the pleura was partly successful in preventing recurrence of the pleural cavity, and CAPD was continued.

In another 51-year-old woman, a large right pleural effusion developed 2 years after she started receiving peritoneal dialysis (214). A radionuclide scan demonstrated a pleural–peritoneal connection. The patient was switched from CAPD to IPD with resolution of the effusion that recurred when she was challenged with CAPD 1 month later. The authors believe that large ultrafiltration volumes with CAPD and prlonged dwell times are more likely to result in pleural effusion rather than the smaller ultrafiltration volumes with IPD in a semisitting position.

Ten patients on CAPD underwent studies of spirography, compliance tests, body plethysmography, and blood oxygen analysis (216). Ventilatory function was compared with the abdomen empty and the abdomen filled with 2 liters of peritoneal dialysis solution. Vital capacity decreased 3.5%, thoracic gas volume increased 7.9%, static absolute compliance decreased 8.8%, and dynamic absolute compliance decreased 6.2%. There were no significant alterations of specific compliance tests or evidence of bronchial obstruction. There was no change in blood oxygen. The authors interpreted the findings as showing mild ventilatory restriction that should produce problems only in patients with diseases of the respiratory tract.

Pulmonary function was measured in eight patients undergoing CAPD (using 2 liters of fluid in all but one patient, who used 3 liters of fluid) (217). Lung volumes were measured by body plethysmographic and helium-dilution techniques; forced vital capacities before and after removal of dialysate fluid were measured. Patients were free of lung disease and were at stable dry weight. Functional residual capacity was significantly higher (mean 590 ml) subsequent to drainage in eight patients using 2 liters of fluid. No significant differences were found in maximum expiratory flow rates. The authors felt there were no detrimental effects on diaphragmatic configuration or function during peritoneal dialysis.

Rebuck speculated that Starling's law applies to the diaphragm as it does to the heart; as distending pressure becomes excessive, the diaphragm will no longer be able to increase its contractile force (218). Hence, depending upon the integrity of the diaphragm and intercostal muscles, larger volumes of abdominal fluid should be tolerated better by some patients than by others.

Osteodystrophy

Studies were performed in 50 patients treated with chronic intermittent peritoneal dialysis for periods ranging from 6 to 37 months (219). Dialysis fluid contained a calcium concentration of 2.25 mmol/liter. Serum calcium normalized from below normal predialytic values. Osteodensitometry performed on 26 patients revealed no significant changes. Serum total alkaline phosphatase and fractioned alkaline phosphatases were increased in 30% of the patients. In only 10% of these patients were increases due to elevated liver isoenzymes. Findings suggested little tendency to develop dialysis associated osteodystrophy in these patients.

Gokal reviewed studies of renal osteodystrophy in CAPD (220). Serum levels of 25-hydroxy vitamin D are frequently low and patients may need cautious vitamin D replacement therapy. He urges additional studies of calcium balance with solutions containing more than 1.5 mmol of calcium per liter. He urges minimal aluminum contamination of peritoneal fluid. He pointed out that in many patients, CAPD appears to achieve adequate control of serum phosphate and of histologic renal osteodystrophy with declining levels of PTH.

Hyperlipidemia

Intravenous fat tolerance tests were performed in control subjects and in uremic patients before and after 6 months on CAPD (221). Serum triglycerides were elevated in the uremic patients before CAPD but no further increase occurred during therapy. Oral carbohydrate intake was restricted to 250 g per 24 hours and the use of hypotonic dialysate was minimized. There were no significant changes in fractional removal rates of lipid. The authors feel that further increases in serum triglycerides in CAPD may be prevented by simple dietary maneuvers.

One study suggested accumulation of remnants of triglyceride-rich lipoproteins in patients with chronic renal failure undergoing peritoneal dialysis or hemodialysis (222).

One review emphasized the risk to patients receiving peritoneal and dialysis of any type from high obligate glucose loads (223). Dietary monitoring to control hyperlipidemia was recommended.

Miscellaneous

Densitometrical analyses of the brain during hemodialysis and peritoneal dialysis suggest increases in brain water with hemodialysis. Changes are not seen with CAPD (224,225).

Acute aluminum intoxication was reported in a patient undergoing CAPD. The particular batch of solutions being used by the patient had been contaminated in production with large amounts of aluminum (226).

Bloody dialysate may be due to a number of causes, including trauma and retrograde menstruation (227).

Five patients showed exacerbation of symptoms of peripheral vascular disease on CAPD (228). This exacerbation was related primarily to overzealous reduction of blood pressure.

Low serum folate levels were reported in four patients undergoing chronic peritoneal dialysis (229). The authors emphasized the importance of adequate folic acid replacement.

An editorial on hepatitis B antigen carriers in peritoneal dialysis units was published (230).

Physical therapy was reviewed as a necessary part of the rehabilitation of patients on chronic peritoneal dialysis (231).

INTERMITTENT PERITONEAL DIALYSIS

Palmer has published a review of the history of peritoneal dialysis emphasizing the important contributions of IPD to the development of peritoneal dialysis in general (232). Other reviews have emphasized the evolution of our concepts about peritoneal dialysis therapy (233,234).

Although CAPD now dominates chronic peritoneal dialysis therapy, there is still a place for chronic intermittent peritoneal dialysis. Also, intermittent peritoneal dialysis is used extensively for the therapy of acute renal failure.

Clinical Results with Chronic Intermittent Peritoneal Dialysis

A comparison of intermittent versus continuous ambulatory peritoneal dialysis involved studies of 12 patients who had been on IPD for an average of 18.3 months and then were switched to CAPD (234). CAPD experience averaged 9.8 months per patient, and 10 remained on CAPD when the report was published. With the change to continuous dialysis there was a fall in serum creatinine, potassium, uric acid, phosphate, and blood urea nitrogen. The total CO_2 rose, and serum calcium rose in nine patients. Mean hematocrit values were higher in most patients on CAPD but fell again after 1 year. Despite an increase in the rate of peritonitis (1 infection/5.9 patient months on CAPD versus 1/12.2 patient months on IPD), CAPD was felt to offer several distinct advantages, especially in the areas of control of uremic acidosis, phosphate retention, blood pressure, and fluid management.

In previous reviews we have described studies of residual peritoneal fluid in IPD patients as an indicator of serum chemistries (236). This past year a comparison of residual fluid and serum values in 53 samples from 16 patients showed a good correlation for blood urea nitrogen, phosphorus, creatinine, uric acid, calcium, and potassium. Correlations for glucose, chloride, bilirubin, osmolality, LDH, bicarbonate, albumin, cholesterol, sodium, globulins, and alkaline phosphatase were poor. Residual fluid values of these latter solutes were not recommended to assess serum concentrations.

Concentrations of plasma middle molecules were determined using high-speed gel filtration combined with ion exchange gradient elution chromatography (237). There were 126 samples from 90 nondialyzed azotemic patients and 210 predialysis samples from 53 regular hemodialysis patients and 24 intermittent peritoneal dialysis patients. Samples were obtained when patients were free from major uremic symptoms and, in addition, when they presented with symptoms or signs of complications such as infection, edema, vomiting, pericarditis, or malnutrition. Patients with infection and malnutrition revealed higher serum middle molecule concentrations, particularly in fraction 7C. In patients with edema, 7A and 7B middle molecule fractions were elevated. Vomiting was not associated with accumulation of middle molecules. The plasma creatinine concentrations did not differ between the groups studied. The authors state that uremic "sickness" is often associated with high plasma, middle molecule concentrations. It is not known whether middle molecules induce symptoms or are elevated secondary to complications of uremia.

Variations on IPD

Twelve patients on chronic IPD were followed a total of 8 months using a high dialysate flow rate (4 liters/hr) and a low dialysate flow rate (2 liters/hr) (238). No significant differences in chemistries or interdialytic weight gain were noted between the two flow rates. The 2 liter/hr dialytic flow rate is less expensive, more convenient for the patient, and, according to these authors, should be the preferred mode of therapy.

The technique of rapid flow, high volume exchanges was studied as an attempt to provide effective peritoneal dialysis over shorter periods (239). Following instillation of 2,000 ml of dialysis fluid, 1,000 ml of fluid were drained and then immediately replaced with the same amount of fresh fluid. Sequential instillation and drainage of 1,000 ml of fluid was maintained at a constant flow rate. Flow rates up to 9.5 liters/hr could be obtained and maintained. The incidence of abdominal pain during dialysis was 28.33%; the authors did not feel these related to the high flow rates. Some of the highest clearances ever reported were listed in this paper. Average creatinine clearances reached 33.4 ml/min and average urea clearances 42.3 ml/min. The authors feel that with their technique dialysis time can be reduced by half.

Other reports describe experiences with rapid cycling of relatively small volumes with a residual reservoir (240–242). This technique mechanically permits rapid cycling and seems to result in very high clearances compared to complete drainage techniques. Automated equipment is necessary.

Experiences were reported with bicarbonate-containing dialysate produced by an automated dialysate delivery machine (243).

CONTINUOUS CYCLING PERITONEAL DIALYSIS

Continuous cycling peritoneal dialysis (CCPD) provides essentially continuous peritoneal dialysis (244–248). However, before bedtime drainage, the peritoneal catheter is connected to a cycler. The cycler is set to deliver three exchanges of 2 liters, each 3 hours in duration. In the morning, following drainage of the third exchange, 2 liters are infused and allowed to dwell for 15 hours. The cycler is disconnected. The solution is drained again that evening after connection to the cycler. Thus, this technique provides 9 hours of automated cycling (three 3 hour exchanges) and 15 hours of a single exchange during the day. Usually dialysis solutions containing 4.25% dextrose are used for the long daytime exchange. This is to prevent net absorption during such a long exchange. 1.5% dextrose dialysis solutions can be used for the shorter night cycles. Glucose concentrations can be increased if more ultrafiltration is necessary.

Table 13. CAPD and CCPD Differences

	CAPD	CCPD
Openings at risk/day	4 spike	4 spike, 2 tubing
Machine	No	Yes
Daytime cycles	3 (4–6 hr)	1 (15 hr)
Nighttime cycles	1 (8 hr)	3 (3 hr)
Nonfree hours/day	2	10
Free hours/day	22	14
Tube change interval	4–8 hr	daily

As of November 1982, there were 66 patients on CCPD registered in the National Registry of CAPD. These CCPD patients are also being followed by the National Registry but are analyzed separately.

CCPD was designed to reduce the high incidence of peritonitis and to eliminate the multiple interruptions created by dialysis exchanges during the day on CAPD. Results show ultrafiltration rates and clearances comparable with those on CAPD, excellent blood pressure control, and reduced infection rates (246,247). Reports of reduced infection rates, however, are not legitimate randomized comparisons of CAPD and CCPD in single units or in multicenter studies. The Registry data on CCPD is nonrandomized, too small, and too preliminary to allow meaningful comparisons of infection rates.

Proposed advantages for CCPD include the assumption that connections should be simpler and easier; connection sessions occur only twice daily. However, counterarguments include the facts that connections involve not only placing spikes in bags, but the connecting of the catheter to the cycler tubing. Thus, although there are fewer connection sessions, there are actually more connections. The fact that only unused sterile spikes are employed could be an advantage, however. Some argue that immediate drainage after cycler connection may provide a washout effect after connections have been made (247). There is no proof, however, that this makes any difference if contamination has occurred. The advantage of complete daytime freedom may be overcome in many patients by 9 hours of forced confinement at night. Table 13 summarizes some of the differences between CAPD and CCPD. Recent kinetic analyses of CAPD and CCPD show very similar daily clearance and ultrafiltration rates (248).

In summary, this continues to be a viable option for chronic peritoneal dialysis, especially in those patients who may need a helper. A helper can often be available twice a day rather than four times a day. The purchase of a cycler and 9 hours of nighttime confinement may be a high price to pay for freedom from two extra exchanges during the day. These factors may primarily depend on life-style and personality. Whether infection rates are lower than in CAPD has yet to be established. Differences in infection rates change as CAPD technologies improve.

CATHETERS AND TEMPORARY BLOOD ACCESS

Preliminary experiences with new catheters and catheter materials has been reported (249–253). Results with 48 Tenckhoff straight catheters were compared with results using 49 curled Tenckhoff catheters in studies in 97 adults undergoing CAPD (252). The cumulative period of treatment was 997 patient months; mean age was 61.1 years. Straight catheters were implanted as the procedure of choice during an 18 month period followed by a 16 month period wherein curled catheters were used. Fifteen straight catheters had to be removed (14 because of symptomatic dislodgment; 1 because of obstruction). Two asymptomatic displacements were observed with the curled catheters. No curled catheters had to be removed. The authors feel that the curled catheter can be easily implanted and has fewer problems with dislodgment.

Studies were performed in 41 patients who required transfer from peritoneal dialysis to hemodialysis (25 temporarily and 16 permanently) (254). The mean duration of temporary transfers was 29.5 days. Subclavian cannulation was used for blood access. Nine patients developed bacteremia attributed to the subclavian cannula, but the morbidity was slight and the mortality nil. All temperature elevations associated with these infections returned to normal within 48 hours after antibiotic therapy and did not recur. The authors feel that the indwelling subclavian cannula permits temporary vascular access with ease and that other types of access that involve blood vessel destruction are not justified for 2–3 weeks of hemodialysis. They also feel that femoral cannulation is a much less attractive alternative in light of the associated patient discomfort and inconvenience to medical and nursing staff.

SPECIAL USES OF PERITONEAL DIALYSIS

Peritoneal Dialysis in Children

Experiences with acute peritoneal dialysis in children were described in multiple reports (254–260). Many of these experiences related to acute renal failure. Dialysis therapy of transient neonatal hyperammonemia was reported (256). Peritoneal dialysis may be helpful during the acute phase treatment of maple syrup urine disease (258).

Chronic peritoneal dialysis is becoming a very common form of chronic dialysis therapy in children (251,261–266). Very small infants are being treated with chronic peritoneal dialysis (270–272).

Specific surgical procedures for inserting pediatric peritoneal catheters have been developed (274). Peritoneography at the time of catheter placement may predict later clinical hernia development and allow early prophylactic repair of subclinical inguinal and umbilical hernias. This series described 101 patient months on CAPD in nine patients without a single catheter failure.

In five uremic children undergoing CAPD for 6–8 months, amino acid losses averaged 10,000 millimicromoles/day (275). Children had uremic profiles of plasma amino acid concentrations that were not altered by CAPD.

Pancreatitis

Renal and peritoneal clearances of amylase and lipase were compared in a patient treated with peritoneal dialysis for acute pancreatitis (277). Amylase clearance by the kidney was better than that by peritoneal dialysis. Lipase, on the other hand, was more efficiently removed by peritoneal dialysis than by the kidney. Absolute levels of plasma clearances of amylase and lipase by peritoneal dialysis are nearly five times those predicted according to their molecular weight. These results suggest direct spilling of pancreatic enzymes into the dialysate from inflamed pancreatic and surrounding tissues.

Thirty patients suffering from acute necrotic hemorrhagic pancreatitis were treated by peritoneal dialysis (278). Peritoneal dialysis appeared to result in early improvement in abdominal and toxemic signs. Of the 30 patients, 19 (63.4%) survived. The authors claim better results if peritoneal dialysis is begun within 7 days of the onset of acute pancreatitis.

Other reports suggest an important role for peritoneal dialysis in the treatment of acute pancreatitis (279,280).

Acute Renal Failure

Peritoneal dialysis continues to have an important role in the dialytic therapy of acute renal failure (281–287). There is growing interest in low-flow continuous peritoneal dialysis for the treatment of acute renal failure (284).

Some hold that peritoneal dialysis, especially slow continuous peritoneal dialysis, is the best method of treating patients with severe head trauma and acute renal failure (287).

Ascites and Liver Disease

In five patients receiving maintenance hemodialysis, ascites refractory to ultrafiltration developed (288). Maintenance peritoneal dialysis was instituted with gradual removal of abdominal fluid. Ascites resolved in all cases. Three patients noted dramatic improvement in appetite after relief of abdominal distention.

Another report supports the efficacy of CAPD in treating dialysis-related ascites (289). Dialysis and ultrafiltration of ascitic fluid has been employed with intraperitoneal reinfusion of the concentrated ascites (290–292). Ascites may be removed via a peritoneal catheter and ultrafiltered using a hemodialyzer (291). The concentrate is continuously returned to the peritoneal space. On the average, 4.8 liters of protein-free ascitic ultrafiltrate was removed without adverse effects over the course of a 3–5 hour procedure (291).

One hundred patients underwent studies by computed tomography to assess the relative distribution of fluid in the greater and lesser peritoneal sacs (293). Patients on peritoneal dialysis had large greater sac collections with little fluid in the lesser sac. Fluid in the lesser sac with little in the greater sac was seen primarily in patients with diseases of organs bordering the lesser sac (pancreatitis and posteriorly penetrating gastric ulcer). Carcinomatosis of the abdomen was associated with fluid in both spaces. The authors suggest that fluid within the lesser sac is not a typical manifestation of generalized peritoneal ascites and its presence should direct a search for pathology in neighboring organs or peritoneal malignancy.

Studies of peritoneal dialysis in the treatment of acute hepatic coma continue (294). There is little to suggest long-term alterations in mortality and morbidity.

Lactic Acidosis

Peritoneal dialysis can be helpful in the treatment of lactic acidosis (295–297). Peritoneal dialysis with bicarbonate-based dialysate appears to be an ideal means of delivering physiologic buffer (296). Peritoneal clearances of lactate were studied in experimental lactic acidosis using two types of dialysis fluid (with and without sodium nitroprusside added) (297). The addition of sodium nitroprusside increased peritoneal clearances of lactate. Alkaline dialysis fluid containing bicarbonate was also associated with higher lactate clearances. The highest clearance values were seen when alkaline dialysis fluid was used together with sodium nitroprusside.

Psoriasis

There continues to be interest in the use of peritoneal dialysis for the treatment of psoriasis (298–301).

Eight patients with 2–32 years of generalized psoriasis vulgaris of the pure plaque type underwent peritoneal dialysis therapy over a period of 1–6 months with an average of eight treatment days (298). In one patient there was a transitory improvement of the skin changes. In five, the picture of the disease remained unchanged. Two showed a deterioration.

One patient treated by peritoneal dialysis for psoriasis showed complete clearing (299). Two treated by hemodialysis gave unsatisfactory results. The authors suggest that solutes in the middle molecular weight range (500–5,000 daltons) are fixed in the epidermis and/or in the walls of the skin capillaries. They also propose that peritoneal dialysis is more effective in removing these substances.

A controlled study was recently completed at our own center (301). Five patients underwent 4 weeks of therapy (40 hr/wk) with real peritoneal dialysis and 4 weeks of therapy with sham peritoneal dialysis in which the same 2 liters of dialysis fluid were repeatedly cycled in and out of the peritoneal cavity. The order of the therapy was randomized and the procedure was blinded so that the patient and the doctors evaluating the skin lesions did not know which type of therapy was being performed. Dramatic clearing resulted from a course of real therapy. No improvements were seen with sham therapy. In those patients in whom real therapy and remission came first, sham therapy was attempted after relapse with no benefit. In those patients in whom sham therapy came first, remission was seen only after the later course of real therapy. These studies are the first attempts to provide controlled results supporting the benefits of peritoneal dialysis for psoriasis.

Peritoneal Dialysis for Drugs, Poisons, and Toxins

Effects of peritoneal dialysis on drug kinetics, overdoses, exogenous poisons, and endogenous poisons were frequently reported (302–314). Experiences reported included the removal of copper in Wilson's disease (302), the treatment of hypercalcemia with CAPD using calcium-free solutions (303), and the treatment of lithium intoxication (304).

Peritoneal clearances of gentamicin, carbon tetrachloride, and other small solutes are usually quite low, resulting in the removal of only small portions of the total body load (305–307).

Clearances of quinine by hemodialysis, peritoneal dialysis, plasmapheresis, and forced diuresis were compared (308). Hemodialysis, peritoneal dialysis, and plasma exchange made only minor contributions to quinine elimination as compared to renal excretion.

Other uses of peritoneal dialysis to treat acute intoxication included mushroom poisoning (309), mannitol intoxication (310), ethylene glycol poisoning (311), thiazide-induced hyponatremia (312), amikacin overdose (313), and assessments of the clearance of quinine (314).

Other Uses

Five patients with accidental hypothermia were rewarmed by peritoneal dialysis with fluid at 37°C (315). Rewarming was rapid, smooth, and free of complications. This continues the annual reporting of the successful treatment of hypothermia with peritoneal dialysis.

Intraperitoneal chemotherapy relates closely to peritoneal dialysis and many of the experiences of peritoneal dialysis may be carried over to the development of intraperitoneal chemotherapy (316).

Whether peritoneal dialysis has specific advantages for the dialytic treatment of pericarditis remains controversial (317). The role of peritoneal dialysis in operative gynecology was reviewed (318). Chronic dialysis in the mentally retarded patient is a challenge and the successful use of CAPD in such a situation was reported (319).

MISCELLANEOUS

Numerous authors have reviewed the care of end-stage renal failure in general and the role of peritoneal dialysis therein (320–333). Mion has reviewed his experiences with chronic IPD and CAPD over a 7 year period (330). Kliger (333) has written a review of current concepts in peritoneal dialysis. He concludes that "the various techniques of performing peritoneal dialysis and improved understanding of the mechanisms of solute clearance and ultrafiltration and the use of systemic and intraperitoneal drugs may offer the dialysis patient of the future the versatility to adapt a treatment regimen to his specific needs. For this reason, peritoneal dialysis may increase in its use and maintain a central role in the treatment of end-stage renal disease."

The employment of medical students in the peritoneal dialysis program at the University of Naples reportedly benefited the program and added greatly to the medical education of the students (334).

Oreopoulos has reviewed the importance of the Artificial Kidney Chronic Uremia Program of the National Institutes of Health as a driving force in the development of peritoneal dialysis (335).

Glycosylated hemoglobin levels were significantly elevated in patients treated by both chronic hemodialysis and chronic peritoneal dialysis (336). Glucose-free hemodialysis did not ameliorate elevated levels over 8 weeks. The authors feel that glycosylated hemoglobin elevation cannot be explained solely by glucose reabsorption from dialysate.

Plasma lecithin cholesterol acetotransferase activity was measured in 43 hemodialysis patients and in 15 CAPD patients (337). Activities were significantly lower than normal in both groups. The cause of the low activities was not ascertained but did not appear to be due to the presence of inhibitors.

Accumulation of inhibitors to fibrinolysis was demonstrated in hemodialysis and peritoneal dialysis patients (338). IPD was considered less effective than hemodialysis in removing such inhibitors. In IPD, protein loss by the peritoneum is also probably responsible for loss of fibrinolytic activators.

Iron absorption was measured in 16 nondialyzed patients, 18 chronic peritoneal dialysis patients, 19 chronic hemodialysis patients, and 14 renal transplant patients (339). The hemodialysis patients had greater blood losses and significantly higher absorption than both nondialysis and peritoneal dialysis patients. The results indicated that regulatory mechanisms that relate iron absorption to body iron stores are intact in patients with chronic uremia.

SUMMARY

The literature on peritoneal dialysis continues to increase in a prolific manner. The interest in peritoneal dialysis has focused on experiences with CAPD.

Several developments during the past year, in my opinion, stand out. First, there is accumulating evidence that the mesothelium may be an important resistant site, and changes in peritoneal transport characteristics may at least in part relate to alterations in mesothelium. In previous years, we focused mainly on the microcirculation of the peritoneum and its influence on peritoneal transport. This year several reports have suggested that there may be two pathways through the mesothelium. Some ultrafiltration and small solute movement may occur through cells, while larger molecules may move primarily through paracellular routes. Alterations in mesothelial intercellular gaps appear to be associated with increased clearances of larger molecules and increased protein losses.

Secondly, we have learned much about ultrafiltration in the past year. Certain conditions such as peritonitis are associated with rapid glucose absorption rates and rapid disappearance of the osmotic gradient.

Reports of certain long-term experiences with CAPD are beginning to come in. Important conclusions in this area do not seem much different from those of previous years. There is much interest in comparisons of CAPD with other types of end-stage renal disease therapy. It is becoming apparent that population characteristics have a marked influence on morbidity, mortality, and hospitalization rates in dialysis populations. This past year the literature mainly emphasizes the lack of data to allow legitimate comparisons. Randomized studies have not been reported and, to my knowledge, are not underway.

REFERENCES

1. Nolph KD, Miller FN, Pyle WK, et al: An hypothesis to explain the ultrafiltration characteristics of peritoneal dialysis. *Kidney Int* 20:543–548, 1981.

2. Rubin J, Ray R, Barnest T, et al: Peritoneal abnormalities during infectious episodes of continuous ambulatory peritoneal dialysis. *Nephron* 29:124–127, 1981.
3. Verger C, Brunschvicg O, Le Charpentier Y, et al: Structural and ultrastructural peritoneal membrane changes and permeability alterations during continuous ambulatory peritoneal dialysis. *Proc Eur Dial Transplant Assoc* 18:199–205, 1981.
4. Verger C, Luger A, Moore HL, et al: Acute changes in peritoneal morphology and transport properties with infectious peritonitis and mechanical injury. *Kidney Int* (in press).
5. Dobbie JW, Zaki M, Wilson L: Ultrastructural studies on the peritoneum with special reference to chronic ambulatory peritoneal dialysis. *Scott Med J* 26:213–223, 1981.
6. McGary TJ, Nolph KD, Kartinos NJ: Polyanions as osmotic agents in a simulated in vitro model of peritoneal dialysis. *Trans Am Soc Artif Intern Organs* 27:314–319, 1981.
7. Rubin J, Klein E, Bower JD: Investigation of the net sieving coefficient of the peritoneal membrane during peritoneal dialysis. *ASAIO* 5:9–15, 1982.
8. Hirszel P, Lasrich M, Maher JF: Arachidonic acid increases peritoneal clearances. *Trans Am Soc Artif Intern Ograns* 27:61–63, 1981.
9. Dunham C, Hak LJ, Null JH, et al: Enhancement of peritoneal dialysis clearance with docusate sodium. *Kidney Int* 20:563–568, 1981.
10. De Santo NG, Capodicasa G, Capasso G, et al: Development of means to augment peritoneal urea clearances: The synergistic effects of combining high dialysate temperature and high dialysate flow rates with dextrose and nitroprusside. *Artif Organs* 5:409–414, 1981.
11. Rubin J, Kirchner K, Bower J: Evaluation of stagnant fluid films during simulated peritoneal dialysis: In vitro and in vivo studies. *Clin Exper Dialysis and Apheresis* 5:285–292, 1981.
12. Miller FN, Nolph KD, Joshua IG, et al: Hyperosmolality, acetate, and lactate: Dilatory factors during peritoneal dialysis. *Kidney Int* 20:397–402, 1981.
13. Alavi N, Lianos E, Andres G, et al: Effect of protamine on the permeability and structure of rat peritoneum. *Kidney Int* 21:44–53, 1982.
14. Rubin J, Adair C, Johnson B, et al: Stereospecific lactate absorption during peritoneal dialysis. *Nephron* 31:224–228, 1982.
15. Rubin J, Rust P, Brown P, et al: A comparison of peritoneal transport in patients with psoriasis and uremia. *Nephron* 29:185–189, 1981.
16. Taraba I, Spustova V, Balas-Eltes A, et al: Peritoneal dialysability of "ureamic substances." *Int Urol Nephrol* 13:193–198, 1981.
17. Anderson KE: Calcium transfer during intermittent peritoneal dialysis. *Nephron* 29:63–67, 1981.
18. Brown GS, Lohr TD, Mayor GH, et al: Peritoneal clearance of theophylline. *Am J Kidney Dis* 1:24–26, 1981.
19. Elzouki AY, Gruskin AB, Baluarte HJ, et al: Development of aspects of peritoneal dialysis kinetics in dogs. *Pediatr Res* 15:853–858, 1981.
20. Gotloib L, Crassweller P, Rodella H, et al: Experimental model for studies of continuous peritoneal dialysis in uremic rabbits. *Nephron* 31:254–259, 1982.
21. Dedrick RL, Flessner MF, Collins, JM, et al: Is the peritoneum a membrane? *ASAIO* 5:1–8, 1982.
22. Legrain M, Rottembourg J: Substitutes for renal function. Technical trends and logistics of treatment. *C R Soc Biol* 175:669–693, 1981.
23. Scheler F: Alternative procedures in the therapy of chronic uremia (hemofiltration, continuing ambulatory peritoneal dialysis). *Verh Dtsch Ges Inn Med* 87:1405–1408, 1981.

24. Pasternack A, Lampainen E, Viranta M, et al: Continuous ambulatory peritoneal dialysis. *Duodecim* 97:1153–1161, 1981.
25. Prowant B, Fruto LV: The continuous ambulatory peritoneal dialysis (CAPD) home training program. *J Am Assoc Nephrol Nurses Tech* 8:18–19, 1981.
26. Arenz R: Continuous ambulatory peritoneal dialysis. *AORN J* 35:946–954, 1982.
27. Levey AS, Harrington JT: Continuous peritoneal dialysis for chronic renal failure. *Medicine* 61:330–339, 1982.
28. Valek A, Kukliik R, Klimova D, et al: Continuous peritoneal dialysis. *Cas Lek Cesk* 120:1457–1462, 1981.
29. Finkelstein FO, Forman BH, Marieb NJ, et al: Continuous ambulatory peritoneal dialysis: Experience with 22 unselected patients with renal failure. *Yale J Biol Med* 54:95–100, 1981.
30. McFarland SC: Protocol management of CAPD complications. *AANNT J* 9:13–15, 1982.
31. Pascoe MD: Continuous peritoneal dialysis. The first 2 years of a programme at Groote Schuur Hospital. *S Afr Med J* 61:19–21, 1982.
32. Prejac M, Antos M, Kovarbascc B: Continuous peritoneal dialysis performed in outpatient departments, a new method of treatment in the terminal stage of chronic renal insufficiency. *Lijec Vjesn* 102:423–426, 1980.
33. Wyszynska T: Peritoneal dialysis in the terminal stage of renal failure. *Pediatr Pol* 56:853–859, 1981.
34. Robeva R, Belovezhdov N: Continuous ambulatory peritoneal dialysis in treating chronic kidney failure. *Vutr Boles* 20:9–13, 1981.
35. Jeffrey JE, Heidenheim AP, Burton HJ, et al: A comparison of home training and problems encountered with initial home dialysis: Hemodialysis vs CAPD. *AANNT J* 9:56–62, 1982.
36. Rigby PJ, Butler JL, Petrie JB: Experience with continuous ambulatory peritoneal dialysis. *Med J Aust* 1:331–335, 1982.
37. Continuous ambulatory peritoneal dialysis. *Lancet* 1:556, 1982.
38. Harrington JT: Chronic ambulatory peritoneal dialysis. *N Engl J Med* 306:670–671, 1982 (editorial).
39. Oreopoulos DG, Khanna R, Williams P, et al: Continuous ambulatory peritoneal dialysis—1981. *Nephron* 30:293–303, 1982.
40. Rottenbourg J, De Groc F, Jacq D, et al: Continuous ambulatory peritoneal dialysis—experience in 100 patients. *Przege Lek* 39:293–297, 1982.
41. Sorrels AJ, Mullins-Blackson C, Moncrief JW: Getting back to reality: Psychosocial adjustments in CAPD. *Nephrol Nurse* 4:22–23, 1982.
42. Boeschoten EW, Krediet RT, Arisz L, et al: A hundred patient months' experience with continuous ambulatory peritoneal dialysis. *Net J Med* 25:65–72, 1982.
43. Watson AJ, Hiliery M, Grant G, et al: Continuous ambulatory peritoneal dialysis—initial experience. *Med J* 74:330–333, 1981.
44. Sandoval M, Parks C: The evolution to CAPD. *Nephrol Nurse* 3:27–32, 1981.
45. Colombi A: What brought us CAPD (continuous ambulatory peritoneal dialysis)? *Praxis* 71:309–312, 1982.
46. Eichsen K: The disabled and the nurse: Continuous ambulatory peritoneal dialysis. *Camp* 38:53–54, 1981.
47. Robertson JA, Wenzl JE: Continuous ambulatory peritoneal dialysis (CAPD). *J Okla State Med Assoc* 74:392–395, 1981.
48. Kincaid-Smith P, Becker G: Continuous ambulatory peritoneal dialysis. *Med J Aust* 1:325–326, 1982 (editorial).

49. Levey AS, Harrington JT: Continuous peritoneal dialysis for chronic renal failure. *Medicine* 61:330–339, 1982.
50. Colombi A, Wyss R, Pfister G, et al: Continuous ambulatory peritoneal dialysis (CAPD). *Ther Umsch* 39:396–401, 1982.
51. Hughes RD: Continuous ambulatory peritoneal dialysis. *J Ark Med Soc* 77:521–524, 1981.
52. Arenz R: Continuous ambulatory peritoneal dialysis. *AORN J* 35:946–954, 1982.
53. Moncrief JW: Continuous ambulatory peritoneal dialysis. Impact on management of patients with end-stage renal disease. *Nephron* 27:226–228, 1981.
54. Wood A: Renal replacement therapy. 4–2. Continuous ambulatory peritoneal dialysis—an alternative approach in maintenance dialysis therapy. *Nurs Times* 78:852–854, 1982.
55. Chan MK, Baillod RA, Chuah P, et al: Three years experience of continuous ambulatory peritoneal dialysis. *Lancet* 1:1409–1412, 1981.
56. Korten G, Kröger E: Observation of the course of 4 year ambulatory peritoneal dialysis in the treatment of chronic uremia. *Z Urol Nephrol* 74:305–310, 1981.
57. Ray R, Samar D: Continuous ambulatory peritoneal dialysis nursing followup: How much times does it take? *J Am Assoc Nephrol Nurses Tech* 8:26–27, 1981.
58. Mehall DL, DeYoung K, DeYoung M: The psychological adjustment of a CAPD patient. *J Am Assoc Nephrol Nurses Tech* 8:23–24, 1981.
59. Harrington JT: Chronic ambulatory peritoneal dialysis *N Engl J Med* 306:670–671, 1982 (editorial).
60. Continuous ambulatory peritoneal dialysis. *Lancet* 1:556, 1982.
61. Feliciangeli G, Coli L, Prandini R, et al: Continuous ambulatory peritoneal dialysis (CAPD) in the substitutive treatment of chronic renal insufficiency. *G Clin Med* 62:280–286, 1981.
62. Khanna R: Thoughts on the future of continuous ambulatory peritoneal dialysis. *Periton Dialys Bull* 1:78–82, 1981.
63. Clayton S: The organization and implementation of a peritoneal dialysis program. *Periton Dialys Bull* 1:134–136, 1981.
64. Fenton SS: Selection criteria for continuous ambulatory peritoneal dialysis. *Periton Dialys Bull* 2:3–7, 1982.
65. Coward RA, Uttley L, Murray Y, et al: The importance of patient selection for CAPD. *Periton Dialys Bull* 2:8–11, 1982.
66. Breckenridge DM, Cupit MC, Raimondo JM: Systematic nursing assessment tool for the CAPD client. *Nephrol Nurse* 4:24–31, 1982.
67. Perras ST, Zappacosta AR: The application of Orem's theory in promoting self-care in a peritoneal dialysis facility. *AANNT J* 9:37–39, 1982.
68. Cote S: "Subsisting" through continuous ambulatory peritoneal dialysis. *Nurs Que* 2:29–31, 1982.
69. Clayton S, Combros N, Zellerman G, et al: Experience with continuous ambulatory peritoneal dialysis. *J Am Assoc Nephrol Nurses Tech* 8:29–31, 1981.
70. Chung HNK: Treatment of chronic renal failure with continuous ambulatory peritoneal dialysis. *Tsa Chih* 20:323–325, 1981.
71. Nolph KD, Boen ST, Farrell PC, et al: Continuous ambulatory peritoneal dialysis in Australia, Europe, and the United States—1981. *Kidney Int* 23:3–8, 1983.
72. Jacobs C, Broyer M, Brunner FP, et al: Combined report on regular dialysis and transplantation in Europe, in BHB Robinson, JB Hawkins, AM Davison (eds): *Proceedings of the European Dialysis and Transplant Association, 18*. London, Pitman Books Ltd, 1981, pp. 4–58.

73. Prowant B, Nolph KD, Dutton S, et al: Actuarial analysis of patient survival and dropout with various end-stage renal disease therapies. *Am J Kid Dis* (in press).
74. Burton HJ, Kaplan De-Nour A, Conley JA, et al: Comparison of psychological adjustment to CAPD and home hemodialysis. *Periton Dialys Bull* 2:76–79, 1982.
75. Bulgin RH: Comparative costs of various dialysis treatments. *Periton Dialys Bull* 1:88–91, 1981.
76. Hutchinson TA, Thomas DC, Macgibbon B: Predicting survival in adults with end-stage renal disease: An age equivalence index. *Ann Intern Med* 96:417–423, 1982.
77. Weller JM, Port FK: Analysis of survival of end-stage renal disease patients. *Kidney Int* 21:78–83, 1982.
78. Bodnar DM: Rationale for nutritional requirements for patients on continuous ambulatory peritoneal dialysis. *J Am Diet Assoc* 80:247–249, 1982.
79. Blumenkrantz MJ, Gahl GM, Kopple JD, et al: Protein losses during peritoneal dialysis. *Kidney Int* 19:593–602, 1981.
80. Lindholm B, Alvestrand A, Furst P, et al: Metabolic effects of continuous ambulatory peritoneal dialysis. *Proc Eur Dial Transplant Assoc* 17:283–290, 1980.
81. von Baeyer H, Gahl GM, Riedinger H, et al: Nutritional behavior of patients on continuous ambulatory peritoneal dialysis. *Proc Eur Dial Transplant Assoc* 18:193–198, 1981.
82. Blumenkrantz MJ, Kopple JD, Moran JK, et al: Nitrogen and urea metabolism during continuous ambulatory peritoneal dialysis. *Kidney Int* 20:78–82, 1981.
83. Blumenkrantz MJ, Kopple JD, Moran JK, et al: Metabolic balance studies and dietary protein requirements in patients undergoing continuous ambulatory peritoneal dialysis. *Kidney Int* 21:849–861, 1982.
84. Lindholm B, Berström J, Karlander SG: Glucose metabolism in patients on continuous ambulatory peritoneal dialysis (CAPD). *Trans Am Soc Artif Intern Organs* 27:58–60, 1981.
85. Grodstein GP, Blumenkrantz MJ, Kopple JD, et al: Glucose absorption during continuous ambulatory peritoneal dialysis. *Kidney Int* 19:564–567, 1981.
86. Kopple JD, Blumenkrantz MJ, Jones MR, et al: Plasma amino acid levels and amino acid losses during continuous ambulatory peritoneal dialysis. *Am J Clin Nutr* 36:395–402, 1982.
87. Williams P, Marliss E, Anderson GH, et al: Amino acid absorption following intraperitoneal administration in CAPD patients. *Periton Dialys Bull* 2:124–130, 1982.
88. Dombros N, Oren A, Marliss EB, et al: Plasma amino acid profiles and amino acid losses in patients undergoing CAPD. *Periton Dialys Bull* 2:27–32, 1982.
89. Roncari DAK, Breckenridge WC, Khanna R, et al: Rise in high density lipoprotein-cholesterol in some patients treated with CAPD. *Periton Dialys Bull* 1:136–138, 1981.
90. Williams P, Kay R, Harrison J, et al: Nutritional and anthropometric assessment of patients on CAPD over one year: Contrasting changes in total body nitrogen and potassium. *Periton Dialys Bull* 1:82–88, 1981.
91. Twardowski Z, Janicka L: Three exchanges with a 2.5 liter volume for continuous ambulatory peritoneal dialysis. *Kidney Int* 20:281–284, 1981.
92. Twardowski Z, Sokolowska G, Bochenska-Nowacka E: Kinetics of continuous ambulatory peritoneal dialysis. I. Ultrafiltration. *Pol Arch Med Wewn* 65:57–63, 1981.
93. Ksiazek A, Twardowski Z, Janicka L, et al: Kinetics of continuous ambulatory peritoneal dialysis. II. Protein and immunoglobulin losses. *Pol Arch Med Wewn* 65:107–114, 1981.
94. Majdan M, Twardowski Z, Milczarska D, et al: Kinetics of continuous ambulatory peritoneal dialysis. III. Urea, creatinine, inulin, sodium, potassium and phosphorus in the blood plasma and dialysate. *Pol Arch Med Wewn* 65:131–140, 1981.

95. Henderson I, Juhasz L, McArdle C, et al: The Glasgow CAPD system. *Int J Artif Organs* 5:25–26, 1982.
96. Bazzato G, Coli U, Landini S, et al: Continuous ambulatory peritoneal dialysis without wearing a bag: Complete freedom of patient and significant reduction of peritonitis. *Proc Eur Dial Transplant Assoc* 17:266–275, 1980.
97. Capodicasa G, De Santo NG, Galione A, et al: CAPD plus hemoperfusion once a week for end-stage renal disease. *Int J Artif Organs* 5:125–129, 1982.
98. Forbes AM, Reed VL, Goldsmith HJ: The adequacy of six liter daily continuous ambulatory peritoneal dialysis. *Proc Eur Dial Transplant Assoc* 17:276–282, 1980.
99. Coli U, Landini S, Lucatello S, et al: 22 months of experience with CAPD with the double-bag system. *Minerva Nefrol* 28:353–358, 1981.
100. Cantarovich F, Loredo JP, Wilberg R, et al: Three daily exchanges on continuous ambulatory peritoneal dialysis. 8 months of treatment in 6 patients. *Nephron* 30:304–309. 1982.
101. Forbes AM, Reed V, Goldsmith HJ: CAPD—A scheme to allow reduction of dialysis bag exchange. *Clin Nephrol* 15:264–266, 1981.
102. Simon P, Moncrief JW, Pyle K: CAPD: Are three exchanges per day adequate? *AANNT J* 9:39–43, 1982.
103. Evans DH, Sorkin MI, Nolph KD, et al: Continuous ambulatory peritoneal dialysis and transplantation. *Trans Am Soc Artif Intern Organs* 27:320–324, 1981.
104. Kennedy JM: CAPD and transplantation. *J Am Assoc Nephrol Nurses Tech* 8:11, 1981.
105. Gokal R, Ramos JM, Veitch P, et al: Renal transplantation in patients on continuous ambulatory peritoneal dialysis. *Proc Eur Dial Transplant Assoc* 18:222–227, 1981.
106. Bandel-Walcer R, Myers C, Malgaonkar S, et al: Intraperitoneal insulin: New alternative for diabetic CAPD patients. *AANNT J* 9:31–35, 1982.
107. Amair P, Khanna R, Leibel B, et al: Continuous ambulatory peritoneal dialysis in diabetics with end-stage renal disease. *N Engl J Med* 18:625–630, 1982.
108. Amair P, Khanna R, Leibel B, et al: Continuous ambulatory peritoneal dialysis in diabetics with end-stage renal disease. *Periton Dialys Bull* 2:S6–S12, 1982.
109. Williams CC, Belvedere D, Cattran D, et al: Experience with CAPD in diabetic patients in Toronto. *Periton Dialys Bull* 2:S12–S15, 1982.
110. Karanicolas S, Thompson D: Intermittent peritoneal dialysis in the treatment of diabetics with end-stage renal disease. *Periton Dialys Bull* 2:S15–S17, 1982.
111. Cordella CJ, Tam PYW, Walker JF, et al: Renal transplantation in diabetes mellitus. *Periton Dialys Bull* 2:S17–S20, 1982.
112. Hanna AK: The importance of blood glucose control in the prevention of diabetic complications. *Periton Dialys Bull* 2:S22–S24, 1982.
113. Zingg W, Shirriff JM, Leibel BS: Experimental routes of insulin administration. *Periton Dialys Bull* 2:S24–S27, 1982.
114. Roscoe JM: Practices of insulin administration. *Periton Dialys Bull* 2:S27–S29, 1982.
115. Singh V, Saiphoo CS, Oreopoulos DG: Psychosocial and sexual aspects of patients on CAPD. *Periton Dialys Bull* 2:S32–S36, 1982.
116. DeMarco V: Psychiatric aspects of diabetics on CAPD. *Periton Dialys Bull* 2:S36–S38, 1982.
117. Clayton S: Training the diabetic patient on continuous ambulatory peritoneal dialysis. *Periton Dialys Bull* 2:S38–S40, 1982.
118. Chisholm L: Evolution of retinopathy in diabetics undergoing CAPD. *Periton Dialys Bull* 2:S42–S44, 1982.
119. Oreopoulos DG, Chisholm L: Discussion on evolution of retinopathy in diabetics undergoing CAPD. *Periton Dialys Bull* 2:S44–S46, 1982.

120. English E: Care of the diabetic foot. *Periton Dialys Bull* 2:S46–S49, 1982.
121. Haber MO, Pettit JM: Nutritional considerations in the diabetic patient on CAPD. *Periton Dialys Bull* 2:S50–S52, 1982.
122. Blair RDG: Electrophysiologic studies in peripheral nerves of diabetics undergoing CAPD. *Periton Dialys Bull* 2:S53–S55, 1982.
123. Madden MA, Zimmerman SW, Simpson DP: Continuous ambulatory peritoneal dialysis in diabetes mellitus. *Am J Nephrol* 2:133–139, 1982.
124. Amair P, Khanna R, Digenis G, et al: Continuous ambulatory peritoneal dialysis (CAPD) in diabetics with end-stage renal disease. *Int J Artif Organs* 5:81–82, 1982.
125. Riambau E, Aubia J, Llorach I, et al: Intraperitoneal insulin in continuous ambulatory peritoneal dialysis. *Rev Clin Esp* 164:333–334, 1982.
126. Adair CM: Intraperitoneal insulin in the diabetic continuous ambulatory peritoneal dialysis (CAPD) patient—nursing management. *AANNT J* 9:62–63, 1982.
127. Anderson KE, Petersen PH: Intraperitoneal administration of insulin during peritoneal dialysis of diabetics with terminal renal failure. *Int J Artif Organs* 4:162–167, 1981.
128. Friedman EA: Diabetic nephropathy: Strategies in prevention and management. *Kidney Int* 21:780–791, 1982.
129. Amair P, Khanna R, Leibel B, et al: Continuous ambulatory peritoneal dialysis in diabetics with end-stage renal disease. *N Engl J Med* 306:625–630, 1982.
130. Cohen IM, Lee S: Diabetes, intraperitoneal insulin, and CAPD. *Clin Exp Dial Apheresis* 5:269–275, 1981.
131. Cable A: Diabetic teaching of the CAPD patient. *AANNT J* 9:21–25, 1982.
132. Flynn CT: Devices to achieve self-care in blind diabetic patients with renal failure. *Int J Artif Organs* 5:137–139, 1982.
133. Bazzato G, Lucatello S, Coli U, et al: Double-bag CAPD with intraperitoneal insulin. Satisfactory management of diabetes and its major complications in uremic patients. *Minerva Nefrol* 28:345–352, 1981.
134. Knotek B: Independence for the visually impaired continuous ambulatory peritoneal dialysis (CAPD) patient. *AANNT J* 9:69–71, 1982.
135. Nolph KD: Issues in nephrology. *NAPHT News* 14:12–14, 1982.
136. Sorkin MI, Luger AM, Prowant B, et al: Histological and functional characteristics of the peritoneal membrane of a diabetic patient after 34 months of CAPD. *Periton Dialys Bull* 2:24–27, 1982.
137. Farrell PC, Randerson DH: Membrane permeability changes in long term CAPD. *Trans Am Soc Artif Intern Organs* 26:197–200, 1980.
138. Zappacosta AR, Caro J, Erslev A: Normalization of hematocrit in patients with end-stage renal disease on continuous ambulatory peritoneal dialysis: the role of erythropoietin. *Am J Med* 72:53–57, 1982.
139. De Paepe M, Laemeire N, Schelstraete K, et al: Changes in red cell mass, plasma volume and hematocrit in patients on continuous ambulatory peritoneal dialysis. *Proc Eur Dial Transplant Assoc* 18:286–289, 1981.
140. Arends JP, Krediet RT, Boeschoten EW, et al: Improvement of bleeding time, platelet aggregation and platelet count during CAPD treatment. *Proc Eur Dial Transplant Assoc* 18:280–285, 1981.
141. Amair P, Gregoriadis A, Rodella H, et al: Serum carnitine in patients on CAPD. *Periton Dialys Bull* 2:11–13, 1982.
142. Gloor HJ, Moore H, Nolph KD: The peritoneal handling of digoxin during CAPD. *Periton Dialys Bull* 2:13–16, 1982.

143. Goodman CE, Husserl FE: Etiology, prevention and treatment of back pain in patients undergoing continuous ambulatory peritoneal dialysis. *Periton Dialys Bull* 1:119–123, 1981.

144. Sorkin MI, Nolph KD, Anderson HO, et al: Aluminum mass transfer during continuous ambulatory peritoneal dialysis. *Periton Dialys Bull* 1:91–94, 1981.

145. Patton TW, Manuel MA, Walker SE: Cimetidine disposition in patients on CAPD. *Periton Dialys Bull* 2:73–76, 1982.

146. Chin TWF, Pancorbo S, Comty C: Quinidine pharmacokinetics in continuous ambulatory peritoneal dialysis. *Clin Exper Dialys Apheresis* 5:391–397, 1981.

147. Delmez JA, Slatopolsky E, Martin KJ, et al: Minerals, vitamin D, and parathyroid hormone in continuous ambulatory peritoneal dialysis. *Kidney Int* 21:862–867, 1982.

148. Slingeneyer A, Mion C, Béraud JJ, et al: Peritonitis, a frequently lethal complication of intermittent and continuous ambulatory peritoneal dialysis. *Proc Eur Dial Transplant Assoc* 18:212–221, 1981.

149. Khanna R, Oreopoulos DG, Vas S, et al: Fungal peritonitis in patients undergoing chronic intermittent or continuous ambulatory peritoneal dialysis. *Proc Eur Dial Transplant Assoc* 17:291–296, 1980.

150. Cheong IK, Lim VK, Ujang K: Bacterial peritonitis in peritoneal dialysis. *Med J Malaysia* 36:17–19, 1981.

151. Gokal R: Peritonitis in continuous ambulatory peritoneal dialysis. *J Antimicrob Chemother* 9:417–420, 1982.

152. Beimel M, Rice R: Early peritonitis in CAPD. *AANNT J* 9:17, 1982.

153. Binswanger U, Keusch G, Bammatter F, et al: Peritonitis during continuous ambulatory peritoneal dialysis: Improving patient defense by type of buffer of dialysate? *Nephron* 28:300–302, 1981.

154. Steurer J, Münch R, Kuhlmann U: Therapy of peritonitis in continuing ambulatory peritoneal dialysis. *Dtsch Med Wochenschr* 107:828–830, 1982.

155. Münch R, Steurer J, Kuhlmann U: Diagnosis of peritonitis in continuing ambulatory peritoneal dialysis. *Dtsch Med Wochenschr* 107:826–833, 1982.

156. Fenton S, Wu G, Cattran D, et al: Clinical aspects of peritonitis in patients on CAPD. *Periton Dialys Bull* 6:S4–S7, 1981.

157. Williams CC, Cattran D, Fenton SS, et al: Peritonitis on CAPD—three years experience in Toronto. *Periton Dialys Bull* 6:S7–S9, 1981.

158. Vas S: Microbiological aspects of peritonitis. *Periton Dialys Bull* 6:S11–S14, 1981.

159. Oreopoulos DG, Williams P, Khanna R, et al: Treatment of peritonitis. *Periton Dialys Bull* 6:S17–S20, 1981.

160. Vas S: Peritonitis during CAPD: A mixed bag. *Periton Dialys Bull* 1:47–49, 1981.

161. Nolph KD, Prowant B, Sorkin MI, et al: The incidence and characteristics of peritonitis in the fourth year of a CAPD program. *Periton Dialys Bull* 1:50–53, 1981.

162. Corey P: An approach to the statistical analysis of peritonitis data from patients on CAPD. *Periton Dialys Bull* 6:S29–S33, 1981.

163. McMahon T, Moriarty MV: Beta Cap technique for CAPD. *Dialysis Transplantation* 10:807–813, 1981.

164. Hemmeloff Andersen KE, Kolmos HJ: Infectious peritonitis. The main complication of intermittent peritoneal dialysis. *Int J Artif Organs* 4:281–285, 1981.

165. Williams P, Pantalony D, Vas SI, et al: The value of dialysate cell count in the diagnosis of peritonitis in patients on CAPD. *Periton Dialys Bull* 1:59–62, 1981.

166. Pierratos A, Amair P, Corey P, et al: Statistical analysis of the incidence of peritonitis on CAPD. *Periton Dialys Bull* 2:32–36, 1982.

167. Karatson A, David MF, Farkas L, et al: Infection of the abdominal cavity and chronic peritoneal dialysis. *Int Urol Nephrol* 13:395–403, 1981.
168. Steiner RW: Clinical observations on the pathogenesis of peritoneal dialysis eosinophilia. *Periton Dialys Bull* 2:118–120, 1982.
169. Gokal R, Ramos JM, Ward MK, et al: "Eosinophilic" peritonitis in continuous ambulatory peritoneal dialysis (CAPD). *Clin Nephrol* 15:328–330, 1981.
170. Nolph KD, Sorkin MI, Prowant B, et al: Case Report: Asymptomatic eosinophilic peritonitis in CAPD. *Dialysis Transplantation* 11:309–315, 1982.
171. Huertas VE, Rosenzweig J, Weller JM: Starch peritonitis following peritoneal dialysis. *Nephron* 30:82–84, 1982.
172. Humayun HM, Ing TS, Daugirdas JT, et al: Peritoneal fluid eosinophilia in patients undergoing maintenance peritoneal dialysis. *Arch Intern Med* 141:1172–1173, 1981.
173. Taylor R, McDonald M, Russ G, et al: Vibrio alginolyticus peritonitis associated with ambulatory peritoneal dialysis *Br Med J* 283:275, 1981.
174. David JD, Ward JI, Fraser DW, et al: Peritonitis due to a myobacterium chelonei-like organism associated with intermittent chronic peritoneal dialysis. *J Infect Dis* 145:9–17, 1982.
175. Holley HP, Tucker CT, Moffatt TL, et al: Tuberculous peritonitis in patients undergoing chronic home peritoneal dialysis. *Am J Kid Dis* 1:222–226, 1982.
176. Berkelman RL, Godley J, Weber L, et al: Pseudomonas cepacia peritonitis associated with contamination of automatic peritoneal dialysis machines. *Ann Intern Med* 96:456–463, 1982.
177. McNeely DJ, Vas SI, Dombros N, et al: Fusarium peritonitis: An uncommon complication of CAPD. *Periton Dialys Bull* 1:94–97, 1981.
178. Goodman W, Gallagher N, Sherrard DJ: Peritoneal dialysis fluid as a source of hepatitis antigen. *Nephron* 29:107–109, 1981.
179. Sewell CM, Clarridge J, Lacke C, et al: Staphylococcal nasal carriage and subsequent infection in peritoneal dialysis patients. *JAMA* 248:1493–1495, 1982.
180. Coward RA, Gokal R, Wise M, et al: Peritonitis associated with vaginal leakage of dialysis fluid in continuous ambulatory peritoneal dialysis. *Br Med J* 284:1529, 1982.
181. Duwe AK, Vas SI, Weatherhead JW: Effects of the composition of peritoneal dialysis fluid on chemiluminescence, phagocytosis, and bactericidal activity in vitro. *Infect Immunol* 33:130–135, 1981.
182. Zaruba K, Oliveri M: Prophylaxis of peritonitis in continuous ambulatory peritoneal dialysis (CAPD) by a simple microbiological patient self-check. *Proc Eur Dial Transplant Assoc* 18:275–279, 1981.
183. Lempert KD, Jones JM: Flucytosine-miconazole treatment of Candida peritonitis. Its use during continuous ambulatory peritoneal dialysis. *Arch Intern Med* 142:577–578, 1982.
184. Shalimov AA, Saenko VF, Dubitskii AE, et al: Current principles of the combined treatment of acute peritonitis. *Klin Khir* 1:1–5, 1982.
185. Schmidt RW, Blumenkrantz M: Peritoneal sclerosis. A 'sword of Democles' for peritoneal dialysis? *Arch Intern Med* 141:1265–1267, 1981.
186. Raja RM, Kramer MS, Rosenbaum JL, et al: Contrasting changes in solute transport and ultrafiltration with peritonitis in CAPD patients. *Trans Am Soc Artif Intern Organs* 27:68–70, 1981.
187. Rubin J, McFarland S, Hellems EW, et al: Peritoneal dialysis during peritonitis. *Kidney Int* 19:460–464, 1981.
188. Thomas U, Boos W, Adam D: Transperitoneal resorption of ampicillin, cefuroxim, and gentamicin in continuous ambulatory peritoneal dialysis. *Med Welt* 33:182–184, 1982.

189. Sewell DL, Golper TA: Stability of antimicrobial agents in peritoneal dialysate. *Antimicrob Agents Chemother* 21:528–529, 1982.
190. De Paepe M, Lamiere N, Ringoir S, et al: Peritoneal pharmacokinetics of gentamicin in man and rabbit, in Gahl KM, Kessel M, Nolph KD (eds): *Advances in Peritoneal Dialysis*. Amsterdam, Excerpta Medica, 1981, pp 99–101.
191. Somani P, Shapiro RS, Stockard H, et al: Undirectional absorption of gentamicin from the peritoneum during continuous ambulatory peritoneal dialysis. *Clin Pharmacol Ther* 32:113–121, 1982.
192. Singlas E, Colin JN, Rottembourg J, et al: Pharmacokinetics of sulfamethoxazole-trimethoprim combination during chronic peritoneal dialysis: Effect of peritonitis. *Eur J Clin Pharmacol* 21:409–415, 1982.
193. Thomas U, Boos W, Adam D: Transperitoneal resorption of oxacillin, azlocillin, and sisomicin in continuous ambulatory peritoneal dialysis in patients with and without peritonitis. *Med Welt* 32:1365–1367, 1981.
194. Pancorbo S, Comty C: Peritoneal transport of vancomyin in 4 patients undergoing continuous ambulatory peritoneal dialysis. *Nephron* 31:37–39, 1982.
195. LaGreca G, Biasioli S, Chiaramonte S, et al: Pharmacokinetics of intravenous and intraperitoneal cefuroxime during peritoneal dialysis. *Int J Clin Pharmacol Ther Toxicol* 20:92–94, 1982.
196. Fish SS, Pancorbo S, Berkseth R: Pharmacokinetics of epsilon-aminocaproic acid during peritoneal dialysis. *J Neurosurg* 54:736–739, 1981.
197. Pancorbo S, Comty C: Pharmacokinetics of gentamicin in patients undergoing continuous ambulatory peritoneal dialysis. *Antimicrob Agents Chemother* 19:605–607, 1981.
198. Appleby DH, John JF: Effect of peritoneal dialysis solution on the antimicrobial activity of cephalosporins. *Nephron* 30:341–344, 1982.
199. Glew RH, Pavuk RA: Stability of vancomycin and aminoglycoside antibiotics in peritoneal dialysis concentrate. *Nephron* 28:241–243, 1981.
200. Luciani L, Gentile MG, Scarduelli B, et al: Multiple hepatic abscesses complicating continuous ambulatory peritoneal dialysis. *Br Med J* 285:543, 1982.
201. Jung N, Schmidt U, Ortmann G, et al: Spontaneous colonic perforation during chronic intermittent peritoneal dialysis. *Dtsch Med Wochenschr* 106:1381–1383, 1981.
202. Francis DM, Schofield I, Veitch PS: Abdominal hernias in patients treated with continuous ambulatory peritoneal dialysis. *Br J Surg* 69:409, 1982.
203. Rubin J, Raju S, Teal N, et al: Abdominal hernia in patients undergoing continuous ambulatory peritoneal dialysis. *Arch Intern Med* 142:1453–1455, 1982.
204. Power DA, Edward N, Catto GR, et al: Richter's hernia: An unrecognized complication of chronic ambulatory peritoneal dialysis. *Br Med J* 283:528, 1981.
205. Lee AB, Waffle CM, Trebbin WM, et al: Clostridial myonecrosis. Origin from an obturator hernia in a dialysis patient. *JAMA* 246:1232–1233, 1981.
206. King C: Hydrocele: A complication of CAPD. *Nephrol Nurse* 3:37–39, 1981.
207. Ramos JM, Burke DA, Veitch PS: Hernia of Morgagni in patients on continuous ambulatory peritoneal dialysis. *Lancet* 1:161–162, 1982 (letter).
208. Digenis GE, Khanna R, Mathews R, et al: Abdominal hernias in patients undergoing CAPD. *Periton Dialys Bull* 2:115–118, 1982.
209. Madden MA, Beirne GJ, Zimmerman SW, et al: Acute bowel obstruction: An unusual complication of chronic peritoneal dialysis. *Am J Kid Dis* 1:219–221, 1982.
210. Wehling M, Jenni R, Steurer J, et al: Ischemic colitis in a patient undergoing CAPD. *Periton Dialys Bull* 2:123–124, 1982.
211. Spadaro JJ, Thakur V, Nolph KD: Technetium-99m-labelled macroaggregated albumin in demonstration of transdiaphragmatic leakage of dialysate in peritoneal dialysis. *Am J Nephrol* 2:36–38, 1982.

212. Scheldewaert R, Bogaerts Y, Pauwels R, et al: Management of a massive hydrothorax in a CAPD patient: A case report and a review of the literature. *Periton Dialys Bull* 2:69–73, 1982.
213. Seebaran AR, Patel PL: Acute massive hydrothorax—a rare complication of peritoneal dialysis. A case report. *S Afr Med J* 60:827–828, 1981.
214. Townsend R, Fragola JA: Hydrothorax in a patient receiving continuous ambulatory peritoneal dialysis: Successful treatment with intermittent peritoneal dialysis. *Arch Intern Med* 142:1571–1572, 1982.
215. Winchester JF, Traveira Da Silva AM: Pulmonary function and peritoneal dialysis. *Int J Artif Organs* 4:267–269, 1981.
216. Thieler H, Riedel E, Pielesch W, et al: Continuous ambulatory peritoneal dialysis and pulmonary function. *Proc Eur Dial Transplant Assoc* 17:333–336, 1980.
217. Epstein SW, Inouye T, Robson M, et al: Effect of peritoneal dialysis fluid on ventilatory function. *Periton Dialys Bull* 2:120–123, 1982.
218. Rebuck AS: Peritoneal dialysis and the mechanics of the diaphragm. *Periton Dialys Bull* 2:109–111, 1982.
219. Hemmeloff Andersen KE, Bengsgaard Pedersen F, Horder M: An assessment of dialysis-associated osteodystrophy in long-term peritoneal dialysis. *Nephron* 30:328–332, 1982.
220. Gokal R: Renal osteodystrophy in continuous ambulatory peritoneal dialysis. *Periton Dialys Bull* 2:111–115, 1982.
221. Turgan C, Feehally J, Bennett S, et al: Accelerated hypertriglyceridemia in patients on continuous ambulatory peritoneal dialysis—a preventable abnormality. *Int J Artif Organs* 4:158–160, 1981.
222. Nestel PJ, Fidge NH, Tan MH: Increased lipoprotein-remnant formation in chronic renal failure. *N Engl J Med* 307:326–333, 1982.
223. Krumlovsky F: Disorders of protein and lipid metabolism associated with chronic renal failure and chronic dialysis. *Ann Clin Lab Sci* 11:350–360, 1981.
224. LaGreca G, Dettori P, Biasioli S, et al: Study on morphological and densitometrical changes in the brain after hemodialysis and peritoneal dialysis. *Trans Am Soc Artif Intern Organs* 27:40–44, 1981.
225. LaGreca G, Biasioli S, Chiaramonte S, et al: Studies on brain density in hemodialysis and peritoneal dialysis. *Nephron* 31:146–150, 1982.
226. Cumming AD, Simpson G, Bell D, et al: Acute aluminum intoxication in patients on continuous ambulatory peritoneal dialysis. *Lancet* 1:103–104, 1982 (letter).
227. Lloyd R, Norwood D: Management of bloody dialysate. *AANNT J* 9:18–19, 1982.
228. Brown PM, Johnston KW, Fenton SS, et al: Symptomatic exacerbation of peripheral vascular disease with chronic ambulatory peritoneal dialysis. *Clin Nephrol* 16:258–261, 1981.
229. Chelazzi G, Bernasconi G, Gastaldi L, et al: Blood folates in chronic uremic patients in dialysis treatment. *Minerva Med* 71:3073–3086, 1980.
230. Vas SI, Oreopoulos DG: Handle with care: Hepatitis B antigen carriers in peritoneal dialysis unit. *Nephron* 29:105–106, 1981.
231. Gray PJ: Management of patients with chronic renal failure. Role of physical therapy. *Phys Ther* 62:173–176, 1982.
232. Palmer RA: As it was in the beginning: A history of peritoneal dialysis. *Periton Dialys Bull* 2:16–24, 1982.
233. Swartz RD: Peritoneal dialysis: New innovations for an old method. *Compr Ther* 7:14–20, 1981.
234. Arisz L, Krediet RT: Peritoneal dialysis today. *Neth J Med* 25:61–64, 1982.

235. Madden MA, Zimmerman SW, Simpson DP: Longitudinal comparison of intermittent versus continuous ambulatory peritoneal dialysis, in the same patients. *Clin Nephrol* 16:293–299, 1981.
236. Selgas Gutierrez R, Lorenzo Aguiar D, Rivero Sanchez, et al: Comparative biochemical study of serum and residual peritoneal fluid in periodic peritoneal maintenance dialysis. *Med Clin* 77:205–208, 1981.
237. Asaba H, Bergström J, Fürst P, et al: Plasma middle molecules in asymptomatic and "sick" uremic patients. *Artif Organs* 4:S137–S142, 1981.
238. Doody PT, Goldberg M: Evaluation of low flow long dwell chronic intermittent peritoneal dialysis. *Clin Exp Dial Apheresis* 6:45–51, 1982.
239. Ratnu KS, Haldia KR, Panicker S, et al: A new technique—semicontinuous rapid flow, high volume exchange—for effective peritoneal dialysis in shorter periods. *Nephron* 31:159–163, 1982.
240. Kron J, Wenkel R, Ohme WD: Automatic semicontinuous peritoneal dialysis with volumetric cycle control. *Z Urol Nephrol* 75:175–179, 1982.
241. Buoncristiani U, Cozzani M, Carobi C, et al: Semicontinuous semiambulatory peritoneal dialysis. *Proc Eur Dial Transplant Assoc* 17:328–332, 1980.
242. Kleint V, Stradtmann H, Klinger H, et al: Semi-continuous peritoneal dialysis—an advantageous modification of the peritoneal dialysis technic. *Z Urol Nephrol* 74:299–304, 1981.
243. Ing TS, Gahdhi VC, Daugiradas JT, et al: Peritoneal dialysis using bicarbonate-containing dialysate produced by automated dialysate delivery machine. *Artif Organs* 6:67–79, 1982.
244. Diaz-Buxo JA, Walker PJ, Farmer CD, et al: Continuous cyclic peritoneal dialysis. *Trans Am Soc Artif Intern Organs* 27:51–54, 1981.
245. Nakagawa D, Price C, Stinebaugh B, et al: Continuous cycling peritoneal dialysis: A viable option in the treatment of chronic renal failure. *Trans Am Soc Artif Intern Organs* 27:55–57, 1981.
246. Diaz-Buxo JA, Farmer CD, Walker PJ, et al: Continuous cyclic peritoneal dialysis: A preliminary report. *Artif Organs* 5:157–161, 1981.
247. Diaz-Buxo JA, Walker PJ, Chandler JT, et al: Continuous cyclic peritoneal dialysis. *Contemp Dialys* 2:23–26,54–55, 1981.
248. Nolph KD, Popovich RP: A comparison of CAPD and CCPD, in Winchester J, Schreiner G (eds): *Controversies in Nephrology*, 1982. (in press).
249. Hernandez EH, Stein JM: Comparison of the Lazarus-Nelson peritoneal lavage catheter with the standard peritoneal dialysis catheter in abdominal trauma. *J Trauma* 22:153–154, 1982.
250. Calderaro V, Mamoli B, Terracciano V, et al: A double chamber catheter for chronic ambulatory peritoneal dialysis (CAPD). *Proc Eur Dial Transplant Assoc* 18:297–299, 1981.
251. Fry AR, Verma K, Chaudhry VP: Evaluation of biocompatibility of polymers for the development of peritoneal dialysis catheter. *Median J Med Res* 74:308–311, 1981.
252. Rottembourg J, Jacq D, Von Panthen M, et al: Straight or curled Tenckhoff peritoneal catheter for continuous ambulatory peritoneal dialysis? *Periton Dialys Bull* 1:123–124, 1981.
253. Uldall R, Williams P: The subclavian cannula: Temporary vascular access for hemodialysis when long-term peritoneal dialysis has to be interrupted. *Periton Dialys Bull* 1:97–100, 1981.
254. Dabbagh S, Chevalier RL, Sturgill BC: Prolonged anuria and aortic insufficiency in a child with Wegener's granulomatosis. *Clin Nephrol* 17:155–159, 1982.
255. Yahav J, Barzilay Z, Aladjem M, et al: Acute peritoneal dialysis in children. *Int J Pediatr Nephrol* 2:33–35, 1981.

256. Rothberg AD, Thomson PD, Andronikou S, et al: Transient neonatal hyperammonaemia. A case report. *S Afr Med J* 62:175–176, 1982.
257. Ellis D, Gartner JC, Galvis AG: Acute renal failure in infants and children: Diagnosis, complications, and treatment. *Crit Care Med* 9:607–617, 1981.
258. Clow CL, Reade TM, Scriver CR: Outcome of early and long-term management of classical maple syrup urine disease. *Pediatrics* 68:856–862, 1981.
259. Wyszynska T, Krynski J: Effectiveness of peritoneal dialysis in acute renal failure in children. *Pediatr Pol* 56:749–754, 1981.
260. Steele BT, Bacheyie GS, Baumal R, et al: Acute renal failure of short duration in minimal lesion nephrotic syndrome of childhood. *Int J Pediatr Nephrol* 3:59–62, 1982.
261. Ishidate T, Iitake K, Yoshida S, et al: Pseudomonas cepacia infection in children. *Int J Pediatr Nephrol* 3:9–102, 1982.
262. McGreal MJ, Vigneux AM, Young J: Continuous ambulatory peritoneal dialysis: Ideal treatment for certain children. *Infirm Can* 24:18–22, 1982.
263. McGreal MJ, Vigneux AM, Young JM: Continuous ambulatory peritoneal dialysis: Treatment of choice for some children. *Can Nurse* 78:21–25, 1982.
264. Yennie KL, Mitchell JC: Management of the patient with juvenile onset diabetes mellitus (JODM) in end-stage renal disease (ESRD) using a variety of dialysis therapies. *AANNT J* 9:27–29, 1982.
265. Guillot M, Lavocat C, Garabedian M, et al: Evaluation of 25(OH)D loss in dialysate of children on continuous ambulatory peritoneal dialysis. *Proc Eur Dial Transplant Assoc* 18:290–292, 1981.
266. Largueche S, Haddad L, Chaabani B, et al: Continuous ambulatory peritoneal dialysis in children. *Tunis Med* 59:281–284, 1981.
267. Potter DE, McDaid TK, McHenry K, et al: Continuous ambulatory peritoneal dialysis (CAPD) in children. *Trans Am Soc Artif Intern Organs* 27:64–67, 1981.
268. Sargeeva TV: Peritoneal dialysis in the treatment of chronic kidney failure in children. *Urol Nefrol* 6:61–64, 1981.
269. Broyer M, Donckerwolcke RA, Brunner FP, et al: Combined report on regular dialysis and transplantation of children in Europe 1980. *Proc Eur Dial Transplant Assoc* 18:60–87, 1981.
270. Hetrick AR, Shah RV: Dietary management of infants on CAPD. *AANNT J* 9:46–48, 1982.
271. Kanarek KS, Root E, Sidebottom RA, et al: Successful peritoneal dialysis in an infant weighing less than 800 grams. *Clin Pediatr* 21:166–169, 1982.
272. Lorentz WB, Hamilton RW, Disher B, et al: Home peritoneal dialysis during infancy. *Clin Nephrol* 15:194–197, 1981.
273. Fielden N, Johnson S: Home-training peritoneal dialysis in pediatric patients. *J Am Assoc Nephrol Nurses Tech* 8:41–43, 1981.
274. Alexander SR, Tank ES: Surgical aspects of continuous ambulatory peritoneal dialysis in infants, children and adolescents. *J Urol* 127:501–504, 1982.
275. Giordano C, De Santo NG, Capodicasa G: Amino acid losses during CAPD in children. *Int J Pediatr Nephrol* 2:85–88, 1981.
276. Irwin MA, Balfe JW, Hardy B: Continuous ambulatory peritoneal dialysis in pediatrics. *J Am Assoc Nephrol Nurses Tech* 8:11–13, 1981.
277. Glenn LD, Nolph KD: Treatment of pancreatitis with peritoneal dialysis. *Periton Dialys Bull* 2:63–69, 1982.
278. Reynaert M, Otte JB, Kestens PJ, et al: Peritoneal dialysis treatment for acute necrotic hemorrhagic pancreatitis. *Acta Chir Belg* 80:363–371, 1981.

279. Carboni M, Negro P, De Bernardinis G, et al: Clinical methodology and therapeutic reality in the treatment of acute pancreatitis. *Minerva Chir* 36:1653–1656, 1981.
280. Hotz J: Therapy of acute pancreatitis. *Dtsch Med Wochenschr* 107:265–267, 1982.
281. Goldfarb JP, Brasitus TA, Cleri DJ: Shigella enterocolitis and acute renal failure. *South Med J* 75:492–493, 1982.
282. Miadinso OO: Challenge of treatment acute renal failure in developing countries. *J Natl Med Assoc* 72:1165–1167, 1980.
283. Rigden SP, Barratt TM, Dillon MJ, et al: Acute renal failure complicating cardiopulmonary bypass surgery. *Arch Dis Child* 57:425–430, 1982.
284. Gastaldi L, Baratelli L, Cassani D, et al: Low flow continuous peritoneal dialysis in acute renal failure. *Nephron* 29:101–102, 1981 (letter).
285. Dapper F, Wizemann V, Moosdorf R, et al: Treatment of renal insufficiency following surgery of the heart. *Med Welt* 33:808–812, 1982.
286. Bende S, Berkessy S, Kellath Z: Hemoperfusion and peritoneal dialysis in endotoxic shock. *Orv Hatil* 122:2785–2787, 1981.
287. Sipkins JH, Kjellstarand CM: Severe head trauma and acute renal failure. *Nephron* 28:36–41, 1981.
288. Ing TS, Daugirdas JT, Popli S, et al: Treatment of refractory hemodialysis ascites with maintenance peritoneal dialysis. *Clin Nephrol* 15:198–202, 1981.
289. Rubin J, Kiley J, Ray R, et al: Continuous ambulatory peritoneal dialysis. Treatment of dialysis-related ascites. *Arch Intern Med* 141:1093–1095, 1981.
290. Adler AJ, Feldman J, Friedman EA, et al: Use of extracorporeal ascites dialysis in combined hepatic and renal failure. *Nephron* 30:31–35, 1982.
291. Hwang ER, Sherman RA, Mehta S, et al: Dialytic ascitic ultrafiltration in refractory ascites. *Am J Gastroenterol* 77:652–654, 1982.
292. Feldman J, Adler AJ, Friedman EA, et al: Extracorporeal recirculating ascites dialysis (EAD) in combined hepatic and renal failure. *Trans Am Soc Artif Intern Organs* 27:563–565, 1981.
293. Gore RM, Callen PW, Filly RA: Lesser sac fluid in predicting the etiology of ascites: CT findings. *AJR* 139:71–74, 1982.
294. Simeonov P: Potentials of purification methods for the treatment of acute hepatic coma. *Vutr Boles* 20:1–6, 1981.
295. Naparstek Y, Friedlaender MM, Rubinger D, et al: Lactic acidosis and peritoneal dialysis. *Isr J Med Sci* 18:513–514, 1982.
296. Warner A, Vaziri ND: Treatment of lactic acidosis. *S Med J* 74:841–847, 1981.
297. Breborowicz A, Szulc R: Removal of endogenous lactates via the peritoneum in experimental lactic acidosis. *Intensive Care Med* 7:297–300, 1981.
298. Stein G, Sperschneider H, Knopf B, et al: Peritoneal dialysis treatment in psoriasis vulgaris. *Z Gesamte Inn Med* 36:938–941, 1981.
299. Hanicki Z, Cichocki T, Klein A, et al: Dialysis for psoriasis—preliminary remarks concerning mode of action. *Arch Dermatol Res* 271:401–405, 1981.
300. Ward RA, Wathen RL: Principles of dialysis: Utilization in nonuremic psoriatic subjects. *Int J Dermatol* 21:154–158, 1982.
301. Whittier FC, Evans DH, Anderson PC, et al: Peritoneal dialysis for psoriasis: A controlled study. *Ann Int Med* (in press).
302. Guerin JM, Raux M, Meresse S, et al: Peritoneal dialysis for eliminating copper in patients with Wilson's disease. *Sem Hop Paris* 58:613–615, 1982.
303. Sorkin MI, Nolph KD, Arfaania D, et al: Case report: Continuous ambulatory peritoneal dialysis for the treatment of hypercalcemia. *Dialysis Transplantation* 10:928–932, 1981.

304. Brown EA, Pawlikowski TR: Lithium intoxication treated by peritoneal dialysis. *Br J Clin Pract* 35:90–91, 1981.
305. Fuquay D, Koup J, Smith AL: Management of neonatal gentamicin overdosage. *J Pediatr* 99:473–476, 1981.
306. Hadi SF, El Mikatti N: Acute carbon tetrachloride poisoning. *Intensive Care Med* 7:203–204, 1981.
307. Rigal D, Parchoux B, Frederich A, et al: Accidental poisoning with gentamicin in an infant. Treatment with peritoneal dialysis. *Arch Fr Pediatr* 38:437–439, 1981.
308. Sabto JK, Pierce RM, West RH, et al: Hemodialysis, peritoneal dialysis, plasmapheresis and forced diuresis for the treatment of quinine overdose. *Clin Nephrol* 16:264–268, 1981.
309. Zulik R: Pathogenesis of amanitin-type mushroom poisoning and therapeutic possibilities. *Orv Hetil* 122:2023–2027, 1981.
310. Borges HF, Hocks J, Kjellstrand CM: Mannitol intoxication in patients with renal failure. *Arch Intern Med* 142:63–66, 1982.
311. Vale JA, Prior JG, O'Hare JP, et al: Treatment of ethylene glycol poisoning with peritoneal dialysis. *Br Med J* 284:557, 1982.
312. Cundy T, Trafford JA: Efficacy of peritoneal dialysis in severe thiazide-induced hyponatraemia. *Postgrad Med J* 57:734–735, 1981.
313. Green FJ, Lavelle KJ, Aronoff GR, et al: Management of amikacin overdose. *Am J Kidney Dis* 1:110–112, 1981.
314. Hall K, Meatherall B, Krahn J, et al: Clearance of quinidine during peritoneal dialysis. *Am Heart J* 104:646–647, 1982.
315. Davis FM, Judson JA: Warm peritoneal dialysis in the management of accidental hypothermia: Report of five cases. *N Z Med J* 94:207–209, 1981.
316. Jenkins JF, Hubbard SM, Howser DM: Managing intraperitoneal chemotherapy: A new assault on ovarian cancer. *Nursing* 12:76–83, 1982.
317. Morlans M, Ballester M, Bartolome J, et al: Diagnosis and management of pericarditis in uremic patients. *Med Clin* 77:269–273, 1981.
318. Szabo A, Nagy ZB, Vasarhelyi B, et al: The role of peritoneal dialysis in operative gynecology. *Orv Hetil* 122:1960–1963, 1981.
319. Kennedy JM: The successful training of a mentally retarded patient for CAPD. *AANNT J* 9:51–55, 1982.
320. Ward MK: Replacement therapy for end-stage renal failure. *Practitioner* 225:1109–1117, 1981.
321. Taraba, Balas EA: Effectiveness of chronic peritoneal dialysis. *Orv Hetil* 122:1899–1902, 1981.
322. Arisz L, Krediet RT: Peritoneal dialysis today. *Neth J Med* 25:61–64, 1982.
323. Gordillo G, Muñoz R, Feiman R: Chronic peritoneal dialysis. *Bol Med Hosp Infant Mex* 38:379–392, 1981.
324. Sorrels AJ: Peritoneal dialysis: A rediscovery. *Nurs Clin North Am* 16:515–529, 1981.
325. Mery JP: State of chronic dialysis in France on 31 December 1979. Chronic hemodialysis, peritoneal dialysis, equipment, number of patients treated. *Nephrologie* 1:121–125, 1980.
326. van Ypersele de Strihou C: Cost and success of the treatment of terminal renal insufficiency in Belgium; from where do we come and where are we going? *Acta Clin Belg* 36:171–177, 1981.
327. Chang M: Peritoneal dialysis: No more needles. *Nurs Mirror* 153:22–25, 1981.
328. Lindsay RM: Adaptation to home dialysis: The use of hemodialysis and peritoneal dialysis. *AANNT J* 9:49–51, 1982.

329. Choudhry VP, Srivastava RN: Peritoneal dialysis. *Indian J Pediatr* 49:79–83, 1982.
330. Mion C: A review of seven years' home peritoneal dialysis. *Proc Eur Dial Transplant Assoc* 18:91–108, 1981.
331. Adequate dialysis. *Lancet* 1:147–148, 1982 (editorial).
332. Graefe U, Dorst K: Individual therapy of chronic terminal kidney failure. *ZFA* 57:1971–1975, 1981.
333. Kliger AS: Current concepts in peritoneal dialysis. *Nephron* 27:209–214, 1981.
334. Giordano C, De Santo NG, Capodicasa G: The employment of medical students in the peritoneal dialysis at the University of Naples during the years 1973–1981. *Periton Dialys Bull* 2:79–82, 1982.
335. Oreopoulos DG: The artificial kidney-chronic uremia program of the National Institutes of Health: A driving force in the development of peritoneal dialysis. *Periton Dialys Bull* 2:105–107, 1982.
336. Hirszel P, Galen MA, Happe T, et al: Glycosylated hemoglobin in patients treated by chronic dialysis. *Int Urol Nephrol* 13:185–191, 1981.
337. Chan MK, Ramdial L, Varghese Z, et al: Plasma lecithin cholesterol acyltransferase activities in uraemic patients. *Clin Chim Acta* 119:65–72, 1982.
338. Canavese C, Stratta P, Pacitti A, et al: Impaired fibrinolysis in uremia: Partial and variable correction by four different dialysis regimens. *Clin Nephrol* 17:82–89, 1982.
339. Milman N: Iron absorption measured by whole body counting and the relation to marrow iron stores in chronic uremia. *Clin Nephrol* 17:77–81, 1982.

CHAPTER 2

Hemodialysis

John C. Van Stone

Hemodialysis was not covered in Volume 6 of *Current Nephrology* and therefore this chapter reviews the hemodialysis-related literature of the last two years.

THE CARDIOVASCULAR RESPONSE TO HEMODIALYSIS

In the past 2 years there has been continued interest in the hemodynamic changes that occur during hemodialysis. Studies indicate that there is a subset of patients who have a high incidence of symptomatic hypotension during their treatments. Degoulet and co-workers (1) reported an epidemologic study of dialysis-induced hypotension. They analyzed data of 1,110 patients treated by chronic hemodialysis in 32 French dialysis centers and found many factors associated with an increased incidence of hypotension. Female sex, diabetic nephropathy, low dialysate osmolarity, low dialysate potassium, high ultrafiltration rates, low predialysis plasma proteins, high predialysis plasma urea concentration, decreased nerve conduction velocity, twice weekly dialysis, and use of coil dialyzers were all found to be significant risk factors for symptomic hypotension. The ultrafiltration rate appeared to be the single most important factor.

The report by Degoulet et al. did not study the relative effects of bicarbonate versus acetate dialysate. However, two recent studies continue to add evidence that acetate in the dialysate is an important contributing factor to hemodialysis-induced hypotension (2, 3). These studies indicate that acetate decreases blood pressure predominantly through reduction in systemic vascular resistance. Schohn and co-workers (2) found a close inverse correlation between plasma acetate concentration and systemic

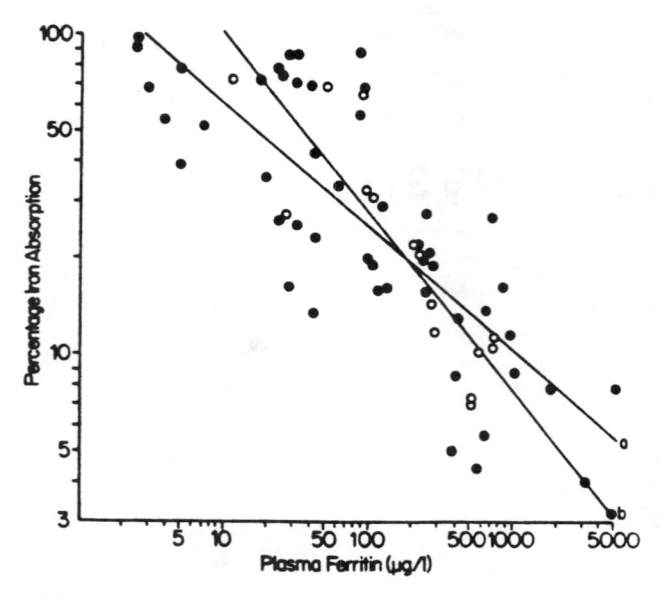

Figure 1. The relationship between the percentage absorption of a 3 mg dose of ferrous iron and the plasma ferritin concentration in a group of 50 subjects with normal renal function (closed circles) and in 15 patients on regular dialysis therapy (open circles). The regression line (a) for the subjects with normal renal function was log ferritin = -0.14 log% iron absorption $+0.40$, while that for the patients on regular dialysis therapy (b) was log ferritin = -0.17 log% iron absorption $+0.44$. Using analysis of variance, there was no significant difference between these two lines. (Bezwoda WR et al: *Nephron* 28:289–293, 1981. Reprinted with permission.)

vascular resistance. (See the following section on dialysate base for a further discussion of the effects of acetate dialysis.)

Wehle and co-workers feel that the dialysate sodium concentration is more important than the dialysate base in the genesis of dialysis-induced hypotension (4). They studied eight patients using five different dialysates that varied with regard to sodium concentration, type of base, and the presence or absence of urea. They found that low sodium (133 mEq/liter) versus high sodium (140 mEq/liter) and acetate versus bicarbonate both induced a fall in blood pressure, whereas urea removal had no effect. However, while acetate in the dialysate with the higher sodium concentration caused more peripheral dilatation than high sodium bicarbonate dialysate, there was little fall in blood pressure with the high sodium acetate dialysate due to a compensatory increase in cardiac output. The study by Man and co-workers (5) supports this contention.

A study by myself and associates (6) suggests that the predominant effect of the dialysate sodium concentration is on the intercompartmental shift of fluid during hemodialysis treatments. We found that if patients were treated with a dialysate whose sodium concentration was below the plasma sodium concentration, fluid shifted from the extracellular compartment into the intracellular compartment, whereas if the dialysate sodium was greater than the plasma sodium, fluid shifted in the opposite direction, from the intracellular compartment into the extracellular compartment. When the dialysate sodium concentration equaled the plasma sodium concentration, there was essentially no change in intracellular compartmental volumes. This occurred whether or not the patients were being ultrafiltered during the dialysis treatment. Essentially all of the fluid removal occurring with ultrafiltration during dialysis comes from the extracellular space. The studies of Swartz et al. (7) also support the contention that higher dialysate sodium concentrations improve vascular stability by altering the movement of body fluid between compartments.

There are several recent studies that examine the autonomic nervous system in hemodialysis patients (8–11). Tests that depend on a change in heart rate, such as the Valsalva maneuver, deep breathing tests, and measures of sinus arrythmia, more often show abnormal results in hemodialysis patients than tests that look at changes in blood pressure, such as postural hypotensive changes, sustained hand grip or the cold pressor test (8,9). This suggests that the cardiac parasympathetic intervention is more frequently abnormal than the vascular sympathetic intervention. The fact that most patients have a normal response to the administration of atropine indicates that the lesion usually involves the afferent limb (9). Mitas and co-workers (12) evaluated the sympathetic nervous system of hemodialysis patients using amyl nitrate inhalation, phenylephrine infusion, and the cold pressor test. Their data confirm that many hemodialysis patients have an autonomic abnormality localized to the afferent limb of the baroreflex arc.

Plasma concentrations of catacholamines are abnormal in most hemodialysis patients (10,11,13). Resting plasma epinephrine and norepinephrine concentrations are higher in hemodialysis patients whether or not they are prone to develop hypotension during dialysis treatments. Standing causes norepinephrine levels to rise significantly in both normotensive and hypotensive prone patients, with the increase similar to that seen in a control nonuremic group(10). This occurs in spite of the fact that patients in the hypotensive prone group have orthostatic hypotension. These results suggest that uremics have normal sympathetic responsiveness and that dialysis-dependent hypotension probably reflects an impairment of the vasoconstrictor response of the vascular wall.

Botey et al. (11) found slightly different results; their hypotensive prone patients had significantly higher plasma norepinephrine levels than the normotensive dialysis patients, both in the basal condition and after standing. They also found that the hypotensive patients had significantly smaller increments in mean arterial blood pressure during norepinephrine

Table 1. Catecholamine Metabolism in Hemodialysis Patients

	Normal	Hemodialysis Patients	p
Plasma epinephrine (pg/ml)	69 ± 5	271 ± 17	<0.05
Plasma norepinephrine (pg/ml)	271 ± 16	468 ± 50	<0.001
Norepinephrine metabolic clearance rate (ml/min/kg)	52 ± 2	83 ± 13	<0.05
Norepinephrine production rate (mg/min/kg)	11 ± 1	31 ± 8	<0.02
Norepinephrine half-life (min)	1.8 ± 0.1	4.0 ± 0.9	<0.02
Apparent volume of norephinephrine distribution (liters/kg)	0.14 ± 0.03	0.52 ± 0.19	<0.05

infusion than did the normotensive group. However, these data also suggest that hemodialysis patients who are prone to hypotension have a defect at the postsynaptic level that prevents the normal increase in blood pressure in response to catecholamines.

Izzo and co-workers (13) attempted to determine norepinephrine production and clearance rates in 24 hemodialysis patients by norepinephrine infusion (Table 1). These studies agree that the chronic hemodialysis patients have elevated circulating levels of norepinephrine. The pharmokinetic studies suggest that there is a marked increase in epinephrine production rate and a fourfold increase in the apparent volume of distribution of norepinephrine. A problem with this study is that it assumes that the endogenously produced epinephrine, which circulates at fairly low serum concentrations, is handled identically to the infused norepinephrine, which results in high serum concentrations.

Effect of Hemodialysis on Myocardial Function

There have been several recent reports on the effect of hemodialysis on myocardial performance (14–17). Both the study by Cine and co-workers (14) and by Ireland and co-workers (15) demonstrate that myocardial function may improve acutely with hemodialysis treatments. This appears to be especially true in patients in whom the cardiac performance is depressed before dialysis, but it may not be true in elderly hemodialysis patients. Thayssen and co-workers (16) found a transient reduction in left ventricular performance occurred in older patients with the hemodialysis treatments.

Chaignon and co-workers (17) suggest that the improved contractility seen during hemodialysis treatments is related to the reduction in serum potassium and/or the increase in serum calcium achieved by hemodialysis. In the same line, Lai and associates (18) found in an uncontrolled study that long-term treatment with cimetidine of hemodialysis patients with active hyperparathyroidism produces a significant increase in cardiac performance, which was associated with an improvement in bone histology. They suggest that the improved cardiac performance is related to suppression of uremic hyperparathyroidism by cimetidine and further suggest that uremic hyperparathyroidism may play an important role in "uremic cardiomyopathy."

Diskin et al. (19) report that hemodialysis causes electrocardiographic changes 30%, 45%, and 75% of the time in the T wave, ST segment, and R wave, respectively. These changes are not correlated significantly with changes in volume during dialysis. The authors conclude that ECG changes that appear to represent ischemia are very common in the postdialysis period and are of uncertain significance.

Angina Pectoris in Hemodialysis Patients with Normal Coronary Arteries

In a series of nine patients undergoing regular maintenance hemodialysis who had coronary angiograms for angina pectoris, Roig and co-workers found four patients who had entirely normal coronary angiograms (20). The patients with normal angiograms were all female, significantly younger, and had more severe hypertension with higher left ventricular wall stress than the patients showing coronary artery lesions. They believe that anemia and increased myocardial oxygen consumption due to high blood pressure may explain the syndrome of angina pectoris in the presence of normal coronary arteries in long-term hemodialysis patients and suggest that this may not be an unusual finding.

Effects of Captopril

The acute effects of 50 mg of captopril on arterial pressure, cardiac output, total peripheral resistance, and plasma renin activity were studied in 14 chronic hemodialysis patients, six of whom were hypertensive (21). Captopril produced a greater than 10% reduction in mean arterial pressure in both the hypertensive and normotensive hemodialysis patients at 30 and 120 minutes. While the change in mean arterial pressure correlated significantly with the change in total peripheral resistance in all patients, it did not correlate with the change in cardiac index or the basal plasma renin activity.

Two separate studies indicate that captopril is very effective in controlling blood pressure in some hemodialysis patients (22,23). It is especially useful in patients with high predialysis plasma renin activity, but as with most antihypertensive medications in hemodialysis patients, it needs to be combined with sodium control. It can control blood pressure in patients who were thought to have otherwise uncontrollable hypertension.

PULMONARY CHANGES IN HEMODIALYSIS PATIENTS

Fairshter and co-workers (24) studied pulmonary pathologic changes in chronic hemodialysis patients by revieweing the autopsy records of 46 chronic hemodialysis patients with end-stage renal disease of various etiologies. Abnormalities were recorded in 45 of the 46 patients. Acute and chronic lung disease were found in 95% and 80% of these subjects, respectively. The most common acute diseases were pulmonary infections and fluid overload; the most common chronic disease process seen was interstitial fibrosis. Other relatively common chronic diseases included pleural fibrosis, pulmonary arteriosclerosis, hemorrhage, thromboembolism, and calcification. The incidence of granulomatous lung disease, pulmonary amyloidosis, and metastatic lung tumor was also higher than expected. There was no relationship between the etiology of chronic renal failure and the different pulmonary diseases.

Szwed and associates (25) studied the effect of hemodialysis on oxygen transport in chronic uremia. They found that the previously described decrease in oxygen affinity that occurs during the hemodialysis treatment is related entirely to changes in plasma phosphate concentration and red blood cell pH. Oxygen delivery is decreased during dialysis because of decreased cardiac output, which was compensated for by an increased tissue extraction of oxygen from the blood. (As discussed later in this chapter, the dialysate base also has definite effects on arterial oxygen concentration during dialysis.)

NEUROLOGY

Two studies in the past year used recently devised electrophysiologic techniques to study peripheral neuropathy in hemodialysis patients (26,27). Ackil et al. (26) performed routine motor nerve conduction studies combined with latency of late responses (H reflex and F response) and sural nerve sensory studies in 17 randomly selected children undergoing hemodialysis. Motor conduction of the peroneal and tibial nerves showed abnormalities in 29%, while sensory conduction was decreased in the medial nerve in only 12%. However, sural nerve sensory potentials were abnormal in 59% of patients. They also found that 59% of patients had abnormal late responses. They suggest that measurement of the late responsiveness and sural nerve sensory potential are sensitive indices of peripheral nephropathy and may be used to quantitatively follow patients whose neuropathy would otherwise be undetectable.

Proximal versus distal slowing of nerve conduction was compared in nine patients undergoing chronic hemodialysis by measuring F-wave conduction (27). Chokroverty found that the values for the F-wave ratio and the differences between the longest and shortest F-wave latencies were significantly longer than control values in 45% of the patients, implying that the proximal peroneal nerve segment is predominantly affected. In the remaining patients, the proximal and distal peroneal nerves were equally affected. Chokroverty feels that the studying of multiple F-wave characteristics is helpful in the complete assessment of peripheral nerve function in chronic hemodialysis patients.

Lowitzsch and co-workers (28) also studied sural nerve conduction in hemodialysis patients. They found that the majority of patients had normal sural conduction velocity, but that before dialysis, 50% of the patients were found to have prolonged refractory periods. After dialysis the refractory period decreased to normal in the vast majority of patients. They suggest that there is a membrane abnormality due to uremic poisoning that causes a prolongation of the refractory period and is reversible by hemodialysis treatment.

A 6% incidence of peripheral entrapment of the medial or ulnar nerve was reported by Delmay et al. (29). The majority of these patients were female and the entrapments were more frequent in extremities with fistulas with abnormally high flow rates. There was no correlation with previous vascular access, duration of hemodialysis, adequacy of dialysis, calcium or phosphorus hemostasis, renal diagnosis, or parathyroid or thyroid function. Surgical intervention was uniformally successful in relieving symptoms, whereas even the return of normal renal function did not spontaneously reverse the disorder.

Immediately before treatment, hemodialysis patients have abnormal cerebral density, as shown by computed tomography (CT) (30). This becomes normal 1–6 hours after the dialysis session. The intermittent nature of chronic hemodialysis treatment is the probable cause of the abnormality, since patients with end-stage renal failure before dialysis and chronic ambulatory hemodialysis (CAPD) patients have normal cerebral densities.

HEMATOLOGY

Anemia

Edmonson et al. (31) studied ferrokinetics, iron status, and serum erythropoietin levels in 28 Asian patients on chronic hemodialysis. They found that these patients seem to have a more severe anemia than their Western counterparts, which appears to be related to decreased bone marrow function. This decreased function may be the result of a relative lack of erythropoietin. Dietary factors and iron deficiency do not appear to be important, but the authors thought it possible that their patients were relatively underdialyzed by Western standards.

A retrospective study of 549 patients on chronic maintenance hemodialysis revealed that 2% of these patients had hematocrits in the normal range (40% or greater) (32). Further studies revealed that the relatively high hematocrit could not be explained by the etiology of renal disease, presence of residual renal function, dialysis prescription, arterial hypoxemia, use of vitamins or anabolic steroids, or amount of parathyroid disease present. Shalhoub et al. (33) report two patients on chronic hemodialysis who developed erythrocytosis. Peripheral serum erythropoitin levels were elevated on radioimmunoassey, and secondary causes were excluded by appropriate clinical studies. Both patients had acquired cystic disease of the kidneys and the authors suggest that the erythrocytosis may have been related to the diseased kidney.

Bezwoda and co-workers (34) studied iron absorption in patients on regular hemodialysis therapy. They found that the rate of iron absorption was normal and inversely related to the serum ferritin level (Fig. 1). Their results suggest that iron deficiency in patients with chronic renal failure undergoing regular hemodialysis treatments can usually be adequately prevented or treated with oral iron therapy.

McCarthy and co-workers suggest that treatment of the iron overloaded hemodialysis patient with hemofiltration and desferrioxamine is better than treatment with routine hemodialysis and desferrioxamine chelation therapy because of the higher filtration coefficient of the hemofiltration membrane (35). They were able to remove 15 mg of iron over $4\frac{1}{2}$ hours of postdilution hemofiltration.

Rembold and co-workers (36) compared the in vitro dialysis of desferrioxamine-bound iron through four different membranes: regenerated cellulose, cellulose acetate, cuprophane, and acrylonitrile. They found that the dialysance through the acrylonitrile membrane (47 ml/min/m^2) to be greater than twice that of any of the other membranes.

Inauen and co-workers (37) studied erythrocyte deformability in 31 uremic patients, 17 of whom were on long-term dialysis and 14 on conservative therapy. They found that erythrocytes of uremic patients were stiffer than normal, and in patients on conservative therapy there was an inverse correlation between erythrocyte deformability and serum creatinine. The dialysis procedure itself did not appear to have any acute or chronic effects on erythrocyte deformability.

Platelets

Remuzzi and co-workers (38) showed that platelets from patients on chronic long-term hemodialysis have biphasic abnormalities in response to arachidonic acid. Low concentrations of arachidonic acid enhance platelet aggregation and prostaglandin formation, but both platelet functions are significantly reduced by high concentrations of arachidonic acid. They suggest that this double functional abnormality of uremic platelets may contribute to the complex coagulation disturbances seen in hemodialysis patients.

Previous studies demonstrating that plasma concentrations of the platelet proteins β-thromboglobulin and platelet factor IV are elevated in chronic hemodialysis patients and increase further with hemodialysis treatments were confirmed by Endo et al. (39). This increase in β-thromboglobulin and platelet factor IV during dialysis can be inhibited by the intravenous administration of 100 mg of indobufen (40).

Berrettini and co-workers (41) compared the effect on platelets of hemodialysis with polyacrylonitrile membranes to hemodialysis with cuprophan membranes. They found that predialysis platelet aggregation abnormalities are completely reversed by hemodialysis with the polyacrylonitrile membranes but not by hemodialysis with cuprophan membranes. They also found that the small but significant decrease in platelet count that is seen during hemodialysis with cuprophan membranes is not found when patients are treated with polyacrylonitrile membranes. They suggest that polyacrylonitrile membranes have better biocompatibility with platelets than cuprophan membranes. Adler and Berlyne report that β-thromboglobulin levels do not increase during dialysis with the AN69 membrane and that predialysis concentrations are lower in patients who are chronically dialyzed with the AN69 dialyzer than in those who are treated with cuprophan or regenerated cellulose (42).

Twardowski and co-workers have demonstrated that the platelet counts in fistula blood are lower than that in venous blood (43). They found a 10–15% decrease in the absolute platelet count of blood obtained from A-V fistulas. They suggest that either there is greater platelet consumption on foreign surfaces in blood taken from the fistula or that uneven distribution of platelets in the rapidly flowing fistula blood may explain these differences.

Leitner and associates (44) found increased concentrations of 6-oxo-prostaglandin $F_{1\alpha}$ (6-oxo-$PGF_{1\alpha}$, the stable metabolite of prostacyclin) during the initial phase of hemodialysis, which occurs coincidently with an increase in the number of platelet microaggregates and a reduction in platelet and leucocyte counts. They suggest that, since prostacyclin is able to resolve platelet microaggregates, this may be a self-protective mechanism against embolization of microaggregates released from the dialyzer into the lung and peripheral vascular systems.

White Blood Cell and Immunologic Studies

There have been several recent studies on the number and function of lymphocytes in chronic hemodialysis patients (45–49). These studies confirm previous reports recording mild decreases both in the absolute number and in the function of lymphocytes in this population. B-lymphocytes appear to be relatively more depressed than T-lymphocytes (47). Although the antibody response to pneumococcal vaccine is less in chronic hemodialysis patients than in a control population with normal renal function, it is large enough to give substantial protection to the majority of hemodialysis patients receiving such vaccination. In view of the serious risk of pneumococcal infection in this group, it is recommended that they receive vaccination (49).

There have been two recent studies of eosinophils in chronic renal failure patients (50, 51). Gabison and co-workers (50) found a progressive increase in the number of bone marrow eosinophils as renal function decreased. Marrow eosinophil count correlated linearly with serum creatinine levels in the predialysis group, and the number of bone marrow eosinophils was highest in patients undergoing hemodialysis. Whereas the peripheral eosinophil count was normal in the uremic group before dialysis therapy, Gabison's group found a distinctive subgroup of hemodialysis patients who showed a marked and progressive peripheral eosinophilia. Spinowitz et al. (51) prospectively studied 144 chronic hemodialysis patients over a 4-month period and found that 57% had significant eosinophilia at some time during the study period. Thirty-four percent of the total population had persistent eosinophilia, with many of the patients always having eosinophil counts greater than 10%. Retrospective studies revealed that the vast majority of these patients had no eosinophilia before beginning chronic hemodialysis. Although only a limited number of dialyzers were used, there was no relationship between the eosinophilia and the type of dialyzers, medications that the patients were receiving, type of vascular access, patient age, or duration of dialysis. These workers did find a higher incidence of hypersensitivitylike symptoms (pruritis and bronchial spasm) in the eosinophilic population. They suggest that there is some as yet undefined aspect of the hemodialysis procedure that causes a hypersensitivity reaction.

Hallgren and co-workers (52) found an increased serum level of the neutrophil protein, lactoferrin, and eosinophil cationic protein soon after the initiation of hemodialysis. These increases were also seen when fresh blood was circulated through the dialyzer without a patient in the circuit, suggesting that there is a local degranulation of neutrophils and eosinophils in the dialyzer itself. Sera obtained at different times during dialysis induced no in vitro release of these granular proteins from isolated granulocytes.

Guerrero and colleagues (53) performed extensive studies of the factor found in patients' plasma early during dialysis treatment which causes the pulmonary sequestration of granulocytes. Their studies and those of others (54) indicate that this factor is probably a biologically active fragment of complement.

COAGULATION AND ANTICOAGULATION

Swartz has recently described a method of measuring heparin sensitivity by using the predialysis thrombin clotting time to determine the initial loading dose of heparin and then following the thrombin clotting time to monitor heparin levels during dialysis (55). He suggests that these procedures will significantly reduce the incidence of hemorrhage in patients at a high risk of bleeding during the hemodialysis procedure. Flicker and co-workers (56) present a method of heparin modeling for hemodialysis by determining heparin sensitivity and heparin degradation using the activated clotting time. Several different reagents for the activated clotting time were compared and the results suggest that the optimized, activated thrombofax is the best reagent to use. The authors feel that heparin modeling is the most logical approach to the assessment of the hemodialysis patient's heparin requirements.

Gunnarsson et al. (57) compared three different heparin regimes in six patients undergoing a 4-hour hemodialysis treatment (1) intravenous heparin loading only, (2) priming of the dialyzers and a continuous infusion of herparin for 2 hours, and (3) intravenous loading and continuous infusion of heparin based on anticoagulation kinetics. Fibrin deposition was monitored with ^{125}I fibrinogen and plasma fibrinopeptide-A concentrations. In all regimens they found a progressive increase in dialyzer fibrin formation; however, they could not find any advantage of the anticoagulation kinetic method over the single loading dose of heparin.

Prostacyclin (prostaglandin I_2) has been studied as an anticoagulant during hemodialysis (58–62). It can be used as the sole anticoagulant, although it is associated with a high incidence of side effects such as hypotension, headache, nausea, and chest pain. Lower doses of prostacyclin cause fewer side effects but an inadequate degree of anticoagulation. It cannot be used as the sole anticoagulant. However, low doses of prostacyclin reduce the amount of heparin needed and may prevent endothelial and platelet damage during dialysis.

Patients with chronic renal failure have an impaired fibrinolytic mechanism (63). Their impairment appears to be due to a small molecular weight toxin. Hemodialysis is a better method of correcting it than either hemofiltration or intermittent peritoneal dialysis. Peritoneal dialysis may actually increase the impairment via the loss of fibrinolytic activators through the peritoneum.

Elson and co-workers (64) report the spontaneous development of mediastinal hemorrhage in two patients undergoing chronic hemodialysis. This was accompanied by the development of cough, dyspnea, and a mediastinal mass on chest roentgenogram. In neither patient was there any spontaneous resolution over a 4-week period, and both required thoracotomy for removal of the clot.

GASTROINTESTINAL DISORDERS

Adams and co-workers (65) report severe bowel dysfunction in 25 of 945 chronic hemodialysis patients during a 10-year period of study. Colonic

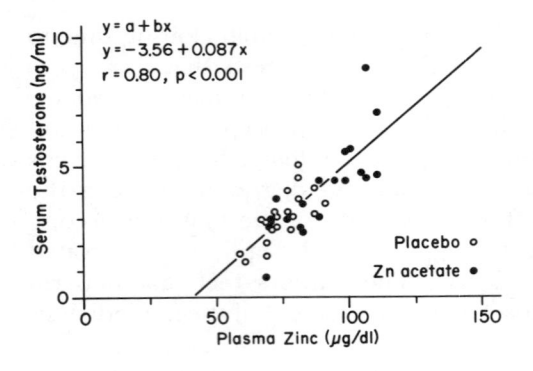

Figure 2. Relation between plasma zinc and serum testosterone in hemodialysis patients before and after zinc and placebo therapy. (Mahajan SK et al: *Ann Intern Med* 97:357–361, 1982. Reprinted with permission.)

perforation occurred in 12 patients, six of whom died due to peritonitis. Ten other patients exhibited prolonged severe adynamic ileus; most were successfully managed by medical decompression although two required surgical intervention. The authors feel that aluminum hydroxide gel, and resultant chronic constipation, is an important etiologic factor. Cunningham describes six cases of multiple gastric telangiectasias in chronic hemodialysis patients that resulted in acute gastrointestinal bleeding (66). The report emphasizes the importance of looking for this source of intestinal hemmorrhage.

ENDOCRINOLOGY

Tourkantonis confirmed previously reported low serum testosterone concentrations with increased follicle stimulating hormone (FSH) and leutenizing hormone (LH) concentrations in men on chronic hemodialysis (67). Most of these men showed normal response of the hypothalamic pituitary system to clomiphene stimulation but a diminished response of the Leydig's cells to human chorionic gonadotropin (HCG), demonstrating predominantly a testicular defect. They could find no effect of hemodialysis on any of these parameters. Mahajan reported that oral zinc therapy increases serum zinc concentrations and is associated with an increase in serum testosterone and improved spermatogenesis, potency, and libido in presumably zinc-depleted men on chronic hemodialysis (Fig. 2)(68). The study supports increasing evidence of a relationship between zinc depletion and end-organ gonadal failure in male dialysis patients. In contrast, Zingraff and co-workers (69) studied pituitary–ovarian function in women on hemodialysis and suggest that the underlying gonadal dysfunction of these women is mainly suprahypophyseal in origin.

Mrinak and colleagues (70) examined repeatedly the functional capacity of the adrenal coretex in 148 patients on long-term hemodialysis. They found a partial insufficiency in 16 cases and total insufficiency in 21 cases. They suggest that the insufficient steriod production may be the result of the long-term loss of cortisol through the dialysis membrane and further imply that this may have an important negative effect on patient survival.

Ramirez and co-workers (71) demonstrated a decreased absorption of oral dexamethasone in hemodialysis patients and warned that this decreased absorption may give a falsely positive low-dose (1 mg) dexamethasone suppression test.

Olgaard et al. (72) studied the effect of calcium infusion on plasma levels of aldosterone, renin activity, and cortisol in six anephric and four nonnephrectomized patients on regular hemodialysis. A significant increase in plasma aldosterone was noted in the nonnephrectomized patients, whereas calcium had no effect on plasma aldosterone in the anephric patients. There was no significant change in plasma cortisol, renin activity, sodium, or potassium in either group. The authors conclude that ionized calcium is a regulatory factor for plasma aldosterone in nonnephrectomized patients undergoing regular hemodialysis.

While patients on hemodialysis frequently have subnormal basal triiodothyronine concentrations and may have low thyroxine concentrations, the vast majority have normal thyroid-stimulating hormone levels, normal pituitary thyrotropin releasing hormone responsiveness, normal thyroid responsiveness to endogenous TSH, and are eumetabolic (73).

CUTANEOUS MANIFESTATIONS

Pruritis is a frequent complaint of chronic hemodialysis patients. Gilchrest and co-workers (74) studied 237 chronic hemodialysis patients by questionnaire and found that 37% of them reported "prolonged bothersome itchiness" at the time surveyed, and an additional 41% had experienced this problem in the past. Two-thirds of the patients reported that the discomfort occurred only during or soon after dialysis or was most severe at these times. Topical and orally administered antipruritics provided relief in less than 20% of the patients. Gilchrest's group did not study the effect of either oral charcoal (75) or ultraviolet radiation (76) both of which have been previously reported to successfully relieve pruritis in more than 50% of hemodialysis patients.

The development of bullous dermatosis as a result of prophyria cutanea tarda in chronic hemodialysis patients is not rare (77,78). Diser and co-workers (78) demonstrated that the plasma porphyrin level can be dramatically reduced by plasma exchange done during the hemodialysis treatments. They found that the decrease was associated with a rapid clinical response, which was maintained for a long period of time without additional therapeutic intervention. They suggest that this form of treatment may be ideal for the patient with porphyria cutanea tarda and chronic renal failure for whom no alternative therapy is available.

There have been two reports of perforating folliculitis occurring in hemodialysis patients (79,80). Early in the course of dialysis these patients develop pruritic, keratotic, perforating follicular papules and nodules. All patients in both reports had insulin-dependent diabetes mellitus, and the skin disease was refractory to all attempts at management. In one patient, however, the eruption cleared completely after a cadaver renal transplant. Histologically, the lesions showed evidence of prurigo nodularis and may be a consequence of pruritis and vigorous rubbing of discrete foci.

INFECTIONS

The most exciting advance relative to infectious complications of hemodialysis patients in the last 2 years is the availability in the United States and Europe of a vaccine effective against hepatitis B (81). This vaccine has been shown to decrease the incidence of hepatitis. It is recommended that both patients and staff of hemodialysis units in which hepatitis antigen-positive patients are being treated should receive the vaccine. The prophylactic administration of hepatitis B immunoglobulins is also effective in patients, relatives, and staff of hemodialysis units, but the need for repeated administration makes this method inferior to active vaccination (82).

Although it is probable that active vaccination will decrease the incidence and importance of hepatitis B in dialysis units in the future, hepatitis B is likely to remain a problem for many years. When attempting to determine the incidence of transfer of hepatitis B in dialysis patients by screening for both antigen and antibody, it is important to note that hepatitis antibody can be passively transferred to hemodialysis patients by blood transfusion (83). Therefore, the development of hepatitis antibody after blood transfusion does not necessarily mean that the patient has been infected with the hepatitis antigen. Both the surface antigen antibody and core antigen antibody can be passively transferred.

The development of chronic hepatitis antigenemia in hemodialysis patients can cause many medical and psychological problems (84–87). Development of chronic hepatitis, hepatic malignancy, and arthritis is possible. Frequently there is also a psychosocial reaction, many hemodialysis patients report that their hepatitis carrier state produces substantially greater restrictions on interpersonal relations and feelings of not being accepted by others than does their renal disease (86). Chronic hepatitis antigenemia is not a contraindication to renal transplantation.

The effects of infectious disease on hemodialysis patients continue to be reported, including an increased incidence of tuberculosis in hemodialysis patients (87–89). This occurs with both typical and atypical mycobacteria. The incidence of systemic infection with coccidioidomycosis in an area where coccidioidomycosis is endemic (Arizona) appears to be increased in hemodialysis patients but is much less than that seen in renal transplantation patients; 0.83% hemodialysis patients are infected, whereas 6.9% of transplant recipients have the disease (91).

Kalweit and co-workers (90) report hemodialysis fistula infection caused by *Legionella pneumophila* in two patients. In both patients the infection followed an acute illness of legionnaires' pneumonia. In one patient, the fistula infection developed 3 weeks after a full course of erythromycin therapy.

Peterson and co-workers (92) have demonstrated that bacterial endotoxin can be leached from both new and reused dialyzers. Although the concentration of endotoxin found in the new dialyzers was substantial, it appears to be a nonpyrogenic variety. Because of the unknown effects of this endotoxin on patients, it is suggested that prime of new kidneys not be administered to the patient. The problem of endotoxin in reused dialyzers can be avoided by using an endotoxin-free disinfectant solution.

OSTEOMALACIA, DIALYSIS ENCEPHALOPATHY, AND ALUMINUM TOXICITY

Increasing evidence is accumulating that the majority of cases of combined osteomalacia and dialysis encephalopathy are caused by aluminum toxicity (93–101). Although the excessive aluminum usually accumulates from the dialysate, at least in some cases it may be related to oral administration of aluminum-containing antacids. There may be some patients who have increased absorption of orally administered aluminum (96). In the aluminum-intoxicated patient's bones, the aluminum is localized mainly at the limit between the osteoid and calcified tissue where bone mineral is normally first deposited (100). These patients have significantly more osteomalacia and significantly less osteofibrosis than dialysis patients who are not aluminum intoxicated (97–100). There is a significant correlation between the dialysate aluminum concentration and the amount of osteomalacia in bone (Fig. 3).

At autopsy the brains of these patients show senile plaques and neurofibrillary tangles similar to lesions found in Alzheimer's disease, a disease known to be associated with increased cerebral aluminum content (101). The electroencephalograms of dialysis dementia patients show a distinctive frontocentral spike-and-wave pattern that can be differentiated from other electroencephalographic changes seen in chronic renal failure (102,103). Preventing the disease by the use of deionized water for dialysate and keeping the aluminum antacid dosage to a minimum by phosphorus restriction is important, but the use of desferrioxamine in patients with the disease seems to help mobilize tissue aluminum and may result in clinical improvement (104,105). Geuillot and co-workers (106) have demonstrated that antacids containing magnesium may be used sparingly to

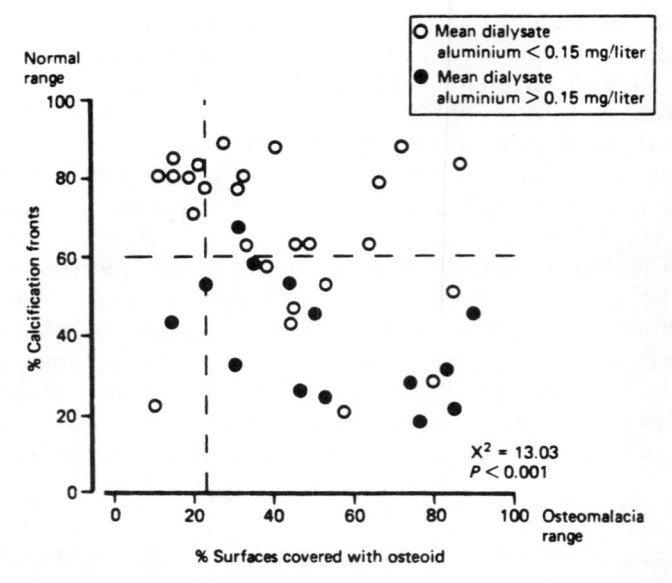

[Figure: scatter plot of % Calcification fronts vs % Surfaces covered with osteoid, showing open circles (Mean dialysate aluminium < 0.15 mg/liter) and filled circles (Mean dialysate aluminium > 0.15 mg/liter); $X^2 = 13.03$, $P < 0.001$.]

Figure 3. Prevalence of osteomalacia and its relationship to mean dialysate aluminum concentration. (Walker GS et al: *Kidney Int* 21:411–415, 1982. Reprinted with permission.)

help control serum phosphate concentration and reduce the dosage of aluminum phosphate binders.

The Redy sorbent cartridge used to regenerate dialysate so that dialysis can be done with a small recirculating volume has recently been shown to release significant amounts of aluminum into the dialysate (107,108). This has been associated with osteomalacia and symptoms of dialysis encephalopathy.

HYPERLIPIDEMIA

There have been several studies in the last 2 years of the lipid abnormalities seen in patients on chronic hemodialysis (109–115). Hemodialysis patients tend to have hypertriglyceridemia with normal total serum cholesterol. However, very low density lipoprotein cholesterol is frequently elevated and high-density lipoprotein cholesterol is uniformally low, causing an increased risk of cardiovascular disease. The hypertriglyceridemia is the result of both defective triglyceride removal (probably the result of insulin resistance) and increased triglyceride production (109). There is also an accumulation of remnants of triglyceride-rich lipoproteins in patients on dialysis (115).

During the dialysis treatment, high-density lipoprotein cholesterol and free fatty acids increase while triglyceride decreases. These effects are probably related to heparin since dialysis using gabexate mesilate in place of heparin is not associated with any significant changes in the plasma lipid pattern (111). Hypertriglyceridemia can be treated successfully with benzafibrate or clofibrate (112). However, the half-life of these drugs is markedly prolonged in dialysis patients and dosages must be severely reduced. The medications need to be administered only every third day.

In both hemodialysis patients and peritoneal dialysis patients there is a significant positive correlation between plasma triglyceride concentration and plasma insulin concentration.

Severini reports that the treatment of hypertriglyceridemic hemodialysis patients with polyacrylonitrile dialysis will decrease the plasma triglyceride to normal range (113). The changes are slow and it takes 4–6 months for normalization of the serum triglyceride. There appears to be no effect on cholesterol or high-density lipoprotein.

NUTRITION

The use of urea kinetics as a guide to nutrition and treatment of renal disease was the topic of a symposium held in Ann Arbor, Michigan. The, reports published in the April 1981 issue of *Dialysis and Transplantation*, demonstrate that many centers have found urea kinetic modeling to be helpful in the treatment of patients with acute or chronic renal failure and especially useful in the treatment of the pediatric hemodialysis patient (116).

Thunberg and co-workers (117) assessed nutrition in 58 nondiabetic chronic hemodialysis patients and suggest that protein–calorie malnutrition is widespread in the stable hemodialysis population. Nutrition was measured by diet survey, anthropometric measurements, and laboratory data. Tricep skin-fold thickness, transferrin, and total lymphocyte counts were subnormal in 72%, 81%, and 69% of patients, respectively. Weight–height ratio, body mass index, arm muscle circumference, and serum albumin were normal in most patients. In the entire group, 62% had greater than three subnormal nutritional measurements and only two patients had all normal measurements. The malnutrition does not, however, appear to be progressive, as sequential measurements revealed little change in patients followed up to 18 months.

These findings are somewhat at variance with the findings of Young and co-workers (118) who assessed hemodialysis patients by measuring nonfasting plasma amino acids and proteins and by anthropometric measurements. They found that apart from two patients with recurrent sepsis, hemodialysis patients of long-standing (1–11 years) were adequately nourished. However, those patients on hemodialysis for less than 15 months, most of whom had previously received peritoneal dialysis, were found to be malnourished. They found that of their measurements, plasma valine concentration had the greatest correlation with the patient's overall nutritional status.

Piraino and co-workers (119) suggest that the administration of glucose with a combination of essential and nonessential amino acids during the dialysis procedure can promote weight gain in previously catabolic chronic hemodialysis patients with inadequate nutritional intake. There was, however, a group of patients with severe metabolic bone disease and myopathy, felt to be due to hyperparathyroidism, who did not respond to the hyperalimentation. Also, if the nonessential amino acids were excluded from the hyperalimentation fluid, the patients developed an abnormal pattern of plasma amino acids, suggesting a deficiency of nonessential amino acids.

The nitrogen balance in hemodialysis patients receiving total parental nutrition can be easily measured by estimating the urea nitrogen accumulation between dialysis from the before and after plasma urea concentrations (120). Nitrogen balance can then be used to determine if amino acid intake is sufficient. Patients with acute renal failure receiving 42.5 g of amino acids and 350 g of glucose have better nitrogen balance than patients receiving 15 g of amino acids and 350 g of dextrose (-0.9 ± 8.5 g/day versus -7.4 ± 7.1 g/day). The rate of rise of BUN was similar in both groups.

Patients lose an average of 8 ± 3 g amino acids during hemodialysis (121). The loss of amino acids results in a decrease in plasma amino acid concentration, which can be prevented by the administration of essential and nonessential amino acids during the dialysis procedure. However, the intravenous or oral supplementation of amino acids during dialysis results in increased dialysis amino acid loss (121,122).

Acchiardo and co-workers (123) demonstrated that chronic oral administration of essential amino acids and calories to stable chronic hemodialysis patients can improve their nutritional status, as manifested by an increase in hematocrit, total protein, serum albumin, transferrin, and total lymphocyte count, as well as an increase in cortical and trabecular bone thickness. Administration of calories without the essential amino acids did not show any beneficial affect.

Ryan-Crowe et al. (124) have reconfirmed previous studies demonstrating that the oral administration of zinc improves taste perception in hemodialysis patients.

Hemodialysis patients have high plasma levels of vitamin A (125,126). The increased vitamin A is entirely bound by retinol-binding protein and the plasma levels of retinyl esters and retinoic acid are not elevated, suggesting that retinyl accumulation is not caused by a deficiency of its oxidative metabolism. Multivitamin supplements containing vitamin A increase the already high plasma concentrations. Kopple and co-workers

(127) evaluated vitamin B_6 deficiency in patients with chronic renal failure and patients undergoing maintenance dialysis by assessing the in vitro activity of erythrocyte glutamic pyruvic transaminase with and without the addition of pyridoxal-phosphate. Patients were then reassessed after the chronic administration of supplemental pyridoxine. Their findings suggest that hemodialysis patients should receive 10 mg per day of pyridoxine hydrochloride, while peritoneal dialysis and predialysis patients should receive 5 mg per day.

DIALYSATE

Dialysate Base

There continues to be a considerable interest in the comparison of bicarbonate dialysate and acetate dialysate. Recent studies support previous observations that suggest that arterial oxygenation is better maintained, hypotension is less frequent, and patients tolerate dialysis better with bicarbonate dialysate (128–134). It appears to be especially helpful in the problem patient.

Pagel and co-workers suggest that it is the presence of acetate rather than the bicarbonate loss that is responsible for patients' intolerance of acetate dialysis (132). They studied blood pressure, frequency of symptoms, and postdialysis task performance in 21 patients undergoing acetate dialysis, bicarbonate dialysis, and dialysis with a dialysate containing both acetate and bicarbonate. They found that dialysis performed with the biocarbonate dialysate resulted in a significantly smaller mean blood pressure drop (Fig. 4), fewer symptoms, and improved task performance as compared to either acetate or the combination dialysis. The toxic effects of acetate, however, were not correlated with the serum acetate level, and patients who were symptomatic on acetate had no more symptoms during bicarbonate dialysis than patients who were symptom-free on acetate dialysate, suggesting that patients symptomatic on acetate dialysis are not simply less tolerant of the process of dialysis, but differed in their response to the presence of acetate. A major criticism of this study is that patients were infused with excessive amounts of base during the combination dialysis, which may itself have caused problems.

At least part of the hypoxia that occurs during acetate dialysis may be related to an increase in oxygen consumption. Eiser and co-workers (133) compared ventilation, oxygen consumption (V_{O_2}), and carbon dioxide production (V_{CO_2}) in patients undergoing acetat and bicarbonate dialysis. They found that V_{CO_2} decreased with both procedures but that V_{O_2} increased with acetate dialysis and decreased with bicarbonate dialysis (Fig. 5). Minute ventilation paralleled V_{CO_2}.

Acetate in the dialysate inhibits the release of growth hormone, both under basal conditions and after stimulation with arginine or insulin

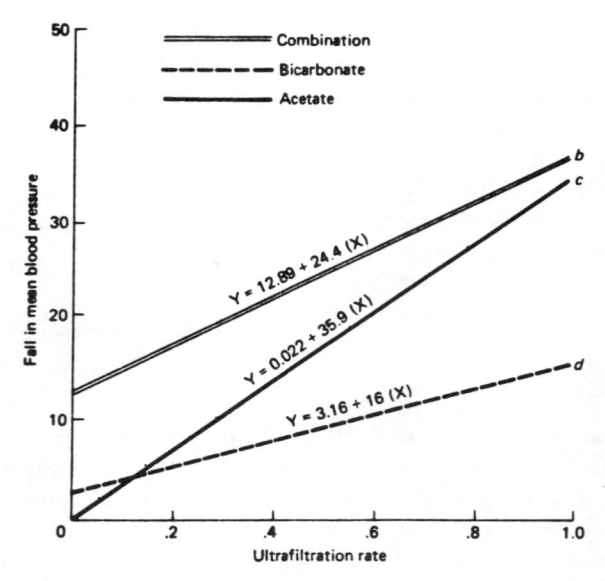

Figure 4. Regression line of fall in mean blood pressure versus rate of ultrafiltration. (b) slope different from zero, $p < 0.050$; (c) slope different from zero, $p < 0.001$; (d) slope different from zero, $p < 0.015$. (Pagel MD et al: *Kidney Int* 21:513-518, 1982. Reprinted with permission.)

(135,136). With acetate dialysate there is also a lack of symptoms during hypoglycemia in diabetics being treated with glucose-free dialysate. This has been hypothesized to be due to the use of acetate as a fuel in the brain (135).

Dialysis with bicarbonate dialysate using the sorbent regenerative system is associated with very high dialysate P_{CO_2} (greater than 200). Most patients tolerate this without difficulty; however, there is a recent report of a 62-year-old woman on a respirator whose arterial blood P_{CO_2} rose from 22 mm Hg before dialysis to 81 mm Hg after the start of dialysis, with a concomitant fall in pH from 7.48 to 7.0. The acid–base and respiratory balance of patients being treated with this system need to be carefully monitored (137).

MIDDLE MOLECULES

There continues to be considerable controversy over the relative toxicity of different molecular weight substances (138–147). Molecules with a molecular weight of 500 to 2,000 (middle molecules) are still being implicated in the etiology of uremic symptoms. However, well-controlled studies are not available, the circumstantial evidence is far from convincing,

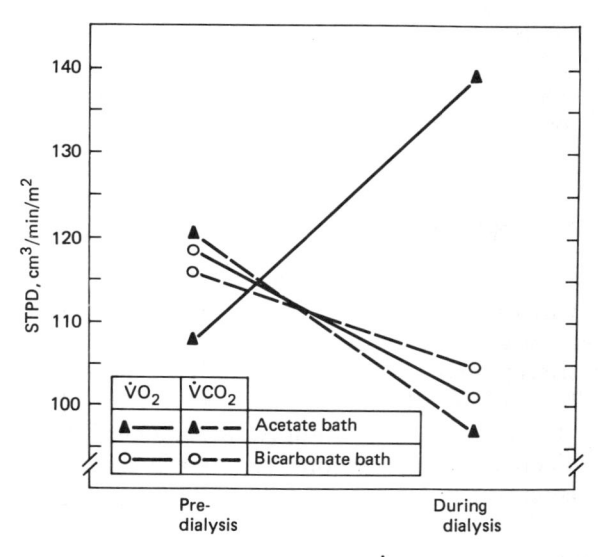

Figure 5. Alterations in oxygen consumption ($\dot{V}_{O_2}$) and CO_2 production ($\dot{V}_{CO_2}$) during acetate and bicarbonate hemodialysis. (Eiser AR et al: *Am J Nephnol* 2:123–127, 1982. Reprinted with permission.)

and properly controlled studies are difficult if not impossible to perform. Various fractions in this molecular weight range isolated from uremic plasma, dialysate, hemofiltrate, or urine have been shown to have in vitro toxicity, but the participation of these substances in the uremic syndrome remains unproven.

The results of a large multicenter national cooperative dialysis study have recently been published (147). In this study 151 patients were placed in four treatment groups divided along two dimensions, dialysis treatment time and mid-week predialysis BUN concentration. Dietary protein was not restricted. Although there was no difference in mortality between the two groups, there was a significant difference in morbidity. Patients in the two high BUN groups had a significantly greater rate of hospitalization time and a higher withdrawal from the study for medical reasons. The dialysis treatment time had no significant effect. Since changing dialysis time affects predominantly middle molecules, this study suggests that small molecule clearance is relatively more important than middle molecule clearance. However, since middle molecule clearance was not modeled for, measured, or estimated, and it is likely that the high BUN groups had some reduction in middle molecule weight clearances as compared to the low BUN groups, the interpretation of this study in relation to the middle molecule theory is inconclusive.

Mitch and Sapir suggest that dialysate frequency may be reduced in patients with residual renal function by means of nutritional therapy

(148). They restricted protein intake to 0.4 g/kg/day and supplemented the patients with 10 g of essential amino acids per day. Patients treated with once weekly hemodialysis had a positive nitrogen balance and increased dry body weight.

HEMODIALYSIS COMPLICATIONS

There has been a host of publications in the last 2 years reporting the contamination of dialysate with various substances, many of which have resulted in serious complications. Webster and co-workers report a group of 23 hemodialysis patients dialyzed against dialysate containing 3 mg/liters of nickel that had entered the dialysate water from a nickel-plated stainless steel water heater tank (149). Symptoms, which included nausea, vomiting, weakness, headache, and palpitations, remitted 3–13 hours after cessation of dialysis. Plasma concentrations of nickel were greater than the dialysate concentrations because of plasma protein binding. Petrie and Roe (150) report the development of severe anemia in patients dialyzed against dialysate containing excessive amounts of zinc obtained from galvanized iron piping or water softeners. Installation of activated carbon filters removed 95–99% of the zinc and returned hemoglobin levels toward previous values.

A 61-year-old woman was accidently hemodialyzed against undiluted sodium hypochlorite (Chlorox) (151). After her blood was exposed to the solution for less than 2 minutes, there was immediate massive hemolysis, hyperkalemia, cyanosis, and cardiopulmonary arrest. The patient received cardiopulmonary resuscitation and was given 5 g sodium thiosulfate as a reducing agent. She subsequently stabilized and recovered 1 week after the incident. Taylor and Price report acute magnesium intoxication and pancreatitis in a patient treated with contaminated dialysate (152). As previously reported, overheated dialysate will cause hemolysis and consumptive coagulopathy (153).

Mulligan et al. (154) report a case of fatal acute hemolysis occurring in a 65-year-old man due to overconcentrated dialysis fluid. Their in vitro studies show that frank hemolysis of blood samples occurs with hemodialysis concentrate at concentrations at or greater than 1:2 dilution. Dialysate concentrate diluted 1:2 results in a 47% hemolysis, and a dilution of 1:1 results in greater than 90% hemolysis.

Lewis and co-workers (155) warn that significant amounts of formaldehyde may remain in formalin-sterilized dialyzers when rinsed by standard techniques. They suggest that the blood compartment be thoroughly rinsed with saline immediately before connection and that the saline left in the dialyzer be discarded at the time of connection. Even with the best of techniques they report that up to 13 mg of formaldehyde is leached slowly from the dialyzer during the dialysis procedure. Recently, a new glutaraldehyde-based disinfectant (Cidex-HD, Surgikos) has been released to replace the use of formaldehyde in hemodialysis system sterilization (156). This disinfectant is effective in killing bacteria, mycobacteria, and viruses (including hepatitis virus). Two cases of death at the same time in one system due to large amounts of formalin in the dialysate were recently reported (157). The major symptom was dyspnea; it is probable that formalin-induced hemolysis decreased oxygen transportation.

Nitrosamines are recognized as potent carcinogens and may be present in deionized water used for dialysate preparation (158). The nitrosamines form in mixed-bed deionizers by some as yet unexplained mechanism. Passing water through an activated carbon charcoal filter before the deionizer prevents nitrosamine formation in the deionizer.

There has recently been considerable interest in release of foreign substances from the dialysis tubing during the dialysis procedure. Most dialysis tubing is treated with the plasticiser di-2-ethylhexyl phthalate (DEHP). Although DEHP is very sparingly soluble in purely aqueous solutions, it is readily lipid soluble and therefore can be leached out of the tubing by blood. During a single dialysis procedure, more than 200 mg of DEHP may be transferred to the patient (159). Fortunately, DEHP has a very low acute toxicity with the LD-50 being greater than 20 g/kg in rats. It is readily metabolized and excreted by both the kidney and the liver. There does not appear to be any chronic toxicity and the carcinogenicity and teratologic effects are of a very low order of magnitude. At this time it appears that the benefits of DEHP appear to outweigh the risks.

Two separate groups have reported the development of foreign body giant cell reaction in the lungs, liver, and spleen of chronic hemodialysis patients, which appears to be secondary to the infusion of silicon during the dialysis procedure (160–163). The silicon was traced to a segment of silicon tubing located in the roller pump of the dialysis machines. Transmission electron microscopy showed the silicon within lysosomal membranes of macrophages found either in groups or singly. The silicon intoxication may be severe enough to cause splenomegaly and resultant pancytopenia.

The low pH of the acidic concentrate used with bicarbonate hemodialysis makes it particularly vulnerable to accidental contamination. Swartz and Maclaren (164) report a case of iron poisoning caused by contaminated acidic concentrate. The concentrate was contaminated by a stainless steel lid that became exposed after a plastic liner broke. The higher pH of the final dialysate caused the precipitation of a rust colored residue in the dialysate lines.

DIALYZER REUSE

Because of the current economic climate, there has been an increased interest in the multiple use of dialyzers. The May, June, and July 1982 issues of *Contemporary Dialysis* present some of the pros and cons of reuse as well as techniques and results of several centers employing reuse (165). An annual saving of $2,000 per patient can be achieved, and some centers have been reusing dialyzers for over 22 years without problems (166). If appropriate safety procedures are established for cleansing, storing, and monitoring, dialyzers can be used many times without an increase in infection, morbidity from any cause, or mortality (166–169). The neutropenia that characteristically occurs early in dialysis is substantially less with reused dialyzers than with new dialyzers, and there may acutally be a reduced incidence of symptoms (chest pain, back pain) with reused dialyzers.

VASCULAR ACCESS

Researchers continue to analyze the patency and complication rates of various types of hemodialysis vascular access (170–176). As in the past the reports consist entirely of retrospective uncontrolled studies and, therefore, are of very limited value in evaluating the different types of access available. In general there is a 50–85% 1-year graft survival and an average survival rate of 2–4 years. Bovine grafts tend to form more aneurysms—usually false aneurysms—than other types of grafts (170). Lynggaard and co-workers report a very poor experience with saphenous loop thigh grafts with many having inadequate blood flow and two of their patients dying from external bleeding episodes (173). Iuchtman and colleagues suggest that patients with chronic pyelonephritis have a decreased graft survival rate as compared to patients with chronic glomerulonephritis (174).

Glutaraldehyde-tanned human umbilical cord vein fistulas appear to be another viable option for internal A-V shunts (176). Preliminary results are similar to those found with bovine and PTFE grafts.

Clotted Brescia A-V fistulas and internal A-V shunts can sometimes be declotted without surgical intervention. Zimmerman describes a technique for nonsurgical declotting of A-V fistulas (177). First, a tight venous tourniquet is placed around the arm to distend the fistula vein down to the vascular anastomosis. The majority of sudden fistula thromboses occur right at the anastomosis, between the artery and the vein. After placing the tourniquet around the arm, the skin directly over the vascular anastomosis is smartly flicked with the fingernail of the second or third finger. This is repeated three or four times and should be done with force. The purpose of this is to dislodge a thrombus from the anastomosis into the distended fistula vein. The area is then kneaded with the thumb for about 10 seconds using a rocking motion in an attempt to milk the fractured clot from the area of the anastomosis into the fistula vein itself. Following this, the venous tourniquet is removed and the fistula inspected for a return of a thrill or bruit. The procedure can be repeated several times. Zimmerman reports 11 successes in 13 clotted Brescia A-V fistulas and one success in five clotted bovine heterografts.

Hart and Oh (178) suggest that intraoperative blood flow measurement is helpful during the placement of bovine grafts. They found that patients with blood flow rates less than 500 ml/min had shortened graft survival and patients with blood flow rates greater than 1,000 ml/min had a high incidence of complications such as steal syndrome and congestive heart failure.

There have been two recent studies of the effect of hemodialysis fistulae on circulatory dynamics and left ventricular function (179,180). Occluding the fistula causes a small but statistically significant increase in vascular resistance, left ventricular systolic diameter, and a decrease in heart rate. There are no changes in left ventricular diastolic dimension or fractional shortening. These changes are probably of little clinical significance in most patients but may be important in patients with decreased cardiac reserve. Intractable angina, left heart failure, and steal syndromes can be dramatically reversed by the reduction of flow through A-V fistulas with banding procedures (181,182).

Angiography is helpful in evaluation of vascular access problems. Glanz and co-workers (183) present the results of angiographic examination of 125 upper extremity internal A-V or graft fistulas. The most frequent problem was venous stenosis at or near the anastomotic site, which occurred in 25% of the cases studied, whereas aneurysms occurred in 18%. Konner and Karnahl report excellect results in evaluating A-V fistulas of hemodialysis patients using transvenous serial xeroarteriography (184). This is performed after intravenous administration of contrast media in the contralateral forearm, which allows adequate visualization of morphologic and functional alterations.

There are two devices now commercially available in the United States for implantation that allow blood access for hemodialysis without the need for skin puncture. These devices appear to have an acceptably low rate of infection, but more experience is needed before they can be recommended for routine use (185,186).

The subclavian catheter and the femoral vein catheter for acute vascular access for hemodialysis have gained popularity and have largely eliminated the need for the acute placement of external A-V shunts (187–192). Dorner performed a retrospective comparison of subclavian catheter placement for hemodialysis to external shunt placement in patients with both acute and chronic renal failure (187). They found that the subclavian vein catheter resulted in a lower incidence of serious infection, hemorrhage, and access thrombosis and fewer replacement procedures were needed. Raja and co-workers (191) compared subclavian catheterization to femoral vein catheterization for acute hemodialysis. They found a similar complication rate with both methods and suggest that the subclavian catheter may be preferable for most patients. The subclavian catheter, however, can result in a compartmental syndrome causing edema and venous congestion of the upper extremities (193), and a fatality due to a subclavian dialysis catheter has recently been reported (194). A catheter can also be easily placed in the internal jugular vein percutaneously by the Seldinger technique for hemodialysis access. This method has an acceptably low rate of complication (195). Excessive recirculation is not infrequent when these catheters are used with single needle devices (191). The double lumen catheters that are now becoming commercially available will largely prevent this problem (189,192).

HEMODIALYSIS AND PREGNANCY

The occurrence of acute renal failure during pregnancy does not necessarily imply the need for termination of the gestation. There is a recent report of acute renal failure developing during the twenty-seventh week of pregnancy in a 21-year-old woman (196). The patient was treated with twice daily hemodialysis for approximately 1 week, after which time renal function spontaneously recovered; the patient delivered a healthy baby 2 months later. The authors suggest that frequent dialysis is needed and that every attempt should be made to keep the BUN level near normal.

USE OF HEMODIALYSIS FOR THE TREATMENT OF NONRENAL DISEASE

Chugh and co-workers (197) compared hemodialysis therapy for psoriasis to sham dialysis, ultrafiltration without dialysis, or systemic heparinization. They found that 15 of 18 patients treated with hemodialysis had regression of the skin lesions, whereas they could demonstrate no effect on the skin lesions of their five control patients, with the exception that the ultrafiltration procedure was followed by a partial regression of psoriasis. The fact that this was not a blinded study and the lack of randomization may explain the difference between this study and the previously controlled study reported by Nissenson (198), which did not find any benefit to hemodialysis. If dialysis is to be tried for psoriasis, peritoneal dialysis appears to be the better choice (199). However, in an uncontrolled study, Steck and co-workers found that six of 11 patients treated by hemofiltration had substantial clearing of their psoriatic lesions; the remaining five patients who had little or no apparent benefit during the course of hemofiltration had dramatic clearing when given previously ineffective topical therapy (200).

Hemodialysis using polyacrylonitrile membranes can be used to remove bile acids from the blood of patients with pruritus of cholestatic disease (201). Clearance rates of 8 ml/min can be obtained with a definite lowering of plasma bile acid concentrations and an improvement in pruritus. The technique compares favorably with alternate techniques such as plasmapheresis or plasma perfusion over activated charcoal.

There continues to be some interest in the use of dialysis for the treatment of schizophrenia. The results indicate that at best there may be some benefit in a small subset of patients but there still is no well-controlled study demonstrating a definite benefit (202–205).

Hemodialysis may have a beneficial effect in patients with familial Mediterranean fever. Ilfeld and co-workers treated a patient with familial Mediterranean fever, amyloidosis, and chronic renal failure with hemodialysis (206). They found that the frequency of febrile attacks was dramatically reduced. No attacks occurred in 21 months of hemodialysis, whereas the patient averaged one attack per month both during conservative medical therapy and during four months on intermittent peritoneal dialysis. Suppressor cell function was significantly better during hemodialysis than during conservative medical therapy or peritoneal dialysis. The authors suggest that suppressor cell deficiency may be associated with the pathogenesis of familial Mediterranean fever and may be corrected by the removal of some unknown substance during hemodialysis. This interesting observation awaits further confirmation.

HEMOFILTRATION

Recently published reports continue to suggest that hemofiltration offers improved cardiovascular stability over hemodialysis (207–212). In contrast to many previously published studies that suggested that the lack of hypotension is related to an improved ability to increase peripheral resistance in response to fluid removal (see *Current Nephrology*, Volume 5), a recent study implicates better maintenance of cardiac output. Chaignon and co-workers compared the hemodynamic effects of hemodialysis and hemofiltration in eight patients (208). They found a similar decrease in body weight, total blood volume, and blood pressure. However, hemodialysis caused a marked decrease in cardiac index and stroke index, whereas these were relatively maintained with hemofiltration. Peripheral resistance was stable after hemodialysis and decreased after hemofiltration. The authors suggest that the major advantage of hemofiltration is the ability of patients to maintain their cardiac output in the face of volume depletion. Both Shaldon and co-workers (211) and Dongradi and co-workers (212) have shown that high-efficiency hemofiltration can be obtained by the use of a large surface area with relatively high blood flows. Treatment time with these techniques can be reduced to less than 3 hours per session with adequate control of uremia. Jeffree and co-workers (213) have demonstrated that hemofiltration efficiency can be increased by pulsing the blood flow over furrowed channels.

Geronemus and associates (214) compared the effect of hemodialysis and hemofiltration on carbohydrate metabolism. While they could find no difference in the mild glucose intolerance between the two treatments, the exaggerated insulin response to glucose infusion was less with hemofiltration. The improvement of carbohydrate metabolism was not related to changes in fasting plasma glucagon, bicarbonate, or potassium concentrations.

One of the most exciting developments in the last 2 years has been the use of continuous A-V hemofiltration for the treatment of acute renal failure (215–217). In this technique, the femoral artery and femoral vein are punctured and blood is allowed to run through a small hemofilter without the use of a blood pump. Ultrafiltration rates of 5–20 ml/min are obtained. The ultrafiltrate is replaced by the continuous infusion of replacement fluid. The treatment is continued 24 hours a day and can be accomplished in an intensive care unit without specialized personnel. Fluid and electrolyte therapy is greatly simplified by this treatment and adequate control of uremia is possible without additional dialysis. There is significant continued loss of amino acids during this procedure; however, hyperalimentation fluid containing amino acids and glucose can be easily infused directly into the venous line (218). The Food and Drug Administration has recently approved the Amicon UF-30 hemofilter for use with this procedure.

REHABILITATION AND ADAPTATION TO DIALYSIS

There has been much recent interest in evaluating and treating psychosocial adaptation to chronic hemodialysis. De-Nour reports that hemodialysis patients have a severe lack of interest in pleasurable leisure activities and suggests that there is a need to devise methods of intervention to improve the quality of life of chronic hemodialysis patients (219). Kutner and Cardanas evaluated medical, vocational, and psychological indicators of rehabilitation in 137 chronic hemodialysis patients (220). Patients aged 25–34 had the best overall adjustment to chronic dialysis but there was a need for improved vocational counseling for patients under age 25 and the need for increased concern for sources of depression among patients 55 and older. Livesley found a high incidence of general distress, anxiety, and sexual problems in 85 patients undergoing chronic hemodialysis who were assessed using a standard questionnaire (221). Psychiatric symptoms were more frequent in women than in men, in those on home dialysis, in those living in rural areas, in the unemployed, and in those with a disturbed nuclear family. Blodgett reviewed the literature of adjustment to hemodialysis and found that there are many factors which are important (222). A very important factor is the premorbid locus of control; patients with an internal locus of control have better overall compliance and lower interdialytic weight gain than patients with an external locus, but there was no significant difference in psychological distress (223).

Eighteen percent of patients entering a home hemodialysis training program were found to suffer major depressive disorders as diagnosed by rigorous clinical criteria (224). The incidence was highest in patients with polycystic kidney disease; there was no association with past or family history of affective disorders. There was no significant difference in intellectual impairment or chemical uremia between the patients with depressive orders and those without. The depressive symptoms had almost invariably remitted during the home dialysis training and had no apparent influence on the outcome. Richman and co-workers (225) studied adaptation to home dialysis in 136 patients followed for more than 18 months. They found some specific physical, psychological, and stress factors that were associated with increased probability of failure on home hemodialysis. In patients under the age of 45, high diastolic blood pressure, congestive heart failure, high levels of stress, insomnia, anxiety, and depression were associated with increased failure. In the older patients, failure was associated with higher levels of depression, self-deprecation, and high levels of stress caused by the fear of death, pain during dialysis, and blood clotting. In both groups, high denial levels were positively correlated with success.

Friedlander and Viederman found that children of dialysis patients also suffer severe psychological problems, frequently having latent aggressive feelings towards the sick parent and exhibiting pseudomature behavior. These problems have a profound impact on the development of these children (226).

Gutman et al. (227) reviewed data from 2,481 patients on maintenance dialysis in order to get a broad overview of their physical status and rehabilitation. Fifty-three percent of their population were over age 50 and 12% were diabetic. They found that 40% of the nondiabetic and 77% of the diabetic patients were not capable of any physical activity beyond that of caring for themselves. They found that only one-quarter of the patients worked outside the home and only an additional third reported any work at home. They concluded that a larger portion of dialysis patients than previously suspected are severely debilitated. The paper does not discuss, however, the large number of negative incentives for rehabilitation that are currently present for the dialysis population in the United States. Johnson and co-workers (228) could not find any difference between the subjective quality of life of patients on chronic hemodialysis and that of patients with successful renal transplantation, whereas patients with a failed transplant showed a definite diminished quality of life.

Because patients are frequently transferred from one mode of therapy to another on a nonrandom basis, comparisons of different types of therapy of end-stage renal disease (ESRD) are difficult. There are three factors that have major effects on survival of ESRD patients: age, duration of diabetes (if present), and the presence or absence of left-sided heart failure (229,230). Hutchinson has developed a method by which survival of individual patients can be predicted by using these factors (230). An analysis of the survival of all patients treated in Michigan suggests that survival is relatively independent of the mode of therapy (229).

Cummings and co-workers found that increased compliance to medical regimes could be obtained through the development of behavioral contacts (with or without the involvement of a family member or friend) (231). Unfortunately, the beneficial effect was rather short-lived, and 3 months after the intervention, patients tended to taper off towards preintervention patterns. Group therapy involving the patient or the patient and the family can be beneficial in helping the patient adjust to ESRD (232–234).

CARNITINE

It has been suggested that carnitine deficiency occurs in hemodialysis patients and may contribute to their hyperlipidemia and muscle weakness. Plasma carnitine levels are low-normal at the beginning of dialysis and fall to subnormal values at the end of dialysis (235,236). Muscle levels of carnitine are markedly reduced and may cause lipid droplets to form in the muscle cells. There are several reports of the effect of administering carnitine to the hemodialysis patient. Bertolli and co-workers (235) report that 50 mg/kg/day of carnitine can result in a significant decrease in plasma triglyceride and increase muscle carnitine content. Suzuki found that 2 g of oral L-carnitine prior to dialysis suppressed the increase in fatty acid levels that occurs during dialysis and decreased the number of premature beats during the hemodialysis treatment (236). Casciani and associates (237) suggest that L-carnitine causes a significant reduction in coronary risk factors by increasing high density lipoproteins and reducing pre-β lipoproteins. In contrast, Chan and co-workers (238) demonstrate no significant effect of the administration of 600 mg or 1.2 of DL carnitine or plasma lipids, but did find an improvement in plasma free fatty acids and lipid clearance after intravenous fat infusion.

HEMOPERFUSION

The present status of hemoperfusion has recently been reviewed by Chang (239). The combined use of both hemodialysis and hemoperfusion to treat chronic uremia underwent a multicenter study in which 39 renal dialysis patients were treated in five centers. The combined treatment proved to be safe and well tolerated and was felt to be effective in improving certain dialysis related problems such as peripheral neuropathy, anorexia, nausea, and relapsing pericarditis. After several weeks of combined therapy there was a marked decrease in the plasma values of urea, uric acid, and creatinine (240,241). These preliminary results await larger, more controlled studies.

THE USE OF DIALYSIS AND HEMOPERFUSION FOR DRUG AND POSION OVERDOSE

For a thorough general discussion of the use of dialysis and hemoperfusion for the treatment of drug and poison overdose, refer to Chapter 10 in Volume 5 of *Current Nephrology*. The present volume summarizes studies published after October 1981 (Table 2). However, it is important to reiterate that dialysis or hemoperfusion is not appropriate for all ingestions. Schreiner (242) has suggested 10 factors that indicate consideration of hemodialysis or hemoperfusion for treating drug overdose:

1. Severe clinical intoxication with abnormal vital signs, often including hypotension despite fluid replacement, apnea, or severe hypothermia
2. Ingestion and probable absorption of a potentially lethal amount of a drug
3. Blood concentration that is in the potentially fatal range
4. Presence of an underlying disease that reduces the normal rate of excretion of the drug
5. Presence of significant quantities of a circulating substance that is metabolized to a more noxious compound.
6. Progressive clinical deterioration while the patient is receiving careful medical therapy
7. Prolonged coma
8. Presence of an underlying disease, such as bronchitis or emphysema, which increases the hazard of coma
9. Development of a significant complication, such as aspiration pneumonitis
10. Poisoning by agents known to produce delayed toxicities, such as paraquat, *Amanita phalloides*, and acetaminophen.

It is also important that the extracorporeal method effectively removes significant quantities from the body and that the clearance of the drug is large enough to significantly increase the total rate of removal from the body. Sufficient quantities of the drug must be in the vascular system and/or the transfer rate from the extravascular compartments into the vascular space must be sufficiently high.

Table 2. Recent References to the Use of Extracorporeal Methods to Remove Toxins

Drug	Treatments Reported	References
Analgesics		
Acetaminophen	HP	243–245
Aspirin	HD,HP,PD	243,246
Phenylbutazone	HP	247,248
Sedatives, tranquilizers, and anticonvulsants		
Barbiturates	HP,HD,PD,HD-HP	245,249,251,252,260,284,285
Benzodiazepines	HD	261
Carbamazepine	HP,PD	258,259
Chloral hydrate	HP	265
Ethylchlorovynol	HP	253,254,260
Lithium	HD	262
Maprotiline	HD(NE)	266
Meprobamate	HP,HD-HP	249,255–257,284
Methaqualone	HD,HP,HD-HP	249,250,284
Methsuximide	HP	263
Phenytoin	HP(NE),PD(NE)	263,264
Triclyclic amines	HP	265
Cardiac Drugs		
Digitalis	HP(NE)	265,270
Disopyramide	HP	271–273
Quinidine	HP	298
Other drugs		
Amikacin	PD(NE)	274
Mannitol	HD	276
Quinine	HD(NE),PD(NE),PE(NE)	267
Theophylline	HP,PD	268,269
Other substances		
Arsenic	HD,HD-HP	277,278,299
Camphor	HP	295
Chlordecone	HP(NE)	294
Ethylene glycol	HD,HP	285–287
Mercury (organic)	HD(NE),HP(NE)	279–282
Methanol	HD	288
Mushroom	PD,HP,HD-HP	265,275,290
Organophosphorus	PD	301
Paraquat	HP	291–293
Pine oil	HD-HP	296
Thallium	HD-HP,PD(NE)	283,284

HD, Hemodialysis; PD, Peritoneal dialysis; HF, Hemofiltration; HD-HF, Simultaneous hemodialysis and hemofiltration; PE, Plasma exchange; (NE), Authors stated technique was not clinically effective.

Analgesics

Acetaminophen
Hemodialysis and hemoperfusion are of questionable benefit in clinical acetaminophen overdose. However, in view of the very high late mortality from liver damage, many recommend the use of charcoal hemoperfusion in acetaminophen overdose (243–245). A retrospective analysis found charcoal hemoperfusion to be associated with a less notable increase in liver enzyme concentrations.

Aspirin
Hemodialysis offers considerable benefit in severe salicylate poisoning and is preferred over hemoperfusion or peritoneal dialysis, since it also rapidly corrects acid–base and electrolyte abnormalities (243). Patients with lesser degrees of intoxication can usually be treated with conservative therapy using forced alkaline diuresis (246).

Pyrasolones (Phenylbutazone, Antipyrine, Aminopyrine)
Acute intoxication with the pyrasolones causes impaired consciousness progressing to coma, sudden apnea, cardiac arrest, and convulsions. Hepatic lesions may develop after a latent period of 12–24 hours. Berlinger and co-workers (247) were able to reduce the half-life of phenylbutazone with both charcoal hemoperfusion and Amberlite hemoperfusion. The half-life without any hemoperfusion was 92 hours as compared to 34 hours with charcoal hemoperfusion and 40 hours with Amberlite hemoperfusion. Charcoal hemoperfusion will remove most other pyrasolones also (248).

Sedatives, Tranquilizers, and Anticonvulsants

Hemodialysis and hemoperfusion have been recommended for treatment of severe intoxication with the barbiturates and many of the commonly used tranquilizers (245,249–260). De Broe and Verpooten suggest that using a procedure combining charcoal hemoperfusion with hemodialysis will increase the clearance rates of many of these drugs over that found with either procedure alone (249). They treated 15 severely intoxicated patients and found that 14 regained consciousness and 12 survived. They feel that combined hemoperfusion and hemodialysis is a safe and efficient procedure. Controlled sequential ultrafiltration is not an effective way to remove these drugs (261). Significant quantities of *methaqualone* can be removed by resin hemoperfusion (250).

Lithium overdose can cause not only neurologic manifestations, but also may result in cardiac manifestations such as atrioventricular block, intraventricular conduction delay and prolonged QT interval. Lithium is effectively removed by hemodialysis (262). Treatment of *phenytoin* overdose with either peritoneal dialysis, hemodialysis, or hemoperfusion does not appear to be effective (263,264). However, *methsuximide* and its major metabolite n-desmethylmethsuximide are removed by charcoal hemoperfusion and rapid clinical improvement was seen during hemoperfusion of a patient with profound central nervous system depression secondary to methsuximide intoxication (263). Heath and co-workers found good clearances of the *tricyclic amines, amitriptyline,* and *nortriptyline* using resin hemoperfusion and feel that this treatment is of definite clinical value in selected, severe cases of self-posioning (265). They also report dramatic effects in one case of severe *chloral hydrate* posioning. Finally, although there is adequate binding of *maprotiline* with the XAD-4 resin hemoperfusion cartridge, treatment by hemoperfusion was found to be ineffective in a case of self-posioning with maprotiline predominately because the drug is tightly tissue-bound and blood concentrations are very low (266).

OTHER DRUGS

A nineteen-year-old youth who had become blind as a result of *quinine* overdose was treated with hemodialysis, peritoneal dialysis, plasma exchanges, and forced diuresis. Minimal amounts of drugs were removed by hemodialysis, peritoneal dialysis, or plasma exchange, none of which appear to have any place in the treatment of quinine overdose. Forced diuresis was felt to be helpful. The patient had some vision return 19 hours after the beginning of treatment, but his vision did not become normal until 5 1/2 months later (267).

Hemoperfusion has been attempted for several cases of drug intoxication. A three-year-old child who accidently received 750 mg of *theophylline* was treated with charcoal hemoperfusion and during a 4-hour period, more than two-thirds of the administered dose was removed. The charcoal column completely removed all of the theophylline from the blood passing through it and saturation did not occur (268). Peritoneal dialysis also removes theophylline, but at significantly lower clearances than hemoperfusion (269). Although the clearance rates of *digitalis* obtained with hemoperfusion are reasonable, the high degree of tissue binding of the drug makes the total amount removed very small. The procedure is probably of very little use in digitalis óverdose (270). Intoxication with *disopyramide* can result in the sudden onset of cardiogenic shock. Both charcoal and resin hemoperfusion are effective in removing the drug and several recent reports suggest that this therapy is useful in treating overdose (271–273).

Peritoneal dialysis was not effective in removing *amikacin*. However, even severe overdose (18 g) can be managed by careful hydration and maintenance of generous diuresis (274). Hemodialysis for eight patients with severe *mannitol* intoxication was recently reported (276). All patients had preexisting renal failure. The manifestations included severe hyponatremia, a large osmolality gap, and fluid overload. Hemodialysis was found to be the treatment of choice as it rapidly removed the mannitol and replaced it with sodium.

Other Substances

Dialysis and perfusion have been used with little success in treating poisoning with metals. Use of hemodialysis or hemoperfusion in acute *arsenic* poisoning appears to be of little value unless the patient has concomitant renal failure, at which time hemodialysis will significantly increase body clearances (277,278). Neither hemodialysis nor hemoperfusion is effective in organic *mercury* intoxication (279,280). However, recent studies using chelating agents encapsulated in microspheres appears promising for future use (281,282). Because of a high degree of tissue binding, neither hemodialysis nor peritoneal dialysis removes significant amounts of the toxic metal *thallium*, and the primary method of treatment remains prompt gastrointestinal decontamination after ingestion (283,284).

Dialysis for poisoning from solvents, toxic mushrooms, herbicides, and pesticides has also been attempted. Hemodialysis with the concomitant administration of ethanol and alkali remain the most effective treatment for severe poisoning of both *ethylene glycol* and *methanol*. Dialysis removes both these substances and their toxic metabolites (285–289). Although not proven beneficial, it is felt by some that hemoperfusion, combined hemodialysis and hemoperfusion, peritoneal dialysis, or plasma exchange may be helpful in preventing the late hepatic damage from the mushroom toxin, *amanitine* (265,275,290). *Paraquat* is efficiently removed from blood by charcoal hemoperfusion and may be of some benefit in paraquat ingestion. However, even with hemoperfusion, the mortality remains high from late respiratory failure resulting from pulmonary fibrosis (291–293). Although there are high blood concentrations and adequate transfer from tissue to blood of the industrial toxin *chlordecone*, hemoperfusion is ineffective because avid binding by plasma proteins prevents adequate removal by the hemoperfusion sorbents. Oral administration of cholestyramine binds chlordecone, increases fecal excretion, and accelerates its disappearance from the body (294).

REFERENCES

1. Degoulet P, Reach I, Di Giulio S, et al: Epidemiology of dialysis induced hypotension. *Proc. Eur Dial Trans Assoc* 18:133–138, 1981.

2. Schohn DC, Klein S, Mitsuishi Y, et al: Correlation between plasma sodium acetate concentration and systemic vascular resistances. Proc Eur Dial Trans Assoc 18:160–168, 1981.
3. Jahn H, Schohn D, Schmitt R: Hemodynamic studies in chronic terminal renal insufficiency—Effects of hemodialysis (Hd), hemofiltration (Hf) and ultrafiltration (Uf) procedures. Nephron 2(2):53–62, 1981.
4. Wehle B, Asaba H, Castenfors J, et al: Influence of dialysate composition on cardiovascular function in insovolaemic haemodialysis. Proc Eur Dial Trans Assoc 18:153–159, 1981.
5. Man NK, Di Giulio S, Zingraff J, et al: The role of sodium in the prevention of vascular instability during haemodialysis. Proc Eur Dial Trans Assoc 18:255–265, 1981.
6. Van Stone JC, Bauer J, Carey J: The effect of dialysate sodium concentration on body fluid compartment volume, plasma renin activity and plasma aldosterone concentration in chronic hemodialysis patients. Am J Kidney Dis 2(1):58–64, 1982.
7. Swartz RD, Somermeyer MG, Hsu CH: Preservation of plasma volume during hemodialysis depends on dialysate osmolality. Am J Nephrol 2:189–194, 1982.
8. Burgess ED: Cardiac vagal denervation in hemodialysis patients. Nephron 30:228–230, 1982.
9. Zoccali C, Ciccarelli M, Maggiore Q: Defective reflex control of heart rate in dialysis patients: Evidence for an afferent autonomic lesion. Clin Sci 63:285–292, 1982.
10. Cannella G, Picotti GB, Movilli E, et al: Plasma catecholamine response to postural stimulation in normotensive and dialysis hypotension-prone uremic patients. Nephron 27:285–291, 1981.
11. Botey A, Gaya J, Montoliu J, et al: Postsynaptic adrenergic unresponsiveness in hypotensive haemodialysis patients. Proc Eur Dial Trans Assoc 18:586–591, 1981.
12. Mitas JW II, O'Connor DT, Stone RA: Evaluation of the neurogenic component of hypertension associated with dialysis and renal insufficiency. ASAIO 4:56–60, 1981.
13. Izzo JL Jr, Izzo MS, Sterns RH, et al: Sympathetic nervous system hyperactivity in maintenance hemodialysis patients. Tran Am Soc Artif Intern Organs 28:604–606, 1982.
14. Cini G, Camici M, Pentimone F, et al: Echocardiographic hemodynamic study during ultrafiltration sequential dialysis. Nephron 30:124–130, 1982.
15. Ireland MA, Mehta BR, Shiu MF: Acute effects of haemodialysis on left heart dimensions and left ventricular function: An echocardiographic study. Nephron 29:73–79, 1981.
16. Thayssen P, Andersen KH, Pindborg T: Non-invasive monitoring of cardiac function during haemodialysis. Scand J Urol Nephrol 15:313–317, 1981.
17. Chaignon M, Chen WT, Tarazi RC, et al: Acute effects of hemodialysis on echographic-determined cardiac performance: Improved contractility resulting from increased serum calcium with reduced potassium despite hypovolemic-reduced cardiac output. Am Heart J 103:374–378, 1982.
18. Lai KN, Fassett RG, Mathew TH: Effect of long-term oral cimetidine treatment on left ventricular function in haemodialysis patients with active hyperparathyroidism. Br J Clin Pharmacol 13:693–697, 1982.
19. Diskin CJ, Salzsieder KH, Solomon RJ, et al: Electrocardiographic changes following dialysis. Nephron 27:94–100, 1981.
20. Roig E, Betriu A, Castaner A, et al: Disabling angina pectoris with normal coronary arteries in patients undergoing long-term hemodialysis. Am J Med 71:431–434, 1981.
21. Iseki K, Onoyama K, Fujimi S, et al: Immediate hemodynamic response to SQ 14225 (Captopril) in hypertensive and normotensive hemodialysis patients. Clin Nephrol 16:137–141, 1981.

22. Wauters JP, Waeber B, Brunner HR, et al: Uncontrollable hypertension in patients on hemodialysis: Long-term treatment with captopril and salt subtraction. *Clin Nephrol* 16:86–92, 1981.
23. Kaneda H, Murata T, Matsumoto J, et al: Effect of captopril on blood pressure and renin-angiotensin-aldosterone system in hypertensive patients on hemodialysis. *Tohoku J Exp Med* 137:21–31, 1982.
24. Fairshter RD, Vaziri ND, Mirahmadi MK: Lung pathology in chronic hemodialysis patients. *Int J Artif Organs* 5:97–100, 1982.
25. Szwed JJ, Handt A, Farber MO, et al: The effect of hemodialysis on oxygen transport in chronic uremics. *Am J Med Sci* 283:50–56, 1982.
26. Ackil AA, Shahani BT, Young RR: Sural nerve conduction studies and late responses in children undergoing hemodialysis. *Arch Phys Med Rehabil* 62:487–491, 1981.
27. Chokroverty S: Proximal vs distal slowing of nerve conduction in chronic renal failure treated by long-term hemodialysis. *Arch Neurol* 39:53–54, 1982.
28. Lowitzsch K, Gohring U, Hecking E, et al: Refractory period, sensory conduction velocity and visual evoked potentials before and after haemodialysis. *J Neurol Neurosurg Psych* 44:121–128, 1981.
29. Delmez JA, Holtmann B, Sicard GA, et al: Peripheral nerve entrapment syndromes in chronic hemodialysis patients. *Nephron* 30:118–123, 1982.
30. Dettori P, La Greca G, Biasioli S, et al: Changes of cerebral density in dialyzed patients. *Neuroradiology* 23:95–99, 1982.
31. Edmondson RP, Ong YW, Chang CH, et al: Studies on the anaemia of Asian patients with chronic renal failure undergoing regular haemodialysis. *Ann Acad Med Singapore* 11:15–23, 1982.
32. Charles G, Lundin AP 3d, Delano BG, et al: Absence of anemia in maintenance hemodialysis. *Int J Artif Organs* 4:277–279, 1981.
33. Shalhoub RJ, Rajan U, Kimm VV, et al: Erythrocytosis in patients on long-term hemodialysis. *Ann Int Med* 97:686–690, 1982.
34. Bezwoda WR, Derman DP, Bothwell TH, et al: Iron absorption in patients on regular dialysis therapy. *Nephron* 28:289–293, 1981.
35. McCarthy JT, Libertin CR, Mitchell JC 3d, et al: Hemosiderosis in a dialysis patient: Treatment with hemofiltration and deferoxamine chelation therapy. *Mayo Clin Proc* 57:439–441, 1982.
36. Rembold CM, Krumlovsky FA, Roxe DM, et al: Treatment of hemodialysis hemosiderosis with desferrioxamine. *Trans Amer Soc Artif Intern Organs* 28:621–626, 1982.
37. Inauen W, Staubli M, Descoeudres C, et al: Erythrocyte deformability in dialysed and non-dialysed uraemic patients. *Eur J Clin Invest* 12:173–176, 1982.
38. Remuzzi G, Benigni A, Dodesini P, et al: Platelet function in patients on maintenance hemodialysis: Depressed or enhanced? *Clin Nephrol* 17:60–63, 1982.
39. Endo Y, Mamiya S, Satoh M, et al: Plasma beta-thromboglobulin and platelet factor 4 in patients with chronic renal failure and effect of hemodialysis. *Tohoku J Exp Med* 135:349–358, 1981.
40. Pogliani EM, Colombi M, Cristoforetti G, et al: Beta-thromboglobulin and platelet factor 4 plasma levels during haemodialysis: effect of indobufen. *Pharmatherapeutica* 3:127–132, 1982.
41. Berrettini M, Buoncristiani U, Parise P, et al: Polyacrilonytrile versus cuprophan membranes for hemodialysis: Evaluation of efficacy and biocompatibility by platelet aggregation studies. *Int J Artif Organs* 4:218–222, 1981.
42. Adler AJ, Berlyne GM: β-Thromboglobulin and platelet factor-4 levels during hemodialysis with polyacrilonitrile. *ASAIO* 4:100–102, 1981.

43. Twardowski Z, Dmoszynska A, Janicka L, et al: Platelet counts in arteriovenous fistula blood are lower than in venous blood. *Dial Transplant* 10:422–426, 1981.
44. Leithner C, Sinzinger H, Silberbauer K, et al: Platelet microaggregates and release of endogenous prostacyclin during the initial phase of haemodialysis. *Proc Eur Dial Trans Assoc* 18:122–125, 1981.
45. Badger AM, Bernard DB, Idelson BA, et al: Depressed spontaneous cellular cytotoxicity associated with normal or enhanced antibody-dependent cellular cytotoxicity in patients on chronic haemodialysis. *Clin Exp Immunol* 45:568–575, 1981.
46. Kerman RH, Floyd M, Van Buren C, et al: Serial measurement of nonspecific immune parameters in chronically hemodialyzed renal failure patients. *J Clin Immunol* 1:163–168, 1981.
47. Hoy WE, Cestero RV, Freeman RB: Lymphocyte populations in maintenance hemodialysis patients—Reassessment and analysis of B cell subtypes. *Clin Exp Dial Apheresis* 5:335–347, 1981.
48. Watson, MA, Hamilton DN, Briggs JD, et al: Cell-mediated immunity during RDT and the outcome of transplantation. *Proc Eur Dial Trans Assoc* 18:387–393, 1981.
49. Linnemann CC Jr, First MR, Schiffman G: Response to pneumococcal vaccine in renal transplant and hemodialysis. *Arch Intern Med* 141:1637–1640, 1981.
50. Gabizon D, Kaufman S, Shaked U, et al: Eosinophilia in uremia. *Nephron* 19:36–39, 1981.
51. Spinowitz BS, Simpson M, Manu P, et al: Dialysis eosinophilia. *Trans Am Soc Artif Intern Organs* 27:161–165, 1981.
52. Hallgren R, Venge P, Wikstrom B: Hemodialysis-induced increase in serum lactoferrin and serum eosinophil cationic protein as signs of local neutrophil and eosinophil degranulation. *Nephon* 29:233–238, 1981.
53. Guerrero IC, Schreiber AD, MacGregor RR: Studies of the plasma factor which induces augmented granulocyte adherence during hemodialysis. *Nephron* 27:79–83, 1981.
54. Kim T, Michael AF, Kjellstrand CM, et al: Complement activation by hemodialysis membranes. *Dial Transplant* 11:265–272, 1982.
55. Swartz RD: Hemorrhage during high-risk hemodialysis using controlled heparinization. *Nephron* 28:65–69, 1981.
56. Flicker W, Russell LW, Farrell PC, et al: Precise anticoagulation—reagents and artifacts. *Dial Transplant* 11:1042–1046, 1980.
57. Gunnarsson B, Asaba H, Dawidson S, et al: The effects of three different heparin regimes on heparin concentrations in plasma and fibrin formation in dialyzers. *Clin Nephrol* 15:135–142, 1981.
58. Gross M, Bush H, McTigue H, et al: Evaluation of prostaglandin D2 (PGD2) as an anticoagulative agent for haemodialysis in comparison with prostaglandin E1 (PGE1). *Proc Eur Dial Trans Assoc* 18:117–121, 1981.
59. Turney JH, Dodd NJ, Williams LC, et al: Prostacyclin prevents endothelial and platelet damage during dialysis. *Proc. Eur Dial Trans Assoc* 18:111–116, 1981.
60. Turney JH, Dodd NJ, Williams LC, et al: Prostacyclin prevents endothelial and platelet damage during dialysis. *Proc Eur Dial Trans Assoc* 18:111–116, 1981.
61. Zusman RM, Rubin RH, Cato AE, et al: Hemodialysis using prostacyclin instead of heparin as the sole antithrombotic agent. *N Engl J Med* 304:934–939, 1981.
62. Smith, MC, Danviriyasup K, Crow JW, et al: Prostacyclin substitution for heparin in long-term hemodialysis. *Am J Med* 73:669–678, 1982.
63. Canavese C, Stratta P, Pacitti A, et al: Impaired fibrinolysis in uremia: Partial and variable correction by four different dialysis regimes. *Clin Nephrol* 17:82–89, 1982.

64. Ellison RT, Corrao WM, Fox MJ, et al: Spontaneous mediastinal hemorrhage in patients on chronic hemodialysis. *Ann Intern Med* 95:704–706, 1981.
65. Adams PL, Rutsky EA, Rostand SG, et al: Lower gastrointestinal tract dysfunction in patients receiving long-term hemodialysis. *Arch Intern Med* 142:303–306, 1982.
66. Cunningham JT: Gastric telangiectasias in chronic hemodialysis patients: A report of six cases. *Gastroenterology* 81:1131–1133, 1981.
67. Tourkantonis A, Spiliopoulos A, Pharmakiotis A, et al: Haemodialysis and hypothalamo-pituitary-testicular axis. *Nephron* 27:271–272, 1981.
68. Mahajan SK, Abbasi AA, Prasad AS, et al: Effect of oral zinc therapy on gonadal function in hemodialysis patients. *Ann Intern Med* 97:357–361, 1982.
69. Zingraff J, Jungers P, Pélissier C, et al: Pituitary and ovarian dysfunctions in women on haemodialysis. *Nephron* 30:149–153, 1982.
70. Mrinak J, Melnicak P, Mrinakova A, et al: Functional capacity of suprarenal cortex in patients on long-term dialysis. *Czech Med* 4:244–251, 1981.
71. Ramirez G, Gomez-Sanchez C, Meikle WA, et al: Evaluation of the hypothalamic hypophyseal adrenal axis in patients receiving long-term hemodialysis. *Arch Intern Med* 142:1448–1452, 1982.
72. Olgaard K, Madsen S, Hammer M, et al: Calcium-dependent aldosterone secretion in anephric and non-nephrectomized patients on regular hemodialysis. *J Clin Endocrinol Metab* 46:740–746, 1978.
73. Davis FB, Spector DA, Davis PJ, et al: Comparison of pituitary-thyroid function in patients with end stage renal disease in in age- and sex-matched controls. *Kidney Int* 21:362–364, 1982.
74. Gilchrest BA, Stern RS, Steinman TI, et al: Clinical features of pruritus among patients undergoing maintenance hemodialysis. *Arch Dermatol* 118:154–156, 1982.
75. Pederson J, Matter B, Czerwinski, et al: Relief of idiopathic generalized pruritus in dialysis patients treated with activated charcoal. *Ann Intern Med* 93:446–448, 1980.
76. Shulz BC, Roenigk HH: Uremic pruritus treated with ultra violet light. *JAMA* 243:1836–1837, 1980.
77. Hanno R, Callen JP: Porphyria cutanea tarda as a cause of bullous dermatosis of hemodialysis. A case report and review of the literature. *Cutis* 28:261–263, 1981.
78. Disler P, Day R, Burman N, et al: Treatment of hemodialysis-related porphyria cutanea tarda with plasma exchange. *Am J Med* 72:989–993, 1982.
79. Hurwitz RM, Melton ME, Creech FT, et al: Perforating folliculitis in association with hemodialysis. *Am J Dermatopathol* 4:101–108, 1982.
80. White CR Jr, Heskel NS, Pokorny DJ: Perforating folliculitis of hemodialysis. *Am J Dermatopathol* 4:109–116, 1982.
81. Crosnier J: Hepatitis B in haemodialysis: Vaccination against HBS antigen. *Proc Eur Dial Trans Assoc* 18:231–240, 1981.
82. Ghio L, Moroni GA, Piccoli P, et al: Hepatitis B prevalence and immunoprophylaxis with hepatitis B immunoglobulins in patients, relatives, and staff of a paediatric haemodialysis unit. *Helv Paediatr Acta* 37:17–26, 1982.
83. Carta JR: Presumed transfer of hepatitis antibody by blood transfusion to chronic hemodialysis patients. *Am J Infect Control* 10:34–36, 1982.
84. Chan MK, Moorhead JF: Hepatitis B and the dialysis and renal transplantation unit. *Nephron* 27:229–232, 1981.
85. Walker WG, Hillis WD, Hillis A, et al: Hepatitis B infection in patients with end stage renal disease: Some characteristics and consequences. *Trans Am Clin Climatol Assoc* 92:142–151, 1980.

86. Kiernan TW, Powers RJ: Hepatitis B virus in patients undergoing hemodialysis: Transmission risks and psychosocial reactions. *Arch Intern Med* 142:51–54, 1982.
87. Leventhal Z, Gafter U, Zevin D, et al: Tuberculosis in patients on hemodialysis. *Isr J Med Sci* 18:245–247, 1982.
88. Azadian BS, Beck A, Curtis JR, et al: Disseminated infection with *Mycobacterium chelonei* in a haemodialysis patient. *Tubercle* 62:281–284, 1981.
89. Smith EC: Tuberculosis in dialysis patients. *Int J Artif Organs* 5:11–12, 1982.
90. Kalweit WH, Winn WC Jr, Rocco TA, et al: Hemodialysis fistula infections caused by *Legionella pneumophila*. *Ann Intern Med* 96:173–175, 1982.
91. Cohen IM, Galgiani JN, Potter D, et al: Coccidioidomycosis in renal replacement therapy. *Arch Intern Med* 142:489–494, 1982.
92. Petersen NJ, Carson LA, Favero MS: Bacterial endotoxin in new and reused hemodialyzers: A potential cause of endotoxemia. *Trans Am Soc Artif Intern Organs* 27:155–160, 1981.
93. Leather HM, Lewin IG, Calder E, et al: Effect of water deionisers on 'fracturing osteodystrophy' and dialysis encephalopathy in Plymouth. *Nephron* 29:80–94, 1981.
94. King SW, Savory J, Wills MR: Aluminum toxicity in relation to kidney disorders. *Ann Clin Lab Sci* 11:337–342, 1981.
95. Milne FJ, Hudson GA, Meyers AM, et al: Healing of fracturing-bone disease occurring in patients on dialysis. A prospective study. *S Afr Med J* 61:955–959, 1982.
96. Fournier G, Gaillard JL, Bourdon R, et al: Spontaneous fracture in a hemodialyzed woman probably associated with the oral intake of aluminium gel. *Nephrologie* 2:23–26, 1981.
97. Walker GS, Aaron JE, Peacock M, et al: Dialysate aluminium concentration and renal bone disease. *Kidney Int J* 21:411–415, 1982.
98. Hodsman AB, Sherrard DJ, Alfrey AC, et al: Bone aluminum and histomorphometric features of renal osteodystrophy. *J Clin Endocrinol Metabol* 54:539–546, 1982.
99. Cournot-Witmer G, Zingraff J, Plachott JJ, et al: Aluminum localization in bone from hemodialyzed patients: Relationship to matrix mineralization. *Kidney Int* 20:375–378, 1981.
100. Prior JC, Cameron EC, Knickerbocker WJ, et al: Dialysis encephalopathy and osteomalacic bone disease: A case-controlled study *Am J Med* 72:33–42, 1982.
101. Brun A, Dictor M: Senile plaques and tangles in dialysis dementia. *Acta Pathol Microbiol Scand* 89:193–198, 1981.
102. Chokroverty S, Gandhi V: Electroencephalograms in patients with progressive dialytic encephalopathy. *Clin Electroencephalography* 13:122–127, 1982.
103. Hughes JR, Schreeder MT: EEG in dialysis encephalopathy. *Neurology* 30:1148–1154, 1980.
104. Brown DJ, Dawborn JK, Ham KN, et al: Treatment of dialysis osteomalacia with desferrioxamine. *Lancet* 2:343–345, 1982.
105. Graf H, Stummvoll Hk, Meisinger V: Desferrioxamine-induced changes of aluminium kinetics during haemodialysis. *Proc Eur Dial Trans Assoc* 18:674–680, 1981.
106. Guillot AP, Hood VL, Runge CF, et al: The use of magnesium-containing phosphate binders in patients with end-stage renal disease on maintenance hemodialysis. *Nephron* 30:114–117, 1982.
107. Mion C, Branger B, Issautier R, et al: Dialysis fracturing osteomalacia without hyperparathyroidism in patients treated with HCO3 rinsed Redy cartridge. *Trans Am Soc Artif Intern Organs* 27:634–638, 1981.
108. Pierides AM, Frohnert PP: Aluminum related dialysis osteomalacia and dementia after prolonged use of the Redy cartridge. *Trans Am Soc Artif Intern Organs* 27:629–633, 1981.

109. Chan MK, Varghese Z, Persaud JW, et al: Hyperlipidemia in patients on maintenance hemo and peritoneal dialysis: The relative pathogenetic roles of triglyceride production and triglyceride removal. *Clin Nephrol* 17:183–190, 1982.

110. Nicholls AJ, Cumming AM, Catto GR, et al: Lipid relationships in dialysis and renal transplant patients. *Q J Med* 50:149–160, 1981.

111. Teraoka J, Matsui N, Nakagawa S, et al: The role of heparin in the changes of lipid patterns during a single hemodialysis. *Clin Nephrol* 17:96–99, 1982.

112. Grutzmacher P, Scheuermann E, Lang W: Improvement of hyperlipidaemia by benzafibrate treatment in RDT patients. *Proc Eur Dial Trans Assoc* 18:169–175, 1981.

113. Severini G, Buongiorno A: Serum triglyceride levels in uremic patients receiving polyacrylonitrile dialysis. *Clin Biochem* 14:71–73, 1981.

114. Krumlovsky FA: Disorders of protein and lipid metabolism associated with chronic renal failure and chronic dialysis. *Ann Clin Lab Sci* 11:350–360, 1981.

115. Nestel PJ, Fidge NH, Tan MH: Increased lipoprotein-remnant formation in chronic renal failure. *N Engl J Med* 307:329–333, 1982.

116. Sargent JA: Introduction to symposium on urea kinetics: A quantitative guide to nutrition and treatment in renal disease. *Dial Transplant* 10:175–276, 1981.

117. Thunberg BJ, Swamy AP, Cestero RV: Cross-sectional and longitudinal nutritional measurements in maintenance hemodialysis patients. *Am J Clin Nutr* 34:2005–2015, 1981.

118. Young GA, Swanepoel CR, Croft MR, et al: Anthropometry and plasma valine, amino acids, and proteins in the nutritional assessment of hemodialysis patients. *Kidney Int* 21:492–499, 1982.

119. Piraino AJ, Firpo JJ, Powers DV: Prolonged hyperalimentation in catabolic chronic dialysis therapy patients. *JPEN* 5:463–477, 1981.

120. Mirtallo JM, Schneider PJ, Ruberg RL, et al: Monitoring protein requirements of the patient receiving hemodialysis and total parenteral nutrition. *Am J Hosp Pharm* 38:1483–1486, 1981.

121. Wolfson M, Jones MR, Kopple JD: Amino acid losses during hemodialysis with infusion of amino acids and glucose. *Kidney Int* 21:500–506, 1982.

122. Tepper T, van der Hem GK, Klip HG, et al: Loss of amino acids during hemodialysis: Effect of oral essential amino acid supplementation. *Mod Probl Pharmacopsychiatry* 17:163–165, 1981.

123. Acchiardo S, Moore L, Cockrell S: Effect of Essential amino acids on chronic hemodialysis patients. *Trans Am Soc Artif Intern Organs* 28:608–613, 1982.

124. Ryan-Crowe VC, Crews MG, Stanbaugh G, et al: Taste acuity response to zinc supplementation in hemodialysis patients. *Dial Transplant* 11:316–320, 1982.

125. Stewart KW, Fleming LW: Plasma retinol and retinol binding protein concentrations in patients on maintenance haemodialysis with and without vitamin A supplements. *Nephron* 30:15–21, 1982.

126. De Bevere VO, De Paepe M, De Leenheer AP, et al: Plasma vitamin A in haemodialysis patients. *Clin Chim Acta* 114:249–256, 1981.

127. Kopple JD, Mercurio K, Blumenkrantz MJ, et al: Daily requirement for pyridoxine supplements in chronic renal failure. *Kidney Int* 19:694–704, 1981.

128. Rohmer D, Nassri M, Sherlock J, et al: A comparison of the respiratory dynamics during hemodialysis using acetate and bicarbonate dialysate in a sorbent regenerative system. *Trans Am Soc Artif Intern Organs* 27:176–178, 1981.

129. Raja RM, Kramer MS, Rosenbaum JL, et al: Hemodialysis associated hypoxemia—Role of acetate and pH in etiology. *Trans Am Soc Artif Intern Organs* 27:180–183, 1981.

130. Raja RM, Kramer MS, Rosenbaum M, et al: Hemodialysis with varying dialysate bicarbonate concentration. *Trans Am Soc Artif Intern Organs* 28:514–516, 1982.
131. Okusa MD, Landwehr DM: Comparison of blood pressure stability with acetate and bicarbonate hemodialysis. *Tran Am Soc Artif Intern Organs* 28:518–521, 1982.
132. Pagel MD, Ahmad S, Vizzo JE, et al: Acetate and bicarbonate fluctuations and acetate intolerance during dialysis. *Kidney Int* 21:513–518, 1982.
133. Eiser AR, Jayamanne D, Kokseng C, et al: Contrasting alterations in pulmonary gas exchange during acetate and bicarbonate hemodialysis. *Am J Nephrol* 2:123–127, 1982.
134. Dolan MJ, Whipp BJ, Davidson WD, et al: Hypopnea associated with acetate hemodialysis: Carbon dioxide-flow-dependent ventilation. *N Engl J Med* 305:72–75, 1981.
135. Orskov H, Hansen AP, Hansen HE, et al: Acetate: Inhibitor of growth hormone hypersecretion in diabetic and non-diabetic uraemic subjects. *Acta Endocrinol* 99:551–558, 1982.
136. Schmitz O, Hansen AP, Hansen HE, et al: Inhibition of arginine- and hypoglycemia-induced growth hormone release by acetate in dialyzed patients. *Clin Nephrol* 17:70–76, 1982.
137. Hamm LL, Lawrence G, DuBose TD Jr: Sorbent regenerative hemodialysis as a potential cause of acute hypercapnia. *Kidney Int* 21:416–418, 1982.
138. Babb AL, Ahmad S, Bergstrom J, et al: The middle molecule hypothesis in perspective. *Am J Kidney Dis* 1:46–50, 1981.
139. Kjellstrand CM: Do middle molecules cause uremic intoxication? *Am J Kidney Dis* 1:51–56, 1981.
140. Valek A, Dzurik R, Spustova V, et al: Concentration of plasma middle molecular weight substances and clinical condition of patients undergoing short-time regular dialysis treatment. *Artif Organs* 4:172–176, 1981.
141. Funck-Brentano JL, Man NK: An overview of clinical implications of middle molecules and their kinetics in uremia. *Artif Organs* 4:125–132, 1981.
142. Cueille G, Man NK, Sausse A, et al: Characterization of sub-peak b4.2, middle molecule. *Artif Organs* 4:28–32, 1981.
143. Le Moel G, Strecker G, Cueille G, et al: Uremic middle molecules: Analytical study of middle molecular weight fractions sub-peak b4-2. *Artif Organs* 4:17–21, 1981.
144. Klein E: Middle molecule definition in terms of membrane permeability. *Artif Organs* 4:46–50, 1981.
145. Brunner J, Mann J, Essers U, et al: Large-scale isolation of middle and higher molecular weight uremic toxins. *Artif Organs* 4:41–45, 1981.
146. Jorstad S, Smeby LC, Wideroe TE: Toxicity of middle molecules: Clinical evaluation using a selective filtration artificial kidney. *Artif Organs* 4:98–102, 1981.
147. Lowrie EG, Laird NM, Parker TF, et al: Effect of the hemodialysis prescription on patient morbidity: Report from the National Cooperative Dialysis Study. *N Engl J Med* 305:1176–1181, 1981.
148. Mitch WE, Sapir DG: Evaluation of reduced dialysis frequency using nutritional therapy. *Kidney Int* 20:122–126, 1981.
149. Webster JD, Parker TJ, Alfrey AC, et al: Acute nickel intoxication by dialysis. *Ann Intern Med* 92:631–633, 1980.
150. Petrie JJ, Row PG: Dialysis anemia caused by subacute zinc toxicity. *Lancet* 1:1178–1180, 1977.
151. Hoy RH: Accidental systemic exposure to sodium hypochlorite (Chlorox) during hemodialysis. *Am J Hosp Pharm* 38:1512–1514, 1981.
152. Taylor PA, Price JD: Acute manganese intoxication and pancreatitis in a patient treated with a contaminated dialysate. *Can Med Assoc J* 126:503–505, 1982.

153. Tielemans CL, Herbaut CR, Geurts JO, et al: Hemolysis and consumption coagulopathy due to overheated dialysate. *Nephron* 30:190–191, 1982.
154. Mulligan I, Parfrey P, Phillips ME, et al: Acute haemolysis due to concentrated dialysis fluid. *Br Med J* 284:1151–1152, 1982.
155. Lewis KJ, Ward MK, Kerr DN: Residual formaldehyde in dialyzers: Quantity, location, and the effect of different methods of rinsing. *Artif Organs* 5:269–277, 1981.
156. Petersen NJ, Carson LA, Doto IL, et al: Microbiologic evaluation of a new glutaraldehyde-based disinfectant for hemodialysis systems. *Tran AM Soc Artif Intern Organs* 28:287–290, 1982.
157. Erkrath KD, Adebahr G, Lloppel A: Lethal intoxication by formalin during dialysis. *Z Rechtsmed* 87:233–236, 1981.
158. Kirkwood, RG, Dunn S, Thomasson L, et al: Generation of the precarcinogen dimethylnitrosamine (DMNA) in dialysate water. *Tran Am Soc Artif Intern Organs* 27:168–170, 1981.
159. Baker RW: Diethylhexyl phthalate as a factor in blood transfusion and haemodialysis. *Toxicology* 9:319–329, 1978.
160. Krempien B, Bommer J, Ritz E: Foreign body giant cell reaction in lungs, liver and spleen. A complication of long-term haemodialysis. *Virchows Arch* 392:73–80, 1981.
161. Bommer J, Waldherr R, Ritz E: Silicone filings in macrophages of viscera: an iatrogenic complication of haemodialysis. *Proc Eur Dial Trans Assoc* 18:731–735, 1981.
162. Leong AS, Disney AP, Gove EW: Spallation and migration of silicone from blood-pump tubing in patients on hemodialysis. *N Engl J Med* 306:135–140, 1982.
163. Bommer J, Ritz E, Waldherr R: Silicone-induced splenomegaly: Treatment of pancytopenia by splenectomy in a patient on hemodialysis. *N Engl J Med* 305:1077–1079, 1981.
164. Swartz RD, Maclaren C: Iron contamination during bicarbonate hemodialysis. *ASAIO* 4:61–64, 1981.
165. Wilson MR: Dialyzer reuse. The controversy over the economics, safety and necessity continues. *Contemporary Dialysis* p12–20, 1982.
166. Shaldon S: 22 years' experience with reuse. *Dial Transplant* 11:569–570, 1982.
167. Mathew TH, Fazzalari RA, Disney AP, et al: Multiple use of dialysers: An Australian view. *Nephron* 27:222–225, 1981.
168. Kant KS, Pollak VE, Cathey M, et al: Multiple use of dialyzers: Safety and efficacy. *Kidney Int* 19:728–738, 1981.
169. Luehmann D, Hirsch D, Carlson G, et al: Dialyzer reuse in a large dialysis program. *Trans Am Soc Artif Intern Organs* 28:76–80, 1982.
170. Shifrin E, Roll D, Anner H, et al: Six-year experience with bovine arterial graft for hemodialysis. *Isr J Med Sci* 17:335–338, 1981.
171. Garvin PJ, Castaneda MA, Codd JE: Etiology and management of bovine graft aneurysms. *Arch Surg* 117:281–284, 1982.
172. Rapaport A, Noon GP, McCollum CH: Polytetrafluoroethylene (PTFE) grafts for haemodialysis in chronic renal failure: Assessment of durability and function at three years. Aust NZ J Surg 51:562–566, 1981.
173. Lynggaard F, Nordling J, Iversen Hansen R: Clinical experience with the saphena loop arteriovenous fistula on the thigh. *Int Urol Nephrol* 13:287–290, 1981.
174. Iuchtman M, Jacob ET, Boner G, et al: Terminal uremia and arteriovenous fistula patency. *Int Surg* 66:241–242, 1981.
175. Doyle DL, Fry PD: Polytetrafluoroethylene and bovine grafts for vascular access in patients on long-term hemodialysis. *Can J Surg* 25:379–382, 1982.

176. Dardik H, Ibrahim IM, Sussman MK, et al: Arteriovenous fistulas: Preliminary clinical experience employing glutaraldehyde-tanned human umbilical cord vein. *ASAIO* 4:64–69, 1981.
177. Zimmerman CE: Bedside manipulation of the clotted arteriovenous fistula. *Dial Transplant* 10:837, 1981.
178. Hart A, Oh HK: Clinical significance of intraoperative flow measurement during bovine heterograft AV fistulae formation. *Trans Am Soc Artif Intern Organs* 27:623–624, 1981.
179. Timis AD, McGonigle RJ, Weston MJ, et al: The influence of hemodialysis fistulas on circulatory dynamics and left ventricular function. *Int J Artif Organs* 5:101–104, 1982.
180. Cooper MW, Stanbaugh GH, Walling SB, et al: Effects of occlusion of fistulae on left ventricular dimensions in hemodialysis patients. *Trans Am Soc Artif Intern Organs* 27:625–628, 1981.
181. Ebeid A, Saranchak HJ; Banding of a PTFE hemodialysis fistula in the treatment of steal syndrome. *Clin Exp Dial Apheresis* 5:251–257, 1981.
182. Sommer I, Knobel B, Robson M, et al: Intractable anginal syndrome and left heart failure due to an arteriovenous dialysis fistula. *Contemporary Dialysis* 3:52–53, 1982.
183. Glanz S, Bashist B, Gordon DH, et al: Angiography of upper extremity access fistulas for dialysis. *Radiology* 143:45–52, 1982.
184. Konner K, Karnahl HM: Transvenous serial xero-arteriography: A new non-invasive angiographic method for AV fistulas in haemodialysis patients. *Proc Eur Dial Transplant Assoc* 18:305–309, 1981.
185. Collins AJ, Shapiro FL, Keshaviah P, et al: Blood access without skin puncture. *Trans Am Soc Artif Intern Organs* 27:308–312, 1981.
186. Nissenson AR, Raible D, Higgins RE, et al: No-needle dialysis: Experience with the new carbon transcutaneous hemodialysis access device. *Clin Nephrol* 15:302–308, 1981.
187. Dorner DB, Stubbs DH, Shadur CA, et al: Percutaneous subclavian vein catheter hemodialysis—Impact on vascular access surgery. *Surgery* 91:712–715, 1982.
188. Smith SB, Wombolt DG, Hurwitz RL, et al: Experience with subclavian vein for vascular access. *Clin Exp Dial Apheresis* 5:293–297, 1981.
189. Connolly TP, Balsys AJ, King EG: Caval catheter haemodialysis. *Intensive Care Med* 6:129–132, 1980.
190. Nidus BD, Neusy AJ: Chronic hemodialysis by repeated femoral vein cannulation. *Nephron* 29:195–197, 1981.
191. Raja RM, Kramer MS, Fernandes M, et al: Subclavian vein and femoral vein chatheterization for hemodialysis—One year comparison. *Trans Am Soc Artif Intern Organs* 28:58–60, 1982.
192. Uldall PR, Joy C, Merchant N: Further experience with a double-lumen subclavian cannula for hemodialysis. *Trans Am Soc Artif Intern Organs* 28:71–75, 1982.
193. Vaz AJ: Compartmental syndrome following subclavian vein hemodialysis. *Clin Exp Dial Apheresis* 6:15–24, 1982.
194. Fine A, Churchill D, Gault H, et al: Fatality due to subclavian dialysis catheter. *Nephron* 29:99–100, 1981.
195. Bambauer R, Jutzler GA: Use of large-bore catheters in the internal jugular vein as an access for acute hemodialysis. *Klin Wochenschr* 60:285–292, 1982.
196. Hensel A, Pauls A, von Herrath D, et al: Successful hemodialysis for acute renal failure in late pregnancy. *Am J Nephrol* 2:98–100, 1982.
197. Chugh KS, Kumar B, Pareek SK, et al: Hemodialysis therapy for psoriasis. *Artif Organs* 6:9–12, 1982.
198. Nissenson AR, Rapaport M, Gordon A, et al: Hemodialysis in the treatment of psoriasis. A controlled study. *Ann Intern Med* 91:76–86, 1979.

199. Hanicki Z, Chichocki T, Klein A, et al: Dialysis for psoriasis—Preliminary remarks concerning mode of action. *Arch Dermatol Res* 271:401–405, 1981.
200. Steck WD, Nakamoto S, Bailin PL, et al: Hemofiltration treatment of psoriasis. *J Am Acad Dermatol* 6:346–349, 1982.
201. Hoek FJ, Grijm R, Sanders GT, et al: Removal of bile acids from the blood by hemodialysis with a polyacrylonitril membrane: Treatment of pruritus of cholestatic disease. *Digestion* 23:135–140, 1982.
202. Splendiani G, Bruno V, D'Alessandro V, et al: Dialysis treatment in schizophrenia: Two years experience. *Artif Organs* 5:175–177, 1981.
203. Gillin JC, Schulz SC, Van Kammen DP, et al: EEG sleep patterns in schizophrenic patients undergoing hemodialysis. *Psychol Res* 5:287–291, 1981.
204. Seidel M, Ernst K, Lindenau K, et al: Treatment trials with hemofiltration/hemodialysis in pernicious catatonia. *Psychiatr Neurol Med Psychol* 34:95–99, 1982.
205. Hombrouckx R, Nefrologie D, Hogerlucht K, et al: Hemodialysis as a treatment for chronic schizophrenia. *Dial Transplant* 11:585–588, 1982.
206. Ilfeld D, Weil S, Kuperman O: Correction of a suppressor cell deficiency and amelioration of familial Mediterranean fever by hemodialysis. *Arthritis Rheum* 25:38–41, 1982.
207. Davison AM, Roberts TG, Mascie-Taylor BH, et al: Haemofiltration for profound dialysis-induced hypotension: removal of sodium and water without blood-pressure change. *Br Med J* 285:87–89, 1982.
208. Chaignon M, Aubert P, Martin MF, et al: Hemodynamic effects of hemodialysis and hemofiltration. *Artif Organs* 6:27–30, 1982.
209. Quellhorst E, Schuenemann B, Hildebrand U: How to prevent vascular instability: Haemofiltration. *Proc Eur Dial Trans Assoc* 18:243–249, 1981.
210. Pierides AM, Schniepp B, Johnson WJ: Two year experience with over 500 sessions of postdilution hemofiltration. *Trans Am Soc Artif Intern Organs* 27:618–624, 1981.
211. Shaldon S, Beau MC, Deschodt G, et al: Mixed hemofiltration (MHF): 18 months experience with ultrashort treatment time. *Trans Am Soc Artif Intern Organs* 27:610–612, 1981.
212. Dongradi G, Haas T, Villeboeuf F, et al: High efficiency haemofiltration (ultrafilration of more than 250 ml/min for two hours) in eight uraemic patients. *Proc Eur Dial Trans Assoc* 18:176–182, 1981.
213. Jeffree MA, Peacock J, Sobey IJ, et al: Gel layer limited haemofiltration rates can be increased by vortex mixing. *Clin Exp Dial Apheresis* 5:373–380, 1981.
214. Geronemus R, Bosch JP, Thornton J, et al: Studies of carbohydrate metabolism after hemodialysis and hemofiltration in uremic patients. *Arch Intern Med* 142:707–710, 1982.
215. Kramer P, Schrader J, Bohnsack W, et al: Continuous arteriovenous haemofiltration. A new kidney replacement therapy. *Proc Eur Dial Trans Assoc* 18:743–749, 1981.
216. Kramer P, Bohler J, Kehr A, et al: Intensive care potential of continuous arteriovenous hemofiltration. *Trans Am Soc Artif Intern Organs* 28:28–32, 1982.
217. Olbricht C, Mueller C, Schurek HJ, et al: Treatment of acute renal failure in patients with multiple organ failure by continuous spontaneous hemofiltration. *Trans Am Soc Artif Intern Organs* 28:33–36, 1982.
218. Paganini EP, Flaque J, Whitman G, et al: Amino acid balance in patients with oliguric acute renal failure undergoing slow continuous ultrafiltration. *Trans Am Soc Artif Intern Organs* 28:615–619, 1982.
219. De-Nour AK: Social adjustment of chronic dialysis patients. *Am J Psychiatr* 139:97–100, 1982.

220. Kutner NG, Cardenas DD: Rehabilitation status of chronic renal disease patients undergoing dialysis: Variations by age category. *Arch Phys Med Rehabil* 62:626–630, 1981.
221. Livesley WJ: Factors associated with psychiatric symptoms in patients undergoing chronic hemodialysis. *Can J Psychiatr* 26:562–566, 1981.
222. Blodgett C: A selected review of the literature of adjustment to hemodialysis. *Int J Psychiatr* 11:97–124, 1981.
223. Zetin M, Plummer MJ, Vaziri ND, et al: Locus of control and adjustment to chronic hemodialysis. *Clin Exp Dial Apheresis* 5:319–334, 1981.
224. Lowry MR, Atcherson E: A short-term follow-up of patients with depressive disorder on entry into home dialysis training. *J Affective Disord* 2:219–227, 1980.
225. Richmond JM, Lindsay RM, Burton HJ, et al: Psychological and physiological factors predicting the outcome on home hemodialysis. *Clin Nephrol* 17:109–113, 1982.
226. Friedlander RJ Jr, Viederman M: Children of dialysis patients. *Am J Psychiatr* 139:100–103, 1982.
227. Gutman RA, Stead WW, Robinson RR: Physical activity and employment status of patients on maintenance dialysis. *N Engl J Med* 304:309–313, 1981.
228. Johnson JP, McCauley CR, Copley JB: The quality of life of hemodialysis and transplant patients. *Kidney Int* 22:286–291, 1982.
229. Weller JM, Port FK, Swartz RD, et al: Analysis of survival of end-stage renal disease patients. *Kidney Int* 21:78–83, 1982.
230. Hutchinson TA, Thomas DC, MacGibbon B: Predicting survival in adults with end-stage renal disease: An age equivalence index. *Ann Intern Med* 96:417–423, 1982.
231. Cummings KM, Becker MH, Kirscht JP, et al: Intervention strategies to improve compliance with medical regimens by ambulatory hemodialysis patients. *J Behav Med* 4:111–127, 1981.
232. Steinglass P, Gonzalez S, Dosovitz I, et al: Discussion groups for chronic hemodialysis patients and their families. *Gen Hosp Psychiatry* 4:7–14, 1982.
233. Campbell DR, Sinha BK: Brief group psychotherapy with chronic hemodialysis patients. *Am J Psychiatr* 137:1234–1237, 1980.
234. Tucker CM, Mulkerne DJ, Ziller RC: An ecological and behavioral approach to outpatient dialysis treatment. *J Chronic Dis* 35:21–27, 1982.
235. Bertoli M, Battistella PA, Vergani L, et al: Carnitine deficiency induced during hemodialysis and hyperlipidemia: Effect of replacement therapy. *Am J Clin Nutr* 34:1496–1500, 1981.
236. Suzuki Y, Narita M, Yamazaki N: Effects of L-carnitine on arrhythmias during hemodialysis. *Jpn Heart J* 23:349–359, 1982.
237. Casciani CU, Caruso U, Cravotto E, et al: L-carnitine in haemodialysed patients. Changes in lipid pattern. *Arzneimittelforsch* 32:293–297, 1982.
238. Chan MK, Persaud JW, Varghese Z, et al: Response patterns to DL-carnitine in patients on maintenance haemodialysis. *Nephron* 30:240–243, 1982.
239. Chang TM: Hemoperfusion in 1981. *Contrib Nephrol* 29:11–22, 1982.
240. Stefoni S, Feliciangeli G, Coli L, et al: Use of combined hemodialysis/hemoperfusion in chronic uremia. *Contrib Nephrol* 29:123–132, 1982.
241. Bonomini V, Stefoni S, Casciani CU, et al: Multicentric experience with combined hemodialysis/hemoperfusion in chronic uremia. *Contrib Nephrol* 19:133–142, 1982.
242. Winchester JF, Gelford MC, Knepshield JH, et al: Dialysis and hemoperfusion of poisons and drugs. *Trans Am Soc Artif Intern Organs* 23:762–842, 1977.
243. Winchester JF, Gelfand MC, Helliwell M, et al: Extracorporeal treatment of salicylate or acetaminophen poisoning—Is there a role? *Arch Intern Med* 141:370–374, 1981.

244. Helliwell M, Essex E: Hemoperfusion in "late" paracetamol poisoning. *Clin Toxicol* 18:1225–1233, 1981.
245. Raper S, Crome P, Vale A, et al: Experience with activated carbon-bead haemoperfusion columns in the treatment of severe drug intoxication. A preliminary report. *Arch Toxicol* 49:303–310, 1982.
246. Temple AR: Acute and chronic effects of aspirin toxicity and their treatment. *Arch Intern Med* 141:364–369, 1981.
247. Berlinger WG, Spector R, Flanigan MJ, et al: Hemoperfusion for phenylbutazone poisoning. Ann Intern Med 96:334–335, 1982.
248. Okonek S: Intoxication with pyrazolones. *Br J Clin Pharmacol* 10:385S–390S, 1980.
249. De Broe ME, Verpooten GA, Christiaens MA, et al: Clinical experience with prolonged combined hemoperfusion-hemodialysis treatment of severe poisoning. *Artif Organs* 5:59–66, 1981.
250. Baggish D, Gray S, Jatlow P, et al: Treatment of methaqualone overdose with resin hemoperfusion. *Yale J Biol Med* 54:147–150, 1981.
251. Darnell A, Garcia M, Bergada E, et al: Long-term hemodialysis in acute barbituate intoxication. *Med Clin* 75:49–53, 1980.
252. de Wolff FA, Smit ND: Analysis of haemoperfusion columns for evaluation of treatment of phenobarbital overdosage. *Arch Toxicol* 43:233–235, 1980.
253. Benowitz N, Abolin C, Tozer T, et al: Resin hemoperfusion in ethychlorvynol overdose. *Clin Pharmacol Ther* 27:236–242, 1980.
254. Zmuda MJ: Resin hemoperfusion in dogs intoxicated with ethychlorvynol. *Kidney Int* 17:303–311, 1980.
255. Hoy WE, Rivero A, Marin MG, et al: Resin hemoperfusion for treatment of a massive meprobamate overdose. *Ann Intern Med* 93:455–456, 1980.
256. Freund LG: Severe meprobamate intoxication treated by hemoperfusion over amberlite resin. *Artif Organs* 5:80–81, 1981.
257. Pontal PG, Bismuth C, Baud F, et al: Respective roles of gastric lavage, haemodialysis, haemoperfusion, diuresis and hepatic metabolism in the elimination of a massive meprobamate overdose. *Nouv Presse Med* 11:1557–1558, 1982.
258. Chan KM, Aguanno JJ, Jansen R, et al: Charcoal hemoperfusion for treatment of carbamazepine poisoning. *Clin Chem* 17:1300–1302, 1981.
259. Montoya-Cabrera MA, Sanchez-Suarez BA, Hernandez-Zamora A, et al: Treatment of acute carbamazepine intoxication according to its pharmacological properties. Preliminary report. *Arch Invest Med* 11:417–424, 1980.
260. Crome P, Hampel G, Widdop B, et al: Experience with cellulose acetate-coated activated charcoal haemoperfusion in the treatment of severe hypnotic drug intoxication. *Postgrad Med J* 56:763–766, 1980.
261. Balogh A, Stein G, Pekkarinen A: Dialysability of benzodiazepines by haemodialysis and controlled sequential ultrafiltration (CSU) in vitro. *Acta Pharmacol Toxicol* 49:174–180, 1981.
262. Mateer Jr, Clark MR: Lithium toxicity with rarely reported ECG manifestations. *Ann Emerg Med* 11:208–211, 1982.
263. Baehler RW, Work J, Smith W, et al: Charcoal hemoperfusion in the therapy for methsuximide and phenytoin overdose. *Arch Intern Med* 140:1466–1468, 1980.
264. Czajka PA, Anderson WH, Christoph RA, et al: A pharmacokinetic evaluation of peritoneal dialysis for phenytoin intoxication. *J Clin Pharmacol* 20:565–569, 1980.
265. Heath A, Delin K, Eden E, et al: Hemoperfusion with Amberlite resin in the treatment of self-poisoning. *Acta Med Scand* 207:455–460, 1980.

266. Hofmann V, Riess W, Descoeudres C, et al: The problem of hemoperfusion in poisonings: Ineffectiveness in maprotiline poisoning. *Schweiz Med Wochenschr* 110:291–294, 1980.
267. Sabto JK, Pierce RM, West RJ, et al: Hemodialysis, peritoneal dialysis, plasmapheresis and forced diuresis for the treatment of quinine overdose. *Clin Nephrol* 16:264–268, 1981.
268. Chang TM, Espinosa-Melendez E, Francoeur TE, et al: Albumin-collodion activated charcoal hemoperfusion in the treatment of severe theophylline intoxication in a 3-year-old patient. *Pediatrics* 65:811–814, 1980.
269. Brown GS, Lohr TO, Mayor GH, et al: Peritoneal clearance of theophylline. *Am J Kidney Dis* 1:24–26, 1981.
270. Clerckx-Braun F, Kadima N, Lesne M, et al: Digoxin acute intoxication: Evaluation of the efficiency of charcoal hemoperfusion. *Clin Toxicol* 15:437–446, 1979.
271. Silberschmidt U: Disopyramide poisoning. *Schweiz Med Wochenschr* 111:681–683, 1981.
272. Gosselin B, Mathieu D, Chopin C, et al: Acute intoxication with diisopyramide: Clinical and experimental study by hemoperfusion an Amberlite XAD 4 resin. *Clin Toxicol* 17:439–449, 1980.
273. Holt DW, Helliwell M, O'Keeffe B, et al: Successful management of serious disopyramide poisoning. *Postgrad Med J* 56:256–260, 1980.
274. Green FJ, Lavelle KJ, Aronoff GR, et al: Management of amikacin overdose. *Am J Kidney Dis* 1:110–112, 1981.
275. Langer M, Vesconi S, Iapichino G, et al: The early removal of amatoxins in the treatment of amanita phalloides poisoning. *Klin Wochenschr* 58:117–123, 1980.
276. Borges HF, Hocks J, Kjellstrand CM: Mannitol intoxication in patients with renal failure. *Arch Intern Med* 142:63–66, 1982.
277. Vaziri ND, Upham T, Barton CH: Hemodialysis clearance of arsenic. *Clin Toxicol* 17:451–456, 1980.
278. Smith SB, Wombolt DG, Venkatesan R: Results of hemodialysis and hemoperfusion in the treatment of acute arsenic ingestion. *Clin Exp Dial Apheresis* 5:399–404, 1981.
279. Keller F, Koeppel C, von Keyserling HJ, et al: Hemoperfusion for organic mercury detoxication? *Klin Wochenschr* 59:865–866, 1981.
280. Bakir F, Rustam J, Tikriti S, et al: Clinical and epidemiological aspects of methylmercury poisoning. *Postgrad Med J* 56:1–10, 1980.
281. Margel S: A novel approach for heavy metal poisoning treatment, a model. Mercury poisoning by means of chelating microspheres: Hemoperfusion and oral administration. *J Med Chem* 24:1263–1266, 1981.
282. Margel S, Hirsh J: Hemoperfusion for detoxification of mercury. A model: Treatment of severe mercury poisoning by encapsulated chelating spheres, Part I. *Biomater Med Devices Artif Organs* 9:107–125, 1981.
283. Koshy KM, Lovejoy FJ Jr: Thallium ingestion with survival: Ineffectiveness of peritoneal dialysis and potassium chloride diuresis. *Clin Toxicol* 18:521–525, 1981.
284. Verpooten GA, DeBroe ME: Prediction of the efficacy of hemoperfusion and hemodialysis in severe poisoning. *Arch Toxicol* 5:304–306, 1982.
285. Adaudi AO, Oehme FW: An activated charcoal hemoperfusion system for the treatment of barbital or ethylene glycol poisoning in dogs. *Clin Toxicol* 18:1105–1115, 1981.
286. Gordon HL, Hunter JM: Ethylene glycol poisoning. A case report. *Anaesthesia* 37:332–338, 1982.
287. Peterson CD, Collins AJ, Himes JM, et al: Ethylene glycol poisoning: Pharmacokinetics during therapy with ethanol and hemodialysis. *N Engl J Med* 304:21–23, 1981.

288. Pappas SC, Silverman M: Treatment of methanol poisoning with ethanol and hemodialysis. *Can Med Assoc J* 126:1291–1294, 1982.
289. Frommer JP, Ayus JC: Acute ethylene glycol intoxication. *Am J Nephrol* 2:1–5, 1982.
290. Masini E, Blandina P, Mannaioni PF: Removal of alpha-amanitin from blood by hemoperfusion over uncoated charcoal. Experimental results. *Contrib Nephrol* 29:76–81, 1982.
291. Tabei K, Asano Y, Hosoda S: Efficacy of charcoal hemoperfusion in paraquat poisoning. *Artif Organs* 6:37–42, 1982.
292. Okonek S, Baldamus CA, Hofmann A: Survival despite potentially fatal plasma paraquat concentrations. *Lancet* 2:589, 1980.
293. Lohmann J, Pott G, Zidek W, et al: Plasma fibronectin in man after a severe paraquat intoxication. *Arch Toxicol* 5:295–297, 1982.
294. Guzelian PS: Therapeutic approaches for chlordecone poisoning in humans. *J Toxicol Environ Health* 8:757–766, 1981.
295. Mascie-Taylor BH, Widdop B, Davidson AM, et al: Camphor intoxication treated by charcoal haemoperfusion. *Postgrad Med J* 57:725–726, 1981.
296. Koppel C, Tenczer J, Tonnesmann U, et al: Acute poisoning with pine oil—Metabolism of monoterpenes. *Arch Toxicol* 49:73–81, 1981.
297. Okonek S: Hemoperfusion in toxicology. Basic considerations of its effectiveness. *Clin Toxicol* 18:1185–1198, 1981.
298. Haapanen EJ, Pellinen TJ: Hemoperfusion in quinidine intoxication. *Acta Med Scand* 210:515–516, 1981.
299. Smith SB, Wombolt DG, Venkatesan R: Results of hemodialysis and hemoperfusion in the treatment of acute arsenic ingestion. *Clin Exp Dial Apheresis* 5:366–404, 1981.
300. Pappas SC, Silverman M: Treatment of methanol poisoning with ethanol and hemodialysis. *Can Med Assoc J* 126:1391–1394, 1982.
301. Kann V, Burgermeister W, Wawschinek O: Standardized forced diuresis and peritoneal dialysis in the therapy of organophosphorous poisoning. *Wien Med Wochenschr* 129:667–669, 1979.

CHAPTER 3

Clinical Transplantation

William J. Flanigan
Gerhard Opelz

Over 50,000 kidney transplants have been done since the first identical twin transplant in 1954 (1). The first successful allografts in the late 1950s heralded a decade of improved graft survival during the 1960s, although patient mortality remained unacceptably high. The expectation in the 1970s of continued improvement in graft survival accompanied by a reduced mortality risk was only partially fulfilled. The latter expectation was achieved. Patients with end stage renal disease (ESRD) were able to undergo transplantation with the expectation that if the graft failed, they could return to dialysis with the reasonable prospect of a second or even a third chance for transplantation. Improved life expectancy was the result of the willingness of transplanters to abandon immunosuppression in instances of inexorable rejection and, to a lesser extent, to improved diagnosis and treatment of infection. However, continued improvement in graft survival remained disappointingly elusive. Nonspecific basic immunosuppression and management of rejection crisis remained fundamentally unchanged until recently; new approaches to the problem were being undertaken but for the most part remained unproven.

During the past 2 years there has been a small but unequivocal improvement in graft survival without sacrificing patient survival. The recognition that multiple blood transfusions afford definite protection against rejection, by mechanisms that are poorly understood, accounts for a significant portion of this improvement. Our previous philosophy of avoiding transfusions in the belief that the immunologic virgin represented the optimum recipient has been reversed. In addition, long-awaited documentation has shown that treatment with antilymphocyte or antithymocyte globulin (ALG, ATG) is effective in delaying early graft rejection and in treating primary rejection crisis.

Considering the fact that transfusion of blood products and administration of ALG have long been known to be highly effective means prolonging graft survival in experimental animals, it is surprising that proof of their clinical applicability in humans has been difficult and so long in coming. The multiplicity of factors, acting either independently or in concert, involved in human transplantation produce an infinite number of variables and subsets within a heterogeneous patient population. These include the presence of cytotoxic antibodies, age, race, sex, blood transfusions, parity, ABO blood type, HLA mismatch, splenectomy, and the primary disease which led to renal failure. When these factors are considered, it becomes less puzzling that maneuvers of proven and reproducible benefit in the laboratory are difficult to document in human transplantation.

RECURRENCE OF DISEASE

One effect of improved early (1–2 year) graft survival has been the increasing concern regarding late deterioration of renal allograft function. Milgran (2) reviewed this problem, emphasizing the role of de novo immunologic processes, including graft rejection, and/or the role of recurrence of the original disease. Evidence that the original "immunologic" disease may recur in the transplanted kidney was highlighted many years ago by Glassock and associates (3,4), who reviewed the outcome of identical twin transplants. These patients were not receiving immunosuppressives and their grafts were not at risk of rejection. There were 18 patients whose primary clinical diagnosis had been unclassified glomerulonephritis. Eleven patients developed clinical signs of a similar disease following placement of the isograft. Kidney biopsy showed deposition of IgG and complement in the glomerular basement membrane, resulting in the loss of seven grafts. At least four broad pathways contribute to late decline in allograft function (5,6):

1. Recurrence of the original glomerular disease in the graft
2. De novo glomerulonephritis unrelated to the nephritogenic process
3. Glomerular changes resulting from rejection processes (transplant glomerulopathy)
4. Glomerular disease present in the donor at the time of transplantation

Evidence that late-occurring glomerular injury is not always the result of recurrent disease is evidenced by the development of allograft lesions characteristic of chronic rejection in patients whose primary illness was nonimmunologic (7,8).

Twenty years ago, Hamburger and associates (9) described "rejection glomerulonephritis," an observation subsequently confirmed by others (10,11). When minimal lesions visible only on electron microscopy are included, no less than 50% of transplanted patients show this kind of glomerular alteration. The commonest immunofluorescent picture is one of deposits of IgM, IgG and C3 within the glomerular basement membrane. Mesangial cell proliferation (often focal) and thickening of the basement membrane are observed on light microscopy. Clinical manifestations are proteinuria, often in the nephrotic range, and microscopic hematuria. Although some patients have progressive deterioration in renal function, others maintain normal renal function for many years following the appearance of "transplant glomerulopathy" (7). The reason that some patients have progressive disease whereas others have a benign clinical course is unknown.

The frequency at which recurrent disease affects the transplanted kidney is difficult to estimate because the kidney's histologic response to any given insult is limited. Obviously, transplantation should not be undertaken in the presence of a known nephritogenic state such as active systemic lupus erythematosus (SLE) or the presence of circulating anti-glomerular basement membrane (GBM) antibodies. Why some patients develop recurrence of their original disease after transplantation, whereas others with what appears to be the identical illness are spared, remains a mystery. It has been argued that the diagnosis of recurrent disease must entail a clinical course and histologic lesion that parallel or mimic those of the original pathologic process. In an excellent review of the issue of recurrent disease, Morzycke and colleagues (6) pointed out that differences in patient outcome with any given renal lesion could be the result of interaction of multiple factors: (*1*) immunosuppression could change the host's immune response and thereby alter both the clinical course and histologic lesion; (*2*) rejection episodes may modify or shorten the life of the graft such that there is insufficient exposure of the kidney to the host environment to permit the native disease to be expressed; (*3*) the nephritogenic stimulus characteristically waxes and wanes during the natural course of the disease; and (*4*) certain phenotypic traits of the host may be present in the transplanted kidney rendering it more susceptible to the humoral pathogen(s). The data presented and cited by these authors indicate a higher incidence of recurrent glomerulonephritis in related donor kidneys as compared to cadaver grafts. These findings would be in accord with the high incidence of recurrent disease in isografts, as cited previously. They also support the findings reported by Noel and associates (13) that in patients with IgA nephropathy (Berger's disease), the risk of recurrent disease after transplantation was significantly higher when the donor was a related HLA identical or haploidentical than when a cadaver graft was used. In this disease, HLA BW35 was significantly increased compared to a control population of patients with glomerulonephritis of other types.

Table 1. Recurrence of Original Disease in Renal Transplants

Disease	Estimated Clinical Recurrence (%)	Reference
Membranoproliferative glomerulonephritis		
Type I	33	15–22
Type II (dense deposit)	75	15–22
Focal glomerulosclerosis	50	23–31
Berger's nephropathy	50	6, 32
Henoch-Schönlein	30	33–35
Idiopathic membranous nephropathy	50	14, 36–40
Hemolytic uremia syndrome	15	41
Scleroderma	15	43–46
Goodpasture's syndrome	rare[a]	47–52
Rapidly progressive nephritis	infrequent	53–55
Amyloidosis	30	58–59

[a] Recurrence rate low after anti-GBM antibodies have disappeared.

The authors suggest that the gene coding for a high frequency of BW35 antigen is not itself involved, but, rather, that a gene in linkage disequilibrium with the B locus gene inside the major histocompatibility complex is involved. The data suggest that the target (mesangial cells) must bear the same specific determinant as that of the recipient's native kidney.

The underlying theme of this discussion is that improved short-term graft survival now permits us to address the general issue of long-term allograft function to define the incidence of recurrence in subsets of glomerulonephritis. The outcome of renal transplant in specific sets of circumstances in the recipient and/or donor is perhaps relevant to the variability in the frequency with which recurrent disease is reported. The clinical characteristics of the major acquired glomerulopathies in which recurrent disease has occurred in the engrafted organ are reviewed. The references cited are not all-inclusive and, in some instances, the diagnostic criteria employed do not fulfill those enumerated above. The estimated frequency of the recurrence of the disease present in the recipient's native kidneys varies considerably. An attempt to summarize the frequency of recurrent disease is presented in Table 1. This is a general estimate based on our review of selected literature. No attempt has been made to separate recipients whose transplant histology demonstrated "pure" recurrent disease from those showing combinations of recurrence, rejection, and transplant glomerulopathy. We have not attempted to correlate duration, age at onset, clinical course, or presence of serologic markers of activity except in instances where it appears likely that these factors are of diagnostic or prognostic significance.

Membranoproliferative Glomerulonephritis

Membranoproliferative glomerulonephritis (MPGN) is the leading immunologic cause of renal failure in children and a less common (although not infrequent) cause of ESRD in adults. MPGN is divided into two subgroups based primarily on morphologic characteristics seen on electron microscopy. Type I is characterized by subendothelial deposits of electron-dense complexes. Type II (dense-deposit disease) is recognized by characteristic ribbonlike deposits within the basement membrane. Despite the similar clinical presentation of nephrosis and hypocomplementemia, the two subgroups appear to be etiologically unrelated. Hypocomplementemia occurs in type I by way of activation of the classic pathway (CIQ, C4). In type II, complement is activated by the alternative (properdin) pathway and is associated with a serum factor capable of cleaving native C3 (nephritic factor). Both types are resistant to therapy. Their clinical courses are marked by deteriorating renal function and ultimate renal failure. Successful renal transplantation has been accomplished in both groups, but recurrent disease is frequent (6,11,14–20). Fortunately, graft loss has been distinctly unusual. The clinical course of patients experiencing recurrent MPGN has generally been indolent. In most reported cases, patients maintained stable renal function for prolonged periods. Interestingly, regression of a documented lesion is occasionally observed (39). The role of immunosuppression in altering the natural history of this (or these) entities is uncertain. Most researchers believe that serum C3 levels tend to return to normal following transplantation and tend to decrease in association with recurrent disease (15,20,22). However, their predictive diagnostic and therapeutic values are low. The consensus is that even though recurrent disease is frequent, renal transplantation is not contraindicated for either type of MPGN.

Focal Glomerulosclerosis

Focal sclerosing glomerulonephritis (FSGN) presents with manifestations of nephrotic syndrome frequently accompanied by hematuria and hypertension. The clinical course in the majority of patients is characterized by rapidly deteriorating renal function. Recurrence of this morphologic entity after transplantation has been reported to occur in the majority of patients (6,23–31). The pattern of recurrence is variable; heavy proteinuria may develop within days or weeks or be delayed for several years (23,25,26). Recurrence coinciding with acute allograft rejection has also been reported (26). The presence or absence of mesangial proliferation provides a valuable clue regarding the likelihood of recurrence. Maizel and colleagues (28) reported 28 recipients whose original disease was FSGN. Recurrent disease was infrequent in the absence of mesangial proliferation but occurred in as many as 50% of patients when this finding was noted on the original biopsy.

Berger's Nephropathy

Berger's syndrome (IgA nephropathy) is characterized by glomerulonephritis in the absence of systemic disease. There are mesangial deposits of immune complexes primarily composed of IgA. Progression to graft failure is distinctly uncommon. The association of this disease with HLA BW35 has previously been cited (13). The typical clinical course is recurrent or persistent painless hematuria, usually without heavy proteinuria. In the majority of patients, there is slow progressive deterioration of renal function that cannot be altered by steroid administration. A remarkable feature of this disease in patients requiring transplantation is the frequency with which it occurs in the grafted organ (6,32). Even though there is histologic evidence of recurrence in over 50% of patients, the majority of them are devoid of clinical disease.

Henoch-Schönlein Syndrome

Henoch-Schönlein syndrome is characterized by nonthrombocytopenic purpura, arthalgias, and abdominal pain. Glomerulonephritis is frequently present and is often the presenting manifestation (33,34). As in Berger's disease, the characteristic immunoflourescent finding on renal biopsy is mesangial deposition of IgA immune complexes. Most patients recover without permanent impairment in renal function, although occasionally there is progressive loss of kidney function. It is estimated that Henoch-Schönlein syndrome is the primary renal disease in approximately 15% of children beginning dialysis. Similar to Berger's syndrome, histologic evidence of recurrence is frequently present after transplantation, but graft loss from recurrence is uncommon. The relationship between isolated IgA nephropathy and Henoch-Schönlein syndrome is an intriguing one, as is the rarity of clinical disease following transplantation. Modification of IgA metabolism incidental to standard immunosuppression and genetic predisposition (i.e., HLA-related factors) could conceivably be important. The possible relationship between these diseases has been reviewed by Weiss and colleagues (35).

Idiopathic Membranous Nephropathy

Idiopathic membranous nephropathy is an immune complex disease characterized by nephrotic syndrome and renal biopsy evidence of subepithelial electron-dense deposits and by a slowly progressing course ultimately leading to renal failure. It is the most common cause of nephrotic syndrome in adults. Its recurrence following transplantation has been thought to be infrequent. However, recent reports indicate that membranous nephropathy is more common in the graft than previously believed. It has been observed as both "recurrent" disease (6,36–38) and in "de novo" nephropathy in patients whose native kidneys were damaged by a different (not immune complex) disease mechanism (39,40). Fortunately, graft loss occurs infrequently (14,37). Rapid progression of the original disease to renal failure appears to indicate a high risk of recurrence after transplantation (38).

Hemolytic Uremic Syndrome

Hemolytic uremic syndrome is characterized by an acute systemic illness accompanied by microangiopathic hemolytic anemia, thrombocytopenia, and acute renal insufficiency. The majority of reports have been in children under the age of 5 years. Supportive care results in recovery in the majority, but a significant percent of patients incur permanent renal damage necessitating transplantation. Like membranous nephropathy, hemolytic uremic syndrome may appear after kidney transplant as "recurrent" disease or as "de novo" nephritis. In the case reported by Folman and colleagues (41), recurrent hemolytic uremic syndrome appeared to be the cause of graft failure in four sequential allografts in a patient whose own kidneys were destroyed by this disease. The etiology of this usually "self-limited" disease is unknown and there are no clinical or serologic markers to indicate which patients might be susceptible to developing recurrent episodes after kidney transplant.

Scleroderma

Progressive systemic sclerosis (scleroderma) is frequently accompanied by renal improvement. Deterioration of kidney function accompanied by severe hypertension is frequently dramatic, necessitating dialysis within weeks or months of onset. In occasional patients, renal failure can be reversed by rigid control of blood pressure even after dialysis is required (42). However, the long-term prognosis is poor because of cardiac, lung, and gastrointestinal involvement. Successful renal transplantation has been reported (43–45). Recurrence of scleroderma happens relatively frequently, often within 1 month of grafting, and usually leads to graft loss (44,46).

Goodpasture's Syndrome

Goodpasture's syndrome is defined as the triad of nephritis, intraalveolar hemorrhage, and the presence of anti-GBM antibodies within the kidney and/or serum. It may exist in a variety of clinical forms. Occasional patients have been described in whom pulmonary hemorrhage is the predominant manifestation (47,48), although coexisting renal failure is more common (49). Renal transplantation has generally been successful if the anti-GBM antibodies have disappeared from the circulation (14,50–52). In the presence of anti-GBM antibodies, histologic evidence of recurrent disease can be anticipated after transplantation, although only a minority of those patients demonstrate evidence of the clinical syndrome (52). Goodpasture's syndrome is a self-limited disease and the consensus is that patients with this syndrome should undergo transplantation only after anti-GBM antibodies have disappeared from the serum.

Rapidly Progressive Nephritis

Idiopathic rapidly progressive glomerulonephritis (crescentric glomerulonephritis) is a common cause of renal failure in adults. Its explosive onset is often heralded by hematuria and symptoms resulting from reduced renal function. The histologic hallmark is the presence of extensive epithelial crescents. In general, the prognosis is poor and appears to be correlated roughly with the percent of glomeruli involved on renal biopsy (53–55).

Crescent formation is a nonspecific response to glomerular injury resulting from a variety of etiologies. It may be seen in association with a variety of systemic illnesses of widely varying prognoses. Examples include subacute nephritis following streptococcal infection, systemic lupus erythematosus, and subacute bacterial endocarditis. When these specific etiologic entities are excluded, there remains a majority of patients in whom the etiology for crescentic or rapidly progressive nephritis cannot be defined. Approximately one-third of this subset has biopsy-demonstrated or circulating evidence of anti-GBM nephritis (Goodpasture's syndrome); in another 30% the granular pattern of immunofluorescence suggests immune complex deposition; the remaining 30% have little or no evidence of circulating antibodies or complexes. With this heterogeneous population it is impossible to ascribe a recurrence rate to rapidly progressive nephritis. Recurrent disease is said to occur in 40% of transplant patients with "non-Goodpasture's anti-GBM nephritis" (49). The frequency of recurrent disease in the remaining patients appears to be relatively small but is undetermined.

Amyloidosis

Amyloidosis is an acquired glomerular disease frequently leading to renal failure. Two types are recognized. In primary amyloidosis and amyloidosis associated with myelomas, tissues are infiltrated with immunoglobulin light chains. In amyloidoses caused by chronic inflammatory disease and familial Mediterranean fever, the infiltrates are derived from a circulating precursor protein unrelated to immunoglobulins. Renal transplantation has been done in both types (56–68) but their 1-year survival is less than that of recipients with other primary disease (59). Recurrence of amyloid deposition has been observed 8 months after transplantation in both types of amyloidosis (56,58,59). Early graft loss is uncommon but later failure must be anticipated unless the stimulus for production of these abnormal proteins can be eliminated or controlled.

IMMUNOSUPPRESSION

Conventional Therapy

The combination of azathioprine (Imuran) and steroids (prednisone or prednisolone) has been the cornerstone of maintenance immunosuppression for two decades. ALG (ATGAM or ATG) can now be added as a third preparation to conventional prophylaxis and management of rejection crisis. In general, both azathioprine and steroids are begun at the time of transplantation, azathioprine dosage being 1.5–3 mg/kg body weight. There is no question that azathioprine alone is a weak immunosuppressant that requires supplemental drugs for clinical effectiveness. Corticosteroids, usually prednisone or methylprednisolone, have occupied the prime spot as adjunctive therapy. The dosing of steroids has been variable from center to center. In the past it was customary to begin relatively large doses of steroids (1.5 mg/kg) in divided doses at the beginning of transplant and to taper them at 2-week intervals. At the end of 3 months, a daily maintenance dose of 0.15–0.2 mg/kg is achieved and continued indefinitely. It has been reported that alternate-day regimens are probably equally effective in preventing acute rejection. It is well documented that alternate-day steroid therapy reduces the complication of iatrogenic Cushing's syndrome, but whether this regimen is as effective as daily steroids for ensuring long-term graft survival remains a question. A significant increase in rejections (as high as 18%) has been reported concurrent with conversion to alternate day therapy (60,61). Naik and colleagues (62) have discontinued all steroid therapy in stable patients after azathioprine was withdrawn. Even after 2 years, there were rejection episodes in four of 10 patients. In a similar report, First and colleagues (63) gradually withdrew steroids 10–21 months after 18 HLA-identical related donor (LRD) transplants. One patient had acute rejection necessitating restarting steroid therapy. In their patients, the frequency of steroid-induced or associated complications was significantly less than in a comparable group maintained on low-dose steroids. Similarly, Steinman and associates (64) withdrew steroids in stable patients (nine LRD, six cadaver donor) while azathioprine was continued (although frequently at a reduced dose because of leukopenia associated with removal of steroid-induced leukocytosis). Two patients were failures (one LRD, one CAD), and one patient with previously normal function lost his graft because of irreversible rejection. It should be emphasized that the long-term effects of steroid withdrawal on graft function have not been ascertained in terms of immunologic damage or in the incidence of recurrent disease.

The interest in discontinuation of all steroid therapy is the result of the justified belief that the majority of posttransplant complications are directly related to chronic steroid administration (and dose) and not to azathioprine. This is clearly the case with cataract formation, aseptic necrosis, hypertension, alterations in serum cholesterol and triglycerides, and probably increased susceptibility to infection. With the exception of the last, these complications are not observed with azathioprine alone. The role of steroids in increasing oncogenesis is probably additive to that of azathioprine. The consensus of most transplant physicians is that in the majority of transplant recipients, steroid therapy is a necessary evil. Long-term steroid therapy should be given at the lowest possible dose to avoid undesirable and serious side effects.

In summary, alternate-day steroid therapy does significantly reduce complications and can be justified in selected patients providing careful monitoring of allograft function is available during the transition phase. This restriction is even more obligatory when withdrawal of all steroid maintenance is proposed.

ATG as a third drug for standard immunosuppression represents a major advance toward the goal of reducing steroid requirements. It appears likely that ATG, given as adjunctive immunosuppression with azathioprine and steroids, improves early graft survival as much as 20%. The fact that such improvement has been difficult to prove even in collaborative multicenter studies is probably a reflection of the relative effectiveness of azathioprine and high-dose steroids in preventing allograft rejection and the multiplicity of factors influencing graft outcome, which were listed earlier. Even with pooled data, the number of subsets are so high that there has simply not been sufficient data to permit meaningful statistical analysis. The work of Cosimi and colleagues (65) documents that the combination of azathioprine, prednisone, and ATG results in fewer early rejection episodes when compared to azathioprine and prednisone alone. Significantly, addition of this third immunosuppressant has resulted in no increase in host infection and there has been a definite reduction in the requirement for steroids. Graft survival was 10–13% higher in the ATG-treated group, an improvement not achieving statistical significance but one that may be clinically significant. Patient survival in both groups was identical. Similar results have been reported by others (66–68). It now appears that ATG, given in combination with azathioprine and lower doses of steroids, improves graft survival, attenuates the number and severity of early graft rejections, decreases steroid-associated complications without increasing the incidence of infection or tumor and, most importantly, does not increase patient mortality.

The treatment of acute rejection crisis has conventionally been intravenous administration of large doses of steroids given as pulsed therapy without alteration in the dose of azathioprine. Customary doses of methylprednisolone have been 10–30 mg/kg given daily or on alternate days for three to six doses. This regimen has been effective in controlling the majority but not all acute allograft rejections. There is a significant number of patients in whom rejection episodes are not amenable to steroid therapy (irreversible [69] or steroid resistant [70]). It is in this group that ATG has demonstrated the legitimacy of its claim as a third partner in immunosuppression. The consensus is that ATG given in a dose of 10–20 mg/kg intravenously for 14–21 days following the diagnosis of rejection is effective in producing more rapid reversal of rejection, fewer and/or temporally more separated second rejection episodes, better long-term graft function, and a marked reduction in steroid requirements (68,72–75). Even in patients having rejection episodes severe enough to necessitate dialysis, a poor prognostic sign when only steroid therapy is used, there is a 70% sustained reversal of rejection after ATG-therapy. Significantly, patient mortality is unchanged despite the addition of increased immunosuppression.

In summary, ATG has proved to be effective in delaying allograft rejection and in reversing rejection when it occurs. "Triple-therapy" combined with blood transfusions (either third-party or donor specific) and HLA D-locus related typing may result in such excellent graft outcome that it may become difficult to demonstrate superior results using other agents. This is particularly true when the multitude of variables and subsets of patient population are considered. The long-term outcome for graft and patient remains to be determined, but one cannot help but believe that with effective prompt control of rejection there will be fewer and/or less severe occurrences of transplant glomerulopathy and, perhaps, fewer recurrences of immunologically mediated nephritis. Prophylactic administration of this agent at the time of transplantation may add 10–15% improvement in graft outcome in recipients of both related living and cadaver donors. The additional 10–15% graft survival in patients with "steroid-resistant" rejection is indeed cause for optimism.

Before leaving the topic of "standard" immunosuppression (which admittedly is nonspecific), it is appropriate to mention the experimental evidence that indicates that under appropriate circumstances administration of ATG may induce specific immunosuppression. This subject was reviewed by Monaco in Volume 6 of *Current Nephrology* (76). To summarize, ATG as currently prescribed provides nonspecific immunosuppression and results in improved graft survival. When donor antigen is given in association with allografting, a specific unresponsiveness to the grafted organ occurs. The donor antigen used may be in the form of cell-free antigen, lymphocytes, tissue extracts, bone marrow, or platelets (77). As emphasized by Monaco, the goal of induction of specific unresponsiveness to allograft should not initially be complete elimination of all nonspecific immunosuppression. Rather, a reduction in nonspecific suppression requirements and improved graft and patient survival would be likely first steps. It is conceivable that this "first step" has serendipitously been taken by the use of ATG in treating acute rejection. The observed improved long-term graft survival and the low incidence of second rejection episodes could conceivably be the result of the donor-specific challenge (rejection) and ATG therapy. Regardless, the prospect of inducing donor specific immunity by deliberate infusion of specific antigen is a potential breakthrough. More clinical trials will undoubtedly be reported soon.

A sophisticated extension of the therapeutic effectiveness of ATG has been reported by Cosimi and co-workers (78), who employed a monoclonal hybridoma antithymocyte globulin for the treatment of acute rejection. Eight patients were treated at the onset of rejection by the intravenous infusion of 1–5 mg of a monoclonal antibody reactive with all mature peripheral lymphocytes. The dose of steroids was not increased. Reversal of rejection was noted in all instances during the 10–20 day course of therapy. Subsequent rejections occurred in five patients and resulted in the loss of two grafts. The hybridoma technique of antibody production permits production of antibodies to specific subsets of lymphocytes, which, in addition to therapy, may provide a valuable tool for in vitro monitoring of lymphocyte populations for the diagnosis of rejection and evaluation of effectiveness of immunosuppressive therapy.

Cyclosporin A

One of the most exciting developments in clinical organ transplantation has been the discovery of what appears to be the most potent immunosuppressive yet described, cyclosporin A. It is an 11-amino acid cyclic peptide derivative of fungal origin. An overall review of the pharmacology and mechanism of action of cyclosporin A has been reviewed by Morris (79). The clinical use of this agent in human renal transplantation was also reviewed in *Current Nephrology,* Volume 6 (76) and by Calne (80,81), who pioneered clinical evaluation of this drug. More than 80% of cadaveric graft survival at 1 year has been achieved using cyclosporin A as the sole immunosuppressant in an uncontrolled, nonrandomized group. Although 1-year graft survival was excellent, there were significant side effects, the most important of which were nephrotoxicity and hepatotoxicity, both of which were dose-related and reversible when therapy was reduced or discontinued. Of particular concern was the development of lymphoma in approximately 10% of these initial patients during the first 12 months of observation. Peroxidase staining of tumor tissue suggested that the lymphomas were of B-cell origin, and in each patient there was an increase in antibody titer to Ebstein-Barr virus. Side effects of lesser significance were hypertrichosis, gingival hypertrophy, and tremor, all of which decreased with lower doses of the drug. Bone marrow suppression was not observed in these original studies.

Conflicting results have been reported in which treatment by cyclosporin A has been inferior to treatment with conventional immunosuppression (82). In contrast to initial reports, bone marrow suppression was observed in the majority of patients.

Within the past year, the preliminary results of a multicenter cooperative study comparing patients treated with cyclosporin A to those treated with azathioprine and steroids has been reported (83). After follow-up from 2 weeks to 11 months, graft survival probability estimates were 73% for the cyclosporin A group as compared to 53% for the "conventional therapy" group. Renal function was similar in both groups of patients, but mortality was three times greater among the conventional therapy group. Blood transfusions and the number of HLA mismatches were the same in both groups. Seventeen percent of the cyclosporin A group were changed to conventional therapy within the first 6 months for a variety of reasons, including nephrotoxicity and excessive steroid dependence. During the period of observation, the incidence of rejection episodes was identical, 2.1 rejections per patient in the cyclosporin A group versus 2 in the controls. Rejection was treated by steroid pulses in both groups with similar results, although irreversible rejection was seen more frequently in the controls. The incidence of bacterial, viral, and fungal infection was identical. In this large series, cyclosporin A appeared convincingly more effective than conventional immunosuppression. The authors advised caution in interpretation of these preliminary results. Ferguson and colleagues from Minnesota compared cyclosporin A with standard immunosuppression in a prospective randomized trial of 100 HLA mismatched related living donor and cadaver donor transplants (84). The 1-year actuarial graft survival was 93% for patients treated with cyclosporin A and prednisone, and 81% for those treated with conventional therapy. In contrast to the European experience, the cyclosporin A treated group experienced fewer rejections and fewer infectious complications. Nephrotoxicity in the cyclosporin A group was frequent but reversible by decreasing the dose of cyclosporin A. Likewise, Starzl and co-workers have reported 42 cadaveric transplant patients, 22 of whom were undergoing transplantation for a second time, for whom cyclosporin A and steroids were used as primary immunosuppression (85). Although the follow-up period was short (2–8 months), the graft survival rate is impressive. Ninety-six percent of primary grafts were functioning at the time of the report, and 85% of second grafts were sustaining life. Preparatory steps prior to primary transplant included mandatory transfusion at least three times (6 units packed cells).

Despite a few discrepant results, the overwhelming affirmation of cyclosporin A as an important, innovative, and highly effective immunosuppressant demands careful attention. All aspects of risk-benefit must be considered. To begin with, the oncogenic potential of cyclosporin A has probably been overemphasized and appears to be dose related. Initial reports indicating a 10% incidence of lymphoma in patients treated with high doses of cyclosporin A (25 mg/kg) and conventional immunosuppression (86) have not been observed in patients in whom azathioprine was omitted and/or the dose of cyclosporin A was reduced to 17 mg/kg/day. The universally acknowledged nephrotoxicity and hepatotoxicity of cyclosporin A raise questions as to its use for "maintenance immunosuppression." Prolonged therapy with a known nephrotoxic drug must be done with caution, particularly in regard to long-term graft outcome. Many observers have reported that patients treated with cyclosporin A have higher serum creatinine values than comparable controls (84,85). The frequency with which commonplace posttransplant complications occur is still undetermined. One approach to the problem of long-term nephrotoxicity has been initial treatment with cyclosporin A followed by gradual substitution of conventional azathioprine and low-dose steroids. Klintmalm and colleagues have cautioned that this transition may induce acute rejection in a previously stable graft (87), a caution supported by the collaborative study cited above (83). The hepatotoxicity and nephrotoxicity of cyclosporin A are said to be reduced by daily determinations of blood levels of cyclosporin A and appropriate adjustment of the dose. The importance of monitoring blood levels of cyclosporin has been emphasized by Kahan and associates (88), who reported a narrow and unpredictable therapeutic window for the dose of the drug. The long-term graft expectancy in all of these initial patients remains to be determined.

In our enthusiasm over encouraging early results with this exciting new potent immunosuppressant we must avoid mistaking the journey for the destination. Considering the length of time that was required to define the role of ATG in the prevention and treatment of acute rejection, it seems likely that several years of carefully designed randomized clinical trials will be required to determine cyclosporin A's role in clinical renal transplantation. Cyclosporin A may have a place in routine immunosuppression. On the other hand, it is conceivable that cyclosporin A may best be used only for limited time periods and/or in high-risk patients (e.g., diabetics, patients undergoing retransplantation). Trials with this agent during the next few years are eagerly anticipated.

HISTOCOMPATIBILITY AND BLOOD TRANSFUSIONS

Typing and matching for HLA-DR antigens has been the major target of clinical histocompatibility research for the last 3 years. Several recent reports from individual transplant centers confirm the previous findings of a significant correlation of HLA-DR matching with graft survival in

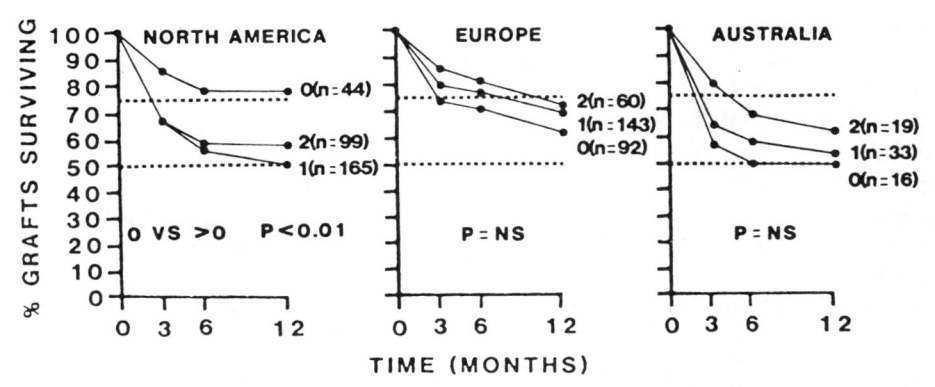

Figure 1. Effect of HLA-DR matching in full house-typed first cadaver transplants. The p value for the North American Transplants was significant by Student's t test for the comparison of 0 versus > 0 mismatches; however, by weighted regression analysis, significance was not reached. (Opelz G et al: *Transplantation* 33:87–95, 1982. Reprinted with permission.)

cadaveric renal transplantation. In light of these very favorable publications, the mildly supportive findings of the Eighth International Histocompatibility Workshop transplant study were somewhat disappointing. With the collaboration of 148 transplant centers in 19 countries, some 2000 cadaver kidney grafts were HLA typed over a period of 2 years. A correlation of HLA-DR matching with graft outcome was found in first cadaver transplants performed in North America; the data submitted by European and Australian centers did not show a correlation (89) (Fig. 1). Thus, the convincing demonstration everyone had hoped for, namely, that HLA-DR matching could be used on a broad scale to improve kidney graft survival, failed to materialize.

Because many outstanding transplant teams independently reported a favorable effect of HLA-DR matching, the results of the international multicenter study must be viewed critically. In particular, the possibility that technical difficulties may have played a significant role must be considered. The Eighth Workshop typings were done in 1980 and 1981, a time when many laboratories had just learned the HLA-DR typing technique. Preparation of sufficiently enriched B-cell targets and selection of suitable batches of rabbit complement caused difficulties at less experienced laboratories. Also, the composition of the typing reagents was of mediocre quality by current standards. Taken together, the possible sources of errors are reason to view the findings of the Eighth Workshop as partial success (after all, correlations were found in certain transplant subsets) or at least as encouragement for further research.

Indeed, the positive response to tissue typing and transplant internationally is demonstrated by the remarkable participation in a new multicenter, the "Collaborative Transplant Study." The coordinating center at the University of Heidelberg, West Germany, has received data on nearly 5000 transplants within a year since January 1982. Thus, participation is approximately four times that of the 1980 Workshop study. For a 1-year period from April 1983 to May 1984 all participants will be using the HLA reagents of the Ninth International Histocompatibility Workshop, a set that includes the best currently available typing sera. Our belief that the current effort will be successful is based primarily on improvements in HLA-DR typing technology. Through national and international workshops and cell and serum exchanges among laboratories, typing laboratories throughout the world have attained a level of expertise that probably surpasses that of the very best laboratories a few years ago. Some 6000 transplants can be expected during the 1-year period for which the Ninth Histocompatibility Workshop reagents will be available. Of course, to test the relevance of matching against the background of modern-day patient management, additional factors, such as transfusions or immunosuppression with cyclosporin A will be considered. Results will become available in 1984.

Perhaps the most stimulating new development in clinical histocompatibility research is the recent claim by Dutch investigators that recipients of HLA-DR type DRW6 are "high responders" as shown by their high kidney graft rejection rate (90) (Fig. 2). According to this claim, the failure rate is reduced if HLA-DRW6 compatible kidneys are grafted. It was suggested further that grafts in which the donor possessed HLA-DRW6 and the recipient was HLA-DRW6 negative (mismatch for DRW6) did particularly well, possibly because of an induction of suppressor cells by the HLA-DRW6 incompatibility. Thus far, the available data are limited to an analysis of patients transplanted in the Netherlands. Certainly, this potentially very important discovery deserves attention; reports on similar analyses by other investigators will be forthcoming within a few months.

Outstanding developments in blood transfusions in relation to renal transplantation were the clear confirmation of the beneficial transfusion effect in first cadaver grafts by the Eighth International Histocompatibility Workshop study (89) and the confirmatory evidence of the improvement effect of donor-specific transfusions in HLA one-haplotype matched LRD transplants, published by Salvatierra et al. (91).

In spite of the multiple variables inherent in the multicenter Workshop study, transfusions were identified as the strongest factor influencing graft success. The effect was dose dependent, although further improvement beyond five transfusions was only small (89) (Fig. 3). The strategy adopted by most transplant centers to transfuse patients a minimum of three to five times before transplantation is quite reasonable in light of these results.

Salvatierra et al. (91) provided data on a series of 132 potential recipients of LRD grafts pretreated with three consecutive donor-specific transfusions. About one-third developed lymphocytotoxic antibodies against the

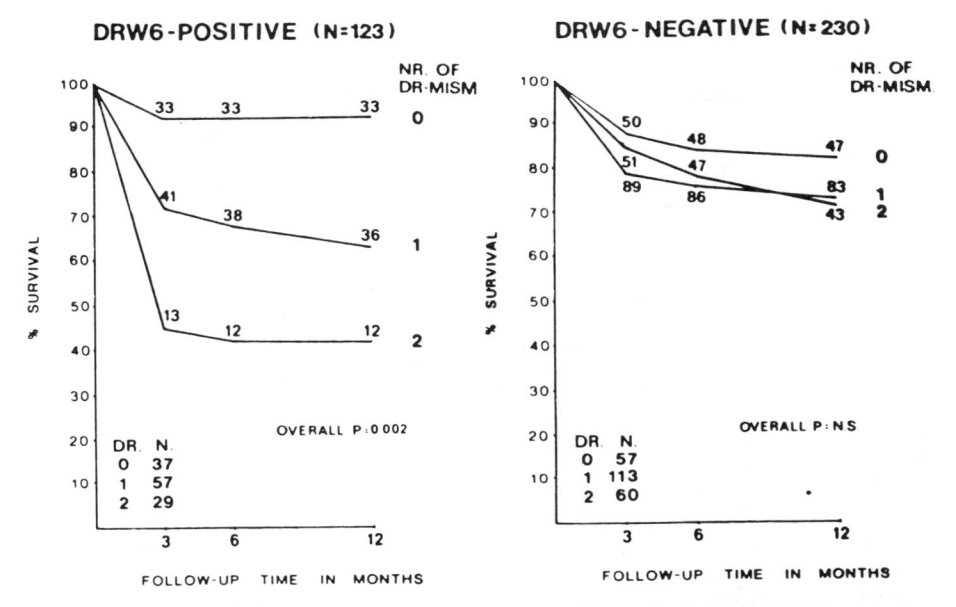

Figure 2. Actuarial survival curve of first renal allografts in 230 DRW6-negative and 123 DRW6-positive recipients in relation to the number of HLA-DR mismatches. (Hendriks GFJ et al: *Dialysis Transplantation* 12:95–96, 1983. Reprinted with permission.)

potential donor. Because of the known risk of hyperacute rejection associated with a positive crossmatch, these patients were eliminated from the LRD program. The remaining 86 patients who were transplanted following the successful completion of the donor-specific transfusion protocol (the crossmatch remained negative) had an excellent graft survival rate of 93% at 2 years, significantly better than the 53% 2-year survival rate in comparable nontransfused controls. Moreover, the clinical course of the grafts was exceptionally benign and barely distinguishable from that of HLA-identical sibling transplants (91).

Whereas the favorable effect on subsequent transplants of donor-specific transfusions appears proven beyond doubt, the high transplantation exclusion rate of about one-third of the patients because of antibody formation remains a major obstacle. Three approaches have been tried to reduce the donor-specific sensitization rate: (*1*) decreasing the immunogenicity of transfusions through the simultaneous administration of immunosuppressive drugs; (*2*) storage of blood prior to transfusion, thereby decreasing the antibody-forming potency of transfused cells, perhaps by decreasing cell viability; and (*3*) administration of random donor blood rather than donor-specific blood.

Administration of azathioprine together with donor-specific transfusions was tried successfully by Anderson et al. (92) in a small series of 24

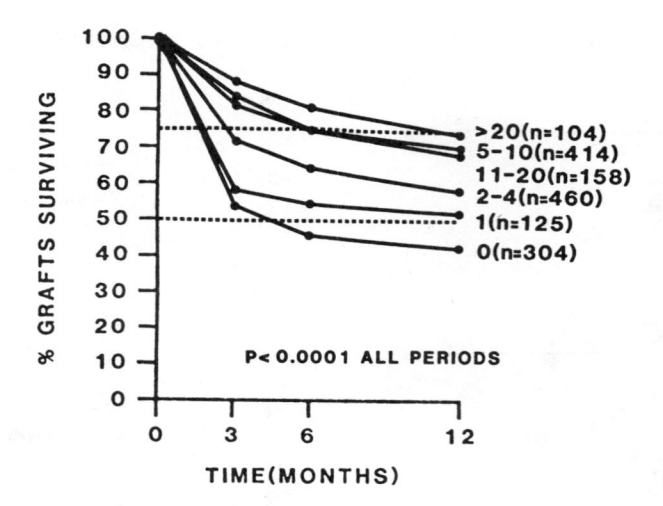

Figure 3. Actuarial graft survival rates of first cadaver donor transplants by the number of transfusions given to the recipients before transplantation. Whole blood, packed cells, washed cells, and frozen blood were combined. Numbers of units transfused are indicated at ends of curves and numbers of patients studied are given in parentheses. (Opelz G et al: *Transplantation* 33:87–95, 1982. Reprinted with permission.)

patients. A reduction in the sensitization rate to 8% was noted. This approach has been adopted by several American transplant centers and information can be expected before long whether sensitization can be reduced without losing the beneficial transfusion effect. Similarly, the administration of stored rather than fresh blood has been carried out with encouraging results in two small series (93,94). Whelchel and co-workers (93) noted a sensitization rate of 8% in a series of 40 patients. The simplest approach has received little attention; rather than donor-specific blood, random blood was administered deliberately by Swedish workers in Gothenburg (95) (Fig. 4). The success rate in 38 patients was lower than that in a series of 27 HLA-identical sibling transplants done at the same center; however, the rate was only about 5% lower than that observed by others with donor-specific transfusions. A similar improvement of HLA one-haplotype matched related donor grafts following random transfusions had been noticed in an earlier multicenter analysis (96). If experienced transplant centers can obtain success rates with random blood similar or only slightly inferior to those obtainable with donor-specific blood, the random blood protocol will be an attractive alternative because of the much lower incidence of sensitization. Only 4% of the patients transfused in Gothenburg developed lymphocytotoxic antibodies and none had to be excluded due to a positive crossmatch.

Which, if any, of the three alternate protocols eventually may replace the donor-specific transfusion schedule introduced by Salvatierra will

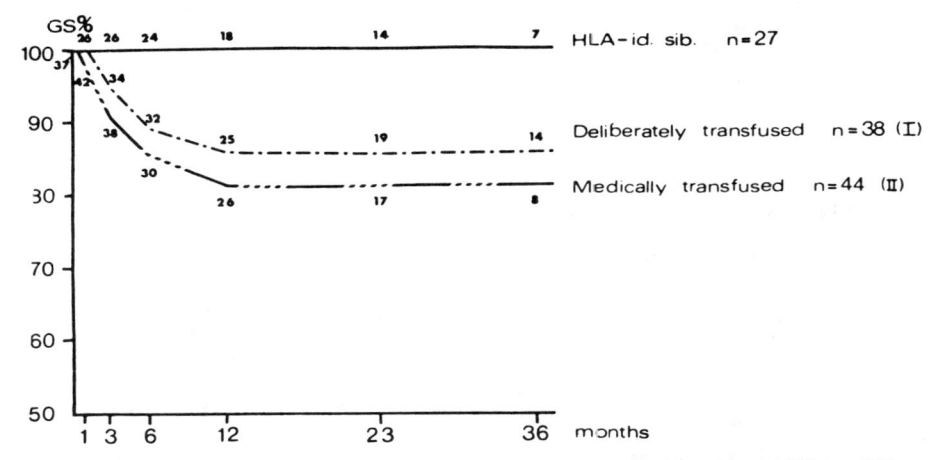

Figure 4. Actuarial graft survival rates in LD transplantations from 1977 to 1981. (Frisk B et al: *Transplantation Proc* 14:386–388, 1982. Reprinted with permission.)

depend on the outcome of studies now underway. Prospective randomized trials may be necessary to provide a conclusive answer.

The mechanism whereby transfusions improve graft survival remains elusive. Data obtained in humans and experimental animals indicate that nonimmunologic effects, such as a possible greater transfusion requirement of patients who *a priori* may have a weak immune system, cannot account for the improved transplant results. Healthy nonuremic animals transfused deliberately show the beneficial transfusion effect. The possibility that "selection of nonresponders" might be the explanation also was ruled out. According to this hypothesis, antibody producers would be sorted out because they frequently would be crossmatch positive against potential donors, and only weak responders (antibody negative patients) would receive transplants. However, prospective transfusion studies showed a sensitization rate that was much too low to support the "selection of nonresponder" hypothesis (97,98). That some selection takes place is generally acknowledged and that a small part of the transfusion effect may be a result thereof cannot be ruled out.

Today, it is widely assumed that a graft-protective immunologic mechanism is induced by transfusions. The mechanism's exact nature, however, is unknown. Current research concentrates on two main possibilities, both of which are supported by experimental data: an induction or activation of suppressor cells (99) and the formation of antireceptor (antiidiotypic) antibodies against the recipient's own immunoreactive lymphocytes (100). While both phenomena clearly can be demonstrated following the administration of transfusions, direct evidence for a connection between their occurrence and improved graft survival still is lacking. Nevertheless, the narrowing focus of investigations provides reason for optimism that the transfusion effect's mechanism will soon be understood.

REFERENCES

1. Rapaport FT: Perspectives in transplantation. *Trans Proc* 13:6–9, 1981.
2. Milgrom F: Late deterioration of renal allografts. *Trans Proc* 1068–1072, 1981.
3. Glassock RJ, Feldman D, Reynolds ES, et al: Recurrent glomerulonephritis in human renal isograft recipients: A clinical and pathologic study. *Proceedings of the First International Congress of Transplantation Society,* Paris, 1967.
4. Glassock RJ, Feldman D, Reynolds ES, et al: Human renal isografts: A clinical and pathologic analysis. *Medicine* 47:411–454, 1968.
5. McPhaul JJ Jr, Lordon RE, Thompson AL Jr: Nephritogenic immunopathologic mechanisms and human renal transplants: The problem of recurrent glomerulonephritis. *Kidney Int* 10:135–138, 1976 (editorial).
6. Morzycka M, Croker BP Jr, Siesler HF: Evaluation of recurrent glomerulonephritis in kidney allografts. *Am J Med* 72:588–598, 1982.
7. Hamburger J, Berger J, Hinglois N, et al: New insights into the pathogenesis of glomerulonephritis afforded by the study of renal allografts. *Clin Nephrol* 1:3–7, 1973.
8. Chiegh JS, Stenzel KJ, Susin M, et al: Kidney transplant nephrotic syndrome. *Am J Med* 57:730–740, 1974.
9. Hamburger J, Crosnier J, Dormont J: Observations in patients with a well-tolerated homo-transplanted kidney. *Ann NY Acad Sci* 120:558–577, 1964.
10. McPhaul JJ Jr, Lordon RE, Thompson AL Jr, et al: Nephritogenic immunopathologic mechanisms and human renal transplants: The problem of recurrent glomerulonephritis. Kidney Int 10:135–138, 1976.
11. Cameron JS, Turner DR: Recurrent glomerulonephritis in allografted kidneys. *Clin Nephrol* 7:47–54, 1977.
12. Descamps B, Noel LH, Hamburger J: The impact of transplantation on nephrology: how the child fostered the mother. *Transplant Proc* 12:800–804, 1980.
13. Noel LH, Descamps B, Jungers P, et al: HLA antigen in three types of glomerulonephritis. *Clin Immunol Immunopathol:* 10:19–23, 1978.
14. Hamburger J, Crosnier J, Noel LH: Recurrent glomerulonephritis after renal transplantation. *Ann Rev Med* 29:67–72, 1978.
15. Curtis JJ, Wyatt RJ, Bhathena D, et al: Renal transplantation for patients with type I and type II membranoproliferative glomerulonephritis. *Am J Med* 66:216–225, 1979.
16. Turner DR, Cameron JS, Bewick M, et al: Transplantation in mesangiocapillary glomerulonephritis with intramembranous dense deposits: Recurrence of disease. *Kidney Int* 9:439–448, 1976.
17. Davis AE, Schneeberger EE, Gruipe WE, et al: Membranoproliferative glomerulonephritis (MPGN type I) and dense deposit disease (DDD) in children. *Clin Nephrol* 9:184–193, 1978.
18. Lamb V, Tisher CC, McCoy RC, et al: Membranoproliferative glomerulonephritis with dense intramembranous alterations. *Lab Invest* 36:607–617, 1977.
19. Beaufils H, Gublen MC, Karam J, et al: Dense deposit disease: Long-term follow-up of three cases of recurrence after transplantation. *Clin Nephrol* 7:31–37, 1977.

20. Leibowitch J, Halbwachs L, Wattel S, et al: Recurrence of dense deposits in transplanted kidney: II. Serum complement and nephritic factor profiles. *Kidney Int* 15:396–403, 1979.
21. Droz D, Zanetti M, Noel LH, et al: Dense deposits disease. *Nephron* 19:1–11, 1977.
22. Leibowitch J, Halbwachs L, Wattel S, et al: Recurrence of dense deposits in transplanted kidneys. II. Serum complement and nephritic factor profiles. *Kidney Int* 15:396–403, 1979.
23. Ellis D, Kapur S, Antonoyych TT, et al: Focal glomeruloscherosis in children: correlation of histology with prognosis. *J Pediatr* 93:762–768, 1978.
24. Velosa JA, Donadio JV, Holley KE: Focal sclerosing glomerulonephropathy: A clinicopathologic study. *Mayo Clin Proc* 50:121–132, 1975.
25. Cameron JS, Turner DR, Ogg CS, et al: The long-term prognosis of patients with focal segmental glomerulosclerosis. *Clin Nephrol* 120:213–218, 1978.
26. Malekzadeh MH, Heuser ET, Ettenger RB, et al: Focal glomerulosclerosis and renal transplantation. *J Pediatr* 95:249–254, 1979.
27. Couser WG, Idelson BA, Stilmant MM, et al: Successful renal transplantation in focal glomerular sclerosis: report of two cases. *Clin Nephrol* 4:62–67, 1975.
28. Maizel S, Sibley R, Horstman J, et al: Incidence and significance of recurrent FGS in renal allographs. Thirteenth Annual Meeting of the American Society of Nephrology, 1980 (abstract).
29. Papadopoulou ZL, Helfrich GB, Turner ME, et al: Recurrence of focal segmental glomerulosclerosis in children following renal transplantation. *Trans Am Soc Certif Int Organs* 27:325–329, 1981.
30. Leumann EP, Briner J, Donckerwolcke RAM, et al: Recurrence of focal segmental glomerulosclerosis in the transplanted kidney. *Nephron* 25:65–71, 1980.
31. Pinto J, Lacerda G, Cameron JS, et al: Recurrence of focal segmental glomerulosclerosis in renal allografts. *Transplantation* 32:83–89, 1981.
32. Berger J, Yaneva H, Nabarra B, et al: Recurrence of mesangial deposition of IgA after renal transplantation. *Kidney Int* 7:232–241, 1975.
33. Cream JJ, Gumpel JM, Peachey RD: Schonlein-Henoch purpura in the adult. *Q J Med* 39:461–483, 1970.
34. Meadow SR: The prognosis of Henoch-Schoenlein nephritis. *Clin Nephrol* 9:87–90, 1978.
35. Weiss JH, Bhathena DB, Curtis JJ, et al: A possible relationship between Henoch-Schoenlein nephritis syndrome and IgA nephropathy (Berger's disease). *Nephron* 22:582–591, 1978.
36. Crosson JT, Wathen R, Raij L, et al: Recurrence of idiopathic membranous nephropathy in a renal allograft. *Arch Intern Med* 135:1102–1106, 1975.
37. Petersen VP, Olsen TS, Kissmeyer-Nielsen F, et al: Late failure of human renal transplants. *Medicine* 54:45–71, 1975.
38. Iskandar SS, Jennette CJ: Recurrence of membranous glomerulopathy in an allograft. *Nephron* 29:270–273, 1981.
39. Dische FE, Herbertson BM, Melcher DH, et al: Membranous nephropathy in transplanted kidneys: Recurrent or de novo disease in four patients. *Clin Nephrol* 15:154–163, 1981.
40. Cosyns JP, Pirson Y, van Ypersele C, et al: Recurrence of de novo graft membranous glomerulonephritis. *Nephron* 29:142–145, 1981.
41. Folman R, Arbus GS, Churchill B, et al: Recurrence of the hemolytic uremic syndrome in a 3½ year old child, 4 months after second renal transplantation. *Clin Nephrol* 10:121–127, 1978.

42. Simon NM, Graham MB, Kyser FA, et al: Resolution of renal failure with malignant hypertension in scleroderma. *Am J Med* 67:533–539, 1979.
43. McKinney TD, McAllister CJ, Stone WJ, et al: Hemodialysis and renal transplantation in progressive systemic sclerosis: Report of 2 cases. *Clin Nephrol* 12:178–185, 1979.
44. Merino GE, Sutherland DE, Kjellstrand CM, et al: Renal transplantation for progressive systemic sclerosis with renal failure. *Am J Surg* 133:745–749, 1977.
45. LeRoy EC, Fleischmann RM: The management of renal scleroderma, experience with dialysis, nephrectomy and transplantation. *Am J Med* 64:974–978, 1978.
46. Woodhall PB, McCoy RC, Gunnels JC, et al: Apparent recurrence of progressive systemic sclerosis in a renal allograft. *JAMA* 236:1032–1034, 1976.
47. Zimmerman SW, Varanasi UR, Hoff B: Goodpasture's syndrome with normal renal function. *Am J Med* 66:163–171, 1979.
48. Mather TH, Hobbs JB, Kalowski S, et al: Goodpasture's syndrome: Normal renal diagnostic findings. *Ann Intern Med* 82:215–218, 1975.
49. Wilson CB, Dixon FJ: Anti-glomerular basement membrane antibody-induced glomerulonephritis. *Kidney Int* 3:74–89, 1973.
50. Bergrem H, Jervell J, Broadwall EK, et al: Goodpasture's syndrome: A report of seven patients including long-term follow-up in three who received a kidney transplant. *Am J Med* 68:54–57, 1980.
51. Teague CA, Doak PB, Simpson IJ, et al: Goodpasture's syndrome: An analysis of 29 cases. *Kidney Int* 13:492–504, 1978.
52. Beliel OM, Coburn JW, Shinaberger JH, et al: Recurrent glomerulonephritis due to anti-glomerular basement membrane-antibodies in two successive allografts. *Clin Nephrol* 1:377–380, 1973.
53. Glassock RJ: A clinical and immunopathologic dissection of rapidly progressive glomerulonephritis. *Nephron* 22:253–264, 1978.
54. Morrin PA, Hinglais N, Nabarra B, et al: Rapidly progressive glomerulonephritis, a clinical and pathologic study. *Am J Med* 65:446–460, 1978.
55. McLeish KR, Jum MN, Luft FC: Rapidly progressive glomerulonephritis in adults: Clinical and histologic correlations. *Clin Nephrol* 10:43–50, 1978.
56. Benson MD, Skinner M, Cohen AS: Amyloid deposition in a renal transplant in familial Mediterranean fever. *Ann Intern Med* 87:31–34, 1977.
57. Kuhlback B, Falck H, Tornroth T, et al: Renal transplantation in amyloidosis. *Acta Med Scand* 205:169–172, 1979.
58. Kennedy CL, Castro JE. Transplantation for renal amyloidosis. *Transplantation* 24:382–385, 1977.
59. Jones NF: Renal amyloidosis: Pathogenesis and therapy. *Clin Nephrol* 6:460–464, 1976.
60. Potter D, Belzer FO, Rames L, et al: The treatment of chronic uremia in childhood: I. Transplantation. *Pediatrics* 45:432–443, 1970.
61. Diethelm A, Sterling WA, Hartley MW, et al: Alternate-day prednisone therapy in recipients of renal allografts. *Arch Surg* 111:867–870, 1976.
62. Naik RB, Abdum H, English J, et al: Prednisolone withdrawal after 2 years in renal transplant patients receiving only this form of immunosuppression. *Transplant Proc* 11:39–44, 1979.
63. First MR, Munda R, Kant KS, et al: Steroid withdrawal following HLA-identical related donor transplantation. *Transplant Proc* 13:319–322, 1981.
64. Steinman TI, Zimmerman CE, Monaco AP, et al: Steroids can be stopped in kidney transplant recipients. *Transplant Proc* 13:323–327, 1981.
65. Cosimi AB. The clinical value of antilymphocyte antibodies. *Transplant Proc* 13:462–468, 1981.

66. Barnes AB, Olivier D: Analysis of NIAID kidney transplant histocompatibility study (KTHS): Factors associated with transplant outcomes. *Transplant Proc* 13:65–72, 1981.
67. Spees EV, Vaughn WK, Niblock G, et al: The effects of blood transfusion on cadaver renal transplantation: A prospective study of the Southeastern Organ Procurement Foundation 1977–1980. *Transplant Proc* 13:155–160, 1981.
68. Novick AC, Braun WE, Steinmuller D, et al: A controlled prospective, randomized double-blind study of antilymphoblast globulin in cadaver renal transplantation. *Transplantation* 34:264–268, 1982.
69. Light JA, Alijans MR, Bigger JA, et al: Antilymphocyte globulin (ALG) reverses "irreversible" allograft rejection. *Transplant Proc* 13:475–481 1981.
70. Hardy MA, Nowygrad R, Elberg A, et al: Use of ATG in treatment of steroid-resistant rejection. *Transplantation* 29:162–167, 1980.
71. Birkeland AG: A controlled clinical trial of treatment with ALG in established rejection of renal allografts. *Acta Med Scand* 198:489–496, 1975.
72. Shield CF III, Cosimi AG, Talkoff-Rubin N, et al: Use of antithymocyte globulin for reversal of acute allograft rejection. *Transplantation* 28:461–464, 1979.
73. Nowygrad G, Appel G, Hardy MA: Use of ATG for reversal of acute allograft rejection. *Transplant Proc* 13:469–472, 1981.
74. Filo RS, Smith EJ, Leapman SB: Reversal of acute renal allograft rejection. *Transplant Proc* 13:482–490, 1981.
75. Howard RJ, Condie RM, Sutherland DER, et al: The use of antilymphoblast globulin in the treatment of renal allograft rejection. *Transplant Proc* 13:473–474, 1981.
76. Monaco AP: Transplantation, in Gonick HC (ed): *Current Nephrology*, vol 6. New York, John Wiley & Sons, 1983, pp. 307–327.
77. Monaco AP, Wood ML: Models of specific unresponsiveness in adult animals: Potential clinical application. *Transplant Proc* 13:547, 1981.
78. Cosimi AB, Burton RC, Calvin RB, et al: Treatment of acute renal allograft rejection with OKT3 monoclonal antibody. *Transplantation* 32:535–539, 1981.
79. Morris PJ: Cyclosporin A. *Transplantation* 32:349–354, 1981.
80. Calne RY: Cyclosporin. *Nephron* 26:57–63, 1980.
81. Calne RY, White DJG: The use of cyclosporin A in clinical organ grafting. *Am Surg* 196:330–336, 1982.
82. Carpenter BJ, Tilney NL, Strom TB, et al: Cyclosporin A in cadaver renal allografts. *Am Soc Nephrol* 13:158, 1980 (abstract).
83. Harder F, Calne RY, Pichlmayr R, et al: Cyclosporin A as sole immunosuppressive agent in recipients of kidney allografts from cadaver donors. Preliminary results of an European multicenter trial. *Lancet* 2:57–60, 1982.
84. Ferguson RM, Rynasiewicz JJ, Sutherland DER, et al: Cyclosporin A in renal transplantation: A prospective randomized trial. *Surgery* 92:175–182, 1982.
85. Starzl TE, Klintmalm GBG, Weill R III, et al: Cyclosporin A and steroid therapy in sixty-six cadaver kidney recipients. *Surg Gynecol Obstet* 153:486–494, 1981.
86. Calne RY, White DJG, Thiru S, et al: Cyclosporin A in patients receiving renal allografts from cadaver donors. *Lancet* 2:1323–1327, 1978.
87. Klintmalm GBG, Iwatzuki S, Starzl TE: Cyclosporin A hepatotoxicity in 66 renal allograft recipients. *Transplantation* 32:488–489, 1981.
88. Kahan BD, Van Buren CT, Boileau M, et al: Cyclosporin A tissue levels in a cadaveric renal allograft recipient. *Transplantation* 35:96–99, 1983.
89. Opelz G, Terasaki PI: International study of histocompatibility in renal transplantation. *Transplantation* 33:87–95, 1982.

90. Hendriks GFJ, Claas FHJ, Persijn GG, et al: Influence of HLA-DRw6 and HLA-DR matching on kidney graft prognosis. *Dialysis and Transplantation* 12:95–96, 1983.
91. Salvatierra O, Iwaki Y, Vincenti F, et al: Update of the University of California at San Francisco experience with donor-specific blood transfusions. *Transplant Proc* 14:363–366, 1982.
92. Anderson CB, Sicard GA, Etheredge EE: Pretreatment of renal allograft recipients with azathioprine and donor-specific blood products. *Surgery* 92:315–321, 1982.
93. Whelchel JD, Shaw JF, Curtis JJ, et al: Effect of pretransplant stored donor-specific blood transfusions on early renal allograft survival in one-haplotype living related transplants. *Transplantation* 34:326–329, 1982.
94. Light JA, Metz S, Oddenino K, et al: Donor specific transfusion with diminished sensitization. *Transplantation* 34:352–355, 1982.
95. Frisk B. Brynger H, Sandberg L: Two random transfusions before primary renal transplantation—four years experience. *Transplant Proc* 14:386–388, 1982.
96. Opelz G, Mickey MR, Terasaki PI: Blood transfusions and kidney transplants: Remaining controversies. *Transplant Proc* 13:136–141, 1981.
97. Opelz G, Graver B, Mickey MR, et al: Lymphocytotoxic antibody responses to transfusions in potential kidney transplant recipients. *Transplantation* 32:177–183, 1982.
98. Opelz G, Graver B, Terasaki PI: Induction of high kidney graft survival rate by multiple transfusions. *Lancet* 1:1223–1225, 1981.
99. Lenhard V, Maassen G, Seifert P, et al: Characterization of transfusion-induced suppressor cells in prospective kidney allograft recipients. *Transplant Proc* 14:329–332, 1982.
100. Singal DP, Joseph S: Role of blood transfusions in induction of antibodies against recognition sites on T-lymphocytes in renal transplant recipients. *Hum Immunol* 4:93–108, 1982.

CHAPTER 4

Pharmacology of Drugs in Renal Failure

Ralph E. Cutler
Stephen C. Forland
Gary M. Davis
Robert T. Misson

Several years have passed since our initial review of this topic in Volume 3 of *Current Nephrology* (1). We have chosen this year to update the previously published data. As an overview to the data contained in the appendices, we will briefly examine some of the principles that influence drug distribution and elimination in patients with renal impairment, ways to modify drug dosage in these patients, and factors that affect drug elimination during dialysis. For a more extensive review of the pertinent pharmacokinetic principles, the reader should read the prior section in Volume 3 or a recent text by Anderson et al., *Clinical Use of Drugs in Patients with Kidney and Liver Disease* (2).

PHARMACOKINETIC PRINCIPLES

Pharmacokinetics is concerned with two general areas. The first is the study and characterization of the time course of drug absorption, distribution, metabolism, and excretion; the second is the relationship of kinetic processes to the intensity and time course of therapeutic and adverse effects of drugs. Pharmacokinetic information can provide a reasonable basis for the design of dosage regimens. It can indicate if dosage adjust-

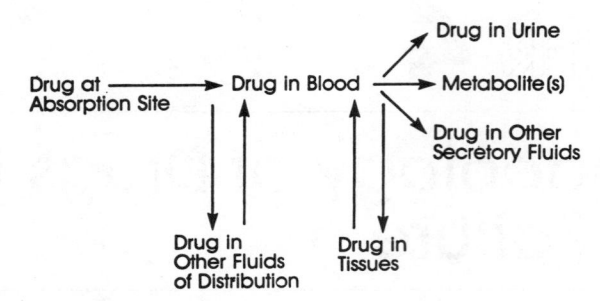

Figure 1. Schematic representation of drug absorption, distribution, and elimination.

ments may be necessary in hepatic or renal impairment, and it may also provide preliminary indications of the likelihood and types of drug interactions that may be encountered.

The response of a patient involves a multiplicity of interacting variables, of which the drug concentration in blood and tissues is only one factor. The end-point of treatment should certainly not be a given drug concentration, unless the concentration of the agent in plasma is used as the immediate target because it correlates well with the effective treatment of a specific disease. The use of pharmacokinetic data, such as the drug–concentration profile in plasma, should not take the place of medical judgment. But the availability of such data does permit the best application of clinical skills by focusing more directly on the disease process and the physiological status of the patients.

Absorption

Bioavailability may be broadly defined as the rate and the amount of drug that is absorbed into the systemic circulation (Fig. 1). The oral route is the most frequently used for administration; it is also the route that gives rise to the most complex kinetics. For a drug to enter the systemic circulation it must first dissolve in the gastrointestinal fluids, be transported through the intestinal wall, and pass through the liver. There are a number of factors that influence this process:

1. *Characteristics of drug*
   Inactivation before gastrointestinal absorption
   Solubility
   Biotransformation in intestinal wall or liver
2. *Formulation of drug product*
   State of the drug (solution, suspension, solid)
   Dosage form (sustained release, enteric coated)

3. *Interaction with other substances in GI tract*
   Food
   Drugs
4. *Patient characteristics*
   Gastrointestinal (pH, motility, perfusion, flora, structure)
   Hepatic function
   Genetic phenotype

If drug release from the dosage form or diffusion of a drug through the gastrointestinal mucosa is too slow, some of the drug will be lost in the stool. In addition, many substances in the diet or other drugs given concomitantly may reduce gut absorption. Milk or other sources of divalent cation, such as antacids, may markedly impair absorption. This is of special concern for the patient with renal failure, who is usually receiving antacids to reduce phosphate absorption. If in doubt, it is important to remember that most drugs are absorbed best in an empty stomach. Examples of drugs that may have reduced bioavailability when given with antacids are digoxin, iron, tetracycline, ampicillin, isoniazid, and sulfonamides.

Another potential source of drug loss is the metabolism, which occurs to various degrees as the drug passes through the intestinal mucosa and the liver. Such a biotransformation is called the *first-pass effect*. When a drug is administered intravenously, it is considered completely bioavailable. If a solution of the same drug is given orally and absorbed rapidly, its metabolism may resemble the plasma time-concentration curve shown in Figure 2. In this example, no substantial first-pass effect can be demonstrated since the plasma curves for both preparations of the agent are similar in both their peak concentrations as well as in their distribution and elimination. Examples of drugs that are subject to extensive first-pass effect after oral absorption are seen in Table 1. It is clear that the parenteral dose of such drugs is considerably smaller than the oral dose.

Distribution and Elimination

The typical time course of a drug concentration in plasma after intravenous and oral administration is shown in Figure 2. Following intravenous injection, the drug becomes mixed in the plasma. It may become partially bound to plasma proteins and adsorbed on blood cells, and it diffuses to various degrees into extravascular tissues. These processes of distribution usually cause a rapid initial decrease of drug concentration in the plasma. Following initial distribution in highly perfused tissues, the subsequent decline of the plasma concentration is caused by the slower elimination of the drug from the body by other processes, such as metabolism, renal excretion, and secretion into other body fluids such as bile.

The relationship between the amount of drug in the body and the plasma concentration after absorption and distribution is expressed by a

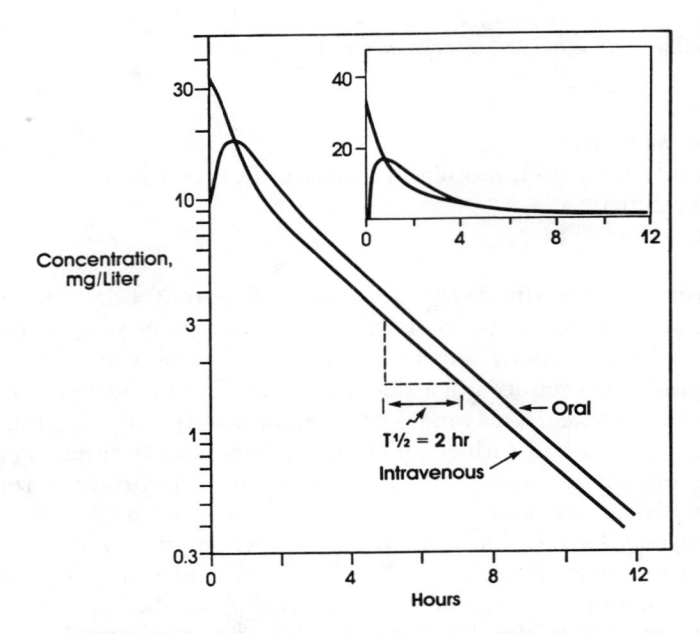

Figure 2. Simulated plasma concentrations after oral or intravenous administration. Concentration scale is logarithmic in main figure and linear in insert.

proportionality constant called the *apparent volume of distribution*. This volume does not necessarily represent a physiological body space. It may be as small as the plasma volume, or it may be as large as several hundred liters, depending on how much of the drug is bound to plasma proteins and tissues, respectively (Fig. 3). Some drugs are displaced from plasma

Table 1. Drugs with Extensive First-Pass Biotransformation

Drug	Usefulness Orally
Amitriptyline	+
L-dopa	+
Isoproterenol	0
Imipramine	+
Lidocaine	0
Meperidine	+
Metoprolol	+
Morphine	0
Organic nitrates	+
Propoxyphene	+
Propranolol	+
Terbutaline	+

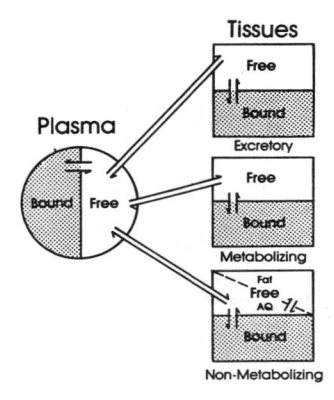

Figure 3. Schematic representation of protein binding of drugs in plasma and tissues. The "free" concentration is the pharmacodynamic fraction that interacts with various receptors.

protein binding sites by other drugs or drug metabolites, resulting in an increase in the apparent volume of distribution. One of the consequences of renal failure is a decrease in the ability of plasma proteins to bind certain drugs. A therapeutic consequence of impaired binding of a drug in renal failure has been noted with phenytoin, digoxin, and disopyramide. With phenytoin, the decreased binding leads to a higher unbound fraction plus an increase in both the elimination rate and apparent volume of distribution. The overall consequence of this perturbation is a low serum plasma concentration and an increase in total body clearance. However, the unbound concentration of phenytoin remains the same, and anticonvulsant effects are maintained with customary doses (Table 2). In the case of digoxin and disopyramide, an interesting decrease in the apparent volume of distribution occurs in renal failure. This is probably related to a change in tissue binding in renal failure. The cause of this decrease in tissue binding has not been revealed by current investigation. However, this decrease is of clinical importance and mandates lower loading doses of the drug in order to avoid toxicity.

Changes in plasma protein binding affect the diffusivity of protein-bound drugs across dialyzer membranes. An increase in the unbound fraction, which occurs in a number of drugs in uremia, increases their clearance during dialysis. The correlation of unbound fraction of a drug to the total quantity of drug extracted from a patient over the course of a single dialysis is, however, not very high. Only when percentage of

Table 2. Phenytoin Pharmacokinetics in Normal and Uremic Subjects

Subjects	Serum Creat (mg/dl)	Phenytoin Conc (mg/dl) Total	Free	Plasma Binding (%) Bound	Free	$T_{1/2}$ (hr)	V_d (L/kg)
Normal	1	10–20	1.0–2.5	88	12	13	0.64
Uremic	15	5–10	1.0–2.5	74	26	8	1.4

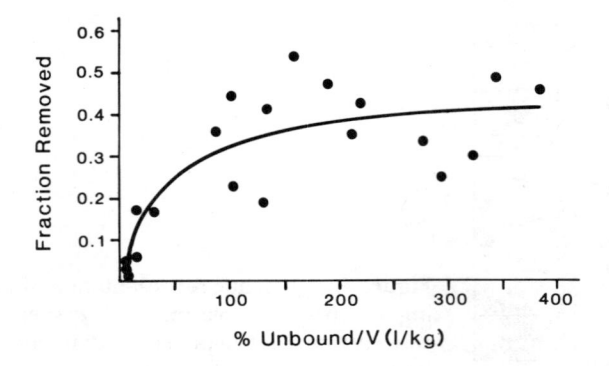

Figure 4. A plot of the fraction of drug in the body (immediately prior to hemodialysis) removed by a 6-hour hemodialysis versus the ratio of the percent of drug in the plasma unbound to plasma proteins to the volume of distribution (V) of the drug. The solid line is the best fit to the data.

unbound drug and volume of distribution are both included in an empiric, nonlinear equation have investigators found a good correlation with hemodializability of drugs (Fig. 4) (3).

Elimination

The concept of "total body clearance" is useful in discussing the relative rates of drug removal. The total body clearance of a drug may be explained by analogy to renal clearance. It is based on the concept of the entire body acting as a drug-eliminating system. The rate of elimination of drug by the body divided by the average plasma concentration of the drug is the total clearance. The sum of all the individual organ (renal, hepatic, pulmonary, etc.) clearances of a drug equals the total body clearance. Because plasma is usually sampled for drug assays, total body clearance is often called plasma clearance (Cl_p). For simplicity, we will express body clearance as the sum of the renal clearance (Cl_r) and the nonrenal clearance (Cl_{nr}). The nonrenal clearance is, of course, the sum of hepatic clearance (Cl_h) and all other routes of elimination (Cl_o). This can be represented symbolically as

$$Cl_p = Cl_r + \overbrace{Cl_h + Cl_o}^{Cl_{nr}} \quad [1]$$

The entry of drugs into the urine occurs by means of a combination of glomerular filtration and tubular transport. Glomerular filtration is unidirectional and permits entry of any dissociated and undissociated drug molecules that are not bound to plasma protein but are small enough to penetrate the glomerular wall. In contrast, tubular transport is bidirec-

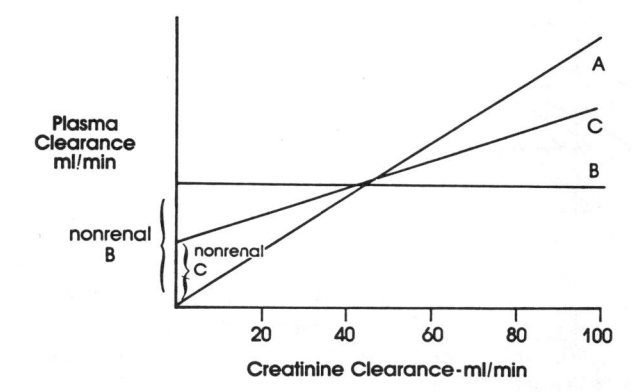

Figure 5. The effect of changes in creatinine renal clearance on the plasma clearance of three prototypical drugs exhibiting renal (drug A), nonrenal (drug B), or a combination of both routes of elimination (drug C).

tional. Many organic acids and bases are both secreted and reabsorbed by carrier-mediated processes located principally in the straight segment of the proximal tubule. Protein binding appears to have little effect on tubular secretion except in those cases where the drug has a low infinity for the carrier-mediated transport system.

Renal clearance is directly proportional to renal plasma flow or glomerular filtration rate. For convenience, drug clearances are usually estimated as some fraction of the creatinine clearance (Cl_{cr}), a convenient endogenous clinical measure of glomerular filtration rate. This can be symbolically represented as follows:

$$Cl_r = k1\,(RPF)$$
$$= k2\,(GFR) \qquad [2]$$
$$= k2\,(Cl_{cr})$$

Therefore, the plasma clearance in Equation 1 can be symbolically rewritten as follows:

$$Cl_p = k(Cl_{cr}) + Cl_{nr} \qquad [3]$$

The effect of changes in renal function on the elimination of three types of drugs is illustrated in Figure 5. It is obvious that drugs A and C have substantial renal elimination and in the absence of renal function their plasma clearance is much impaired. However, drug B is eliminated by nonrenal routes and is not influenced in its plasma clearance by changes in creatinine clearance. Drugs A and C differ in the degree of nonrenal elimination present. Drug A has little elimination in the absence of renal function, but drug C continues to be removed at a reasonable rate even in the anephric subject.

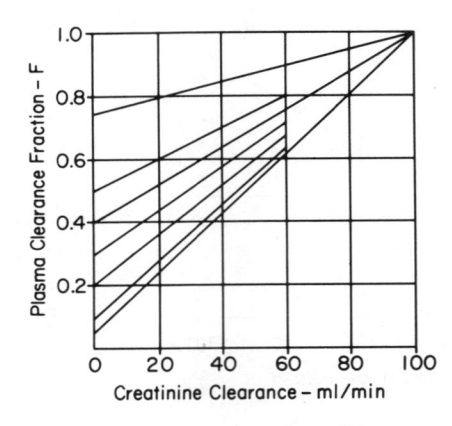

Figure 6. Nomogram for the graphic determination of individual plasma clearance rate fraction (F) of drugs in patients with renal failure.

These effects may also be expressed in terms of the change in biologic half-life, since total clearance of a drug is inversely proportional to half-life. Specifically,

$$Cl_p = (0.693)(V_d)/T_{\frac{1}{2}} \qquad [4]$$

where V_d is the apparent volume distribution, and $T_{\frac{1}{2}}$ is the biologic half-life. The numerical constant 0.693 results from the logarithmic transformation required in the mathematical derivation of this equation.

Examples of type A (mainly renal excretion) drugs are aminoglycosides, vancomycin, certain cephalosporins, (cefamandole, cefazolin, cefoxitin, cephalexin, cephradine), some penicillins (amoxicillin, ampicillin, carbenicillin, methicillin, penicillin G, ticarcillin), tetracycline, methotrexate, and lithium carbonate. Type B drugs (both excreted and metabolized to a significant degree) include digoxin, disopyramide, procainamide, methyldopa, isoniazid, cephalothin, cloxacillin, and cimetidine. Type C drugs (largely metabolized) include digitoxin, propranolol, quinidine, acetaminophen, phenytoin, chloramphenicol, theophylline, and doxycycline.

Principles of Dosage Modification

For drugs that are mainly eliminated by the renal route, dosage calculations must be individualized when the patient has renal insufficiency. This estimate is often made by grouping the degree of renal dysfunction to mild, moderate, and severe categories with suggested modification of dosage for each level of creatinine clearance. However, this approach is simplistic and does not enhance an understanding of the drug kinetics involved. The description given in this section is similar to that outlined by Dettli (4). The analysis is reasonably simple and should enhance the comprehension of the pharmacokinetic principles involved.

In order to simplify the estimating process, a dosing nomogram (Fig. 6) is used, allowing a graphic estimation of plasma clearance in any patient with renal failure. The nomogram is based on changes in the plasma clearance fraction (F) as a linear function of the creatinine clearance. F is called the plasma clearance fraction because it describes the plasma clearance as a fraction of the mean plasma clearance in subjects who have normal renal function (Cl_r = 100 ml/min; F = 1). In the anuric patient (Cl_r = 0 ml/min), F is specifically designed as F_0 and represents a fraction of the plasma clearance that is removed by nonrenal routes:

$$F = Cl_{nr}/Cl_p \qquad [5]$$

Because of these relationships, the dosing curve for a specific drug is made by drawing a line between its F_0 value on the ordinate, at left, and the right upper corner of the nomogram. A line drawn from the patient's creatinine clearance rate (abscissa) will intersect the dosing curve at the drug's estimated plasma clearance fraction, F, which is found on the ordinate. The values of F_0 for various drugs, calculated according to Equation 5, are listed in Appendices 1–8.

As an example, for a patient receiving atenolol, we might ask: How much change must be made in the maintenance dose or dosing interval for atenolol in this patient whose creatinine clearance is 50 ml/min? Calculation of the fractional value, F, gives the answer to that question. First, turn to Appendix 5 and find the F_0 value. For atenolol this number is 0.08, indicating that the plasma clearance in an anephric patient is 8% of that seen in patients with normal renal function. Thus, 8% of the plasma clearance of atenolol occurs through nonrenal routes. The value 0.08 is then plotted on the ordinate of the dosing nomogram (Fig. 6) and this point is connected by a line to the right upper corner of the nomogram. Next, the creatinine clearance of interest is found on the abscissa, in this case, 50 ml/min. The point of intersection between the Cl_{cr} and the dosing curve for atenolol as read on the ordinate equals the individual clearance rate fraction, F. The value in this particular case is 0.54, indicating that the plasma clearance for atenolol in a patient with creatinine clearance of 50 ml/min is 54% of that in a patient with a Cl_{cr} of 100 ml/min. Further use of this plasma clearance fraction is illustrated below.

Use of Dosing Nomogram

The dosing nomogram can be used to modify a normal dosing regimen in stable renal failure. Four arithmetic values are required for calculation:

1. Normal dosage regimen
2. Fractional rate of elimination in anuria, F_0
3. Current creatinine clearance
4. Elimination rate fraction, F, for the current Cl_{cr}

For example, what changes may be made in the dosage regimen for gentamicin in a 60-year-old patient weighing 75 kg with a creatinine clearance of 21 ml/min?

1. The normal dosage regimen is 1–2 mg/kg every 8 hours: 1 mg/kg × 75 kg = 75 mg
2. The F_0 value (Appendix 1, gentamicin) is 0.03. This value is plotted on the ordinate and then connected to the right upper corner of the nomogram.
3. The current Cl_{cr} is measured or estimated by the Cockroft and Gault formula:

$$Cl_{cr} = \frac{(140-\text{age, yr})(\text{body weight, kg})}{72 \times \text{serum creatinine, mg/dL}}$$

4. The point of intersection of a Cl_{cr} of 21 ml/min with the dosing line for gentamicin is F = 0.24.

Based on these values, the following modifications are possible:

1. Change the dosing interval (T): T (failure) = 8 hr/0.24 = 33 hr
2. Change the maintenance dose (D): D (failure) = 75 mg × 0.24 = 18 mg
3. Change rate of administration (D/T): D/T (failure) = 75 mg/8 hr × 0.24 (or 2.3 mg/hr or 25 mg/12 hr)

In this patient, an initial loading dose of 75 mg (2 mg/kg) can be followed by any of the previously mentioned modifications. Modification of the dosing interval is the most common technique used for aminoglycoside drugs in renal failure because it appears to be the safest. It gives high peaks and low troughs since most of the drug is excreted before the next dose is given. Thus, the risk of renal toxicity and ototoxicity from high sustained tissue and plasma concentrations of the drug is lessened with this method.

Changing the maintenance dose of aminoglycoside drugs by method 2, or the rate of administration by method 3, gives a plateau effect with moderate oscillation of the plasma concentration around the mean. It has not been proven whether this technique is more effective for antimicrobial therapy, but it may be more toxic with drugs that have a narrow therapeutic:toxic ratio. However, for certain agents, such as the antiarrhythmic and anticonvulsant drugs, the maintenance of a relatively constant plasma concentration is desirable, and, if drug modification is needed, dosage or rate modification rather than interval changes should be used.

Drug Dosage Modification During Dialysis Treatment

Drug removal during dialysis can be predicted by the addition of dialysis clearance (Cl_d) to the overall clearance described by equation 1:

$$Cl_p = Cl_r + Cl_{nr} + Cl_d \qquad [6]$$

Several techniques have been used to calculate Cl_d. Methods 1 and 2 are clearly superior to method 3:

Method 1.
$$Cl_d = \frac{A_d \, _{t1}^{t2}}{AUC \, _{t1}^{t2}}$$

where A_d equals the dose removed in dialysate between time t1 and t2, and AUC equals the area under serum concentration-time curve between time t1 and t2.

Method 2.
$$Cl_d = \frac{Q_d \times C_d}{C_A}$$

where Q_d equals the dialysate flow rate, C_d equals the dialysate drug concentration, and C_A equals the arterial (inflow) drug concentration.

Method 3.
$$Cl_d = \frac{Q(A - V)}{A}$$

where Q equals the dialysis blood flow, A equals the arterial (inflow) drug concentration, and V equals the venous (outflow) drug concentration.

Although a drug may have a relatively high dialyzer clearance with current hemodialyzer equipment, the fractional removal of a drug during a standard 4-hour dialysis procedure is only clinically significant if two factors are present: (*1*) the Cl_d is at least 50% or more of the interdialytic Cl_p, and (*2*) the volume of drug distribution does not exceed 1 L/kg body weight. The following examples may clarify this important, and largely neglected, concept:

- *Digoxin.* The pharmacokinetic data for digoxin is in Appendix 5. Although the Cl_d is 20 ml/min, a value close to 60% of the interdialytic Cl_p of 35 ml/min, the drug distribution is so large (4.2 liter/kg) that only an insignificant fraction of the drug is removed during dialysis.
- *Procainamide.* The Cl_d of procainamide drug is 65 ml/min, but the Cl_p without dialysis is 200 ml/min (Appendix 5). Thus, almost three times as much drug is lost by nonrenal routes as can be achieved by the hemodialyzer. This fact plus a large distribution volume means that the fractional removal of this drug during hemodialysis is trivial and no supplemental dosage is needed.
- *Aminoglycosides.* The Cl_d for the aminoglycosides is 15–30 ml/min, the distribution volume is about 0.25 L/kg, and the interdialytic Cl_p is 3 ml/

Table 3. Common Drugs Requiring Posthemodialysis Dosage

Analgesic	Acetylsalicylic acid
Antihypertensive	Atenolol, captopril, diazoxide, nadolol
Antimicrobial	
Antifungal	Flucytosine
Antitubercular	Ethambutol
Aminoglycosides	Amikacin, gentamicin, kanamycin, streptomycin, tobramycin
Cephalosporins	Cefadroxil, cefazolin, cefoxitin, cephalexin, cephradine, moxalactam
Penicillins	Amoxicillin, ampicillin, carbenicillin pencillin G, piperacillin, ticarcillin, sulfamethoxazole, trimethoprin
Antineoplastic	Cyclophosphamide, methotrexate
Cardiovascular	Disopyramide
Psychotropic	Lithium, meprobamate, phenobarbital

min (Appendix 1). Thus, all conditions are favorable for substantial drug removal during dialysis. Clinical experience demonstrates that a postdialysis dose that is 50–75% as large as the initial loading dose will be necessary to restore body stores to a level comparable to those prior to dialysis.

The drugs that have substantial fractional removal during hemodialysis and that require postdialysis dosing are shown in Table 3. It is difficult to estimate a precise postdialysis dose because of the many variables present. Extant pharmacokinetic data suggest that a dose that is 50–75% of the initial loading dose or of the maintenance dose is probably safe and may be adequate. However, if plasma concentration is critical because of a narrow therapeutic:toxic ratio (e.g., for eminoglycosides or disopyramide), then plasma monitoring will be necessary for optimal safety and effectiveness. When necessary it is best to check plasma drug concentrations before, rather than immediately after, hemodialysis, since equilibration from extravascular sites may take place over several hours following dialysis.

DRUG DATA TABLES

In order to apply the previously described pharmacokinetic principles to drug treatment of individuals with renal failure, we have prepared tables of commonly used drugs (see p. 159) with the available pharmacokinetic data that seem relevant to dosage modification in renal failure (Appendicies 1–8). Unfortunately, the pharmacokinetic data base for many of these agents is incomplete (2,5). In addition, many of the values chosen are averages from a small patient population and may not accurately reflect drug handling in certain individuals. Therefore, it is mandatory that these data be used carefully in guiding therapy. Drugs that require the most attention in renal failure are those having a small dose range between therapeutic and toxic levels, an F_0 less than 0.30, and a clinical effect that is not easily monitored. Whenever possible, plasma peak and trough measurements should be obtained to further aid in dosage adjustment.

Antiinfective Drugs (Appendix 1)

Some antimicrobial agents require little or no dosage modification in patients with renal failure. These drugs are either eliminated primarily by nonrenal routes or their margin of safety is so wide that moderate drug accumulation does not produce adverse effects.

Antifungal Agents

Amphotericin B, flucytosine, ketoconazole, miconazole, and griseofulvin are the most common antifungal agents used for systemic mycoses. The pharmacokinetics of these agents have been recently reviewed (6).

Amphotericin B is mainly eliminated by nonrenal routes. Dosage adjustment is not necessary for patients with renal failure, and dialysis does not remove significant fractions of the drug from plasma. Sodium depletion may enhance nephrotoxicity. Mannitol does not protect patients from, and may contribute to, renal vascular pathology (7). Recent studies in dogs suggest that dopamine and saralasin may reduce renal damage when amphotericin B is given (8). Dosage adjustment in patients with severe liver failure may be necessary. The drug is nephrotoxic, and it may produce tubular dysfunction in patients with residual renal function. The combination of amphotericin B and gentamicin may produce synergistic nephrotoxicity (9).

Flucytosine is eliminated mainly by the kidney and requires a significant reduction in dose in renal insufficiency because of potential bone marrow toxicity. Significant quantities of the drug are removed by dialysis, and supplemental postdialysis dosage is necessary.

Griseofulvin has a large volume of distribution, multicompartment kinetics, and slow elimination. It does not require dosage adjustment in renal failure since elimination is mainly by hepatic metabolism. Activity and toxicity of the metabolites is unknown. It is not known if dialysis removes significant quantities of the drug.

Ketoconazole is well absorbed orally and eliminated mainly through hepatic mechanisms. The rate of elimination is probably dose dependent. Most of the drug is metabolized, and none of the identified metabolites has antifungal activity. Pharmacokinetic studies have been hampered by lack of an intravenous preparation. No dosing changes are necessary in patients with renal failure. An important drug interaction with cimetidine is a decrease in AUC of ketoconazole (10). This can be avoided if cimetidine is given two or more hours after ketoconazole.

Miconazole is poorly absorbed from the gastrointestinal tract. The drug is often used topically for mycotic gastrointestinal or skin infections. Therapy of systemic infections requires parenteral administration. The distribution of the drug is very large with penetration into many tissues but not into the cerebrospinal fluid. The drug is rapidly metabolized by hepatic oxidative routes and excreted into the gut. The drug kinetics are unchanged in renal failure or during hemodialysis. Toxic effects appear not to be dose related. An antagonism with amphotericin B is recognized, and the two agents should not be given together (11).

Antitubercular Agents

Isoniazid, ethambutol, and rifampin are the most common agents used for treatment of tuberculosis. The elimination of all of these agents is substantially nonrenal, and customary treatment can be given to patients with renal failure. Slow acetylators of isoniazid may require reduction in dosage to prevent drug accumulation. Significant removal of isoniazid by dialysis is unlikely except in the slow acetylator.

Ethambutol is largely eliminated through the kidneys. However, in renal failure the drug is substantially metabolized, with accumulation of metabolites. The toxicity of these metabolites has not been adequately evaluated. Because of potential drug toxicity, it is important to reduce the dose in renal insufficiency. Substantial amounts of ethambutol, and possibly its metabolites, are removed by dialysis so that postdialysis doses are suggested.

Rifampin is principally eliminated through nonrenal routes, and dosage modification in renal insufficiency seems unnecessary. Dialysis removal has not been reported but will be much less than the fraction of the drug that is metabolized. Therefore, no postdialysis supplementation is required.

Antiviral Agents

Amantadine and acyclovir are potentially useful antiviral agents. Acyclovir, a recently introduced drug for the treatment of herpes simplex, is largely excreted by the kidneys and requires dosage modification in advanced renal failure. Dialyzer clearance is substantial but less than 50% as rapid as the nonrenal routes of elimination. Therefore, postdialysis supplementation following dialysis does not seem necessary.

Amantadine is eliminated predominantly through renal mechanisms and it has a very extended half-life in end-stage renal disease (ESRD). Its use in renal failure has been inadequately studied; however, accumulation and possible toxicity from the drug would be anticipated, and reduced dosage or an increased dosage interval should be considered. Although hemodialysis clearance is substantial, the fraction removed by this route is trivial because of the large distribution volume. Therefore, drug supplementation following dialysis is not indicated.

Aminoglycosides
The aminoglycoside antibiotics (amikacin, gentamicin, kanamycin, streptomycin, and tobramycin) are extensively used for treatment of serious gram-negative infections. These drugs are not metabolized and have very little nonrenal elimination. In addition, they have a narrow therapeutic:toxic ratio. Therefore, modification of dosage in renal failure is an important consideration. Although toxicity of various agents differs, the primary adverse effects are ototoxicity and nephrotoxicity. A recent report concerning experimental gentamicin nephrotoxicity in rats concluded that renal damage could be reduced by increasing urinary calcium excretion by dietary loading (12). High urinary calcium decreased gentamicin uptake by the renal tubular cells, thereby reducing tubular injury. Studies need to be done in humans to establish application of this technique in the prevention of clinical nephrotoxicity. Because substantial amounts of these drugs are removed during dialysis, supplemental doses after dialysis are suggested. For patients receiving alternate-day hemodialysis, a postdialysis dose that is 50–75% of the initial loading dose is usually adequate and safe.

Because aminoglycosides are frequently given with other broad-spectrum antimicrobials, a recently noted drug interaction with the penicillins is potentially important. It has been shown previously that a combination of aminoglycosides (gentamicin, tobramycin) and carbenicillin or ticarcillin in solution results in rapid loss of antimicrobial activity. The possibility exists that such an interaction would occur in patients with ESRD where elimination rates are greatly reduced and the two types of drugs would be present in plasma for an extended period. Recent studies have shown that the usually prolonged half-life (60–80 hours) of gentamicin or tobramycin in ESRD was reduced to less than 24 hours when these agents were administered along with either carbenicillin or ticarcillin (13,14). It is of clinical interest that a comparable interaction with amikacin has not been found. A similar, but smaller, decrease in elimination half-life is noted with gentamicin and tobramycin when the new acylamino penicillins (azlocillin, mezlocillin, piperacillin) are used (13).

Cephalosporins
Although these drugs have substantial renal elimination, and accumulation may occur in renal failure, they are relatively safe and have created few recognized clinical problems even when accumulation occurs. Several of these agents are extensively metabolized (cephalothin, cephapirin, cefotaxime) (5). Although their desacetyl metabolites are less active than the parent drug, they do accumulate to high concentrations in ESRD, suggesting that dosing of the parent drug should be reduced in renal failure. Fortunately, the metabolites are apparently not very toxic and no harmful effects have been reported even when dosage is not reduced in ESRD.

However, the dosage or dosage interval of the other cephalosporins should be changed when moderate to severe renal insufficiency is present. Because substantial amounts of cefadroxil, cefamandole, cefazolin, cefoxitin, cephalexin, cephradine, and moxalactam are removed during dialysis, postdialysis doses are suggested.

Penicillins
Except for the isoxazolyl derivatives (cloxacillin, dicloxacillin, oxacillin, nafcillin), the penicillins are excreted primarily by the kidneys. Because there is a wide range between therapeutic and toxic levels with all of these agents, modification of dosage is rarely necessary except in severe renal failure. The toxic effects of the penicillins resulting from high plasma concentrations include a syndrome of altered sensorium, myoclonic movements, and seizures.

Penicillin G, ampicillin, amoxicillin, carbenicillin, ticarcillin, mezlocillin, azlocillin, and piperacillin all require dosage modification in advanced renal insufficiency. Such modification is rarely necessary until the estimated creatinine clearance is less than 10 ml/min. At that point the usual plan is to give a customary maintenance dose every 12 hours. In patients receiving dialysis, large amounts of these drugs may be removed, and a postdialysis dose is advised. For patients receiving chronic peritoneal dialysis, it is likely that customary doses can be given safely, but the total daily dose of penicillin G should not exceed 10–12 million units.

Sulfonamides and Trimethoprim
About 20–35% of sulfamethoxazole and 50–70% of sulfisoxazole are eliminated in the urine as unchanged drug. For patients with severe renal insufficiency, the dosage of these drugs should be modified. Because sulfonamides are principally used in treating urinary tract infections, less toxic agents with greater transport into urine, such as the penicillins and cephalosporins, should be prescribed for urinary tract infections in renal failure. When sulfamethoxazole along with trimethoprim is used to treat systemic infections in ESRD, supplemental postdialysis dosages are advised because of significant removal by this route.

Trimethoprim is almost exclusively removed by the kidneys. Substantial modification of dosage is therefore required in renal insufficiency. In patients with an estimated creatinine clearance of less than 10 ml/min, the dosage interval should be increased to every 24 hours. Because of the extensive removal of this drug by dialysis, supplemental doses will be required to restore body fluid levels.

Tetracyclines
With the exception of doxycycline and minocycline, all tetracyclines are relatively contraindicated in patients with mild to moderate renal insufficiency. In patients with severe renal insufficiency, tetracyclines accelerate

protein metabolism causing increased production of urea and exaggeration of azotemia and metabolic acidosis. In addition, these drugs may have direct nephrotoxic effects in patients with cirrhosis. Because only small amounts of minocycline and doxycycline are removed by dialysis, no supplemental postdialysis dosage is necessary.

Miscellaneous
Chloramphenicol is principally eliminated by nonrenal routes. An accumulation of the glucuronidated conjugate occurs in renal insufficiency but appears to cause little difficulty. Because of the potential effect of this agent and its metabolites on erythropoiesis, it should be avoided whenever possible in the anemic patient with renal failure. Compared to nonrenal clearance, hemodialysis removal is small and supplemental postdialysis dosing is not required.

Erythromycin, clindamycin, and lincomycin are eliminated mainly by nonrenal routes, and only mild changes in their rate of elimination occur in renal insufficiency. Little toxicity has been reported with these agents in renal failure. The fractional removal of the drugs during dialysis is insignificant, and no supplemental dosage is required.

Nalidixic acid, nitrofurantoin, and methenamine have been used mainly in the treatment of urinary tract infections. In the presence of renal failure, these drugs do not enter the urine in sufficient amounts to be effective. In addition, they have significant toxicity. This is particularly true of nitrofurantoin, which has produced polyneuropathy, principally in patients with severe renal failure. Although hemodialysis clearance of these drugs is significant, the fractional removal is low when compared to nonrenal routes.

Vancomycin is primarily excreted by the kidneys. The normal half-life of approximately 7 hours is expanded to an average of 240 hours in renal insufficiency. Because of the large size of the agent, little is removed by dialysis. The antistaphylococcal spectrum of the agent and its long persistence in renal insufficiency even during dialysis has led to its frequent use for the treatment of staphylococcal soft tissue infections. Good results have been obtained when the drug is administered in loading doses of 1g intravenously approximately every 7–10 days.

Antiarthritic Drugs (Appendix 2)

For the acute treatment of gout or inflammatory arthritis, the short-term use of customary doses of nonsteroidal antiinflammatory drugs (fenoprofen, ibuprofen, indomethacin, naproxen, phenybutazone, piroxicam, salicylates, sulindac) or colchicine can be used in renal failure. All of the nonsteroidal antiinflammatory drugs (NSAIDs) inhibit synthesis of prostaglandins that help regulate renal blood flow, glomerular filtration, and renal sodium and water excretion. NSAIDs can cause fluid retention and diminish sodium excretion, followed by prerenal azotemia, hyperkalemia, oliguria, and anuria (15). This type of renal toxicity is more likely in patients with renal disease, lupus erythematosus, heart failure, cirrhosis, or hypertension treated with diuretics; it can occur after only a few days of therapy and is generally reversible when the drug is stopped, but fatal hyperkalemia has been reported. In addition, acute interstitial nephritis, sometimes presenting as a nephrotic syndrome, has been described in patients taking NSAIDs, particularly fenoprofen (15). This effect, which appears to be idiosyncratic and not related to prostaglandins, generally takes weeks or months to develop. Acute papillary necrosis has occurred in patients taking these drugs, as well as in patients taking aspirin. Although the NSAIDs are generally well tolerated, they can also cause hepatic, gastrointestinal, and hematologic toxicity. Available data are not sufficient to recommend any one of these agents as safer than the others. Patients taking these drugs should probably have periodic determinations of white blood cell counts, serum creatinine concentration, and hepatic enzyme activities.

The treatment of hyperuricemia in renal failure is probably not required unless symptomatic gout occurs. The drug of choice is allopurinol, which along with its major metabolite, oxypurinol, is a potent inhibitor of xanthine oxidase and is effective in controlling hyperuricemia. Allopurinol is almost exclusively metabolized to oxypurinol, the latter being eliminated mainly through the kidney. Therefore, patients with decreased renal function may have an adequate therapeutic effect with lower doses of allopurinol. However, the effects of the drug are easily monitored by following the serum urate. Although substantial amounts of oxypurinol are removed during dialysis, postdialysis supplementation is not required.

Because uricosuric agents such as probenicid and sulfinpyrazone are ineffective in the presence of renal failure, they should not be used.

Anticoagulant and Antihistamine Drugs (Appendix 3)

Anticoagulants
Both heparin and warfarin are eliminated by nonrenal mechanisms, and conventional doses can be used in renal failure. Because advanced renal failure is associated with impaired hemostasis, such drugs should be used cautiously. The removal of these drugs by dialysis is insignificant.

Antihistamines
The conventional H_1-receptor antagonists, such as chlorpheniramine, diphenhydramine, and hydroxyzine, are often used in patients with renal failure for their antipruritic or antiemetic properties. They are metabolized extensively and appear to have no significant adverse effects when given in conventional doses in uremic patients.

The H_2-receptor antagonist, cimetidine, has been useful in treating various gastrointestinal diseases that improve with the reduction of gastric secretion of hydrogen ion produced by this agent. As an organic base that is secreted by the kidney, it competes with the secretory transport pathway for creatinine and may produce slight elevations of the serum creatinine concentration. Although this agent has substantial renal elimination, it is extensively metabolized to a product that has low toxicity in uremic patients. However, when adverse effects such as sedation and confusion have been noted, it is usually in patients with impaired renal function. Therefore, the dosage of the drug should be decreased in patients with renal insufficiency. Although the drug is readily dialyzed, the fractional removal by this route is insignificant compared to the nonrenal routes of elimination, and postdialysis supplemental doses are not required.

Several important drug interactions with cimetidine have been described based on two possible mechanisms: (1) inhibition of microsomal enzymes or (2) reduction of hepatic blood flow (20). Interactions with warfarin, phenytoin, theophylline, propranolol, and metoprolol are probably clinically significant. The reduction of microsomal metabolism induced by cimetidine produces a marked slowing of the plasma clearance of warfarin, phenytoin, and theophylline. Thus, dosage reduction of these agents would be needed to prevent toxicity during combined therapy. Potentiation of the anticoagulant effect of warfarin and elevation of phenytoin and theophylline serum concentrations have been reported (16). Drugs with a high hepatic extraction may show a reduced plasma clearance when hepatic blood flow is decreased. Cimetidine has been shown to reduce hepatic blood flow by 25–30% and lidocaine clearance by a similar degree. Resting pulse rates were reported to be significantly lower after propranolol plus cimetidine than after propranolol alone.

Antineoplastic and Immunosuppressive Agents (Appendix 4)

The metabolism and elimination of adrenocorticosteroids is not substantially changed in uremia, and the dose prescribed is individualized depending upon the drug being used and the disease being treated. Removal during dialysis is insignificant. Renal insufficiency in patients receiving cytotoxic drugs for malignancy may be the result of direct tumor invasion, the results of tumor-derived nephrotoxic metabolites, or as a direct complication of tumor chemotherapy. Many of the currently used cytotoxic and immunosuppressive drugs (bleomycin, cisplatin, methotrexate) are substantially excreted by the kidney and their dosage may require significant modification when renal failure is present.

Based on current data, bleomycin and methotrexate should be given in modified doses in the presence of renal failure. Although it has been suggested that cisplatin should be given in reduced doses in renal failure, anecdotal experience in patients with testicular carcinoma and severe obstructive uropathy suggests that this agent should be used at full dosage and that no unusual toxicities are encountered. The only drugs in this class removed significantly during dialysis are cyclophosphamide and methotrexate, and supplemental postdialysis doses may be required.

Although dosages of busulfan, mithramycin, nitrosoureas, and streptozotocin do not require substantial modification in renal failure, these drugs must be used with caution because of the high frequency of nephrotoxicity associated with these agents.

Cardiovascular Drugs (Appendix 5)

Antiarrhythmic Agents

Lidocaine, quinidine, nifedipine, diltiazam, and verapamil can be administered in standard doses in patients with renal failure. However, bretylium, disopyramide, and procainamide must be given in reduced dosages when renal insufficiency is significant. One of the difficulties in using procainamide in renal failure is the unpredictable accumulation of its active metabolite, N-acetylprocainamide (NAPA), which has antiarrhythmic effect similar to that of procainamide. The metabolite is only eliminated by renal excretion and may accumulate and reach toxic levels in severe renal failure. Since NAPA accumulates in patients with poor renal function, plasma concentration of both NAPA and procainamide should be monitored. Although substantial procainamide is removed during dialysis, this amount is trivial compared to its metabolic elimination. However, the removal of NAPA is substantial and important, and a postdialysis dose of the drug may be necessary but should be monitored by plasma measurements of procainamide and NAPA.

The data concerning bretylium and disopyramide suggest that dosage must be reduced in patients with renal insufficiency. Although clinical experience has not yet been reported, in vitro data suggest that hemodialysis can remove substantial amounts of disopyramide and that postdialysis supplemental dosing will probably be required. Because there is marked variation in protein binding of this drug within the plasma concentration range commonly found in clinical practice, this drug may be difficult to use in renal insufficiency where variations in protein binding may be even larger.

Antilipemic Drugs

Clofibrate is converted rapidly to its active metabolite, chlorophenoxyisobutyric acid, then conjugated and excreted in the urine as the glucuronide. Its slow elimination in uremia suggests that the kidney may be the main site of conjugation. This drug has been associated with substantial myopathy in renal disease, particularly in patients with hypoproteinemia, for whom the free fraction of drug and metabolite are increased. Furthermore, clinical trials using this drug for prolonged periods of time have shown an increased incidence of gastrointestinal tumors and cholelithiasis. Dialysis is a route of substantial elimination of the drug in renal failure.

Cardiac Glycosides

Because of potential toxicity, it is best to avoid the use of digitalis whenever possible in uremic patients. Although digoxin is more commonly used for digitalization, its rate of elimination is much more affected by decreases in renal function than is that of digitoxin. The half-life, serum concentration, and volume of distribution of digitoxin are not significantly affected by renal failure. Thus, standard digitalizing and maintenance doses of digitoxin can be used in patients with renal failure. Although digitoxin is not removed substantially by hemodialysis because of a high level of protein binding, hemoperfusion is an effective way of removing digitoxin in cases of toxicity.

Digoxin, on the other hand, undergoes little metabolism and is mainly excreted by the kidney. Its rate of elimination is directly proportional to changes in GFR. Thus, the maintenance dose must be significantly reduced in renal insufficiency. Since considerable decreases in the volume of distribution of digoxin may occur with uremia, a 40–50% decrease in the usual loading dose of digoxin is suggested. Although the hemodialysis clearance of digoxin is close to that of plasma clearance in uremic patients, the large volume of distribution means that the fractional removal by hemodialysis is insignificant. Thus, supplemental doses after dialysis are not required.

Based on the foregoing, it is suggested that 5–10 µg/kg body weight of digoxin be given as a loading dose when acute digitalization is required, and then a maintenance dose of 0.125 mg be given on alternate days or 5 days per week. For digitoxin a 10 µg/kg loading dose followed by 0.1 mg daily or 5 days per week is reasonable. These dosage levels will result in a low, therapeutic, nontoxic serum concentration for digoxin of 0.84 ± 0.05 ng/ml and 19 ± 1 ng/ml for digitoxin.

One of the debates over therapy in the medical literature has been whether digoxin or digitoxin is the preferred glycoside in renal failure. Obviously, digitoxin is less altered by renal failure. However, digoxin is altered in a reasonably predictable manner. Thus, there is no definite preference if these agents are used cautiously.

There are several important drug interactions that have been described in recent years. For both digoxin and digitoxin, impaired absorption with resulting decrease in serum concentrations may occur with concomitant use of antacids, kaolin-pectin suspensions, sulfasalazine, neomycin, cholestyramine, or colestipol. Because of changes in distribution volume, increased concentrations of digoxin may be seen when quinidine is given concomitantly. On the other hand, decreased serum concentrations of digitoxin may be seen due to accelerated hepatic metabolism when phenobarbitol, other barbiturates, phenytoin, or phenylbutazone are being given.

Antihypertensive Agents
The use of antihypertensive agents is rarely complicated in the azotemic patient because the end-point of drug action—changes in blood pressure—is readily measurable. However, special precautions should be taken with several of these agents because of their decreased elimination in the azotemic patient. Particular attention is called to dosage reduction or increased interval administration with atenolol, captopril, guanethidine, hydralazine, and nadalol. Because of large volumes of distribution or substantial plasma protein binding, insignificant fractional removal of these drugs occurs during dialysis. Because hypertension is commonly extracellular-volume-dependent in patients with renal failure, every effort should be made to control hypertension by sodium restriction, diuretics, or dialysis in ESRD to control hypertension without the use of other agents. When this is not possible, any of these agents can be used for control of hypertension. However, because of different pharmacodynamic actions on cardiac output and peripheral vascular resistance, these drugs should be used selectively to modify hemodynamic parameters in the most appropriate way.

Central Nervous System Drugs (Appendix 6)

Analgesics
Acetaminophen, aspirin, codeine, meperidine, methadone, morphine, pentazocine, and propoxyphene can be administered in customary doses for the short-term treatment of pain in renal failure. With chronic use of meperidine or propoxyphene, a metabolite accumulates in uremic patients that has a toxic effect on the nervous system. Studies in animals have shown that the *N*-demethylated metabolite has half the analgesic potency but twice the convulsant potency. Uremic patients may also be somewhat more susceptible to the analgesic and sedative effects of all of these agents and should be titrated initially with small doses and monitored carefully. Although the short-term effects of salicylates are well tolerated, chronic use should be avoided because of their irritant effect on the gastrointestinal mucosa and the abnormalities in platelet function that are induced.

Anticonvulsant Agents
Current data suggest that no modification of the dosage of these drugs is required in treating uremic patients. The decreased plasma binding of phenytoin is associated with more rapid elimination; thus, the therapeutic concentration of the drug in the uremic patient is 5–10 mg/liter. Lack of appreciation of this reduction in the therapeutic level can produce toxicity if the dosage is increased in the uremic patient.

Since elimination of phenobarbitol is decreased in patients with severe renal failure, accumulation of the drug may occur with conventional doses. Furthermore, since these patients are probably more sensitive to the effects of barbiturates, lower doses should be used initially, and increased gradually until the desired effect in plasma concentration is attained or side effects are noted. A supplemental dose after dialysis may be needed.

Antiemetic Drugs
A new agent, metoclopramide, a dopamine antagonist, has recently been introduced in intravenous and oral formulations. It has powerful centrally acting antiemetic properties and a direct effect on gastrointestinal smooth muscle. It is approved as an adjunct to tube placement into the stomach and small bowel, to accelerate small bowel transit during fluoroscopic studies, to treat diabetic gastric stasis, and for short-term use in gastroesophageal reflux. The drug is well-absorbed, has a half-life of about 3 hours, and is mainly excreted unchanged in the urine or as a conjugate in the bile. It is weakly bound to plasma proteins and readily removed by conventional hemodialysis, but its large distribution volume prevents much drug removal during a conventional 4-hour hemodialysis session. Impaired renal function prolongs elimination and the half-life in ESRD is 14 hours. Therefore, dosage modification should be used in renal failure by increasing the interval between doses; for example, in ESRD a dose every 12 hours is appropriate. Postdialysis supplementation is not necessary.

Psychotherapeutic Drugs
Phenothiazines, benzodiazepines, and tricyclic agents are eliminated from the body by many metabolic pathways. They have all been used safely in patients with renal failure when given in customary doses. Lithium carbonate, useful in manic-depressive disorders, is excreted principally by the kidney and requires dosage reduction in uremic patients. Because of its low molecular weight and lack of plasma protein binding, significant fractional removal occurs during dialysis, and supplemental doses are necessary. Lithium should be avoided whenever possible and used only in extraordinary circumstances because of the risk of toxicity. If lithium is required, the plasma level should be maintained in the range of 0.6–1.2 mEq/liter. Most patients receiving chronic maintenance hemodialysis can be controlled with a single dose of 300–600 mg of lithium carbonate after each dialysis.

Hypnotics and Sedatives
Chloral hydrate, etchlorvynol, glutethimide, meprobamate, methaqualone, benzodiazepines (chlordiazepoxide, diazepam, flurazepam, lorazepam, oxazepam), and short-acting barbiturates are eliminated principally by nonrenal routes and can be given in customary doses to patients with renal failure. With the exception of some of the benzodiazepines and the

short-acting barbiturates, the pharmacokinetics of these drugs have not been studied in renal failure. Although several of them have high dialyzer clearances, only meprobamate and phenobarbital are significantly removed during hemodialysis therapy.

Diuretic Agents (Appendix 7)

Because of the marked reduction in GFR and filtered sodium, diuretic agents are much less effective in patients with decreased renal function. Practically speaking, thiazides are not useful when the endogenous creatinine clearance is less than 20 ml/min. However, more potent agents, such as furosemide and ethacrynic acid, may continue to be effective in high doses at this level of renal impairment. Patients who do not respond adequately to high doses of the loop diuretics may diurese if an agent such as metolazone, thiazide, or spironolactone is added; diuresis then occurs as a result of blockade of sodium transport at more distal sites in the nephron.

When the GFR is less than 30 ml/min, furosemide is the most effective diuretic. Daily doses up to 5 mg/kg body weight in divided doses may be required for adequate diuresis in some patients. Little toxicity is seen with the drug, except for transient tinnitus or decreased hearing. On the other hand, ethacrynic acid, another loop diuretic, exhibits no therapeutic advantages over furosemide but may have disadvantages in terms of toxicity. The alleged efficacy of ethacrynic acid in cases of furosemide resistance is more anecdotal than factual. Gastrointestinal symptoms as well as ototoxicity are more commonly observed with the use of ethacrynic acid than with furosemide.

The potassium-sparing diuretics—spironolactone, triamterene, and amiloride—should be administered with extreme caution, if at all, to patients with renal failure because of the danger of severe hyperkalemia.

Antidiabetic Drugs (Appendix 8)

Many uremic patients exhibit mild glucose intolerance caused by multiple defects in carbohydrate metabolism. Where antidiabetic drugs are required to adequately control blood glucose concentrations, insulin is probably the drug of choice. There is increasing evidence that better control of the blood glucose concentration may slow the progression of vascular disease and the concomitant development of retinopathy and nephropathy. Patients receiving CAPD for treatment of renal failure appear to do better when their insulin is administered in the peritoneal dialysis solution.

If hypoglycemic agents other than insulin are used, tolbutamide may be the safest because its elimination is principally nonrenal. However, other agents have been used successfully because the end-point, the blood glucose concentration, can be monitored easily.

REFERENCES

1. Cutler RE, Krichman KH, Blair AD: Pharmacology of drugs in renal failure, in Gonick HC (ed): *Current Nephrology*, vol 3. Boston, Houghton Mifflin, 1979, pp 397–435.
2. Anderson RJ, Schrier RW, Gambertoglio JG: *Clinical Use of Drugs in Patients with Kidney and Liver Disease*. Philadelphia, WB Saunders, 1981.
3. Gwilt PR, Perrier D: Plasma protein binding and distribution characteristics of drugs as indicies of their hemodialyzability. *Clin Pharmacol Ther* 24:154–161, 1978.
4. Dettli L: Elimination kinetics and dosage adjustments of drugs in patients with kidney disease. *Prog Pharmacol* 1:1–34, 1977.
5. *USP Dispensing Information*. Maryland, United States Pharmacopeial Convention, 1982.
6. Daneshmend TK, Warnock DW: Clinical pharmacokinetics of systemic antifungal drugs. *Clin Pharmacokin* 8:17–42, 1983.
7. Bullock WE, Luke RG, Nuttall CE, et al: Can mannitol reduce amphotericin B nephrotoxicity? Double-blind study and description of a new vascular lesion in the kidneys. *Antimicrob Agents Chemother* 10:555–563, 1976.
8. Reiner NE, Thompson WL: Dopamine and saralasin antagonist of renal vasoconstriction and oliguria caused by amphotericin B in dogs. *J Inf Dis* 140:564–575, 1979.
9. Churchill DN, Seely J: Nephrotoxicity associated with combined amphotericin B-gentamicin therapy. *Nephron* 19:176–181, 1977.
10. van der Meer JWM, Keuning JJ, Scheijgrond HW, et al: The influence of gastric acidity on the bio-availability of ketoconazole. *J Antimicrob Chemother* 6:552–554, 1980.
11. Schacter LP, Owellen RJ, Rathbun HK, et al: Antagonism between miconazole and amphotericin B. *Lancet* 2:318, 1976.
12. Bennett Wm, Elliott WC, Houghton DC, et al: Reduction of experimental gentamicin nephrotoxicity in rats by dietary calcium loading. *Antimicrob Agents Chemother* 22:508–512, 1982.
13. Thompson IB, Russo ME, Saxon BJ, et al: Gentamicin inactivation by piperacillin or carbenicillin in patients with end-stage renal disease. *Antimicrob Agents Chemother* 21:268–273, 1982.
14. Blair DC, Duggan DO, Schroeder ET: Inactivation of amikacin and gentamicin by carbenicillin patients with end-stage renal failure. *Antimicrob Agents Chemother* 22:376–379, 1982.
15. Forland SC, Cutler RE: Drugs in the kidney, in Gonick HC (ed): *Current Nephrology*, vol 6. New York, John Wiley & Sons, 1983, pp 115–150.
16. Freston JW: Cimetidine. II. Adverse reactions and patterns of use. *Ann Intern Med* 97:728–734, 1982.
17. Albibi R, McCallum RW: Metoclopramide pharmacology and clinical application. *Ann Intern Med* 98:86–95, 1983.
18. Laskin OL, Longstreth JA, Whelton A, et al: Acyclovir kinetics in end-stage renal disease. *Clin Pharmacol Ther* 31:594–601, 1982.
19. Miranda P, Good SS, Laskin OL, et al: Disposition of intravenous radioactive acyclovir. *Clin Pharmacol Ther* 30:662–672, 1981.
20. Soung L-S, Ing TS, Daugirdas JT, et al: Amantadine hydrochloride pharmacokinetics in hemodialysis patients. *Ann Intern Med* 93:46–49, 1980.
21. Horadam VW, Sharp JG, Smilack JD, et al: Pharmacokinetics of amantadine hydrochloride in subjects with normal and impaired renal function. *Ann Intern Med* 94:454–458, 1981.
22. Spyker DA, Gober LL, Scheld WM, et al: Pharmacokinetics of cefaclor in renal failure: Effects of multiple doses and hemodialysis. *Antimicrob Agents Chemother* 21:278–281, 1982.

23. Barriere SL, Gambertoglio JG, Alexander DP, et al: Pharmacokinetics of cefonicid in patients with renal insufficiency on hemodialysis. *J Inf Dis* (in press).
24. Pitkin D, Dubb J, Actor P, et al: Kinetics and renal handling of cefonicid. *Clin Pharmacol Ther* 30:587–593, 1981.
25. Barriere SL, Hatheway GJ, Gambertoglio JG, et al: Pharmacokinetics of cefonicid, a new broad-spectrum cephalosporin. *Antimicrob Agents Chemother* 21:935–938, 1982.
26. Bolton WK, Scheld WM, Spyker DA, et al: Pharmacokinetics of cefoperazone in normal volunteers and subjects with renal insufficiency. *Antimicrob Agents Chemother* 19:821–825, 1981.
27. Ings RMJ, Fillastre JP, Godin M, et al: The pharmacokinetics of cefotaxime and its metabolites in subjects with normal and impaired renal function. *Rev Inf Dis* 4:S379–S391, 1982.
28. Bolton WK, Scheld MW, Spyker DA, et al: Pharmacokinetics of moxalactam in subjects with various degrees of renal dysfunction. *Antimicrob Agents Chemother* 18:933–938, 1980.
29. Leroy A, Humbert G, Fillastre JP: Pharmacokinetics of moxalactam in subjects with normal and impaired renal function. *Antimicrob Agents Chemother* 19:965–971, 1981.
30. Aronoff GR, Sloan RS, Luft FC: Pharmacokinetics of moxalactam in patients with normal and impaired renal function. *J Inf Dis* 145:365–369, 1982.
31. Aronoff GR, Sloan RS, Mong SA, et al: Moxalactam pharmacokinetics during hemodialysis. *Antimicrob Agents Chemother* 19:575–577, 1981.
32. Peterson LR, Bean B, Fasching CE, et al: Pharmacokinetics, protein binding, and predicted extravascular distribution of moxalactam in normal and renal failure subjects. *Antimicrob Agents Chemother* 20:378–381, 1981.
33. Lam M, Manion CV, Czerwinski AW: Pharmacokinetics of moxalactam in patients with renal insufficiency. *Antimicrob Agents Chemother* 19:462–464, 1981.
34. Srinivasan S, Neu HC: Pharmacokinetics of moxalactam in patients with renal failure and during hemodialysis. *Antimicrob Agents Chemother* 20:398–400, 1981.
35. Luthy R, Blaser J, Bonetti A, et al: Comparative multiple-dose pharmacokinetics of cefotaxime, moxalactam, and ceftazidime. *Antimicrob Agents Chemother* 20:567–575, 1981.
36. Scheld M, Spyker DA, Donowitz GR, et al: Moxalactam and cefazolin: Comparative pharmacokinetics in normal subjects. *Antimicrob Agents Chemother* 19:613–619, 1981.
37. Leroy A, Humbert G, Godin M, et al: Pharmacokinetics of azlocillin in subjects with normal and impaired renal function. *Antimicrob Agents Chemother* 17:344–349, 1980.
38. Fiegel P, Becker K: Pharmacokinetics of azlocillin in persons with normal and impaired renal functions. *Antimicrob Agents Chemother* 14:288–291, 1978.
39. Aletta JM, Francke EF, Neu HC: Intravenous azlocillin kinetics in patients on long-term hemodialysis. *Clin Pharmacol Ther* 27:563–566, 1980.
40. Aronoff GR: Mezlocillin elimination in patients with impaired renal function. *J Antimicron Chemother* 9:77S–79S, 1982.
41. Bergan T, Brodwall EK, Wiik-Larsen E: Mezlocillin pharmacokinetics in patients with normal and impaired renal functions. *Antimicrob Agents Chemother* 16:651–654, 1979.
42. Mangione A, Janicke DM, Boudinot FD, et al: Dose-dependent pharmacokinetics of mezlocillin in subjects with normal and impaired renal function. *J Antimicrob Chemother* 9:81S–85S, 1982.
43. Janicke DM, Mangione A, Schultz RW, et al: Mezlocillin disposition in chronic hemodialysis patients. *Antimicrob Agents Chemother* 20:590–594, 1981.
44. Aronoff GR, Sloan RS, Luft FC, et al: Mezlocillin pharmacokinetics in renal impairment. *Clin Pharmacol Ther* 28:523–528, 1980.
45. Francke E, Mehta S, Neu HC, et al: Kinetics of intravenous mezlocillin in chronic hemodialysis patients. *Clin Pharmacol Ther* 26:228–231, 1979.

46. Bergan T, Williams JD: Dose dependence of piperacillin pharmacokinetics. *Chemother* 28:153–159, 1982.
47. Batra VK, Morrison JA, Lasseter KC, et al: Piperacillin kinetics. *Clin Pharmacol Ther* 26:41–53, 1979.
48. Thompson MIB, Russo ME, Matsen JM, et al: Piperacillin pharmacokinetics in subjects with chronic renal failure. *Antimicrob Agents Chemother* 19:450–453, 1981.
49. Gabriel R, Page CM, Weller IVD, et al: The pharmacokinetics of metronidazole in patients with chronic renal failure. Proceedings of the Second International Symposium of Anaerobic Infections, Geneva, 1979.
50. Ralph ED, Clarke JT, Libke RD, et al: Pharmacokinetics of metronidazole as determined by bioassay. *Antimicrob Agents Chemother* 6:691–696, 1974.
51. Tocco DJ, Breault GO, Zacchei AG, et al: Physiological disposition and metabolism of 5-(2,4-difluorophenyl)salicylic acid, a new salicylate. *Drug Metab Dispos* 3:453–466, 1975.
52. Verbeeck RK, DeSchepper PJ: Influence of chronic renal failure and hemodialysis on diflunisal plasma protein binding. *Clin Pharmacol Ther* 27:628–635, 1980.
53. Verbeeck R, Tijandromaga TB, Mullie A, et al: Biotransformation of diflunisal and renal excretion of its glucuronides in renal insufficiency. *Br J Clin Pharmacol* 7:273–282, 1979.
54. Wiseman EH, Hobbs DC: Review of pharmacokinetic studies with piroxicam. *Am J Med* 72:9–17, 1982.
55. Hobbs DC, Twomey TM: Piroxicam pharmacokinetics in man: aspirin and antacid interaction studies. *J Clin Pharmacol* 19:270–281, 1979.
56. Ishizaki T, Nomura T, Abe T: Pharmacokinetics of piroxicam, a new nonsteroidal anti-inflammatory agent, under fasting and postprandial states in man. *J Pharmacokinet Biopharm* 7:369–381, 1979.
57. Fouda HG, Hobbs DC, Stambaugh JE: Sensitive assay for determination of hydroxyzine in plasma and its human pharmacokinetics. *J Pharm Sci* 68:1456–1458, 1979.
58. Droz JP, Macquet JP: Kinetics of cisplatin in an anuric patient undergoing hemofiltration dialysis. *Cancer Treatment Rep* 65:665–668, 1981.
59. LeRoy A, Bachur NR, Wiernik PH: High-dose cisplatin therapy using mannitol versus furosemide diuresis: Comparative pharmacokinetics and toxicity. *Cancer Treatment Rep* 65:73–78, 1981.
60. Narang PK, Adir J, Josselson J, et al: Pharmacokinetics of bretylium in man after intravenous administration. *J Pharmacokinet Biopharm* 8:363–372, 1980.
61. Anderson JL, Patterson E, Wagner JG, et al: Oral and intravenous bretylium disposition. *Clin Pharmacol Ther* 28:468–478, 1980.
62. Connolly SJ, Kates RE: Clinical pharmacokinetics of N-acetylprocainamide. *Clin Pharmacokin* 7:206–220, 1982.
63. Stec GP, Atkinson AF Jr, Nevin MJ, et al: N-acetylprocainamide pharmacokinetics in functionally anephric patients before and after perturbation by hemodialysis. *Clin Pharmacol Ther* 26:681–682, 1979.
64. Meier J: Pharmacokinetic comparison of pindolol with other beta-adrenoceptor-blocking agents. *Am Heart J* 104:364–373, 1982.
65. Flouvat B, Decourt S, Aubert P, et al: Pharmacokinetics of atenolol in patients with terminal renal failure and influence of haemodialysis. *Br J Clin Pharmacol* 9:379–385, 1980.
66. Heel RC, Brogden TM, Speight TM, et al: Captopril: A preliminary review of its pharmacological properties and therapeutic efficacy. *Drugs* 20:409–452, 1980.
67. Johnson G, Regardh CG, Sulvell L: Combined pharmacokinetic and pharmacodynamic studies in man of the adrenergic β-receptor antagonist metoprolol. *Acta Pharmacol Toxicol* 36:31–44, 1975.

68. Seiler KU, Schuster KJ, Meyer GJ, et al: The pharmacokinetics of metoprolol and its metabolites in dialysis patients. *Clin Pharmacokinet* 5:192–198, 1980.
69. Jordo L, Attman PO, Aurell M, et al: Pharmacokinetic and pharmacodynamic properties of metoprolol in patients with impaired renal function. *Clin Pharmacokinet* 5:169–180, 1980.
70. Gottlieb TB, Thomas RC, Chidsey CA: Pharmacokinetic studies of minoxidil. *Clin Pharmacol Ther* 13:436–441, 1972.
71. Lowenthal DT, Onesti G, Mutterperl R, et al: Long-term clinical effects, bioavailability, and kinetics of minoxidil, a new antihypertensive agent. *J Clin Pharmacol* 18:500–508, 1978.
72. Dreyfuss J, Brannick LJ, Vukovich RA, et al: Metabolic studies in patients with nadolol: Oral and intravenous administration. *J Clin Pharmacol* 17:300–307, 1977.
73. Frishman W: Clinical pharmacology of the new beta-adrenergic blocking drugs. Part 9. Nadolol: A new long-acting beta-adrenoceptor blocking drug. *Am Heart J* 99:124–128, 1980.
74. Herrera J, Vukovich RA, Griffith DL: Elimination of nadolol by patients with renal impairment. *Br J Clin Pharmacol* 7:227S–231S, 1979.
75. Chau NP, Weiss YA, Safar ME, et al: Pindolol availability in hypertensive patients with normal and impaired renal function. *Clin Pharmacol Ther* 22:505–510, 1977.
76. Lavene D, Weiss YA, Safar ME, et al: Pharmacokinetics and hepatic extraction ratio of pindolol in hypertensive patients with normal and impaired renal function. *J Clin Pharmacol* 17:501–508, 1977.
77. Lowenthal DT, Pitone JM, Affrime MB, et al: Timolol kinetics in chronic renal insufficiency. *Clin Pharmacol Ther* 23:606–615, 1978.
78. Tocco DJ, Duncan AEW, DeLuna FA, et al: Physiological disposition and metabolism of timolol in man and laboratory animals. *Drug Metab Dispos* 3:361–370, 1975.
79. Eichelbaum M: Clinical pharmacokinetics of calcium ion antagonists. *Clin Invest Med* 3:13–17, 1980.
80. McAuley BJ, Schroeder JS: The use of diltiazem hydrochloride in cardiovascular disorders. *Pharmacotherapy* 2:121–131, 1982.
81. Zelis RF, Kinney E: The pharmacokinetics of diltiazem in healthy American men. *Am J Cardiol* 40:529–532, 1982.
82. Ross-Lee LM, Eadie MJ, Hooper WD, et al: Single-dose pharmacokinetics of metoclopramide. *Eur J Clin Pharmacol* 20:465–471, 1981.
83. Bateman DN, Gokal R, Dodd TR, et al: The pharmacokinetics of single doses of metoclopramide in renal failure. *Eur J Clin Pharmacol* 19:437–441, 1981.

Generic Names and Proprietary Equivalents of Frequently Used Drugs

acetaminophen (many choices)
acetazolamide (Diamox, Hydrazol)
acetylsalicylic acid (aspirin)
acyclovir (Zovirax)
allopurinol (Zyloprim)
amantadine (Symmetrel)
amikacin (Amikin)
amitriptyline (Elavil, Endep, SK-Amitriptyline)
amoxicillin (Amoxil, Larotid, Polymax, Trimox, Wymox)
amphotericin B (Fungizone)
ampicillin (Amcill, Omnipen, Pfizerpen-A, Polycillin, SK-Ampicillin)
atenolol (Tenormin)
azathioprine (Imuran)
azlocillin (Azlin)

bleomycin (Blenoxane)
bretylium (Bretylol)
bumetanide

captopril (Capoten)
carbamazepine (Tegretol)
carbenicillin (Geopen, Pyopen)
cefaclor (Ceclor)
cefadroxil (Duricef, Ultracef)
cefamandole (Mandol)
cefazolin (Ancef, Kefzol)
cefonicid
cefoperazone (Cefobid)
cefotaxime (Claforan)
cefoxitin (Mefoxin)
cephalexin (Ceporex, Keflex)
cephaloridine (Ceporin, Loridine)
cephalothin (Keflin)
cephapirin (Cefadyl)
cephradine (Anspor, Eskacef, Velosef)
chloral hydrate (Noctec, SK-Chloral Hydrate)
chloramphenicol (Amphicol, Chlorcetin, Chloromycetin, Econochlor, Kemicetine, Paraxin)
chlordiazepoxide (A-poxide, Libritabs, Librium, Menrium, Screen, SK-Lygen)
chlorpheniramine (many choices)

chlorpromazine (Thorazine)
chlorthalidone (Hygroton)
cimetidine (Tagamet)
cisplatin (Platinol)
clindamycin (Cleocin)
clofibrate (Atromid-S)
clonazepam (Clonopin)
clonidine (Catapres)
cloxacillin (Cloxapen, Tegopen)
colchicine
colistimethate (Coly-Mycin-M)
cyclophosphamide (Cytoxan)
cytosine arabinoside (Cytarabine HCl)

dapsone (Avlosulfon)
demeclocycline (Declomycin, Declostatin)
desipramine (Norpramin, Pertofrane)
diazepam (Valium)
diazoxide (Hyperstat, Proglem)
dicloxacillin (Dynapen, Pathocil, Veracillin)
diflunisal (Dolobid)
digitoxin (Crystodigin, De-Tone, Digitaline Nativelle, Maso-Toxin, Purodigin)
digoxin (Lanoxin, Masoxin, SK-Digoxin)
diltiazem (Cardizem)
diphenhydramine (many choices)
disopyramide (Norpace)
doxorubicin (Adriamycin)
doxycycline (Doxycycline, Vibramycin, Vibra-Tabs)

erythromycin (Dowmycin, E-Mycin, Erythrocin, Ethril 500, Ilotycin, Robimycin, RP-Mycin)
ethacrynic acid (Edecrin)
ethambutol (Myambutol)
ethchlorvynol (Arvynol, Placidyl, Serensil)
ethosuximide (Zarontin)

fenoprofen (Nalfon)
flucytosine (Ancobon)
fluorouracil (Adrucil, Fluorouracil)

(continued)

Generic Names and Proprietary Equivalents of Frequently Used Drugs

flurazepam (Dalmane)
furosemide (Furosemide, Lasix, SK-Furosemide)

gentamicin (Garamycin)
glutethimide (Dorimide, Doriden, Rolathimide)
griseofulvin (Fulcin, Fulvicin, Grifulvin, Grisactin, Grisowen, Gris-Peg)
guanethidine (Ismelin)

haloperidol (Haldol)
heparin (Hepathrom, Heprinar, Lipo-Hepin, Liquaemin, Panheprin)
hydralazine (Apresoline, Apresazide, Hydralazide, Unipres)
hydrochlorothiazide (many choices)
hydroxyzine (Atarax, Hyzine, Vistarex, Vistazine, Vistaril)

ibuprofen (Brufen, Motrin)
imipramine (Imavate, Janimine, Presamine, SK-Pramine, Tofranil)
indomethacin (Indocin)
isoniazid (INH, Laniazid, Niconyl, Nydrazid, Rolazid, Teebaconin, Triniad, Uniad)

kanamycin (Kantrex, Klebcil)
ketoconazole (Nizoral)

lidocaine (many choices)
lincomycin (Lincocin)
lithium carbonate (Eskalith, Lithane, Lithobid, Lithonate, Lithotabs)

meclofenamate (Meclomen)
mefenamic acid (Ponstel)
meperidine (Demerol, Mepergan)
meprobamate (Arcoban, Equanil, Meprocon, Meprotabs, Miltown, SK-Bamate)
methadone (Dolophine, Methadone)
methaqualone (Mequin, Parest, Quaalude)
methenamine (Cystitol, Lanased, Uramine, Uricide, Urised, Urostat Forte)

methicillin (Staphcillin)
methotrexate (Amethopterin)
methyldopa (Aldomet, Aldoclor, Aldoril)
metoclopramide (Reglan)
metolazone (Zaroxolyn, Diulo)
metoprolol (Lopressor)
metronidazole (Flagyl, Metryl, Satric)
mezlocillin (Mezlin)
miconazole (Monistat)
minocycline (Minocin, Vectrin)
minoxidil (Loniten)
morphine
moxalactam (Moxam)

nadolol (Corgard)
nafcillin (Nafcil, Unipen)
nalidixic acid (Neggram)
naproxen (Anaprox, Naprosyn)
nifedipine (Procardia)
nitrofurantoin (Cyantin, Furadantin, Furalan, Furantoin, Nitrofor-50, Urotoin)
nortriptyline (Aventyl, Pamelor)

oxacillin
oxazepam (Serax)
oxytetracycline (Oxymycin, Terramycin, Urobiotic)

penicillin G (many choices)
pentazocine (Talwin)
pentobarbital (Nembutal)
phenobarbital (many choices)
phenylbutazone (Azolid, Butazolidin)
phenytoin (Dihycon, Dilantin, Di-Phenyl, Toin)
pindolol (Visken)
piperacillin (Pipracil)
piroxicam (Feldene)
prazosin (Minipress)
primidone (Mysoline, Primidone)
probenecid (Benacen, Benemid, Benn, Probalan, Robenecid)
procainamide (Pronestyl, Sub-Quin)
propoxyphene (Darvon, Dolene, Myopaz, Progesic, Pro-Pox, Ropoxy, Scrip-Dyne)
propranolol (Inderal)

(continued)

Generic Names and Proprietary Equivalents of Frequently Used Drugs

quinidine (Cin-Quin, Maso-Quin, Quinidex, Quinora, SK-Quinidine)

reserpine (many choices)
rifampin (Rifomycin, Rimactane, Rimactazid)

secobarbital (many choices)
spironolactone (Aldactone)
streptomycin
sulfamethoxazole (Bactrim, Gantanol, Septra)
sulfinpyrazone (Anturane)
sulfisoxazole (Barazole, Gantrisin, G-Sox, Rosoxol, SK-Soxazole, Sulfizin, Urizole)
sulindac (Clinoril)

tetracycline (many choices)
ticarcillin (Ticar)
timolol (Blocadren)
tobramycin sulfate (Nebcin)
tolbutamide (Orinase, SK-Tolbutamide)
tolmetin (Tolectin)
triamterene (Dyrenium, Dyazide)
trimethoprim (Bactrim, Septra)

valproic acid (Depakene, Labazene)
vancomycin (Vancocin)
verapamil (Calan, Isoptin)
viomycin sulfate (Viocin)

warfarin (Coumadin, Panwarfin)

zomepirac (Zomax)

Appendix 1. Antiinfective Drugs

Drug Name	Apparent VD (L/kg)	Terminal Half-Life (hr) NL	Terminal Half-Life (hr) ESRD	F_0	Plasma Clearance (ml/min) NL	Plasma Clearance (ml/min) ESRD	Percent Excreted Unchanged[a]	Percent Protein Bound[a]	Dialyzer Clearance (ml/min)	Reference
Antifungal drugs										
Amphotericin B	0.46[b]	24	40	0.6	15	9	2–5	90–95	NS	1, 2, 5
Flucytosine	0.70	5	85	0.07	113	7	76–107	4	110	1, 2, 5
Griseofulvin	1.6	14	20	0.7	95	65	1	—	—	1, 2, 5
Ketoconazole	—	8[c]	—	—	—	—	2–4	99	NS	6
Miconazole	21	24	24	1.0	700	700	1	92	NS	6
Antitubercular drugs										
Ethambutol	1.6	3	10	0.3	435	130	50–65	20–30	50	1, 2, 5
Isoniazid	0.60	1[d]	4	0.25[d]	485[d]	120	7[d]	1–10	50	1, 2, 5
	—	3[e]	4	0.75[e]	160[e]	—	37[e]	1–10	50	1, 2, 5
Rifampin	0.93	4	4	1.0	215	215	5–15	60–90	NS	1, 2, 5
Antiviral drugs										
Acyclovir	0.6	2–3	19.5	0.1	300	—	60–90	15.4	82	18, 19
Amantadine	4.5	12	192	0.06	306	20	90	—	67	20, 21
Aminoglycosides										
Amikacin	0.25	2.5	70	0.04	90	3	81–98	<10	18	1, 2, 5
Gentamicin	0.24	2	60	0.03	95	2	80–90	<10	24	1, 2, 5
Kanamycin	0.23	2	80	0.03	95	2	84–90	<10	25	1, 2, 5
Streptomycin	0.26	2.5	80	0.03	85	3	41–87	35	22	1, 2, 5
Tobramycin	0.23	2.5	60	0.04	80	3	80–90	<10	27	1, 2, 5
Cephalosporins										
Cefaclor	0.24	0.8	2.8	0.3	240	69	—	24	60	22
Cefadroxil	0.26	1.5	17	0.09	142	10	88–93	20	35	1, 2, 5
Cefamandole	0.16	0.7	15	0.05	109	9	65–85	67–80	9	1, 2, 5

Cefazolin	0.14	1.8	27	0.07	60	5	80–90	70–85	10	1, 2, 5
Cefonicid	0.11	5	70	0.07	18	1	88	98	3	23–25
Cefoperazone	0.22	1.8	2.0	0.9	100	90	20–30	65–90	—	26
Cefotaxime	0.28	1	2.5	0.4	322	135	40–60	36	81	27
	—	1.3[f]	15[f]	0.09[f]	—	—	—	—	[g]	27
Cefoxitin	0.30	0.9	22	0.04	290	12	80–90	50–60	—	1, 2, 5
Cephalexin	0.26	0.8	20	0.04	263	10	90–98	10–15	70	1, 2, 5
Cephaloridine	0.23	1.5	20	0.08	128	9	56–68	10–30	34	1, 2, 5
Cephalothin	0.26	0.6	10	0.06	350	21	60–70	60–65	—	1, 2, 5
Cephapirin	0.23	0.6	2	0.3	310	93	50–70	44–54	—	1, 2, 5
Cephradine	0.31	1.0	12	0.08	323	20	78–96	8–20	—	1, 2, 5
Moxalactam	0.3	2.5	20	0.13	97	12	70–90	50	45	28–36
Penicillins										
Amoxicillin	0.2	1	9	0.1	160	25	50–70	15–25	23	1, 2, 5
Ampicillin	0.48	1.2	14	0.09	325	30	50–90	16–20	46	1, 2, 5
Azlocillin	0.22	1	6	0.17	175	40	60–70	28	50	37–39
Carbenicillin	0.19	1.0	15	0.07	155	10	82	50	18	1, 2, 5
Cloxacillin	0.15	0.6	0.8	0.75	220	115	62–78	85–95	NS	1, 2, 5
Dicloxacillin	0.20	0.7	1.0	0.7	225	160	73–90	97	NS	1, 2, 5
Methicillin	0.31	0.5	5	0.1	495	50	50–70	28–49	—	1, 2, 5
Mezlocillin	0.2	1	3.6	0.27	250	50	45–70	16–42	60	40–45
Nafcillin	0.32	0.5	1.2	0.4	520	215	35–40	90	NS	1, 2, 5
Oxacillin	0.21	0.5	1.0	0.5	335	170	40–55	93	NS	1, 2, 5
Penicillin G	0.18	0.7	13	0.05	205	10	75–90	65	12	1, 2, 5
Piperacillin	0.21	1	3.3	0.3	188	57	50–70	21	50	46–48
Ticarcillin	0.21	1.2	11	0.1	140	15	90–100	45	35	1, 2, 5
Sulfonamides										
Sulfamethoxazole	0.36	10	35	0.29	30	10	16–33	60–68	16	1, 2, 5
Sulfisoxazole	0.20	6	12	0.5	30	15	50–70	40–90	—	1, 2, 5

Appendix 1. (*continued*)

Drug Name	Apparent VD (L/kg)	Terminal Half-Life (hr) NL	Terminal Half-Life (hr) ESRD	F_0	Plasma Clearance (ml/min) NL	Plasma Clearance (ml/min) ESRD	Percent Excreted Unchanged[a]	Percent Protein Bound[a]	Dialyzer Clearance (ml/min)	Reference
Tetracyclines										
Demeclocycline	1.8	12	50	0.24	121	29	40–50	75–91	—	1, 2, 5
Doxycycline	0.7	20	20	1.0	29	29	15–35	80–93	—	1, 2, 5
Minocycline	0.40	18	16	1.0	40	40	5–15	75	—	1, 2, 5
Oxytetracycline	1.4	9	60	0.15	125	19	70	27–35	—	1, 2, 5
Tetracycline	1.5	9	80	0.11	131	14	48–60	25–65	—	1, 2, 5
Chloramphenicol	0.9	3	5	0.06	245	147	5–10	25–60	NS	1, 2, 5
Miscellaneous										
Clindamycin	0.7	2.3	4	0.6	250	150	10–28	94	NS	1, 2, 5
Colistimethate	0.47	6	15	0.4	70	25	60–75	—	—	1, 2, 5
Erythromycin	0.57	2	5	0.4	310	90	15	73–93	NS	1, 2, 5
Lincomycin	0.44	5	10	0.5	72	35	9–30	72	NS	1, 2, 5
Metronidazole	0.7	7	7	1.0	82	82	20	20	—	49, 50
Nalidixic acid	0.4	2	2	1.0	163	163	2–3	93	60	1, 2, 5
Nitrofurantoin	0.5	0.3	1	0.3	1360	408	30–50	60	60	1, 2, 5
Trimethoprim	2.0	13	25	0.5	125	65	80–90	40–70	100	1, 2, 5
Vancomycin	0.47	7	240	0.03	55	2	90–100	10	NS	1, 2, 5

[a] In normal humans.
[b] Reported by one investigator.
[c] The rapid elimination half-life as reported by most authors is 1.5–2 hours.
[d] Rapid acetylators.
[e] Slow acetylators.
[f] Desacetyl cefotaxime.
[g] Half-life decreased from 14 hours to 3 hours during dialysis.
NS, No significant removal but actual clearance unknown.

Appendix 2. Antiarthritic Drugs

Drug Name	Apparent VD (L/kg)	Terminal Half-Life (hr) NL	Terminal Half-Life (hr) ESRD	F_0	Plasma Clearance (ml/min) NL	Plasma Clearance (ml/min) ESRD	Percent Excreted Unchanged[a]	Percent Protein Bound[a]	Dialyzer Clearance (ml/min)	Reference
Allopurinol	0.6	5	—	—	245	—	30	0	—	1, 2, 5
	—	24[b]	—	—	—	—	60	0[b]	100[b]	1, 2, 5
Colchicine	2.1	0.3	0.7	0.43	5650	2420	20–50	0	NS	1, 2, 5
Diflunisal	7.5	11	115	0.09	8	2	3	99.9	NS	51–53
Fenoprofen	0.15	3	—	—	—	—	<5	>90	NS	1, 2, 5
Ibuprofen	—	2.0	—	—	—	—	<5	>90	NS	1, 2, 5
Indomethacin	1.0	5	5	1.0	163	163	10–20	>90	NS	1, 2, 5
Meclofenamate	—	3	—	—	—	—	66	>90	NS	1, 2, 5
Mefenamic acid	—	3	—	—	—	—	—	>90	NS	1, 2, 5
Naproxen	0.1	14	14	1.0	6	6	<10	>90	NS	1, 2, 5
Piroxicam	0.14	38	[c]	—	3	[c]	2–5	99	NS	54–56
Phenylbutazone	0.17	84	60	1.4	2	3	<5	90	NS	1, 2, 5
Probenecid	0.13	7[d]	—	—	15	—	4–13	83–94	NS	1, 2, 5
Sulindac	—	8	—	—	—	—	20–50	>90	NS	1, 2, 5
	—	16[e]	—	—	—	—	—	—	—	1, 2, 5
Tolmetin	—	1	—	—	—	—	17	>90	NS	1, 2, 5
Zomepirac	—	10	—	—	—	—	—	>90	NS	1, 2, 5

[a] In normal humans.
[b] Oxypurinol.
[c] Reported to be normal.
[d] Dose dependent.
[e] Half-life of active sulfide metabolite.
NS, no significant removal but actual clearance unknown.

Appendix 3. Anticoagulant and Antihistamine Drugs

Drug Name	Apparent VD (L/kg)	Terminal Half-Life (hr) NL	Terminal Half-Life (hr) ESRD	F_0	Plasma Clearance (ml/min) NL	Plasma Clearance (ml/min) ESRD	Percent Excreted Unchanged[a]	Percent Protein Bound[a]	Dialyzer Clearance (ml/min)	Reference
Anticoagulants										
Heparin	0.06	1.5[b]	1.5	1	30	30	50[c]	>90	NS	1, 2, 5
Warfarin	0.11	33	30	1.1	3	3	<1	97	NS	1, 2, 5
Antihistamines										
Cimetidine	0.81	2	5	0.4	330	132	45–75	13–25	50	1, 2, 5
Chlorpheniramine	2.5	13	—	—	155	—	—	72	NS	1, 2, 5
Diphenhydramine	3.7	5.2	—	—	575	—	<4	98	NS	1, 2, 5
Hydroxyzine	—	3.0	—	—	—	—	—	—	—	57

[a] In normal humans.
[b] Increases with dose: 100 U/kg = 1.0 hours; 200 U/kg = 1.5 hours; 400 U/kg = 2.5 hours.
[c] Usually excreted as a metabolite; unchanged drug appears at high doses only.
NS, no significant removal but actual clearance unknown.

Appendix 4. Antineoplastic and Immunosuppresive Drugs

Drug Name	Apparent VD (L/kg)	Terminal Half-Life (hr) NL	Terminal Half-Life (hr) ESRD	F_0	Plasma Clearance (ml/min) NL	Plasma Clearance (ml/min) ESRD	Percent Excreted Unchanged[a]	Percent Protein Bound[a]	Dialyzer Clearance (ml/min)	Reference
Adriamycin	—	30	—	—	—	—	3.4–5	—	NS	1, 2, 5
Azathioprine	0.6	3	—	—	—	—	10	30	—	1, 2, 5
Bleomycin	0.35	0.5	>21[b]	0.02	565	—	31–88	—	NS	1, 2, 5
Cisplatin	—	225	120[c]	1.0	—	—	—	NS	NS	58, 59
Cyclophosphamide	0.64	6.5	6.5	1.0	56	56	21–45	13	78	1, 2, 5
Cytosine arabinose	—	2	—	—	—	—	10	—	—	1, 2, 5
5-Fluorouracil	0.63	0.3	—	—	—	—	20	—	—	1, 2, 5
Methotrexate	0.64[d]	10[e]	64	0.16	52	5	76–80	50–70	—	1, 2, 5

[a] In normal humans.
[b] Data on one person with Cl_{cr} = 11 ml/min.
[c] Report of one investigator.
[d] Volume of distribution reduced to 0.42 L/kg in ESRD.
[e] Following high-dose treatment.
NS, no significant removal but actual clearance unknown.

Appendix 5. Cardiovascular Drugs

Drug Name	Apparent VD (L/kg)	Terminal Half-Life (hr) NL	Terminal Half-Life (hr) ESRD	F_o	Plasma Clearance (ml/min) NL	Plasma Clearance (ml/min) ESRD	Percent Excreted Unchanged[a]	Percent Protein Bound[a]	Dialyzer Clearance (ml/min)	Reference
Antiarrhythmic drugs										
Bretylium	7.0	7.8	—	—	725	—	77	0–1	—	60, 61
Disopyramide	0.48	7	30	0.23	55	13	40–60	5–65[b]	30	1, 2, 5
Lidocaine	1.2	2	2	1.0	606	606	<10	66	NS	1, 2, 5
Procainamide	2.0	2	8	0.25	810	200	40–54	15	65	1, 2, 5
	1.5[c]	6[c]	42[c]	0.14[c]	200[c]	29[c]	59–89[c]	10[c]	97[c]	62, 63
Quinidine	2.0	6	6	1.0	270	270	10–50	80–85	<10	1, 2, 5
Antihypertensive drugs										
Atenolol	1.2	5.5	73.4	0.07	176	13	—	<5	29–39	64–65
Captopril	3.0	1.9	35	0.05	1277	69	50	25–30	120	66[d]
Clonidine	3.2	8	—	—	315	—	—	—	—	1, 2, 5
Diazoxide	0.12	25	56	0.45	7	3	50	94[e]	25	1, 2, 5
Guanethidine	60	120	245	0.5	400	200	35–50	0	NS	1, 2, 5
Hydralazine	1.6	3	>16	0.19	431	<80	3–14	87	NS	1, 2, 5
Methyldopa	0.69	2	5	0.4	280	104	24	0	—	1, 2, 5
Metoprolol	4.5	3.5	4	0.75	1000	1000	3–10	12	NS	67–69
Minoxidil	2.5	4.2	—	—	588	—	10	0	—	70, 71
Nadolol	2.0	10–14	44.7	0.22	—	—	70	20–30	46–102	72–74

Pindolol	2.0	3–4	—	—	538	—	—	40	—	64, 75, 76
Prazosin	0.94	3	—	—	255	—	—	97	NS	1, 2, 5
Propranolol	3.0	3.5	3.5	1.0	695	695	0	93	0	1, 2, 5
Reserpine	1.7	60	185	0.32	23	7	1	40	—	1, 2, 5
Timolol	3.5	3.5	3.5	1.0	225	—	20	10	NS	64, 74, 75
Antilipemic drugs										
Clofibrate	0.12[f]	8.6	80	0.11	11	2	32	96	<10	1, 2, 5
Calcium blocking drugs										
Diltiazem	—	5	—	—	—	—	2	80–85	—	79–81
Nifedipine	—	2	—	—	—	—	[g]	—	—	79
Verapamil	5	3.7	—	—	1000	—	3	90	—	79
Cardiac glycosides										
Digitoxin	0.5	145	200	0.73	3	2	8–30	90[h]	NS	1, 2, 5
Digoxin	7.1[h]	36	100	0.36	160	35	>90	20–30	20	1, 2, 5

[a] In normal men.
[b] Binding is concentration dependent.
[c] N-acetylprocainamide.
[d] Duchin K: personal communication; data on file at Squibb.
[e] Binding is 84% in ESRD.
[f] Vd = 0.22 liters/kg in uremic patients.
[g] Binding is 86%–89% in ESRD.
[h] Vd = 4.2 liters/kg in uremic patients.
NS, no significant removal but actual clearance unknown.

Appendix 6. Central Nervous System Drugs

Drug Name	Apparent VD (L/kg)	Terminal Half-Life (hr) NL	Terminal Half-Life (hr) ESRD	F_0	Plasma Clearance (ml/min) NL	Plasma Clearance (ml/min) ESRD	Percent Excreted Unchanged[a]	Percent Protein Bound[a]	Dialyzer Clearance (ml/min)	Reference
Analgesics										
Acetaminophen	1.0	2	2	1.0	400	400	2–3	10–21[b]	120	1, 2, 5
Aspirin	0.21	2–19[c]	2–19[c]	1.0	9–85	9–85	5–85[d]	73–94	100	1, 2, 5
Meperidine	3.8	3.6	[e]	—	835	—	2	40–60	—	1, 2, 5
Methadone	—	15	—	—	—	—	15.5–29.9	71–87	—	1, 2, 5
Morphine	3.2	3	—	1.0	860	—	10–12	35	—	1, 2, 5
Pentazocine	—	2	2	—	—	—	1.7–12.6	50–75	—	1, 2, 5
Propoxyphene	—	12	[f]	—	—	—	0.8–4.5	78	—	1, 2, 5
Anticonvulsant drugs										
Carbamazepine	1.1	15	—	—	59	—	1	70–80	NS	1, 2, 5
Clonazepam	2.0	25	—	—	65	—	2	47–82	NS	1, 2, 5
Ethosuximide	0.7	60	—	—	10	—	20	0	—	1, 2, 5
Phenytoin	0.57[g]	18	9	2.0[h]	25	125	5	87–93	0	1, 2, 5
Primidone	0.6	12	—	—	40	—	1	0	—	1, 2, 5
Sodium Valproate	0.15	12	—	—	10	—	—	—	—	1, 2, 5
Antiemetic drugs										
Metoclopramide	3.4	3	14	0.2	916	196	20	—	—	82, 83
Psychotherapeutic drugs										
Amitriptyline	—	25	—	—	—	—	—	96	NS	1, 2, 5
Chlordiazepoxide	0.3	10	0	—	25	0	0	86–93	NS	1, 2, 5
Chlorpromazine	—	15	—	—	—	—	—	90	NS	1, 2, 5
Desipramine	—	17	—	—	—	—	—	69–76	NS	1, 2, 5

Diazepam	0.74[i]	20	20	1.0	35	90	1	98	0	1, 2, 5
Haloperidol	23	14	—	—	1330	—	—	90	NS	1, 2, 5
Imipramine	—	10	—	—	20	—	—	86–96	18	1, 2, 5
Lithium carbonate	0.79	30	640	0.05	20	0	89–98	0	150	1, 2, 5
Nortriptyline	21	23	—	—	740	—	0.7–3.6	94	NS	1, 2, 5
Sedative-hypnotics										
Chloral hydrate[j]	6.0	8	—	—	600	—	—	70–80	120	1, 2, 5
Ethchlorvynol	2.8	25	—	—	90	—	—	30–50	64	1, 2, 5
Flurazepam	—	75	—	—	—	—	—	—	NS	1, 2, 5
Glutethimide	2.7	12	—	—	180	—	1.65	45	50	1, 2, 5
Meprobamate	0.75	10	—	—	60	—	10–20	0–20	60	1, 2, 5
Methaqualone	6.0	35	—	—	140	—	—	80	23	1, 2, 5
Pentobarbital	0.99	22	22	1.0	36	36	—	66	—	1, 2, 5
Phenobarbital	0.75	70	100	0.7	9	6	—	25–60	80	1, 2, 5
Secobarbital	1.42	25	—	—	46	—	—	70	NS	1, 2, 5

[a] In normal humans.
[b] Concentration dependent.
[c] Increases with dose: 2 hours with 0.25 g; 19 hours with 10–20 g.
[d] Excretion variable dependent on dose and urine pH.
[e] Normeperidine, a metabolite, accumulates in renal failure.
[f] Norpropoxyphene, a metabolite accumulates in renal failure.
[g] Increases in uremia to 1.4 L/kg.
[h] Fractional clearance is greater then normal in ESRD but dosing is unchanged because of an increase in active unbound drug (see text).
[i] Increased in uremics: VD = 2.2 L/kg.
[j] Data are for the metabolite trichloroethanol.
NS, no significant removal but actual clearance unknown.

Appendix 7. Diuretic Drugs

Drug Name	Apparent VD (L/kg)	Terminal Half-Life (hr) NL	Terminal Half-Life (hr) ESRD	F_0	Plasma Clearance (ml/min) NL	Plasma Clearance (ml/min) ESRD	Percent Excreted Unchanged[a]	Percent Protein Bound[a]	Dialyzer Clearance (ml/min)	Reference
Acetazolamide	0.3	8	—	—	30	—	90	70–90	—	1, 2, 5
Bumetanide	—	0.9	—	—	—	32.5	85–95	—	3	1, 2, 5
Chlorthalidone	—	54	—	—	—	—	—	90	—	1, 2, 5
Ethacrynic acid	—	3	—	—	—	—	—	—	—	1, 2, 5
Furosemide	0.12	0.5	1.35	0.4	162	105	40–95	95	NS	1, 2, 5
Hydrochlorthiazide	—	9	—	—	—	—	35–60	60	—	1, 2, 5
Metolazone	—	8	—	—	—	—	—	90	—	1, 2, 5
Spironolactone	—	19	—	—	—	—	1	98	—	1, 2, 5
Triamterene	—	2	—	—	—	—	15–30	40–70	—	1, 2, 5

[a] In normal humans.

NS, no significant removal but actual clearance unknown.

Appendix 8. Antidiabetic Drugs

Drug Name	Apparent VD (L/kg)	Terminal Half-Life (hr) NL	Terminal Half-Life (hr) ESRD	F_0	Plasma Clearance (ml/min) NL	Plasma Clearance (ml/min) ESRD	Percent Excreted Unchanged[a]	Percent Protein Bound[a]	Dialyzer Clearance (ml/min)	Reference
Acetohexamide	0.2	2[b]	30	0.07	80	5	—	65–90	—	1, 2, 5
Chlorpropamide	0.18	33	65	0.5	4	2	20	60–90	—	1, 2, 5
Tolazamide	—	7	—	—	—	—	—	—	—	1, 2, 5
Tolbutamide	0.2	6	6	1	27	27	—	80–95	NS	1, 2, 5

[a] In normal humans.
[b] Half-life of active metabolite = 5 hours.
NS, no significant removal but actual clearance unknown.

CHAPTER 5

Parenteral Nutrition in the Treatment of Acute Renal Failure

Eben I. Feinstein
Marsha Wolfson
Joel D. Kopple

The use of parenteral nutrition has become an accepted part of the therapeutic approach to the patient with acute renal failure. The increasing recognition that malnutrition and catabolism often accompany the acutely uremic state has paralleled the growing perception that nutritional disorders may contribute to morbidity, and possibly mortality, in a variety of acute and chronic illnesses. Unfortunately, it has not been possible to demonstrate unequivocally that total parenteral nutrition (TPN) produces consistent, statistically significant, and clinically important improvement in either the rate of recovery of renal function or of overall patient survival. Investigations in rats with acute renal failure have also shown variable results. Despite evidence that phospholipid and protein synthesis in renal cortical slices is increased with administration of amino acids, suggesting enhanced renal cellular regeneration, improvement in the rate of recovery of renal function and survival has not been consistently shown. Recent clinical studies concerned with nutritional management of acute renal failure have focused on several issues: the catabolism and wasting frequently exhibited by patients with acute renal failure; comparison of the effects of treatment using hypertonic dextrose and essential amino acids with treatment using hypertonic dextrose and essential and nonessential amino acids on the metabolic status and clinical outcome of patients; and modifications in the dialytic management of the patients so as to minimize the large fluctuations in fluid volume that are entailed by TPN.

The aims of parenteral nutrition in acute renal failure are to reduce the catabolic response, morbidity, and mortality and, if possible, to facilitate the regeneration of renal tissue and recovery of renal function. Each of these therapeutic goals is dealt with in this review; however, several preliminary observations to provide background are in order.

It is clear that acute renal failure encompasses a wide range of specific diseases. We do not discuss acute renal failure due to glomerulonephritis, vascular lesions, other inflammatory disorders, or obstructive uropathy. Our focus is upon potentially reversible acute renal failure that is of the acute tubular necrosis type. Patients with acute tubular necrosis are not a homogeneous group. Some patients may be expected to recover with only conservative therapy or with several dialytic treatments. These patients are less likely to exhibit high rates of protein catabolism and may be able to receive adequate nutrition through the gastrointestinal tract. Such an example would be the diabetic patient with acute renal failure precipitated by receiving a radiocontrast agent. Another category of patients is the previously healthy individual who develops acute tubular necrosis in association with a self-limited stressful event that engenders a short-lived hypercatabolic state. Typical is the patient with nontraumatic rhabdomyolysis following drug-induced coma. Although these patients are hypercatabolic, the prognosis for recovery of renal function and survival is very good. Finally, there is the group of patients who develop acute renal failure as a result of, or in association with, systemic illnesses that cause pervasive traumatic or metabolic insults. These include sepsis, traumatic injuries, extensive surgery, or vascular catastrophies. These patients may have been in good health before the renal insult or may have had preexisting illnesses, which can complicate their clinical course. Hypercatabolism and grave prognosis are common in this group, particularly if hypotension or sepsis was the cause of acute renal failure. It is this group of patients that has contributed most to the continuing high morbidity and mortality of acute renal failure.

A number of reports have called attention to the lack of significant improvement in the outcome of acute renal failure since the early 1960s when the availability of hemodialysis became widespread (1,2). Kjellstrand et al. recently reviewed their experience at the University of Minnesota with 432 cases of acute tubular necrosis (3). The overall mortality rate was 69%. Mortality was higher in those patients who had renal failure associated with gastrointestinal surgery (78%) or cardiovascular surgery (73%). Almost half of the patients were 50 years of age or older, and they had an increased mortality rate in comparison to patients 21 to 50 years old (3).

There are several reasons for the lack of improvement in outcome during the past 20 years. Butkus has pointed out that one difficulty lies in the use of historic controls (4). Certainly, we see patients with renal failure today who, two decades ago, would not have survived their initial traumatic insult long enough to become uremic. Also, high-risk patients, such as the elderly and those with significant cardiovascular disease, now undergo surgical procedures for which they would not have been candidates in the past. Therefore, that the survival statistics are not better may reflect a changing patient population.

Another possible reason for the persisting poor outcome for patients with acute renal failure lies in the poor nutritional status of many patients. It is well established that malnutrition leads to impaired function of the immune system and normal healing (5-7). Law et al. (5) and Bistrian et al. (6) have demonstrated depressed responses of thymus-dependent cellular immunity in nonuremic patients with protein–calorie malnutrition. Parenteral nutrition with dextrose and amino acids led to significant improvement in cellular immune function (5). Wound healing is also delayed in patients with malnutrition (7). In nonuremic sick patients, a direct correlation has been described between the degree of abnormality of several parameters of nutritional status and survival. These considerations support the notion that treatment of the malnutrition seen in acute renal failure might decrease the protein catabolism and associated morbidity and improve the recovery of renal function and survival.

CLINICAL EXPERIENCE WITH TPN IN ACUTE RENAL FAILURE

Many clinical investigations of parenteral nutrition in acute renal failure have examined the effects of amounts and types of amino acids on the course of this condition. Dudrick and co-workers showed that in the experimental animal and in humans (8-10), intravenous administration of glucose (50% or 70% dextrose/water) and essential amino acids could reduce the rate of rise of serum urea nitrogen. The choice of essential amino acids alone was based on the experience with feeding diets containing small amounts of essential amino acids to patients with stable chronic renal failure (11,12). Such diets resulted in reduced net synthesis of urea (urea nitrogen appearance, UNA) and a fall in serum urea nitrogen to low levels (11); however, negative nitrogen balance often occurred (13). Originally, such formulations were thought to reduce UNA by enhancing reincorporation of the amino groups in urea into amino acids; recent studies suggest that, at least in the clinically uremic patient, UNA falls when essential amino acids are administered because of reduced urea synthesis.

When small amounts of eight essential amino acids were given to patients with acute renal failure, improved wound healing, better control of

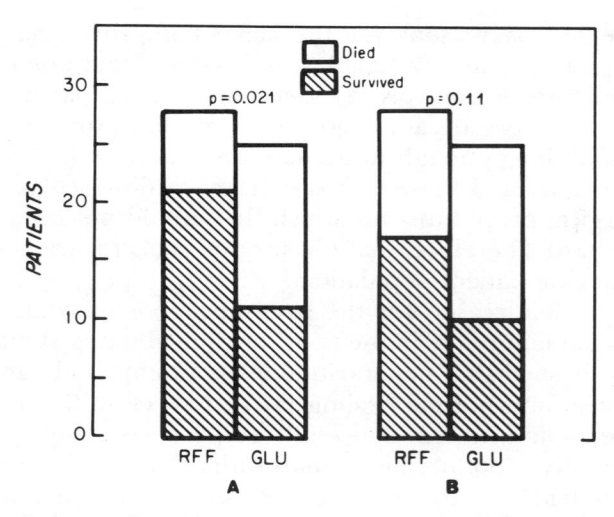

Figure 1. Survival rates from acute renal failure (A) and overall hospital mortality rates (B) in 53 patients treated with either essential L-amino acids and hypertonic glucose (RFF) or hypertonic glucose alone (GLU). (Abel RM et al: *N Engl J Med* 288:695–699, 1973. Used with permission.)

hyperkalemia and hyperphosphatemia, and less negative nitrogen balance were reported. Abel et al. described a decrease in serum potassium, phosphate, and magnesium with infusion of glucose and essential amino acids that could not be ascribed to dialysis therapy (14).

In order to determine the effects of glucose and essential amino acids on the course and outcome of acute renal failure, Abel et al. conducted a prospective, randomized, double-blind trial in 53 patients (15). Twenty-eight patients received hypertonic dextrose and about 13 g/day of eight essential amino acids (excluding histidine). A control group was given hypertonic dextrose alone. The mean caloric intake was 1426 kcal/day in the amino acid group and 1641 kcal/day in the control group. Recovery of renal function was significantly greater in the amino acid group, 75%, as compared to 44% in the controls, but overall hospital survival was not significantly increased (Fig. 1). However, in the most severely ill patients, those with pneumonia, sepsis, or gastrointestinal hemorrhage, there was a significant improvement in survival in the patients receiving essential amino acids and glucose. Serum urea nitrogen was lower in the amino acid group. Of interest was the observation that in the patients who survived, the peak serum creatinine seemed to decline sooner in the essential amino acid group as compared to controls, although the difference from the control group was not statistically significant. Abel interpreted this to indicate a more rapid recovery of renal function (16).

The studies of Abel and co-workers were very influential. Essential amino acid formulations came into widespread use for the treatment of acute renal failure. However, other investigators subsequently questioned whether giving small amounts of only essential amino acids was adequate nutritional therapy. In a prospective, single-blind study, Leonard and associates (17) randomly assigned 20 patients with acute renal failure to receive treatment with 47% dextrose or with 47% dextrose and 1.75% essential amino acids. Despite the nitrogen intake, the amino acid group had a marked negative nitrogen balance (-10 g/day) similar to that of the dextrose only group. Finally there was no difference in recovery of renal function or survival between the two groups (17). The patients receiving amino acids displayed a reduction in the rate of rise of serum urea nitrogen.

McMurray et al. (18) reported that in patients with acute renal failure who had multiple complications, the survival rate was higher in those who received a nitrogen intake of about 12 g/day (from essential and nonessential amino acids) with hypertonic dextrose as compared to those who received only dextrose. However, the study was retrospective; the two groups of patients were not treated concurrently, and the observations therefore cannot be considered conclusive.

Several investigators studied the effects of amino acids and varying energy intakes on the degree of negative nitrogen balance. Abitbol and Holliday (19) found that infusions of essential amino acids and glucose could produce neutral or possibly positive nitrogen balance, as assessed from the UNA, in six anuric children with acute or chronic renal failure. Furthermore, as caloric intake was raised from 20 to 70 kcal/kg/day the negative nitrogen balance decreased. The children in this study were all malnourished; their diagnoses were systemic lupus erythematosus, hemolytic uremic syndrome, and congenital nephrosis. Thus, the results of the study may not be fully applicable to adult patients with acute tubular necrosis.

Blackburn and co-workers reported the effects of varying amino acid and calorie intakes in two groups of patients with acute renal failure (20). In one group, there was a treatment crossover in each patient between 2% essential and nonessential amino acids and 37.5% dextrose and either 2.1% essential and nonessential amino acids and 52.5% dextrose of 1.2% essential amino acids alone and 37.5% dextrose. The authors found a decline in serum urea nitrogen with all three treatments, which was accelerated when higher energy intake was provided. Nitrogen balance approached neutrality when nitrogen intake was 4–5 g/day. A second group of patients with acute renal failure and multiple organ failure was given between 1% and 3% essential and nonessential amino acids and 5% or 47% dextrose. Although in two patients the average nitrogen balance was positive, the overall mean nitrogen balance was -2.5 g/day, and mortality rate was 62.5%. Interpretation of these data is limited by the lack of a randomized protocol and the fact that patients also received oral nutrients. However, the authors did observe that infusion of both essential and nonessential amino acids may lead to increased urea appearance, and they argued that this increase was acceptable if the increased nitrogen intake improved nitrogen balance (20).

Spreiter et al. (21) also addressed the question of the requirements for calorie and amino acid intake in 14 patients with acute renal failure. They estimated nitrogen balance from the difference between nitrogen intake and rate of urea generation. There was a direct correlation between nitrogen balance and both calorie intake and nitrogen intake, provided in the form of essential and nonessential amino acids. Positive nitrogen balance was attained when calorie intake equaled or exceeded 50 kcal/kg/day and nitrogen intake was greater than 1 g/kg/day. This quantity of amino acid nitrogen is greater than that administered by Abel et al. (15) or Leonard et al. (17), and provides further support for the need for a higher nitrogen intake in acute renal failure. This study does not shed light on the role of caloric intake per se in improving nitrogen balance, since the amounts of calories and amino acids administered were changed simultaneously. Moreover, the lowest nitrogen and calorie intakes were administered at the beginning of treatment in each patient when the patients might have been more catabolic; the largest amino acid and energy intakes were given near the end of treatment when the patients may have been less refractory to nutritional therapy. Finally, despite the increased amount of nutrients given to these patients, only two patients survived (21).

Rainford compared survival rates in patients with trauma and acute renal failure treated during three time periods (22). Contrary to the reports of others, this investigator reported improvement in survival over the past 22 years: 48% during 1958–1964, 58% during 1965–1975, and 71% during 1976–1980. Rainford attributes the difference between the first two periods to the use of daily dialysis, and the improvement between the last two periods to the use of TPN. This consisted of essential and nonessential amino acids, about 9 g of nitrogen per day, and hypertonic dextrose. Calorie intake was 3000 kcal/day. The report gives almost no information about the patients and, in addition, has the usual drawbacks of retrospective analyses.

In the report of Lopez-Martinez et al. (23), patients in the polyuric phase of acute renal failure were treated with either essential amino acids and 2000 kcal/day, or essential and nonessential amino acids, 15 g/day and 3000 kcal/day. Patients receiving the higher nitrogen and calorie intake demonstrated improvement in nitrogen balance (23). Many of the subjects in this study did not seem severely ill. Also, this report does not address the issue of the treatment of patients in the oliguric phase of acute renal failure, when catabolism is usually greatest.

Several conclusions are suggested by these foregoing studies. The great majority of patients with acute renal failure who are unable to be nourished through the enteral tract exhibit negative nitrogen balance, which may be marked and which is not corrected by small amounts of essential amino acids. Moreover, with the exception of Abel's study (15), the survival rate of these patients was not improved in comparison to that of individuals given hypertonic glucose and slightly larger quantities (e.g., up to 42 g/day) of essential and nonessential amino acids. Several arguments have been raised against the use of essential amino acids as the sole nitrogen source in renal failure. The use of small amounts of essential amino acids alone was based on the perception that urea nitrogen could be reused for the synthesis of nonessential amino acids and protein (11,24). This recycling of urea has been shown to occur only to a minimal extent (25) that is not of major nutritional importance. The low UNA with essential amino acids appears to be due to decreased entrance of amino acids into the urea cycle rather than to enhanced reutilization of urea. It is likely that the use of small amounts of essential amino acids may not provide sufficient amino acids or nitrogen to maintain nitrogen balance. Also, both essential and nonessential amino acids are required to synthesize protein, and it is not clear that each of the nonessential amino acids can be synthesized in sufficient quantities for optimal protein synthesis.

AMINO ACID INFUSIONS IN EXPERIMENTAL ACUTE RENAL FAILURE

In the experimental animal, improved growth is observed when nonessential amino acids are included in the diet. Pennisi and associates (26) tested three diets in chronically uremic rats. One diet provided only essential amino acids, whereas the other two contained either essential and nonessential amino acids or casein. Although all three treatment groups received the same amount of nitrogen, the rats receiving nonessential amino acids displayed increased growth. Humans who are ingesting a low nitrogen diet appear to maintain nitrogen balance better when they are given nonessential amino acids than when they are given diammonium citrate and either glycine or a mixture of glycine and glutamic acid (27).

Toback and co-workers investigated the effects of infusing essential and nonessential amino acids in rats with acute renal failure produced by injection of mercuric chloride (28–30). Treatment with the amino acids was compared with infusion of glucose and with no treatment. The mean serum creatinine concentration was significantly lower in the group treated with amino acids as compared to the glucose and control groups (28). This finding may indicate that the essential and nonessential amino acids engendered less renal injury or enhanced healing of the renal lesion and recovery of renal function. That the difference in serum creatinine may be due to improved regeneration of renal tubular cells is suggested by studies of renal protein and phospholipid synthesis. The leucine levels in renal cortical slices were decreased in control kidneys, and infusion of amino acids corrected this abnormality. The rate of protein synthesis in

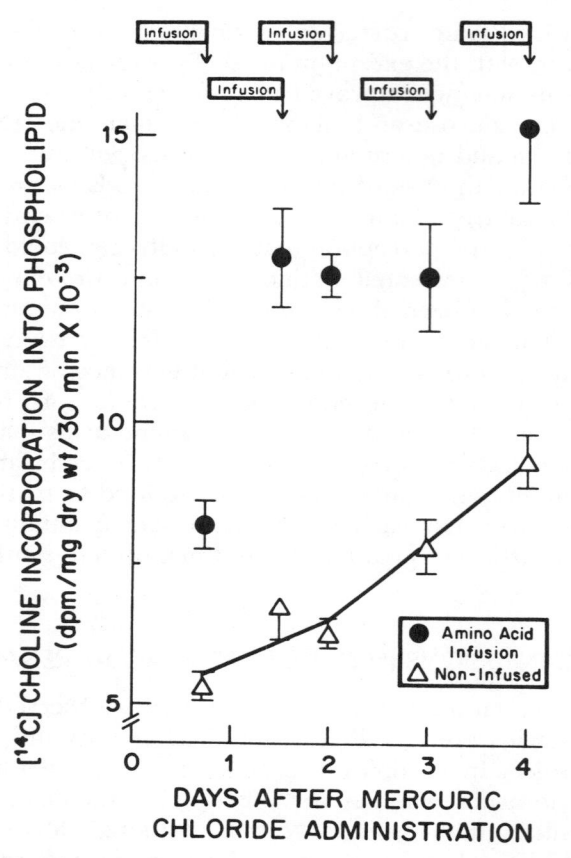

Figure 2. Rate of (^{14}C)-choline incorporation into phospholipid in the kidney of rats made uremic with mercuric chloride. The values are expressed as mean ± SEM and are greater in the amino acid infused than in noninfused animals at each time. (Toback FG: *Kidney Int* 12:193–198, 1977. Used with permission.)

the renal cortex was assessed by measuring incorporation of ^{14}C-labeled leucine into protein (29). Protein synthesis increased in the acutely uremic animals after they received infusions of amino acids. Incorporation of ^{14}C-labeled choline into renal phospholipids was used as an indicator of the formation of new cellular membranes. In one experiment, animals received either amino acids and glucose or an isocaloric infusion of dextrose alone. Incorporation of labeled choline into renal cortical slices was increased after the amino acid infusion in comparison to noninfused animals or those that had received glucose infusion (Fig. 2) (28). In another experiment, renal tissue incubated with amino acids without dextrose demonstrated improved synthesis of phosphatidylcholine, a key phospholipid constituent of the cell membrane. The amino acids seemed to act by increasing available substrate for the phospholipid synthetic pathway (30). The improved protein and lipid synthesis in renal cortical slices that occurred with administration of essential and nonessential amino acids was taken as biochemical evidence for cellular healing and regeneration, presumably in the proximal tubule.

In contrast to Toback et al. (28), Oken et al. (31) could not demonstrate beneficial effects of amino acid infusions in rats with acute renal failure produced by injections of either mercuric chloride or glycerol. They compared the effects of administration of varying quantities of essential or essential and nonessential amino acids as compared to glucose alone. In general, the results showed no advantage to treatment with amino acids as compared to glucose alone with regard to recovery of renal function or survival. In fact, the rats receiving the larger quantities of amino acids had higher serum urea nitrogen levels. The authors' data are subject to another interpretation, however. It is possible that the rats needed both larger quantities of essential and nonessential amino acids to improve nutritional status and facilitate healing, as well as some means of removing the greater quantity of toxic metabolic products that will accumulate with this treatment. Since the rats did not receive dialysis treatment, the potential advantages of large amounts of amino acids were counteracted by the development of uremic toxicity.

Controlled Studies of TPN with EAA versus EAA and NEAA

Based on earlier reports of high morbidity and mortality in patients with acute renal failure who were treated with essential amino acids and glucose, and the theoretical considerations that small amounts of essential amino acids might not provide sufficient nutrition, Feinstein and co-workers began a series of studies to evaluate the potential advantage of infusion of larger amounts of essential and nonessential amino acids (32).

In an initial study, patients with acute renal failure were randomly assigned in a double-blind manner to receive hypertonic dextrose alone; dextrose and 21 g/day of essential amino acids (EAA) (Aminosyn-RF, Abbott Laboratories); or dextrose, 21.2 g of EAA, and 20.9 g of nonessential amino acids (ENAA) (Aminosyn, Abbott Laboratories). None of the patients were able to receive adequate nutrition through the gastrointestinal tract and no oral or enteral feeding was given during the study period. In addition, to compensate for losses of amino acids during dialysis, supplemental infusions of the three solutions were given during dialysis treatments.

Thirty patients were studied; all, except one, were men. There was no significant difference in the incidence of recovery of renal function or survival among the three groups (Table 1). Poor prognostic factors included hypotension or sepsis as the cause of renal failure, for which recovery of renal function and the survival rate were each 17%, as

Table 1. Characteristics of Patients with Acute Renal Failure

	Treatment group		
	Glucose	Glucose + EAA	Glucose + ENAA
No. of subjects	7	11	12
Age (years)[a]	40 ± 19	55 ± 23	38 ± 21
Duration of TPN (days)[a]	17 ± 13	6.9 ± 2.7	6.3 ± 2.3
Causes of renal failure (recovered renal function, survived)[b]			
Hypotension	5(0,0)	4(1,1)	7(2,2)
Sepsis	—	1(0,0)	1(0,0)
Rhabdomyolysis	1(1,1)	2(2,2)	3(1,1)
Antibiotics	1(1,1)	2(2,1)	1(1,0)
Radiocontrast material	—	1(1,1)	—
Unknown	—	1(1,1)	—
TOTAL[b]	7(2,2)	11(7,6)	12(4,3)

SOURCE: Kopple JD, Feinstein EI, in Johnston IDA (ed): *Advances in Clinical Nutrition.* Lancaster, MTP Press, 1983, pp 113–121. (Reprinted by permission.)

[a] Mean ± standard deviation

[b] In the parentheses, the first number indicates the number of patients who recovered from renal failure, the second number indicates those who survived.

compared to renal failure due to other causes, for which the recovery of renal function was 83% and the survival rate was 67%. There was a tendency toward slightly greater recovery of renal function and survival in the patients receiving essential amino acids alone. However, the incidence of hypotension or sepsis as the cause of renal failure, which were indicators of poor prognosis, was somewhat lower in this group. Thus, although six of 11 patients in the EAA group survived as opposed to three of 12 patients in the ENAA group, only five of the EAA group had hypotension or sepsis-related renal failure, as compared to eight in the ENAA group. Two of seven patients who received the glucose infusions survived. Patients with coexistent surgical illnesses had a survival rate of 22%; in those patients who needed dialysis therapy, survival was also 22%. The mean energy intake did not differ among the three groups (2678 ± 744 kcal/day for the dextrose group; 2265 ± 598 kcal/day for the EAA group; 2445 ± 720 kcal/day for the ENAA group). However, the mean energy intake was higher in surviving patients, 40 ± 10 kcal/kg/day versus 32 ± 7 kcal/kg/day in nonsurvivors. This may reflect the fact that the patients who were healthier and more likely to survive received more energy because they were better able to tolerate the great water intake. Marked elevations in UNA were found in members of all three groups. The ENAA group had a higher overall mean UNA, 14 ± 8 g of nitrogen per day, as compared to the EAA group, 6.7 ± 7.2 g per day (Table 2). The mean value for the maximum UNA in individual patients was also

Table 2. Urea Nitrogen Appearance and Estimated Nitrogen Balance in Patients with Acute Renal Failure

	Treatment Group		
	Glucose	Glucose + EAA	Glucose + ENAA
No. of subjects	7	11	11
Urea nitrogen appearance (g/day)[a]			
Maximum	14.9 ± 5.6[b]	10.1 ± 10.0[c]	20.5 ± 12.3
Mean[d]	10.4 ± 5.9	6.7 ± 7.2[c]	14.0 ± 8.0
Estimated mean total nitrogen output (g/day)[d,e]	12.0 ± 5.7	8.4 ± 7.0[c]	15.5 ± 7.7
Mean nitrogen intake minus estimated mean nitrogen output[d]	12.0 ± 5.7[f]	6.2 ± 7.0[g]	10.2 ± 7.7[f]

SOURCE: Kopple JD, Feinstein EI, in Johnston IDA (ed): *Advances in Clinical Nutrition.* Lancaster, MTP Press, 1983, pp 113–121. (Reprinted by permission.)

[a] Calculated during the interdialytic interval as previously described (34)

[b] Mean ± standard deviation

[c] Probability that estimated nitrogen balance does not differ from the glucose + ENAA group; $p < 0.05$

[d] Grand mean of the mean values for the entire period of study in each patient

[e] Calculated from the equation, total nitrogen output (g/day) = 0.7 × (urea nitrogen appearance) + 1.93 (34)

[f] Probability that estimated nitrogen balance does not differ from zero; $p < 0.05$

[g] Probability that estimated nitrogen balance does not differ from zero; $p < 0.02$

higher among those receiving ENAA as compared to those receiving EAA, 20.5 ± 12.3 g/day versus 10.1 ± 10 g/day. Nitrogen balance was estimated from the difference between the mean total nitrogen output and the mean nitrogen intake (33). The mean estimated nitrogen balance was markedly negative in all three groups and did not differ among the groups. There were several patients who had low levels of UNA; when these individuals received either of the two amino acid regimens, several attained neutral or near neutral nitrogen balance. In one-third of the patients, estimated net protein degradation, averaged throughout the period of study in individual patients, ranged between 102 and 209 g/day. These marked protein losses may explain why striking protein wasting may occur within several weeks after the onset of acute renal failure.

Serum protein and plasma amino acid concentrations also indicated that patients had been hypercatabolic. The average levels of serum total protein, albumin, and transferrin were low in each group before parenteral nutrition was begun. Despite the nutritional therapy, and the administration of large volumes of blood and albumin, the concentrations of these proteins remained significantly decreased in comparison to normal values. There was a significant decline in serum albumin during the study in the most catabolic patients from all three groups (i.e., those patients with a UNA greater than 10 g/day).

The plasma concentrations of many individual amino acids, total EAA, total NEAA, and total amino acids were decreased in each of the three groups at the end of treatment as compared to normal control subjects or nondialyzed chronically uremic patients who were ingesting 40 g/day of protein. These differences were observed even though the EAA and ENAA patients were receiving intravenous amino acids at the time of blood drawing and blood was obtained from the normal control subjects and chronically uremic patients after an overnight fast.

The glucose group showed declines in nearly all plasma amino acids during the course of treatment. The EAA group showed a rise in phenylalanine and a fall in asparagine, ornithine, and cystine during parenteral nutrition. The essential amino acids, leucine and isoleucine, fell in the ENAA group while the glycine level rose during therapy. Despite the infusion of different amounts of amino acids in the three groups and the assessment of the final plasma amino acids while the patients were still receiving their treatment regimen, there were no significant differences in the total essential, total nonessential, or total amino acid levels among the three groups.

Several conclusions may be drawn from this study. Many patients with acute renal failure are in a hypercatabolic state and exhibit evidence of severe malnutrition. Recovery of renal function and survival of the patients depended more on the underlying cause of renal failure (i.e., the presence or absence of hypotension or sepsis) than on the type of nutritional therapy given.

Since most patients were hypercatabolic and wasted with each of the three treatment regimens, we reasoned that infusion of energy and a larger quantity of amino acids might improve nutritional status and possibly lower morbidity and mortality. Other reports had suggested that larger amounts of essential and nonessential amino acid nitrogen might be beneficial (18,21), but these conclusions were based upon retrospective analyses. Accordingly, we embarked upon a randomized prospective study of two treatment regimens (35). One group of patients received about 21 g/day of the nine essential amino acids (Nephramine, McGaw Laboratories). In the other group, the goal was to administer an amount of essential and nonessential amino acids that would equal or exceed by 2 g/day the daily UNA. The maximum amount of daily nitrogen given would not exceed 15 g. All patients were given between 30 and 35 kcal/kg/day, mostly provided by 70% dextrose in water. The essential and nonessential solution was the same one used in the previous protocol.

Preliminary results obtained from the first 11 patients have been reported (35). All patients were treated on the surgical service of the Los Angeles County-University of Southern California Medical Center. Renal failure was caused by hypotension in 10 patients, was secondary to trauma

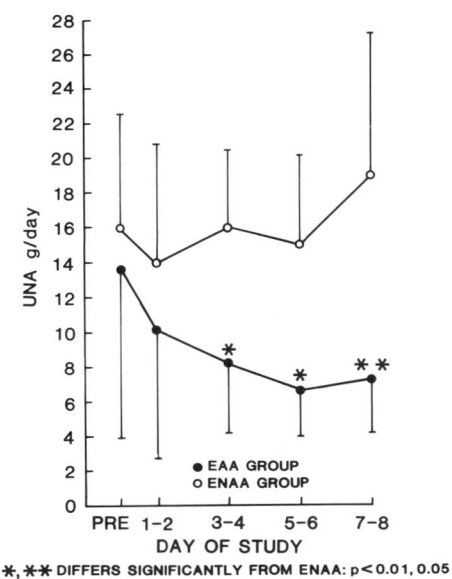

Figure 3. Urea nitrogen appearances (UNA) for patients with acute renal failure receiving glucose and essential amino acids (closed circles) or glucose and essential and nonessential amino acids (open circles). In each group values shown are the mean ± SD of the UNA for the day before starting TPN (PRE) and for each 2-day interval during the first 8 days of treatment. (Feinstein EI et al: *Kidney Int*, in press.)

*,** DIFFERS SIGNIFICANTLY FROM ENAA: p<0.01, 0.05

in eight patients, and was caused by intestinal infarction in two patients. Five patients received the EAA infusion, of whom three recovered renal function and two left the hospital alive. None of the six patients who received the ENAA treatment recovered renal function or survived, although in two patients urine output was increasing at the time of death. Mean daily nitrogen intake was 11.3 ± 1.9 g in the ENAA group versus 2.3 ± 0.3 g in the EAA group. Mean daily calorie intake was not different and averaged between 2500 and 2600 kcal/day. The ENAA group exhibited a significantly higher grand mean UNA (mean of the mean values from each patient), 14.0 ± 4.7 g/day versus 7.5 ± 3.0 g/day, $p < 0.02$. In three patients receiving the ENAA regimen, nitrogen balance, estimated from the difference between nitrogen intake and UNA, became neutral or positive for several days during the course of treatment. However, the overall mean of protein nitrogen balance did not differ significantly and was −3.0 ± 4.0 g/day with ENAA treatment and −5.2 ± 2.9 g/day with EAA therapy. It should be emphasized that this method of estimating nitrogen balance probably underestimates the degree of negative nitrogen balance by about 2 g/day.

Analysis of the UNA and protein nitrogen balance for the first 8 days of the study revealed that the UNA before starting treatment did not differ between the two groups. This suggests that both groups were similar in their degree of catabolism at the beginning of the study. From the third to eighth day of study, the UNA was significantly higher with the ENAA therapy as compared to the EAA regimen (Fig. 3).

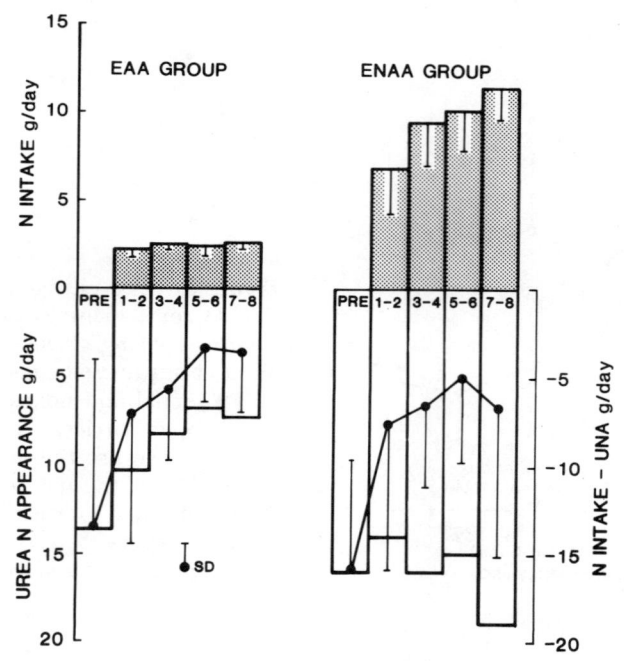

Figure 4. Mean nitrogen intake (shaded bars), mean urea nitrogen appearance (open bars), and mean estimated protein nitrogen balance (N intake–UNA) (solid lines) in patients with acute renal failure receiving glucose and essential amino acids (EAA) and glucose and essential and nonessential amino acids (ENAA). Notations in the open bars refer to the day before TPN was started (PRE) and to each 2-day interval for the first 8 days of treatment. (Feinstein EI et al: *Kidney Int*, in press.)

On the other hand, the estimated daily nitrogen balance for each of the first 8 days did not differ between the two groups, even though the daily nitrogen intake was higher in the ENAA group (Fig. 4). These findings imply that a large proportion of the administered amino acids in the ENAA group was degraded to urea, and very little was used for anabolism. The small sample size in this study does not allow us to conclude whether treatment of acute renal failure with 21 g/day of EAA leads to improved survival. However, since none of the patients receiving the ENAA treatment survived, it seems unlikely that this regimen could be shown to have major advantages over the EAA treatment, even if the sample size was much larger. The fact that the UNA remained high and that estimated protein nitrogen balance was negative in the ENAA group points to the need for other approaches to the problem.

One might consider, for example, infusions with larger quantities of EAA alone (i.e., greater than 40 g/day). However, current evidence suggests that this is hazardous, since at least some patients with acute renal failure appear to have difficulty in metabolizing such a load of essential amino acids. In the pediatric patients reported by Motil et al. (36), elevated plasma ammonia and methionine concentrations developed after intravenous treatment with a large quantity of eight essential amino acids. There was also a fall in plasma histidine, ornithine, citrulline, and arginine, which was corrected when essential and nonessential amino acids were infused. We have also observed bizarre amino acid patterns in adult patients with acute renal failure who were given infusions with glucose and up to 75 g/day of essential amino acids.

ALTERED LIVER AND MUSCLE METABOLISM IN ACUTE RENAL FAILURE

There is a growing body of data that suggests that acute renal failure is associated with altered hepatic and muscle metabolism, which underlies and tends to maintain the catabolic response. Frohlich et al. demonstrated increased release of urea and glucose from the perfused liver of bilaterally nephrectomized rats (37). When amino acids were added to the liver perfusate, urea and glucose synthesis increased further. Flugel-Link et al. examined protein synthesis and degradation and amino acid metabolism in the hemicorpus of rats made acutely uremic by bilateral nephrectomy (38). The animals were fasted for 30 hours after surgery, except for gavage with sodium bicarbonate, and the hemicorpus was then perfused with albumin and erythrocytes during the experiments. Protein degradation was increased in the hemicorpus of the acutely uremic animals. Protein synthesis was also reduced in the hemicorpus of the uremic rats although the difference from the sham-operated controls was not statistically significant. However, more recent studies by Inadomi and coworkers in our laboratory have demonstrated increased protein degradation and reduced protein synthesis, both statistically significant, in the hemicorpus of this acutely uremic rat model (unpublished observations).

The acutely uremic rats also displayed increased net release of phenylalanine, tyrosine, alanine, total NEAA, total amino acids, potassium, and phosphorus from the perfused hemicorpus. Increased degradation of the amino acids released from the catabolized muscle protein was suggested by the significantly increased UNA in the uremic animals and the low plasma and muscle intracellular amino acid concentrations. The levels of the proteases cathepsins B_1 and D and alkaline protease were not different in the muscle of the uremic and control rats. Acute uremia therefore appears to be a condition in which the liver is predisposed toward increased urea and glucose production from amino acids derived from proteolysis in muscle and possibly other tissues.

The altered hormonal milieu in the stressed uremic patient may also contribute to the catabolic state of these patients. Such individuals may have increased circulating levels of catecholamines, glucagon, cortisol, and parathyroid hormone, all catabolic agents. Moreover, there is often resistance to insulin, normally a potent anabolic hormone.

There are data from human studies that suggest a role for circulating proteases in the hypercatabolism of acute uremia (39,40). In two patients with hypercatabolic renal failure, Hörl and Heidland (39) isolated fractions from the sera that degraded subunits of the enzyme phosphorylase kinase. Sera from these patients also caused a pH-dependent digestion of bovine serum albumin. They speculated that the proteases in the patients' sera had molecular weights of 5000 daltons or higher. The authors suggested that a decrease in circulating protease inhibitors could be responsible for the enhanced serum protease activity in acute renal failure.

More recent reports have characterized a circulating peptide, found in the plasma of nonuremic patients with trauma or sepsis, that possesses proteolytic activity. The protease activity was demonstrated by incubation with rat or normal human skeletal muscle (40). This peptide is thought to have a molecular weight of 4274 daltons and to contain 33 amino acids in addition to sialic acid. Plasma levels of the peptide (measured by bioassay) were correlated with the rate of peripheral amino acid release in a group of patients with varying degrees of trauma and sepsis. Although the renal function of these patients was not mentioned in this report, it is quite possible that similar peptides may be present in the circulation of hypercatabolic patients with acute renal failure.

Other factors that have been implicated in the increased protein degradation of nonuremic septic patients include prostaglandin E_2 and a leukocyte pyrogen, interleukin-1. Baracos et al. reported that human leukocyte pyrogen stimulates protein degradation (41). Indomethacin caused a marked decrease in proteolysis, which supports a role for prostaglandins in the proteolytic process.

The contribution of altered hormonal concentrations and activities, proteases, and other mediators of protein wasting to the hypercatabolic state of patients with renal failure should be a fruitful area for investigation. If these factors are operative in renal failure, it would seem appropriate to examine methods for controlling their deleterious effects.

RECENT ADVANCES IN DIALYSIS THERAPY THAT FACILITATE TPN

Another promising development for the management of acute renal failure are newer techniques that facilitate the safe administration of parenteral nutrition to patients who are frequently severely oliguric.

Large volumes of fluid are often necessary to provide adequate calories to the hypercatabolic patient; 30–35 kcal/kg body weight/day or more are believed to be required for the septic or traumatized patient. We have used 70% dextrose in water as the main source of calories in our patients.

This solution is calculated to provide about 2.3 kcal/ml, assuming 3.75 kcal/g glucose and making allowance for the fact that glucose monohydrate (90% anhydrous glucose) is used in parenteral solutions. Thus a minimum of 1 liter per day of 70% glucose is required in a 70 kg patient. Moreover, more recent experience suggests that patients with acute or chronic renal failure have metabolic needs for lipids and that intravenous infusions of lipids are well tolerated. A 20% lipid emulsion provides 2.0 kcal/ml, while a 10% lipid emulsion provides 1.1 kcal/ml. The most concentrated solutions of amino acids available are 10% solutions. Thus at least 500 ml to one liter are required to provide 50–100 g/day of amino acids. From these considerations, it is clear that TPN in these patients obligates infusion of about 2 liters of fluid daily. In fact, total daily input is frequently even higher due to the intravenous infusions of blood, albumin, antibiotics, and other medications.

It is clear that prevention of fluid overload and dilutional hyponatremia will require frequent, often daily, conventional hemodialysis. Many patients undergo daily fluctuations in fluid volume as a result. One technique to surmount this problem, continuous arteriovenous hemofiltration (CAVH), has been advocated by Kramer et al. (42). His technique consists of extracorporeal circulation of blood from an artery to a vein across a highly permeable polysulfone membrane (Amicon hemofilter). The ultrafiltration coefficient is very high, and even at low blood flow rates (no blood pump is used) removal of large amounts of fluid (up to 20 liters/day) are possible. The treatment may be performed continuously for 24 hours. Careful monitoring of the quantity of fluid removed is mandatory to prevent rapid volume depletion. In patients with hypotension, vasopressor agents have been infused intravenously to allow continued hemofiltration.

The ultrafiltrate that is produced by CAVH contains urea, creatinine, potassium, and amino acids in concentrations similar to the patient's plasma. If blood is diluted by replacement fluid before it enters the ultrafilter, concentrations in the ultrafiltrate may be somewhat lower than in plasma. Kramer and co-workers measured a loss of 2 g/24 h of amino acids while 100 g of amino acids were given intravenously over the same period (43). These amino acid losses seem lower than would be predicted and other investigators have reported a daily loss of 10% of administered EAA (44). In comparison, during conventional hemodialysis, losses of amino acids during amino acid infusion may be as high as 12.6 g over a 5 hour period (45).

The reported experience with CAVH in patients with acute renal failure indicates that maintenance of fluid balance and control of azotemia can be accomplished (43). Unfortunately, no dramatic improvement in mortality has been reported with this technique. In fact, survival of two of 32 surgical patients with multiple organ system failure (43) is a lower rate than reported in other series of surgical patients with acute renal failure. In another series, six of 20 patients with associated trauma, sepsis, or recent abdominal surgery survived (46). The lower survival in these patients may be related to the selection of sicker patients; a number of patients were under CAVH while they received pressor agents to maintain blood pressure. CAVH is generally viewed as a promising new technique and will probably be used increasingly in the United States now that the CAVH filters are commercially available.

Another new method for administering parenteral nutrition to patients with acute renal failure is called continuous slow hemodialysis (47). Patients undergo hemodialysis using a dialysate that contains glucose and amino acids. In order to allow efficient and economical uptake of the nutrients from the dialysate, the flow rate of dialysate is decreased from the usual 500 ml/min to approximate 50 ml/min. The amount of glucose taken up with this technique varies with the dialysis flow rate. Using a dialysate glucose concentration of 5%, the glucose absorbed (g/min) = 1.4 × dialysate flow rate (ml/min) + 18.3. The creatinine and urea clearances are approximately the same as the dialysis flow rate. In four patients who received this treatment for 3–5 hours, with dialysis flow rate reduced to about 25 ml/min and dialysate glucose and amino acid concentrations of 5 g/dl and 0.5 g/dl, respectively, the mean glucose and amino acids absorbed were 50 g/hr and 4 g/hr, respectively. The percent uptake for each nutrient was about 79% of the amount delivered in the dialysate with this regimen. The patients received an average of 181 kcal/hr from the dialysate (48). To provide substantially larger amounts of calories or amino acids, it would be necessary to increase the concentrations of these nutrients or to increase the duration of the treatment. We foresee that this technique, used for 10–12 hours daily, will deliver adequate nutrition without fluid administration and simultaneously provide necessary hemodialysis. Currently, an advantage to CAVH that is not present with continuous slow hemodialysis is that, after training, CAVH can be performed by intensive care nurses while they perform their other duties. In contrast, continuous slow hemodialysis still requires the more costly use of hemodialysis nurses.

In conclusion, the optimal formulations for parenteral nutrition in patients with acute renal failure who are unable to receive adequate enteral nutrition remains unsettled. Many patients with acute renal failure show signs of hypercatabolism with wasting and malnutrition.

DIRECTIONS FOR FUTURE RESEARCH

In the future, nutritional management of the hypercatabolic patient with acute renal failure will likely require pharmacological therapy (1) to control the factor(s) promoting protein breakdown, and (2) to enhance net accrual in the body of proteins and other biologically valuable compounds. Further research into the nature and role of tissue and circulating proteases should allow development of agents to counteract these substances. Other approaches to the problem of catabolism may involve therapy with hormones, or hormone antagonists. For example, insulin has been shown to decrease protein breakdown in nonuremic patients after trauma (49).

Continuing efforts are also needed to develop a more rational approach to the administration of amino acids and other nutrients in patients with acute renal failure. It is possible that different degrees of catabolic response require different nutritional therapies. Patients who show only mild catabolic stress (e.g., with UNA of 5 g/day or less) may benefit from treatment with infusions of glucose and small amounts of EAA. Patients with augmented net protein breakdown are likely to require more amino acids, both essential and nonessential. Newer amino acid formulations, with higher proportions of branched chain amino acids, are reported to stimulate protein synthesis and decrease protein degradation in nonuremic postoperative patients (50). Therapeutic trials of such amino acid formulations for patients with acute renal failure are clearly needed.

REFERENCES

1. Scott RB, Cameron JS, Ogg CS, et al: Why the persistently high mortality in acute renal failure? *Lancet* 2:75–78, 1972.
2. Lordon RE, Burton JR: Post-traumatic renal failure in military personnel in Southeast Asia. *Am J Med* 53:137–147, 1972.
3. Kjellstrand CM, Ebben J, Davin T: Time of death, recovery of renal function, development of chronic renal failure and need for chronic hemodialysis in patients with acute tubular necrosis. *Trans Am Soc Artif Intern Organs* 27:45–50, 1981.
4. Butkuss D: Persistent high mortality in acute renal failure. *Arch Int Med* 143:209–212, 1983 (editorial).
5. Law DK, Dudrick SJ, Abdou N: Immunocompetence of patients with protein-calorie malnutrition. *Ann Intern Med* 79:545–550, 1973.
6. Bistrian BR, Blackburn GL, Scrimshaw MD, et al: Cellular immunity in semi-starved states in hospitalized adults. *Am J Clin Nutr* 28:1148–1155, 1975.
7. Bozzetti F, Terno G, Longoni C: Parenteral hyperalimentation and wound healing. *Surg Gynecol Obstet* 141:712–714, 1975.
8. Wilmore DW, Dudrick SJ: Treatment of acute renal failure with intravenous essential L-amino acids. *Arch Surg* 99:669–673, 1969.
9. Dudrick SJ, Steiger E, Long JM: Renal failure in surgical patients. Treatment with intravenous essential amino acids and hypertonic glucose. *Surgery* 68:180–186, 1970.
10. VanBuren CT, Dudrick SJ, Dworkin L, et al: Effects of intravenous essential L-amino acids and hypertonic dextrose on anephric beagles. *Surg Forum* 23:83–85, 1972.
11. Giordano C: Use of exogenous and endogenous urea for protein synthesis in normal and uremic subjects. *J Lab Clin Med* 62:231–246, 1963.
12. Giovanetti S, Maggiore Q: A low-nitrogen diet with proteins of high biological value for severe chronic uremia. *Lancet* 1:1000–1002, 1964.
13. Kopple JD, Coburn J: Metabolic studies of low protein diets in uremia, I: Nitrogen and potassium. *Medicine* 52:583–595, 1973.

14. Abel RM, Abbott WM, Fischer JE: Intravenous essential L-amino acids and hypertonic dextrose in patients with acute renal failure. Effects on serum potassium, phosphate, and magnesium. *Am J Surg* 123:632–638, 1972.
15. Abel RM, Beck CH Jr, Abbott WM, et al: Improved survival from acute renal failure after treatment with intravenous essential L-amino acids and glucose. Results of a prospective double-blind study. *N Engl J Med* 288:695–699, 1973.
16. Abel RM: Parenteral nutrition in the treatment of renal failure, in Fischer JE (ed): *Total Parenteral Nutrition*. Boston, Little, Brown, 1976, pp 143–170.
17. Leonard CD, Luke RG, Siegel RR: Parenteral essential amino acids in acute renal failure. *Urology* 6:154–157, 1976.
18. McMurray SD, Luft FC, Maxwell DR, et al: Prevailing patterns and predictor variables in patients with acute tubular necrosis. *Arch Intern Med* 139:950–955, 1978.
19. Abitol CL, Holliday MA: Total parenteral nutrition in anuric children. *Clin Nephrol* 5:153–158, 1976.
20. Blackburn GL, Etter G, Mackenzie T: Criteria for choosing amino acid therapy in acute renal failure. *Am J Clin Nutr* 31:1841–1853, 1978.
21. Spreiter SC, Myers BD, Swenson RS: Protein-energy requirements in subjects with acute renal failure receiving intermittent hemodialysis. *Am J Clin Nutr* 33:1433–1437, 1980.
22. Rainford DJ: Nutritional management of acute renal failure. *Acta Chim Scand* 507(Suppl):327–330, 1980.
23. Lopez-Martinez J, Caparros T, Perez-Picouto F, et al: Nutricion parenteral en enfermos septicos con fracaso renal agudo en fase poliurica. *Rev Clin Exp* 157:171–177, 1980.
24. Giordano C, DePascal C, Balestrieri C, et al: Incorporation of urea ^{15}N in amino acids of patients with chronic renal failure on a low nitrogen diet. *Am J Clin Nutr* 21:394–404, 1968.
25. Varcoe R, Holliday D, Carson ER, et al: Efficiency of utilization of urea nitrogen for albumin synthesis by chronically uremic and normal man. *Clin Sci Mol Med* 48:379–390, 1975.
26. Pennisi AJ, Wang M, Kopple JD: Effects of protein and amino acid diets in chronically uremic and control rats. *Kidney Int* 13:472–479, 1978.
27. Swendseid ME, Harris CL, Tuttle SG: The effect of sources of nonessential nitrogen on nitrogen balance in young adults. *J Nutr* 71:105–108, 1960.
28. Toback FG: Amino acid enhancement of renal regeneration after acute tubular necrosis. *Kidney Int* 12:193–198, 1977.
29. Toback FG, Dodd RC, Maier ER, et al: Amino acid enhancement of renal protein synthesis during regeneration after acute tubular necrosis. *Clin Res* 27:432a, 1979.
30. Toback FG, Teegarden DE, Havener LJ: Amino acid-mediated stimulation of renal phospholipid biosynthesis after acute tubular necrosis. *Kidney Int* 15:542–547, 1979.
31. Oken DE, Sprinkle FM, Kirshbaum BB, et al: Amino acid therapy in the treatment of experimental renal failure in the rat. *Kidney Int* 17:14–23, 1980.
32. Feinstein EI, Blumenkrantz MJ, Healy M, et al: Clinical and metabolic responses to parenteral nutrition in acute renal failure—a controlled double-blind study. *Medicine* 60:124–137, 1981.
33. Kopple JD, Feinstein EI: Nutritional therapy for patients with acute renal failure, in Johnson IDA (ed.): *Advances in Clinical Nutrition*. Lancaster: MTP Press, 1983, pp 113–121.
34. Kopple JD: Nutritional therapy in kidney failure. *Nutr Rev* 39:193–201, 1981.
35. Feinstein EI, Kopple JD, Silberman H, et al: Total parenteral nutrition with high or low nitrogen intake in patients with acute renal failure. *Kidney Int* (in press).

36. Motil KJ, Harmon WE, Grupe WE: Complications of essential amino acid hyperalimentation in children with acute renal failure. *JPEN* 4:32–35, 1980.
37. Frohlich J, Hoppe-Seyler G, Schollmeyer P, et al: Possible sites of interaction of acute renal failure with amino acid utilization for gluconeogenesis in isolated perfused rat liver. *Eur J Clin Invest* 7:261–268, 1977.
38. Flugel-Link RM, Salusky I, Jones M, et al: Altered muscle protein and amino acid metabolism in rats with acute renal failure. *Kidney Int* (in press).
39. Horl WH, Heidland A: Enhanced proteolytic activity—cause of protein catabolism in acute renal failure. *Am J Clin Nutr* 33:1423–1427, 1980.
40. Clowes GHA Jr, George BC, Villee CA Jr, et al: Muscle proteolysis induced by a circulating peptide in patients with sepsis or trauma. *N Engl J Med* 308:545–552, 1983.
41. Baracos V, Rodermann HP, Dinarello CA, et al: Stimulation of muscle protein degradation and prostaglandin E_2 release by leukocyte pyrogen: A mechanism for the increased degradation of muscle proteins during fever. *N Engl J Med* 308:553–558, 1983.
42. Kramer P, Wiggin W, Rieger J, et al: Arteriovenous hemofiltration: A new simple method for treatment of overhydrated patients resistant to diuretics. *Klin Wschr* 55:121–124, 1977.
43. Kramer P, Bohler J, Kehr A, et al: Intensive care potential of continuous arteriovenous hemofiltration. *Trans Am Soc Artif Intern Organs* 28:28–32, 1982.
44. Paganini EP, Flaque J, Whitman G, et al: Amino acid balance in patients with oliguric renal failure undergoing slow continuous ultrafiltration. *Trans Am Soc Artif Intern Organs* 28:615–620, 1982.
45. Wolfson M, Jones MR, Kopple JD: Amino acid losses during hemodialysis with infusion of amino acids and glucose. *Kidney Int* 21:500–506, 1982.
46. Olbricht C, Mueller C, Schwek HJ, Et al: Treatment of acute renal failure in patients with multiple organ failure by continuous spontaneous hemofiltration. *Trans Am Soc Artif Intern Organs* 28:33–37, 1982.
47. Feinstein E, Collins J, Blumenkrantz M, et al: Parenteral nutrition via hemodialysis. 20:in press, 1983 (abstract).
48. Feinstein E, Collins J, Blumenkrantz M, et al: Nutritional hemodialysis. Artif Organs (abstract, in press).
49. Woolfson AMJ, Healthey RV, Allison SP: Insulin to inhibit protein catabolism after injury. *N Engl J Med* 300:14–17, 1979.
50. Cerra FB, Upson D, Angelico R, et al: Branched chains support post-operative protein synthesis. *Surgery* 92:192–198, 1982.

ACKNOWLEDGMENTS

This work was supported in part by a grant from Abbott Laboratories, Inc., and a contract with the USPHS-NIH AM 3-2210 and NIH-7R01-AM 324 39-1. The author wishes to gratefully acknowledge the valuable assistance of Miss Morgan Bailey, Miss Riva Kussmaul, and Miss Patti Kentor.

CHAPTER 6

Glomerulonephritis and Nephrotic Syndrome

John A. Bertolatus
Lawrence G. Hunsicker

In the last few years, there has been a resurgence of interest in the mechanisms of glomerular injury with rapid advances in our understanding of them, as evidenced by the ever-increasing literature on glomerular disorders. The student of glomerular disorders, traditionally grounded in pathology and deeply involved with immunology, must now extend his interests still further. He must study biochemistry and physical chemistry to understand the nature of fixed glomerular anions and their role in glomerular permselectivity and immune complex deposition. He must renew his acquaintance with physiology in order to study the basis for glomerular hyperfiltration in renal insufficiency and its role in progression of renal failure. The increased attention paid to the glomerulus and the broadened basis for studying glomerular disorders has led to the emergence of yet another specialist in nephrology, the "glomerulologist," who is equally at home in all of these disciplines, but focuses his attention on this first, most frequently injured, portion of the nephron. This chapter will attempt to review some of the results and hypotheses in the new discipline of "glomerulology."

FUNDAMENTAL INVESTIGATIONS

Introduction

Investigation of the immunopathogenesis of glomerulonephritis continues to be guided by the basic concepts, elaborated several decades ago, of deposition within the glomerulus either of antibodies against glomerular basement membrane (GBM) antigens or of immune complexes of antibody plus nonglomerular antigen. These concepts, however, have been extended considerably by new studies. Recent work has also further clarified the mechanisms by which immune reactants within the glomerulus lead to glomerular injury and progressive renal insufficiency. A very thoughtful review of these new developments has recently been published by Cameron (1).

Formation of Glomerular Immune Complexes

Recent studies continue to support the relatively new idea that the in situ reaction of circulating free antibody with native glomerular antigens or exogenous ("planted") antigens is the principal mechanism responsible for the formation of subepithelial immune deposits within the GBM. Native GBM antigens involved in the formation of these subepithelial immune deposits are clearly different from the antigens participating in classical anti-GBM antibody diseases, such as Goodpasture's syndrome, since immunofluorescence microscopy in the former case shows a granular pattern of antibody deposition typical of membranous nephropathy, and there is no cross-reactivity between antibodies mediating these different diseases.

The best defined example of in situ immune complex formation with a native glomerular antigen continues to by Heymann nephritis (HN), also called experimental membranous nephropathy because of the resemblance of this experimental model to human membranous glomerulopathy. In current investigations, this disease is produced either by active immunization of animals with a purified renal tubular brush border antigen, designated Fx1A, or by passive administration of purified anti-Fx1A antibodies obtained from the serum or kidneys of actively immunized nephritic animals.

A recent study by Neale and Wilson examined the nature of the glomerular antigen responsible for in situ complex formation in rat HN (2). They examined by indirect immunofluorescence the reactivity of serum antibodies and antibodies eluted from HN kidneys with normal target kidney sections. The eluted antibodies produced a strong granular pattern of deposition in the glomeruli of the targets, while serum antibodies showed much weaker but still detectable reactivity with glomeruli. Ultrastructural studies with immunoperoxidase staining showed the HN antigen to be in a subepithelial location. Pretreatment of target kidney sections with "classic" anti-GBM antisera or neuraminidase did not affect subsequent binding of HN antibody, but nitrous acid treatment, known to digest heparin sulfate, abolished the reactivity of the targets with HN antisera, suggesting to the authors that the antigen mediating HN is a GBM proteoglycan. In addition to possessing reactivity with normal target glomeruli in sections, eluted HN antibodies have also been shown to bind specifically to glomeruli and to form the typical subepithelial deposits when perfused into isolated kidneys (3). This establishes even more firmly the in situ mechanism of deposit formation in this model. Another group (4) has shown that in active HN, the development of the membranous lesion proceeds with a high level of free circulating anti-Fx1A antibody but without circulating immune complexes.

Much current attention is directed to the role of glomerular anionic sites in mediating glomerular deposition of exogenous immune reactants. These negatively charged sites were initially recognized because of the role they played in maintaining normal glomerular permselectivity. More recently, the GBM anions have also been recognized as being able to bind circulating cationic macromolecules. For example, Border et al. (5) employed a chemically modified cationic bovine albumin (BSA) instead of the traditional anionic BSA as the injected antigen in a rabbit model of serum sickness nephritis. Unlike anionic BSA, the cationic BSA bound to glomeruli *prior* to development of an anti-BSA antibody response in the rabbits. This supports a role for antigen charge in glomerular deposition and provides further evidence for the in situ mechanism of immune complex deposition. The model also differed from "classic" serum sickness in that glomerular injury developed more rapidly and immune deposits formed in a subepithelial, rather than subendothelial, location. Another group (6) has also demonstrated, by immunofluorescence, that not only cationic albumin but also a wide variety of cationic protein antigens show affinity for GBM. When cationized ferritin was infused followed by antiferritin antibodies, subepithelial GBM immune complex formation resulted, again presumably by an in situ mechanism.

Isaacs and Miller (7) reported an additional demonstration of the role of antigen charge and defined a new class of exogenous antigens able to produce glomerular injury. They injected various charged or neutral derivatives of the polysaccharide dextran into mice. Animals given the various dextran derivatives developed different morphologic patterns of glomerular IgA deposition as assessed by immunofluorescence. However, the dextrans of all charges produced primarily mesangial IgA deposits, rather than the subepithelial deposits more typical of cationic protein antigens. The reason for the divergent behavior of the protein and polysaccharide antigens is unclear, but it is presumably related to their differing chemical natures. As noted, most of the antidextran antibodies in serum and the immunoglobulin in glomerular deposits of these animals were of the IgA class. To date, this is the only animal model of glomerulonephritis involving predominately an IgA immunoglobulin response. The authors note the similarity of the morphology produced by dextran administration (Fig. 1) to that of IgA nephropathy in man, raising the question of a possible role in that disorder for a polysaccharide antigen, perhaps related to bacterial cell walls.

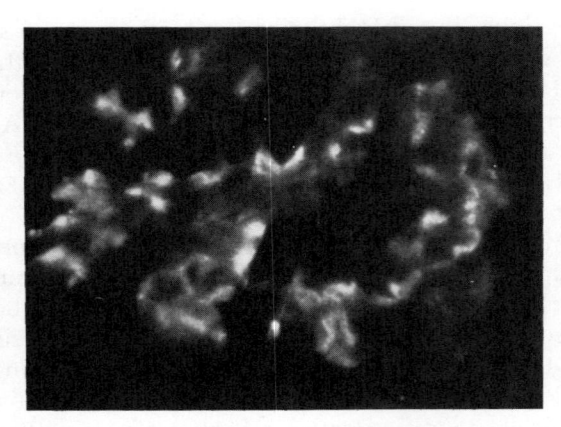

Figure 1. Immunofluorescence micrograph of kidney from mouse treated with cationic DEAE-dextran for 10 weeks. Note mesangial pattern of immunoglobulin deposition revealed by staining with rabbit antimouse IgA, similar in pattern to human IgA nephropathy. (×220) (Isaacs KL, Miller F: *Lab Invest* 47:198–205, 1982. Used with permission.)

Although the studies discussed in the preceding paragraphs have emphasized the attention being given to antigenic charge and in situ immune complex formation, it is important to point out that these factors have been most frequently described in relation to formation of subepithelial deposits. Deposits within other sites of the glomerulus probably occur by other mechanisms, such as trapping of circulating soluble immune complexes, which has been the "traditional" explanation. In this area, interest continues to focus on those factors intrinsic to circulating complexes that promote glomerular deposition. Haakenstad et al. (8) have challenged the notion that it is mainly small soluble antigen-antibody complexes, such as those formed in marked antigen excess, that are deposited in glomerular capillaries. They injected into mice preformed human albumin-antialbumin complexes, made either in marked antigen excess (small soluble complexes) or in approximate equivalence (large soluble complexes). The smaller complexes, which consisted primarily of one to two antibody and antigen molecules per complex, were not deposited in the glomeruli, whereas substantial quantities of the larger complexes were. The exact size of the larger complexes was not determined. Studies of preformed immune complexes injected into animals have come under close scrutiny because of the possibility of dissociation of complexes, deposition of free antigen, and re-formation of complexes in situ in the GBM. However, it seems unlikely that the marked difference in glomerular complex deposition observed in this study could have occurred by this route, since the same antibody, in roughly equivalent total amounts, was injected into the different groups. Only the size of the complexes differed.

Antibody affinity is another factor influencing the pattern of immune complex formation in the GBM. Steward et al. (9) showed that mice genetically selected to produce low affinity antibody developed high levels of circulating immune complexes and a subepithelial pattern of immune deposits in the GBM when immunized with human albumin. In contrast, mice producing high affinity antibody had few circulating immune complexes and a subendothelial or mesangial pattern of glomerular immune deposits. In this case, it seems quite likely that the low affinity antibody may have promoted subepithelial deposit formation by dissociating from antigen in the circulation and combining with antigen in situ in the subepithelial space.

Glomerular immune complex deposition is also influenced by factors controlling access of the complexes to the GBM. One such factor is the level of circulating immune complexes, which is in turn a function of the rate of removal of complexes by the reticuloendothelial system. Raij et al. (10) injected rats with radiolabeled aggregated IgG as model immune complexes. Animals whose reticuloendothelial systems had been stimulated with zymosan had much more rapid clearance of aggregated IgG from their circulation and consequently much less glomerular deposition of the aggregates. In addition, the deposition of circulating immune complexes in glomeruli may be promoted by the presence of factors that increase vascular permeability. The release of an IgE-dependent platelet activating factor from sensitized basophils, with subsequent release of permeability-altering vasoactive amines from the activated platelets, may constitute such a mechanism. Recently, Camussi et al. (11) have shown that immune complex deposition in acute serum sickness nephritis in rabbits is preceded by degranulation of basophils in vivo, and development of antigen specific basophil sensitivity to bovine albumin in vitro. Basophils from rabbits presensitized to horseradish peroxidase and then given albumin to induce serum sickness showed loss of in vitro basophil sensitivity to the original horseradish peroxidase antigen, implying that the basophils had already been activated and degranulated at the time glomerular immune deposits developed. Measurable platelet-activating factor was detectable in the circulation of some, but not all, of the nephritic rabbits.

Finally, there is also evidence that the clearance of material deposited in the GBM in glomerulonephritis may be impaired, as if the mechanisms for clearing the GBM were overloaded. Sharon et al. (12) have demonstrated that in HN, the normally rapid clearance of protamine-heparin aggregates from the subepithelial GBM region by epithelial cell endocytosis is markedly reduced. The reduced clearance of the aggregates was noted in regions of immune deposit formation; in other areas, clearance appeared to proceed normally.

Anti-GBM Disease

With regard to the anti-GBM antibody mechanism of glomerular injury, interest has centered upon the variety of antigens within the GBM that can be recognized by antibodies mediating nephritis. As discussed earlier, studies on HN have shown that there is a "nonclassic" GBM antigen residing in a subepithelial location that binds HN antibodies in a granular pattern. In addition, Abrahamson and Caulfield (13) have shown that passively administered, heterologous, affinity purified antibodies to the protein laminin bind specifically to rat GBM. On immunoflorescence, the antibody appears in a linear pattern and is seen ultrastructurally throughout the thickness of the GBM. Animals receiving antilaminin antibody developed GBM thickening, C3 deposition, and mild proteinuria, with minimal hypercellularity. A role for this antigen in spontaneously occurring anti-GBM disease has yet to be demonstrated.

Mediators of Glomerular Injury

The now classic studies of the heterologous phase of anti-GBM nephritis in animals established the following sequence of events as mediating glomerular injury. First, heterologous anti-GBM immunoglobulin attaches to the GBM. The antibody deposits result in activation and deposition of complement components that are chemotactic for neutrophils. The neutrophils release degradative enzymes that digest GBM and other glomerular components, leading to manifestations of injury, such as proteinuria, hematuria, and glomerular sclerosis. Recent studies have not firmly established any new categories of mediators, but rather have offered insight into modes of glomerular injury by antibodies, complement components, and inflammatory cells, which are not included in the above sequence of events.

For example, in the sequence of events described for anti-GBM disease, the role of antibody is to trigger later mediators of the inflammatory response. One recent study shows that an antibody can cause proteinuria directly. Salant and co-workers (14) developed a model of proteinuria produced in rats by passive administration $F(ab')_2$ or Fab' fragments of HN antibodies. In addition to proteinuria, the animals developed typical subepithelial lesions of HN. The injury produced by the fragments, however, was not prevented by prior depletion of complement or inflammatory cells. The authors indicate that the antibody fragments probably combine with a subepithelial GBM component and directly alter permselectivity as a result of this interaction, without participation of complement or inflammatory cells.

Another example of a familiar mediator that may work in a newly appreciated way comes from a study by Biesecker et al. (15) on the role of terminal complement components in the glomerular injury of lupus nephritis in man. They utilized a fluorescein-labeled antibody specific for the assembled membrane attack complex (MAC) of the complement cascade to examine renal tissue from lupus patients. The majority of the specimens examined showed definite evidence of MAC deposition in glomeruli and in peritubular regions. In particular, there was definite glomerular capillary wall staining for MAC in several instances, suggesting the presence of the assembled complex within the GBM. The MAC damages cell membranes such as those of the erythrocyte by disrupting osmoregulation leading to cell lysis. However, it is at present unclear how the MAC might damage GBM, which is quite different from the erythrocyte membrane, how such damage might lead to proteinuria, or how universal this mechanism of injury might be.

In the final stage of GBM injury in the classic sequence of events, the major perpetrator of damage is the neutrophil. Recent studies indicate that other inflammatory cells participate in immune glomerular injury. Specifically, marrow-derived circulating monocytes have been recognized as a major component of the glomerular hypercellularity of proliferative types of nephritis. Three recently reported studies confirm earlier observations on the role of monocytes in proliferative glomerulonephritis. First, Sterzel and Pabst (16) studied the kinetics of glomerular cell proliferation, identifying dividing cells by autoradiography of kidney sections after tritiated thymidine pulse labeling, in a model of accelerated autologous phase anti-GBM nephritis in rats. In this mildly proliferative, proteinuric nephritis, there was initial proliferation of intrinsic glomerular cells on the first day. However, this was followed on subsequent days by an influx of histologically identified monocytes into the glomeruli. The infiltration of glomeruli by the monocytes coincided with the peak of protein excretion in these animals, supporting a role for the monocytes in glomerular injury. Second, Cattell and Arlidge (17) administered anti-GBM serum to rabbits and compared in the same animal hypercellularity of crescents and glomerular tufts in a control kidney with that in the contralateral kidney, locally irradiated to suppress division of intrinsic glomerular cells. Despite the fact that division of intrinsic renal cells, as assessed by mitotic activity of renal tubular cells, was suppressed by irradiation, the two kidneys developed equal intra- and extracapillary proliferation, implicating infiltration of extrarenal cells as the cause of hypercellularity. These authors did not specifically identify monocytes as the infiltrating cells. Finally, in a different type of proliferative nephritis occurring in rabbits infected with trypanosomes, Nagle et al. (18) identified monocytes as a principal contributor to glomerular hypercellularity. Studies such as these demonstrate that circulating monocytes may act as mediators of glomerular injury and that inflammatory cell participation in glomerulonephritis is not limited to the neutrophil.

Circulating monocytes may not be the only cells of the macrophage series involved in the immunopathogenesis of glomerulonephritis. Schreiner and co-workers (19) have recently characterized a population of resident glomerular mesangial cells in the rat that bear type II surface histocompatibility antigens designated Ia antigens in the rat. These are therefore designated Ia-positive cells. These cells comprise approximately

2% of the normal glomerular cell population and are distinct from the previously recognized mesangial cell population possessing contractile elements. The Ia-positive cells are phagocytic and bear receptors for the Fc portion of immunoglobulin. The importance of these cells lies in the observation that they are capable of processing antigen and are probably necessary for initiation of cellular and humoral responses by lymphocytes. Their role in disease states remains to be defined.

While the role of B-cell-mediated humoral immunity in glomerular injury seems well established, there is still little strong evidence for a role for cell-mediated immunity in renal injury. Recently, two groups of Japanese investigators (20,21) have employed the T-cell deficient nude mouse as an experimental test of the importance of the T-cell system in development of anti-GBM disease. There was no difference in the severity of injury as judged histologically or by presence of proteinuria between the nude mice and their normal controls. These results suggest that although T-cells may participate in this model of nephritis, their presence is not mandatory for glomerular injury.

Mechanisms of Proteinuria

It is now clear that the GBM, the principle protein filtration barrier of the glomerulus, restricts molecules on the basis of both size and charge. The restriction of anionic molecules probably results from the presence within the GBM of fixed anionic sites, which, as described earlier, also influence the deposition of cationic antigens and subsequent in situ formation of immune complexes. The role of these anionic sites in maintaining normal glomerular permselectivity to proteins has been demonstrated by the fact that in vivo neutralization of the GBM anions by infusion of polycations leads to acute reversible proteinuria. These observations have recently been confirmed by Vehaskari et al. (22) who infused the polycations protamine, polylysine, or hexadimethrine systemically or intrarenally in the rat and demonstrated increased urinary albumin excretion bilaterally or unilaterally, respectively. Hemodynamic alterations and systemic toxicity could not explain the proteinuria observed, which was associated in general with decreased glomerular anionic sites as revealed by colloidal iron staining.

In another model of proteinuria, Bertani et al. (23) administered doxorubicin (Adriamycin) to rats that subsequently developed nephrotic syndrome, histologic changes identical to those seen in the older model of proteinuria produced by puromycin aminonucleoside, and loss of glomerular anions as assessed by colloidal iron staining. The basis for proteinuria in this model has not yet been established, but the loss of colloidal iron staining suggests that loss of glomerular charges may be a factor.

There is as yet little evidence implicating circulating polycations as the mediators of proteinuria in immunologic renal disease. However, some provocative experiments have recently been reported by Bakker and colleagues (24,25). These authors showed that incubation of normal rat or human kidney sections with mitogen-stimulated normal human mononuclear cells in vitro led to loss of colloidal iron staining in the incubated sections. Unstimulated mononuclear cells did not affect the kidney sections. Mononuclear cells from donors with renal disease were not evaluated. These preliminary results suggest that activated lymphocytes may, by direct toxicity or by production of a soluble factor, reduce glomerular anionic sites and lead to proteinuria.

Melnick et al. (26) employed cationized ferritin as a marker of GBM anionic sites to examine possible alterations in these sites in lupus nephritis in mice. They found that focal loss of GBM anions, shown by loss of cationic ferritin binding, occurred as the mice reached the age at which they generally developed proteinuria. At this time, the mice usually had few immune deposits. The authors postulate that loss of GBM anions, by an unspecified mechanism, leads to altered glomerular permeability and proteinuria, which then enhances deposition of immune complexes.

Progression of Renal Disease

Considerable attention has been paid to the hypothesis (27–29) (Fig. 2) that the compensatory hyperfiltration and glomerular hypertension in intact nephrons occurring after a reduction in nephron mass may lead to progressive damage to these remaining "overloaded" nephrons, regardless of the nature or activity of the process causing the initial loss of nephrons. Thus, if immunologic mediators cause an initial reduction of functioning nephrons sufficient to induce compensatory hyperfiltration, the renal damage may progress even if therapy or the natural history of the process removes the immunologic mediators. The implications for therapy and prevention of immunologic renal disease are obvious.

A recent experimental demonstration of the effects of compensatory hyperfiltration has been reported by Olson et al. (30). These authors examined glomerular permselectivity and histopathology in a model of marked nephron reduction—a rat that had a five-sixths nephrectomy. In this 2-week study, animals undergoing renal ablation developed albuminuria and progressive glomerular sclerosis. Tracer studies demonstrated the presence of a defect in both the size- and charge-selective properties of the glomerular barrier. Dietary protein restriction, shown previously to prevent hyperfiltration in the residual nephrons after renal ablation, prevented development both of albuminuria and glomerular sclerosis. The authors postulate that the altered permselectivity in the "overloaded" residual nephrons may contribute to mesangial accumulation of protein and, in turn, to progressive glomerulosclerosis. Although provocative, this

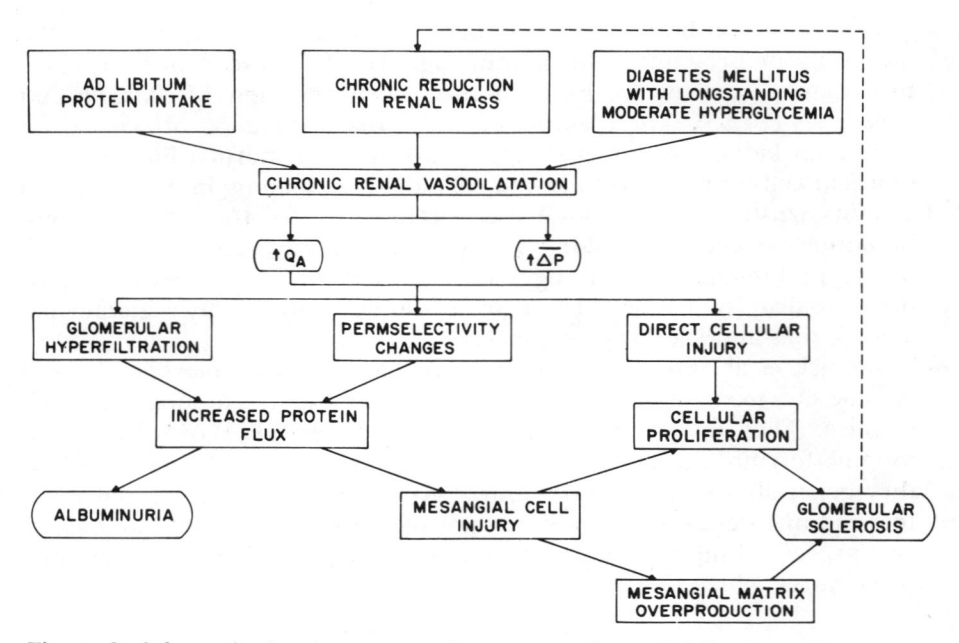

Figure 2. Schematic showing proposed sequence of events following reduction in renal mass. Compensatory increases in afferent arteriolar blood flow (Q_A) and net glomerular capillary ultrafiltration pressure (ΔP) lead to glomerular hyperfiltration in remaining nephrons, permselectivity changes, and direct cell injury. Hyperfiltration and altered permselectivity result in increased protein flux into the tubule (albuminuria) and into the mesangium, which may eventually lead to glomerular sclerosis. As indicated by the dashed line, this hypothetical sequence could become self-perpetuating because of the further reduction in renal mass due to glomerular sclerosis. (Brenner BM et al: *N Engl J Med* 307:642–649, 1982. Used with permission.)

study employed a model of severe reduction in nephron mass. It remains unknown what critical number of lost nephrons must be lost before hyperfiltration in the remaining nephrons initiates the pathogenetic sequence demonstrated in these rats. Other questions to be resolved are the nature of the intrarenal events occurring after slowly progressive, rather than acute, nephron loss, and the effects of dietary protein restriction on compensatory hyperfiltration in other species and other types of renal injury.

The progression of renal disease is hastened by systemic, as well as glomerular, hypertension. This was recently reemphasized by the study of Neugarten et al. (31) who demonstrated that glomerular sclerosis, vascular sclerosis, and proteinuria were much more severe in rats with nephrotoxic serum nephritis that were also rendered hypertensive by unilateral renal artery stenosis.

Laboratory Studies of the Treatment of Nephritis

Laboratory studies of the management of glomerular disorders this year have centered on the remarkable antiinflammatory actions of the prostaglandins and on the efforts discussed above to prevent by dietary manipulations the progression of glomerular damage related to hyperfiltration. Prostaglandins of the E series (PGEs) are known to have multiple effects on the immune system in vitro and have previously been shown to ameliorate dramatically experimental immune complex glomerulonephritis. Because PGEs are known to inhibit antibody synthesis in vitro, McLeish et al. (32) have studied the effects of in vivo administration of PGEs on apoferritin antibody levels, plaque-forming cells (PFCs), and glomerular histology in the model of apoferritin-induced immune complex glomerulonephritis. They confirmed a marked reduction in glomerular damage, associated with a shift in the pattern of immune complex deposition from the peripheral capillary loops to the mesangium, and significant decrease in serum antiapoferritin levels. There was, however, no change in the frequency of splenic antiapoferritin PFCs, suggesting that the PGEs might be regulating the quantity of antibody synthesis by individual cells. This is not the only mechanism by which PGEs may reduce glomerular damage. Kunkel et al. (33) studied the effect of administration of PGE_1 to rats with heterologous anti-GBM nephritis. PGE_1 administration suppressed both glomerular cellularity and proteinuria without affecting at all the binding of specific anti-GBM antibody to the GBM. Presumably in this case the PGE_1 served to reduce the inflammatory response to the glomerular bound antibody.

HUMAN GLOMERULAR DISEASE

Hematuria is one of the cardinal signs of glomerular disease, but it may also result from disease of the urinary collecting system. In the past, only when hematuria has been associated with red cell casts has it been possible to be sure of a renal source of hematuria, and patients with hematuria but no red cell casts are usually subjected to cystocopy to exclude disease such as tumors and stones. Two recent publications (34,35) suggest that glomerular hematuria can be distinguished from urinary tract bleeding by examination of the urinary red cells with phase contrast microscopy. Red cells entering the urine within the kidney are dysmorphic, with variations in size and shape, some showing fragmentation or having bleblike extrusions of cytoplasm (35). Erythrocytes entering the urinary collecting system, on the other hand, generally have normal morphology. Fasset and co-workers (34) examined the urine of 303 patients while still unaware of the clinical diagnosis. The patients were correctly classified into groups with glomerular or collecting system bleeding in 85% of the cases. In 11% of the cases, the urine contained both normal and dysmorphic red cells so that no diagnosis could be made. An incorrect diagnosis was made in only 4% of the patients. Another group (36) report that those who do not have phase microscopes easily available can get the same information by using a simple stain of the urinary sediment. Use of these techniques may help to assure that patients with disease of the collecting system are referred promptly to urologists and that patients with glomerular diseases are spared unnecessary urological instrumentation.

The clinical nephrologist is frequently faced with the practical question of whether a patient with evidence of renal disease will benefit from a renal biopsy. A recent review (37) offers an excellent summary of the literature regarding the risks of percutaneous renal biopsy. A companion article (38) reviews the indications for renal biopsy in various settings. The major indication at this time seems to be nephrotic syndrome in the adult. The need for biopsy in other situations remains more controversial. In particular, the usefulness of renal biopsy in the management of lupus nephritis will be discussed later in this chapter.

Investigators continue to explore the mechanism of formation of glomerular immune deposits in human glomerulonephritis, as well as in the animal models described earlier (39,40). Cairns et al. (39) employed four different assays to examine sera from 134 patients with either minimal change disease, membranous nephropathy, mesangial proliferative glomerulonephritis, or Henoch-Schönlein syndrome. As in prior studies reported by others, most patients (approximately 80%) had detectable circulating immune complexes by at least one test at some time during their course. However, there was little evidence for a general relationship between the circulating complexes and the renal immune deposits (or absence thereof). For example, there was no correlation between the immunoglobulin classes (IgG, IgA, or IgM) present in the circulating complexes and the classes present in glomerular deposits. In addition, there was no correlation between disease activity and the level of circulating complexes. Finally, 60% of patients with minimal change disease had circulating complexes in levels similar to those present in other categories, despite the fact that, by definition, in this study these patients had biopsy results that showed no immunoglobulin deposition. This study emphasizes the difficulty in explaining glomerular immune deposits by passive deposition of circulating complexes and has strengthened the case for in situ complex formation mechanisms.

Other recent investigations have demonstrated a variety of immunologic abnormalities in primary glomerulonephritis, including evidence of T-cell sensitization to glomerular antigens in patients with glomerulonephritis, as evidenced by inhibition of mononuclear cell migration in vitro (41) and alterations in the populations of B-cells bearing particular IgG classes on their surfaces (42). There are also several new reports of immunologic alterations in patients with nephrotic syndrome of diverse histologies, including defects in B-cell function as measured by decreased immunoglobulin synthesis in vitro (43) defects in T-cell function as measured by in vitro tests (44–46), and increased levels of concanavalin-A inducible suppressor T-cells (47–49). It remains unclear whether these alterations are part of the process causing the disease, a side effect of the nephrotic syndrome, or, in some cases, the result of therapy.

A recently reported series (50) describes the renal pathology and clinical picture in 76 patients over age 60 with nephrotic syndrome. Not surprisingly, 40% of patients had membranous nephropathy; 10 of the patients with membranous nephropathy had a systemic illness, and seven of the 10 had a malignancy. The authors emphasize that despite the age of their patients, 14 patients (20%) had minimal change disease, which was generally steroid responsive. Forty percent of the total group had some systemic disease. Frequent diagnoses were amyloidosis (13%) and neoplasia (8%).

Drugs continue to be recognized as a cause of nephrotic syndrome. Recent case reports document nephrotic syndrome due to lithium (51), tolmetin (52), and fenoprofen (53). In these three cases, renal biopsy showed normal glomeruli by light microscopy. The fenoprofen-induced nephropathy was characterized by interstitial accumulations of T-lymphocytes, leading the authors to speculate that the nephrotic syndrome had a basis in disordered cell-mediated immunity.

PRIMARY GLOMERULOPATHIES

Minimal Change Nephrotic Syndrome (MCNS) and Related Syndromes

Although the glomeruli in MCNS are customarily described as normal by light microscopic examination, it has been recognized that some patients with otherwise typical MCNS have minor glomerular histologic changes, such as mild mesangial hypercellularity (Fig. 3) and focal glomerular obsolescence. Although such patients have generally been included within the MCNS category, it has been proposed that they represent a subgroup within MCNS. A recent report from the International Study of Kidney Disease in Children (54) addressed this question in a group of 389 patients with MCNS followed (in most cases) for 2 years in a multicenter study. The major finding was that patients with focal tubular changes or mesangial hypercellularity were significantly more likely to be initially unresponsive to steroid therapy. However, as the authors point out, most patients even in the category with mild histologic changes were responders, and many of the early nonresponders did remit at later follow-up. The authors appropriately conclude that the finding of mild histologic changes in MCNS should not alter therapy for this disorder. A second series (55), involving 68 patients with a longer follow-up period (6 years), showed that positive immunofluorescence microscopy, as well as mesangial hyper-

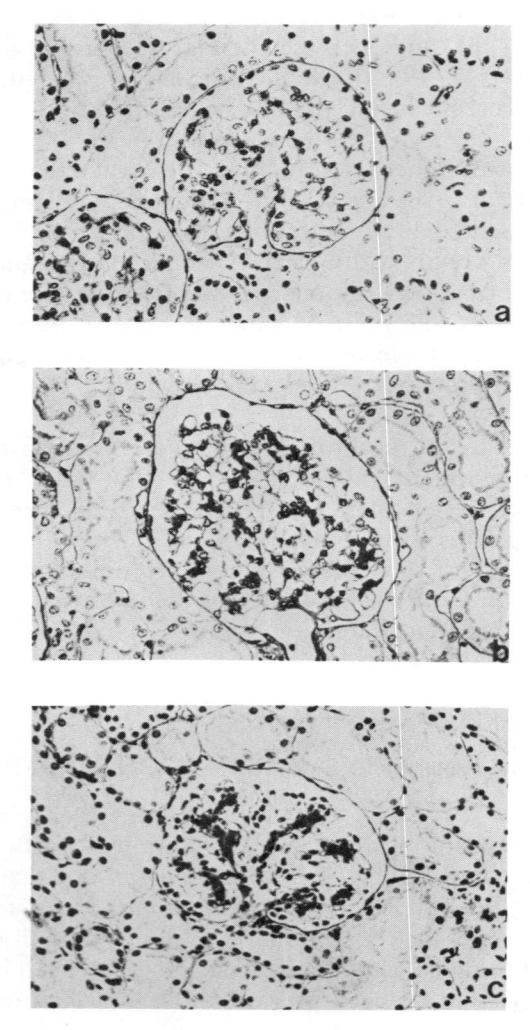

Figure 3. Variations in mesangial hypercellularity in minimal change nephrotic syndrome (MCNS). (*a*) normal mesangial cellularity, (*b*) mild mesangial hypercellularity, and (*c*) more pronounced mesangial hypercellularity. The changes present in (*b*) and (*c*) predict a lower likelihood of steroid responsiveness. (Periodic acid Schiff stains. ×180) (International Study of Kidney Disease in Children: *Kidney Int* 20:765–771, 1981. Used with permission.)

cellularity, is predictive of an increased likelihood of initial steroid unresponsiveness, but that the long-term outcome is not detectably altered.

Similarly, four recently published studies (56–59) have described a clinical entity characterized by nephrotic syndrome, mild to moderate mesangial hypercellularity, and mesangial deposition of IgM without other immunoglobulins. Of the total of 57 patients described in these four reports, only three had hypertension and four had reduced creatinine clearance. Almost all of these patients had remission of nephrotic syndrome after steroid therapy. The clinical and laboratory data suggest that this entity represents another subgroup of patients with minimal change nephrotic syndrome. In fact, in two of these series (57,58) the cases of mesangial hypercellularity with IgM deposition were identified by reviewing a larger group of MCNS patients. Approximately 25% fell into this newly described histopathological subgroup. The authors of these reports concur that there is no indication so far that the course of these patients with respect to treatment, response, or prognosis is different from other MCNS patients lacking mesangial IgM deposits.

The pathogenesis of MCNS and its related syndromes remains obscure. One clue to a possible origin lies in the association (60) between clinical atopy, manifested as allergic rhinitis or asthma, and idiopathic nephrotic syndrome. A recent study by Pirotzky et al. (61) examined patients with typical MCNS for evidence of atopic sensitivity as measured in vitro by basophil degranulation after allergen exposure. Basophils from 57% of patients with MCNS and 78% of patients with focal glomerulosclerosis, underwent degranulation after allergen exposure, as compared to only 17% and 9% of patients with other glomerulonephritides and normal controls, respectively. These findings add to those of other studies to suggest that some product released by basophils or other activated inflammatory cells leads to altered glomerular permselectivity, although the identity of the mediator/mediators eludes us.

Focal Segmental Glomerulosclerosis

The most significant recent development regarding focal segmental glomerulosclerosis (FGS) has been the recognition that it can result in experimental animals from reductions in nephron mass and the subsequent compensatory hyperfiltration in the remnant nephrons. Evidence that this mechanism is clinically relevant comes from a recent survey of autopsy and surgical pathology specimens displaying FGS (62). The authors of this paper demonstrated a significant association between FGS and solitary kidneys due to renal agenesis or nephrectomy. A number of these patients with FGS had clinical features commonly associated with that histopathology, such as nephrotic grade proteinuria and progressive renal insufficiency. Of course, this study leaves unanswered the crucial question of how frequently such severe functional consequences follow unilateral nephrectomy and what fraction of human FGS results from the mechanism of compensatory hyperfiltration.

Membranous Glomerulopathy

As previously discussed in this chapter the major development in the understanding of membranous nephropathy has been the mounting evidence that the characteristic subepithelial immune deposits are formed by in situ combination of antibody and antigen. Evidence that a mechanism similar to that seen in HN accounts for at least one case of human membranous nephropathy has been presented by Douglas et al. (63) who performed immunohistologic studies on serum and renal tissue from a patient with typical membranous nephropathy. The patient's serum contained an antibody reactive with the tubular brush border in normal human kidney sections. This reactivity could be abolished by preincubation of the normal targets with heterologous rabbit anti-Fx1A antiserum or by absorption of the patient's serum with a human Fx1A antigen preparation. After elution of the patient's renal biopsy specimen with a chaotropic buffer designed to dissociate preexisting bound antibodies, the authors found that heterologous anti-Fx1A bound to glomerular capillary walls with the same pattern seen in the original immunofluorescence performed with antihuman IgG. These immunohistological studies suggest that the subepithelial deposits of membranous nephropathy in this patient were formed, at least in part, by combination of anti-Fx1A antibody and Fx1A or cross-reactive antigen. This study does not determine whether the complexes of Fx1A and corresponding antibody form in situ or are deposited from the circulation. The authors point out that the peritubular immunoglobulin deposits seen in this case are atypical for membranous nephropathy. It should be noted that extensive prior studies have found no similar case of human "Heymann nephritis," which must therefore be a rare cause of human membranous nephropathy.

Other recent clinical observations concerning membranous glomerulopathy include a possible association with sarcoidosis (64) as well as the implication of immunologic mechanisms in mercury-induced membranous nephropathy (65).

IgA Nephropathy

There continues to be lively discussion about the molecular form of the IgA deposited in the glomeruli in IgA nephropathy and related diseases. It is now fairly well accepted that a high molecular weight form of IgA can be found in the circulation of patients with these disorders, but there is disagreement whether this represents normal serum IgA in immune complexes or whether it is a polymeric IgA, similar to secretory IgA, normally found only in secretions. Lesavre et al. (66) have now shown that 68% of patients with IgA nephropathy have circulating IgA-containing aggregates that can be detected by the Raji cell binding assay, implying the ability to fix C3 through the alternative complement pathway. Most of this complement-fixing IgA coeluted from gel filtration columns with native monomeric IgA, with a smaller amount having a higher molecular weight. None of the circulating IgA bore secretory piece, and the large molecular weight fraction of IgA failed to bind to solid phase secretory piece as would have been expected of polymeric IgA. The authors concluded therefore that the complement-binding IgA represented IgA immune complexes and not polymeric IgA. Similarly, Sancho et al. (67) have studied the IgA-containing immune complexes found in patients with alcoholic cirrhosis, a condition frequently associated with elevated plasma IgA levels and IgA nephropathy. They found that 55% of plasma IgA in these patients was of high molecular weight. Acid dissociation reduced most of the plasma IgA to monomeric form, but approximately 25% remained in the 9–13 S fraction, consistent with true polymeric IgA. Furthermore, these sera were able to bind free secretory piece. These authors obtained similar results in studies of IgA eluted from autopsy kidneys of patients dying from alcoholic liver disease with IgA nephropathy, suggesting that polymeric IgA not only circulates in these patients, but is trapped in the mesangial deposits as well, presumably contributing to glomerular injury. Other investigators have also obtained strong evidence of the presence of polymeric IgA in the glomerular mesangium of patients with idiopathic IgA nephropathy by demonstrating the specific mesangial binding of purified secretory piece (68), by demonstrating mesangial deposits of J chain (68,69) and by demonstrating both J chain and high molecular weight IgA in acid eluates of renal biopsy specimens. However, in other studies (70) the latter group of investigators has also provided strong evidence that the glomerular IgA is present as immune complexes. Eluted IgA bound specifically to persistent antigens in autologous, acid-treated renal tissue, but not to normal renal tissue. There was a limited, but not complete, cross-reactivity of eluted IgA with renal tissue from other patients with IgA nephropathy. The nature of the antigen involved is unknown. It appears, then, that both theories are correct: that patients with IgA nephropathy have both circulating and glomerular immune complexes containing IgA, some of which is polymeric.

In the past, it has been suggested that IgA nephropathy might result from a failure of suppressor cell function, leading to overproduction, especially of polymeric IgA normally found only in secretions. Egido et al. (71) have recently reported that pokeweed mitogen-stimulated peripheral blood lymphocytes from patients with IgA nephropathy synthesized significantly more IgA, especially of high molecular weight, than lymphocytes from control subjects. The high molecular weight material appeared to be true polymeric IgA as evidenced by its ability to bind secretory piece and by its stability in dissociating acid buffers. On the other hand, other investigators (72) have been unable to confirm any difference in IgA synthesis of lymphocytes from patients with IgA nephropathy and normals. This debate will undoubtedly continue.

IgA nephropathy and the related condition, Henoch-Schönlein purpura (HSP), are rather unpredictable diseases, benign in most patients but progressing to renal insufficiency in others. In the past, neither clinical criteria nor glomerular histology have been very useful in predicting which patients would do poorly. Three papers this year have addressed themselves to this difficulty (73–75). Two papers call attention to the importance of tubulointerstitial immune deposits and interstitial disease, in addition to glomerulosclerosis and crescents, in determining outcome (73,74). A third paper (75) describes unusual dense round microparticles, 30–80 nm in diameter, termed *lead shot* deposits, that were strongly associated with progressive disease (nine of 16 patients) in children with HSP.

Poststreptococcal Glomerulonephritis

Although poststreptococcal glomerulonephritis appears to be a benign disease in the short and intermediate term for the large majority of patients, it has recently been suggested that there may be a significant incidence of late progression to renal failure. The publication this year of three studies of long-term (10–17 years) follow-up of patients after episodes of acute poststreptococcal nephritis clarifies this issue. Potter et al. (76) report on 534 of an original 760 patients from Trinidad, followed 12–17 years after their original episode of nephritis. Only two patients appear to have died of renal failure since their original report, and both had persistent urinary abnormalities on previous follow-up. Of the surviving patients, only 3.6% had an abnormal urine (proteinuria and/or hematuria) and only 3.6% had hypertension. No surviving patient had a serum creatinine higher than 1.2 mg/dl. Drachman et al. (77) report on 80 of an original 155 children from Israel 11–12 years after their acute disease. No patient in this series had a persistently abnormal urine, and all patients had normal blood pressure and plasma creatinine. An additional 55 patients had been examined 2–10 years after their illness. None of this group had any evidence of renal damage. Singhal et al. (78) report on the long-term outcome of an epidemic of severe poststreptococcal glomerulonephritis in Chandigarh, India. Twenty-five of 144 patients in this series died within 2 years of their acute episode of rapidly progressive disease, and six others had established renal insufficiency. In the next 8 years, only six other patients have developed renal insufficiency, and only three of the total of 12 patients with renal insufficiency have progressed to renal failure. The adverse course of these 12 patients was correlated with persistence of nephrotic syndrome, hypertension, and renal insufficiency after the original attack, and with glomerular crescents on renal histology. As has been found in other series, the prognosis for affected children was substantially better than for affected adults. It appears from these three studies that it is distinctly uncommon for a patient who has had a clinical recovery from an episode of acute poststreptococcal glomerulonephritis to develop later a delayed progressive renal disease.

Membranoproliferative Glomerulonephritis (MPGN)

Reports in the recent literature have dealt with the possible clinical significance of variations in renal pathology in MPGN (79–81). Strife et al. (79) present data on six cases out of a total of 61 children with MPGN who presented with focal and segmental, rather than diffuse, glomerular changes. Most of these patients had type I MPGN (subendothelial deposits by electron microscopy). They were younger and had less severe evidence of clinical renal disease, suggesting that they were perhaps cases that were caught early in development of the lesion prior to diffuse glomerular involvement. However, it was the authors' impression that even during follow-up, these cases pursued a more benign course than the rest of their MPGN population.

Abreo and Moorthy (80) report on long-term follow-up (4–15 years) of nine patients with type III MPGN; the category is defined by presence of subendothelial and subepithelial GBM deposits. Their data indicate that, in this small series, the clinical course of type III patients was no different from or slightly more favorable than that of type I patients.

Rapidly Progressive Glomerulonephritis

This glomerular lesion was recently reviewed in depth by Couser (82). Idiopathic rapidly progressive glomerulonephritis (RPGN) is characterized histologically by the presence of "crescents," comprised of proliferating cells in Bowman's space surrounding the glomerular tuft. Experimental studies in animals with crescentic glomerulonephritis, such as those discussed earlier in this chapter, have shown that infiltrating peripheral blood monocytes account for a substantial proportion of the hypercellularity of the crescents. In a recent study of biopsy findings from 14 patients with idiopathic RPGN, Magil and Wadsworth (83) provide evidence that monocytes also contribute to crescent formation in humans. Monocytes were identified in biopsy specimens by means of nonspecific esterase staining, lysozyme content, and electron microscopy. Interestingly, only the patients with RPGN due to an anti-GBM antibody mechanism (defined by linear immunofluorescence staining for immunoglobulins) had prominent monocytes in their crescentic lesions. The patients with granular immunofluorescence and deposits on electron microscopy, categorized as "immune complex RPGN," did not have monocytes.

Treatment of Primary Glomerulopathies

Beyond the universally accepted observation that steroid therapy can induce remissions in a large fraction of patients with MCNS, therapy for glomerulonephritis has been associated with uncertainty and frustration. This is largely due to the fact that no therapy is strikingly effective, and that the great variety of glomerular lesions and the relative infrequency of the disease make controlled trials very difficult to perform. The few successful controlled trials are therefore very important. The APN, a collaborative group of German pediatricians, has studied the vexing question of when to use cytotoxic therapy for frequently relapsing MCNS. They report (84) that steroid-dependent patients (those relapsing during the steroid taper or immediately after its completion) also had early relapses after 8 weeks of therapy with either cyclophosphamide or chlorambucil. In contrast, those patients whose relapses occurred 2 or more weeks after cessation of steroid therapy had long-lasting remissions following cytotoxic therapy. Cyclophosphamide and chlorambucil were equally effective in producing this result. Although this study does not exclude the possibility that a higher dose or a longer period of therapy with cytotoxic agents might be more effective in steroid-dependent patients, it does suggest that, pending new information, such patients should be spared cytotoxic drugs.

There continues to be controversy about the place of steroid therapy in idiopathic membranous glomerulopathy. This topic has been reviewed in a thorough and balanced way in a coordinated series of "Fiat Lux" articles (85–87). Our conclusion is that the best available information, while certainly not conclusive, suggests that the progression to renal failure may be slowed in some patients. There is no evidence to suggest prolongation of life. Such information would be extremely difficult to obtain, though another controlled trial has been initiated. Another group (88) has published a small nonrandomized trial of steroid therapy in nonnephrotic patients with membranous nephropathy. Eight of nine treated patients had a complete remission of proteinuria after an average of 2.4 months of therapy, and the findings of all five repeat biopsies showed definite regression of the pathological lesions. None of the nine contemporaneous nontreated patients had remission of proteinuria within a year. Given the high rate of spontaneous remission of mild membranous nephropathy seen by other investigators and the generally benign nature of this lesion, it is difficult to know what conclusions can be made as a result of this trial.

The unresponsiveness of proliferative forms of glomerulonephritis to conventional therapies continues to lead to exploratory, usually uncontrolled, trials of new approaches. This year, preliminary but uncontrolled trials of dipyridamole therapy (89), pulse methylprednisolone (90), and plasmapheresis (91) in proliferative glomerulonephritis have been published. In each case, the side effects and complications of therapy were minimal and the results promising, suggesting that future controlled trials might be warranted.

GLOMERULONEPHRITIS IN MULTISYSTEM DISEASE
Lupus Erythematosus

Through the years, more has been written about systemic lupus erythematosus (SLE) and its renal manifestations than about any other form of glomerulonephritis. This year, two major published symposia (92,93) have summarized and consolidated the recent advances in understanding SLE and lupus nephritis. They serve as excellent resources for those interested in more detailed review.

Genetic and immunologic factors are most frequently identified as the most likely etiologies for SLE. Winchester and Nuñez-Roldan (94) have reviewed the evidence for a genetic basis for human lupus. Studies of twins have revealed concordance for SLE in 69% of identical twin pairs, indicating a strong but not unique role for a genetic background. However, fraternal twins had only a 3% concordance for lupus, indicating that as many as four separately segregating genes might be involved in the genetic predisposition to lupus. The fairly frequent occurrence of parent-child pairs suggests that at least some of these genetic traits are dominant. Further evidence for a genetic factor in lupus has come from studies of the HLA gene products (95,96). There is an increased frequency of the HLA specificities DR2, DR3, and MB1 among patients with SLE compared with control populations. These data indicate that at least one of the genes for SLE susceptibility resides in or close to the HLA gene complex on the short arm of chromosome 6. The linkage of SLE susceptibility to HLA may also explain the association of deficiency of the early complement components C2 and C4 with SLE (96). The genes for both of these deficiencies are HLA-linked, and C2 deficiency, in particular, is linked with DR2. Further, the C2 heterozygous state, in which there is no functional complement defect, is associated with SLE (and DR2). There continue to be reports of the association of other complement component deficiencies with lupuslike states (97), so there may be other functional bases for the association between complement deficiency and lupus. However, there is a real possibility of ascertainment bias in these reports. Complement assays are most frequently performed in patients with collagen vascular diseases so that a high frequency of patients with SLE would not be surprising. The frequency of these other complement component deficiencies is not high enough to permit the kind of population studies that firmly demonstrated the C2 deficiency SLE link.

The search for a single basic immunological defect responsible for the manifestations of SLE has not yet provided a convincing result. Though

B-cell hyperreactivity is the most obvious abnormality in lupus, most investigators believe that this results from abnormal T-cell regulation. Steinberg et al. (98) have reviewed the current state of confusion in this area. Many patients with SLE have defects in their suppressor cell function that might explain the B-cell hyperreactivity, but some do not. A defect in the autologous mixed lymphocyte response (AMLR) is characteristic of patients with SLE, but the significance of this abnormality is not clear, since the AMLR may give rise to suppressor or helper functions. Finally, the abnormalities in T-cell regulation may result from the presence of lymphocytotoxic antibodies, raising again the possibility of a primary B-cell abnormality. Studies in lupus mice suggest the presence of independent abnormalities both of B-cells and of T-cells.

Although SLE is notoriously variable in its clinical manifestations, it has usually been assumed that there would prove to be a common etiologic factor responsible for the disease in all patients. This assumption is increasingly questioned. It is now realized (99) that the phenotypically similar lupuslike syndromes seen in different strains of mice may have entirely different genetic and immunological causes, all converging in hyperactivity of the B-cells. If there is etiologic diversity among mice, there may also be etiologic diversity among groups of human patients who may have differing clinical characteristics and who may respond to different therapies (99). There continue to be efforts to define subsets of lupus based upon various immunological parameters. Steinberg et al. (99) have found that there is a substantially different pattern of disease in those patients with high ratios of circulating helper/suppressor T-cells (multisystem disease, sicca syndrome, myalgias, Raynaud's syndrome, lung disease) compared with those having low ratios of helpers/suppressors (renal disease, lymphopenia, thrombocytopenia, no widespread systemic involvement). Similarly, Ahearn et al. (95) found that patients with HLA-DR2 or DR3 had a higher frequency of seroreactivity (anti-Ro, anti-DNA, rheumatoid factor, hyperglobulinemia) than patients lacking these antigens. Sharp (100) found that SLE patients with Sm, RNP, and/or anti-La antibodies had less central nervous system (CNS) and renal disease and generally a milder course, while those with anti-Ro antibodies more frequently had high titers of anti-DNA antibodies and severe renal disease. On the other hand, Barada et al. (101) found no difference in renal or CNS disease or general disease severity between Sm positive and Sm negative patients. Finally, Ballou and Kushner (102) found that patients lacking antibodies to double-stranded DNA had less frequent clinical renal disease than did patients with this antibody. There were no other significant clinical differences between the two groups. Since anti-DNA antibodies are the predominant immunoglobulin in the glomeruli of patients with progressive renal failure, this difference may reflect only the direct pathogenicity of this particular antibody.

While immunologic tests such as those discussed above may help distinguish different subgroups of SLE, it is less clear that they are helpful in monitoring disease activity or in predicting outcome. Morrow et al. (103) studied the correlation between clinical estimation of disease activity and levels of circulating immune complexes, anti-DNA antibody, complement levels, lymphocyte and platelet counts, plasma IgG and albumin levels, and erythrocyte sedimentation rate. No single test distinguished reliably between the three defined levels of disease activity, and even the optimum combination of four tests permitted the correct placement of only 44% of patients into the correct category, which is little better than chance. These authors concluded that better methods for monitoring the course of SLE were needed.

Patients with active SLE virtually all have circulating immune complexes. Since large quantities of DNA–anti-DNA complexes are found in the kidneys of patients with progressive renal disease, it was originally expected that they would also be found in the circulation. Surprisingly, it turned out to be very difficult to detect them. Now, finally, these complexes have been reliably detected by several groups (104–107). The complexes tend to be rather small (104,105), probably because the DNA itself is most frequently a small fragment (~25,000 daltons, ~30–40 base pairs) (106). Emlen and Mannik (108) have found that immune complexes containing large molecular weight DNA are removed from plasma very rapidly, more rapidly even than aggregated IgG. However, the IgG from these cleared immune complexes is subsequently released into the circulation as monomers which may be complexed to small DNA fragments similar to those found in the circulation of SLE patients. The small fragments of DNA are rich in guanine-cytosine content, which may be the basis for their antigenicity (106). Circulating DNA–anti-DNA cold precipitable complexes from SLE patients have been shown to be biologically active in complement activation and neutrophil chemotaxis (107). Interestingly, the titer of these complexes correlates very poorly with standard assays for immune complexes (104,105), suggesting either that the standard assays do not detect these complexes well or that other antigen-antibody systems are responsible for most of the circulating complexes in lupus (105). Certainly DNA–anti-DNA complexes are not the only ones important in SLE nephritis. Given the hyperresponsiveness of all B-cell clones in SLE, one might expect complexes containing any persistent antigen. Looi and Prathap (109) have reported that in Malaysia, where there is a high prevalence of hepatitis B infection, 30 of 43 patients with lupus nephritis had hepatitis B antigen in immune deposits within their glomeruli in the absence of clinical liver disease. Deposits of hepatitis B antigen were uncommon (4%) in patients with other forms of glomerulopathy.

The relationship between the circulating immune complexes seen in SLE and the development of renal diseases remains unclear. As discussed above, it seems increasingly likely that subepithelial glomerular immune complexes are formed in situ from circulating antibody and free antigen, whereas mesangial deposits seem most likely to result from trapping of circulating immune complexes (110). However, the source of the large subendothelial immune complexes associated with severe proliferative lupus nephritis is not clear. Cameron (1) has made a strong argument that these complexes result from the precipitation within the glomeruli of preformed, circulating immune complexes of large size. These complexes are normally cleared from the circulation very rapidly by the reticuloendothelial system. It has been proposed that dysfunction of the reticuloendothelial system (RES) function in SLE permits these complexes to circulate for longer periods of time, contributing to their deposition in the glomeruli. The NIH group have continued their studies of defective RES Fc receptor function in SLE (111), finding that the defect existed in most patients at presentation, improved in those with clinical improvement, and worsened in one patient with a flare. There was significant correlation of the defect with disease activity. The CR_1 complement receptor on the human erythrocyte provides another recently recognized mechanism for the sequestering of these large complexes (112), binding up to 70% of the immune complexes added to whole blood. In SLE, the average number of these receptors on erythrocytes is reduced by more than 50% (113), possibly contributing to the persistence in the circulation of the large molecular weight complexes that may be responsible for the subendothelial deposits. This defect was also partially corrected during remissions from SLE. It may be that these receptor defects are only manifestations of the high levels of circulating immune complexes in SLE since both defects were in fact highly correlated with assays for circulating immune complexes (111,113). However, it has also been reported (114) that the CR_1 complement receptor normally found on glomerular podocytes is completely absent in patients with severe proliferative lupus nephritis (and focally absent in patients with focal segmental glomerulosclerosis), while it is normal in quantity and distribution on podocytes from patients with all other forms of proliferative, membranous, and mesangial nephritis. This suggests the possibility of a specific defect of CR_1 receptor synthesis or turnover in SLE and focal glomerulosclerosis.

However the glomerular immune complexes are formed, complement deficiency induced by the circulating immune complexes may be a factor favoring persistence of large glomerular immune deposits. Aguado et al. (115) have shown that SLE patients with low serum complement levels have a decreased ability to solubilize immune complexes in vitro, an increased incidence of renal disease, and a worse evolution of their disease. It is possible that the acquired complement deficiency in these patients may impair a normal mechanism for removal of complexes, leading to worsening of the disease.

There are several mechanisms by which glomerular immune complexes may cause injury. It has long been recognized that there were deposits of the early complement components in the glomeruli of patients with lupus nephritis, thought to result from complement activation by the glomerular immune complexes. The MAC of complement has now been demonstrated in the glomeruli, vessels, and peritubular regions of patients with lupus nephritis (15) in a distribution correlating with membrane damage and inflammation. It is unclear how the MAC, an ion channel that kills cells by disrupting osmoregulation, could itself mediate damage to glomerular or tubular basement membrane, but its presence is evidence of intense complement activation with release of chemotactic factors and other mediators of inflammation, and it correlates with tissue injury in other sites such as skin. Glomerular immune complexes can also initiate inflammation by binding and activating monocytes through the antibody Fc regions. Recently, monocytes have been identified in the glomeruli of patients with proliferative lupus nephritis (116). The monocytes correlated both with endocapillary hypercellularity and with proteinuria, suggesting that they were responsible both for inflammation and for glomerular damage. Both glomerular and circulating immune complexes may contribute to a pathogenetic mechanism newly postulated by Camussi and colleagues (117). This group has reported that in patients with lupus nephritis, immune complexes induce circulating and possibly glomerular neutrophils to release their cationic proteins, which then become localized to the anionic sites of the glomerular filter, with resulting loss of stainable anions and appearance of proteinuria.

Over the past 20 years, innumerable papers have been published on the description, classification, and clinical utility of renal biopsies. Practicing nephrologists and rheumatologists now perform renal biopsies almost uniformly on patients with lupus and anything more than the most trivial manifestations of nephritis (118). Despite this wealth of information and widespread practice, however, substantial questions remain about the interpretation and utility of renal biopsies in lupus nephritis. Robert McCluskey has published this year (119) a very thoughtful review of the current status of renal biopsy in lupus nephritis that should be read by everyone who deals with lupus patients. He questions whether the universally used World Health Organization (WHO) classification of lupus nephritis (Table 1) can be used consistently to classify lupus nephritis, whether the WHO classification is in fact consistently used by current investigators, whether transitions from one form of lupus nephritis to another are too frequent to make any one-time biopsy helpful, whether the classification assists in establishing prognosis or choosing treatment, and whether there may be other ways of interpreting biopsy results in lupus that may give more useful information. These questions form a good framework for reviewing this year's literature on renal biopsy in lupus nephritis.

There is uniform agreement (120–122) that classification of lupus nephritis should not be based solely upon light microscopy, as the original

WHO criteria implied. It is recognized that the extent and distribution of immune deposits, as revealed by immunofluorescence (120) or electron (121) microscopy, may be as important as the light microscopic appearance in understanding the pathophysiology and predicting the course of lupus nephritis. Thus, modifications of the WHO classification have appeared (122) (Table 1) that include information from all three histological techniques. Though these classifications are fairly successful in permitting a consistent classification of lupus nephritis, a problem remains when there is a mixture of proliferative glomerular changes, associated primarily with subendothelial or mesangial deposits, and membranous changes, associated with subepithelial deposits (119). There has been no consistent way of handling these cases. The approach often taken of further subdividing the classification of lupus nephritis, as in Table 1, has the tendency to reduce the classification to no more than an extended description. Even excluding the problem of mixed membranous and proliferative lesions, it has not been possible to achieve consistency in interpretation of biopsy results of lupus nephritis from laboratory to laboratory. The main problem has been the distinction between focal segmental (class III) and diffuse (class IV) lupus nephritis. Some laboratories (123) define focal lesions in a very restrictive way, find a small fraction of biopsy results fitting into this classification, and report a very benign course for these patients. Others (124) doubt any qualitative difference between focal and diffuse disease, find a higher fraction of patients with class III lesions, and fail to find a significant difference in the courses of patients with class III and class IV lesions.

Although initially it appeared that transitions in lupus nephritis from one form of lupus nephritis to another were infrequent, a later series of reports suggested that the frequency of transitions was much higher. A consensus now appears to be emerging that transitions appear in perhaps one of six patients. Baldwin (125) has recently compiled the results of seven series, reporting a total of 475 patients. Transitions from mesangial (class II) lesions to focal or diffuse proliferative (class III or IV) lesions occurred in 15% of patients, and from focal (class III) to diffuse (class IV) lesions in 18% of patients. Transitions from membranous lesions (class V) to focal or diffuse proliferative lesions occurred in 7% of patients. Thus, a past biopsy result in a patient with lupus nephritis is reasonably likely, but not certain, to reflect present or future disease.

An assumption underlying the widespread use of renal biopsy in the management of patients with lupus nephritis is that the patient's clinical course, and perhaps the response to therapy, can be better predicted if the underlying renal pathology is known. This assumption has come increasingly into question in recent years. This is partially the result of the questions raised above about the consistency with which diagnostic criteria can be applied and about the frequency with which transitions in the type of renal pathology have appeared. Recently, the utility of renal

Table 1. Modified WHO Classification of Lupus Nephritis

	Immunofluorescence		Electron Microscopy		
Class (Light Microscopy)	Peripheral	Mesangial	Mesangial	Endothelial	Epithelial
I. Normal					
A. No mesangial deposits	0	0	0	0	0
B. With mesangial deposits	0	+	+	0	0
II. Pure mesangial glomerulopathy					
A. Mild	0	+	+	0	0
B. Moderate	0	+	+	0	0
III. Focal and segmental glomerulonephritis (Mild: <20%; Mod: 20–50%; Sev: ≥50%)					
A. Active	+	++	++	+	±
B. Active and Sclerotic					
C. Sclerotic					
IV. Diffuse glomerulonephritis					
A. Pure	++	++	++	++	±
B. With sclerosis					
V. Membranous glomerulopathy					
A. Pure	+	0	0	0	++
B. With mesangial glomerulopathy	+	+	+	0	++
C. With focal and segmental glomerulopathy	+	+	+	±	++
D. With diffuse glomerulonephritis	+	+	+	+	++
VI. Advanced sclerosing glomerulonephritis	±	±	±	±	±

SOURCE: Modified from Kashgarian M: *Am J Kidney Dis* 2:164–169, 1982. Reprinted with permission.

biopsy has been more formally evaluated in terms of the degree to which information derived from the biopsy improves the ability to predict clinical outcome. Specifically, it is asked whether information from renal biopsy improves the predictions based on other clinical information available from history, physical examination, and noninvasive tests—that is, whether the biopsy contributes "marginally useful information." Previous studies have suggested that renal biopsy does not improve the prediction of death in lupus patients. Whiting-O'Keefe and associates (126) recently asked whether information from renal biopsy findings could at least improve prediction of changes in renal function over a period of 1 year. They concluded that renal biopsy findings did contain marginally useful information; specifically, they found that the percent glomerular sclerosis and the extent of subendothelial immune deposits added significantly to the predictive power of the model based on clinical information alone. However, even after addition of information obtained from biopsy, only about one-third of the total variability in outcome was attributable to measured clinical or histologic variables, and the biopsy information accounted for only about 8% of total variability. These authors found that knowledge of the WHO biopsy classification per se added nothing to predictive value. In a companion paper (127), these same authors asked whether addition of information obtained from biopsy to clinical information actually improved the predictions of a group of 197 experienced academic rheumatologists and whether it influenced their choice of therapy. They found, as did Knutsen (118), that biopsy information had a substantial impact on the therapy chosen, but it had no effect at all on the predictive accuracy of the rheumatologists. The authors concluded that the potentially useful information from the biopsy was not well utilized even by experienced clinicians, and that renal biopsy as currently used added no marginally useful information to that available from clinical information alone. Further evidence for the secondary value of biopsy information in predicting outcome has come from studies of patients with minimal clinical evidences of renal disease who were found on renal biopsy to have diffuse proliferative nephritis. The observation that a patient with minimal clinical disease might prove to have severe disease upon biopsy has been used in the past as an argument for more widespread use of renal biopsy in lupus. However, two reports (128,129) indicate that such patients have, in fact, a good prognosis; the clinical data correlated better with outcome than the WHO histological grade.

The failure of the WHO biopsy classification to add significantly to clinical data in prognostication does not imply that the biopsy is inherently of little value, but only that we have not yet learned how to extract useful information from it. Whiting-O'Keefe et al. (126) analyzed 19 previously studied biopsy variables, in addition to the WHO classification, in order to find the two that added useful information to clinical data. More attention must be paid now to newly described distinctions in biopsy results between groups of lupus patients. Kant et al. (130) have recently called attention to glomerular thrombosis in lupus nephritis as an important predictor of subsequent progression of glomerulosclerosis. They emphasize the importance of looking for capillary thrombi by light microscopy (using the Lendrum stain) in addition to immunofluorescence, since they may be only focally distributed and missed on the smaller frozen blocks. Glomerular thrombosis correlated well with proliferative pathology, either focal or diffuse, and was often associated with a circulating anticoagulant and mild thrombocytopenia, suggesting accelerated platelet destruction. The association of glomerular thrombi and evidence of platelet destruction with progressive glomerulosclerosis, frequently in the absence of significant abnormalities of complement or anti-DNA antibodies, suggested to these authors that coagulation mechanisms might be an important contributor to progressive renal insufficiency in lupus nephritis. It should be noted, however, that other authors (121) have found glomerular thrombosis to be an uncommon finding. Schwartz et al. (131) have recently differentiated two types of subepithelial dense deposits (SED) found on biopsy of lupus patients. Type I SEDs (Fig. 4a) were regular in size and shape, had a homogeneous electron density, and were distributed uniformly along all the basement membranes. These deposits were associated with membranous lupus nephropathy in patients with mild serological disease and slow loss of renal function. Type II SEDs (Fig. 4b) were irregular in size, shape, and electron density, tended to be quite large, were fewer in number, and were irregularly distributed in the glomerular capillary loops. These deposits were associated with diffuse proliferative nephritis in patients with more severe clinical and serological disease, with a more rapid decline in renal function. Patients with type II SED could not be distinguished clinically or serologically from other patients with proliferative lupus nephritis. The authors propose that the pathogenesis of the two types of SED are probably entirely different. Bhathena et al. (132) have reemphasized the importance of noninflammatory renal vascular lesions, similar to those seen in malignant hypertension and thrombotic microangiopathy, which may be important contributors to progressive renal damage, and Schwartz and associates (133) have reemphasized the importance of tubulointerstitial lesions. It is to be hoped that increased recognition of these and other newly described abnormalities in biopsy findings will improve the utility of renal biopsy in predicting the clinical course of patients with lupus nephritis.

The long-term prognosis of SLE and lupus nephritis has been much more solidly established this year with the publication of reports of two large series, one a multicenter study of 1,103 patients with various forms of SLE (134,135), and the other a single center study of 230 patients specifically with lupus nephritis (136). The presence of nephritis is clearly the most important factor affecting outcome in SLE. Patients wtihout nephritis have 5- and 10-year survivals of 90%, whereas those with nephritis

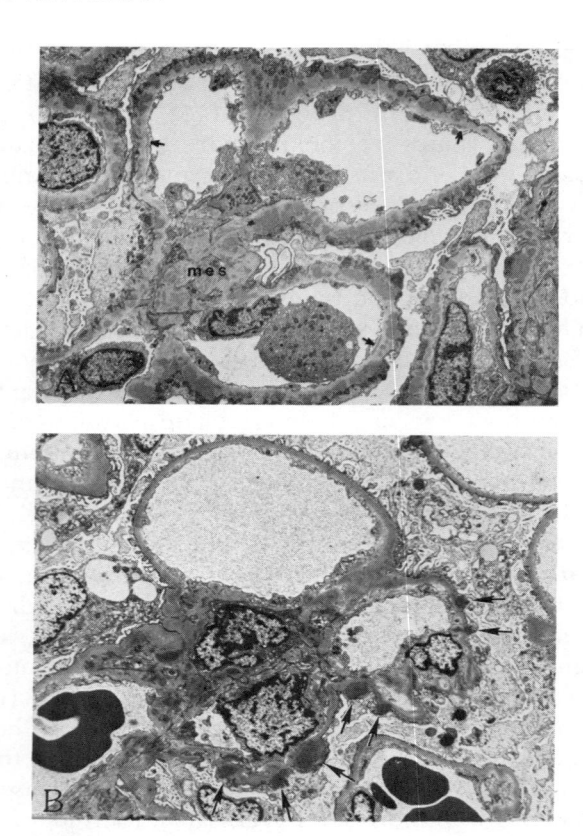

Figure 4. Subepithelial deposits (SED) in glomeruli of patients with lupus nephritis. (a) Type I SED are distributed diffusely around all capillary loops. They are of comparable size and homogeneous electron density. Mesangial electron-dense deposit (mes) and small focal subendothelial deposits are also present (arrows). (×2100) (b) Type II SED are irregularly distributed throughout the glomerulus (arrows), with some loops having several deposits while other loops (top) are free of deposits. Deposits differ in size and electron density. (×2100) (Schwartz MM et al: *Ultrastruct Pathol* 3:105–118, 1982. Used with permission.)

have 5- and 10-year survivals of about 75% and 65%, respectively (134,136). Not surprisingly, those with elevated serum creatinine at or prior to study entry had the worst prognosis; those with a serum creatinine in excess of 3.0 mg/dl at any time prior to study entry had 5- and 10-year survivals of only 29% and 12% (134). About half of the patients in the single center study (136) had a remission of their renal disease during follow-up, generally within the first year or two, and this subgroup had a substantially better prognosis than those whose nephritis persisted (5- and 10-year survivals were 90% and 77% versus 70% and 34%, respectively). Renal disease and infection were the most common causes of death in both studies (135,136), each accounting for about 25% of the deaths. It appears that death from infection has become more frequent in recent years (136), possibly due to use of more intensive therapy. Death from cardiovascular disease or from central nervous system lupus were relatively uncommon, each accounting for about 5% of deaths. Age of onset of SLE has previously been thought to have a major influence on prognosis, with disease in children thought to be more severe and disease in the elderly thought to be milder. Three recent studies suggest that age may have less influence on outcome than previously thought. Two studies of SLE in children (137,138), almost all with renal involvement and half to two-thirds with impaired renal clearance at presentation, showed 10-year survivals of 75% and 85%, respectively, apparently better than those reported for adults with lupus nephritis. Another study (139) comparing SLE in older (age > 55) and younger adults found few differences in the manifestations of the disease and no difference in 5-year survival (72% and 79%, respectively) as a function of age.

Hayslett (140) has reviewed the interactions of SLE and pregnancy in nine large series, and Jungers et al. (141) have added another large series. These authors confirm that a patient who becomes pregnant during or shortly after a period of clinical lupus activity has an increased likelihood of disease exacerbation and a markedly reduced likelihood of successful completion of pregnancy. More importantly, however, they have found that pregnancies in patients whose SLE has been quiescent for 6 months or more are usually not associated with exacerbation. The rate of live births in such patients, even if they previously have had evidence of severe nephropathy, is not detectably different from that of normal women, and one should not be overly pessimistic with such patients about the chances for a successful pregnancy.

Therapy for lupus nephritis has been thoroughly reviewed in articles included in the two major symposia on SLE referred to above (92,93). Most impressive about these articles is the extent to which skepticism about the value of current steroid and cytotoxic therapy has replaced an earlier enthusiasm or at least cautious optimism. Decker (142) and Pollak (143) discuss the difficulty of evaluating the results of steroid therapy and the difficulty of formulating an appropriate therapeutic plan for their use in the absence of any controlled studies. Though Wallace et al. (136) were impressed with the efficacy of nitrogen mustard in an uncontrolled trial in 44 patients, the NIH group (144) have been unable to demonstrate a significant improvement in renal outcome by addition of either cyclophosphamide or azathioprine. Donadio (145) concludes that while survival of patients with lupus nephritis has improved since 1970, the improvement cannot be attributed to the use of azathioprine or cyclophosphamide. The use of cyclophosphamide has been further challenged with the description of two lupus patients who developed bladder cancer after its use (146).

In this setting, it is not surprising that there continues to be interest in new therapeutic approaches. The use of methylprednisolone pulse therapy, popularized over the last few years, has been studied by two groups. Ponticelli et al. (147) reported an uncontrolled series of 25 patients with diffuse proliferative lupus nephritis who were treated with 1g methylprednisolone pulses daily for three days. Extrarenal symptoms disappeared in all patients, and all but four had a rapid and sustained improvement of their serum creatinines, with lessening proteinuria and serological improvement. On the other hand, Barron et al. (148) reported on a series of 15 children with lupus nephritis treated with pulse methylprednisolone, compared with a control group of seven patients with similar renal disease who were treated with conventional doses of steroids. They found no difference between the two groups in side effects, relapse rate, or long-term outcome, though the pulse steroid treated group had a more rapid initial improvement in glomerular filtration rate (GFR). In addition, two other groups have reported their initial results with plasmapheresis (142,149). Sharon et al. (149) reported an uncontrolled trial of plasmapheresis in 10 patients with severe lupus nephritis. These authors found rapid initial and long-term improvement in immune complex levels, anti-DNA antibodies, and serum creatinine, and concluded that the therapy was probably beneficial. However, two patients died within 6 months of treatment, and the authors caution that it is not clear that the long-term outcome of lupus nephritis is changed by plasmapheresis. The NIH group (142) performed a small double-blind trial of plasmapheresis, compared to sham apheresis, in a group of patients with predominantly rheumatological symptoms of the disease. They also noted a rapid improvement in serological parameters with apheresis, but this improvement disappeared as soon as the series of apheresis treatments were completed. Plasmapheresis was associated with no clinical benefit at any time, and they have abandoned this approach. Finally, Pollak and associates (150), because they suspect that glomerular thrombosis may be an important contributor to progressive glomerular sclerosis (130), have treated five patients with glomerulonephritis and glomerular fibrin deposits (four with lupus nephritis) with the defibrinating agent ancrod. There were no significant complications of therapy and all patients had improvement of renal function with disappearance of glomerular thrombi. Obviously, more studies need to be done to establish the effectiveness and safety of this agent. The search for a new approach to therapy for SLE has not yet revealed a convincing alternative to standard therapy.

Goodpasture's Syndrome and Anti-GBM Nephritis

Efforts continue to identify and characterize the GBM antigen involved in spontaneous human anti-GBM nephritis. Hunt et al. (151) passed solubilized GBM over affinity columns to which they had bound antibodies

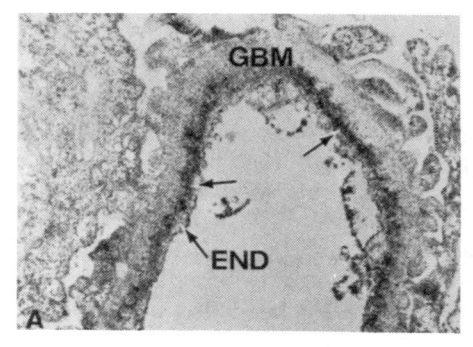

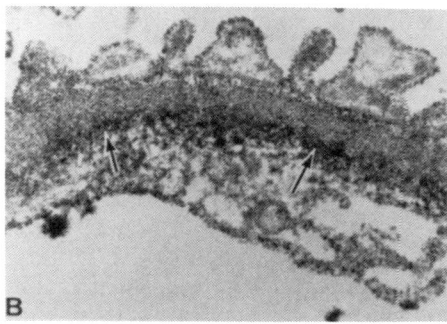

Figure 5. (*a*) Normal human kidney, incubated with IgG eluted from the kidney of a patient with Goodpasture's syndrome, followed by treatment with peroxidase-labeled antihuman IgG. The antibody, recognized by the electron-dense peroxidase reaction product, localizes exclusively to the subendothelial region and the lamina rara of the GBM (arrows) and to the surface of endothelial cells (END). ($\times$ 7,300) (*b*) Normal human kidney treated as in (*a*), except that IgG eluted from a different Goodpasture's patient was employed. Reaction product again localizes to the lamina rara interna (arrows). ($\times$ 17,300) (Sisson S et al: *Clin Immunol Immunopathol* 23:414–429, 1982. Used with permission.)

eluted from the kidney of a patient with Goodpasture's syndrome. The bound antigen fractions were then eluted, studied by electrophoresis, and analyzed for amino acid and carbohydrate content. Four major protein bands were identified. The authors concluded, in agreement with others studying this question, that the nephritogenic antigens are noncollagenous glycoproteins. Sisson et al. (152) have examined the distribution of the nephritogenic antigen by immunoelectron microscopy. When renal tissues from four patients with Goodpasture's syndrome were stained with peroxidase-labeled antihuman IgG and examined by electron microscopy, the peroxidase reaction product was confined to the lamina rara interna of the GBM. Furthermore, when eluates from the kidneys of two of the patients were used in an immunoperoxidase stain of normal human kidneys, the reaction product was similarly confined to the lamina rara interna (Fig. 5). Thus, the nephritogenic antigen appears to be a specific component of the lamina rara interna, distinct from laminin, fibronectin, and collagen.

Jennette et al. (153) have reported a curious finding in one of their patients with Goodpasture's syndrome. There appeared to be concurrent linear and granular epimembranous deposits of IgG in the glomeruli, suggesting both anti-GBM and immune complex disease. Since the IgG subclass restriction of both the linear and granular deposits was the same (predominantly IgG1 and IgG4), they hypothesized that the granular deposits resulted from reaction of anti-GBM antibodies with antigens released from the GBM by the inflammatory reaction.

From the clinical point of view, one of the major points made this year is that not all patients with glomerulonephritis and pulmonary hemorrhage have Goodpasture's syndrome. Leatherman et al. (154) reported on nine such patients who represented half of all patients seen with glomerulonephritis and lung hemorrhage at their institution. Ultimate diagnoses were Wegener's granulomatosis, rheumatoid arthritis with vasculitis, and crescentic glomerulonephritis with negative immunofluorescence, each in two patients, and polyarteritis nodosa, Henoch-Schönlein purpura, and mixed connective tissue disease in one patient each. These authors emphasized the difficulty of differentiating these conditions from Goodpasture's syndrome, and the importance of making a specific immunological diagnosis by immunopathology and assays of anti-GBM antibodies. The same point has been made in three other case reports that appeared this year (155–157).

Peters et al. (158) have reviewed several aspects of their experience with anti-GBM nephritis, now totaling 41 patients. They continue to find a strong genetic association between anti-GBM nephritis and HLA-DR2 (32 of 36 patients, with a relative risk of 33.7 compared to the general population). Those patients also bearing the HLA-B7 antigen, which is in linkage disequilibrium with DR2, seemed to do particularly poorly, with 11 of 12 progressing to end-stage renal failure compared to five of 13 bearing DR2 only. These authors find little evidence of a relationship between Goodpasture's syndrome and hydrocarbon exposure in their patients, but have noted a strong relationship between smoking and lung hemorrhage; 32 of 35 smokers had lung hemorrhage but only three of 11 nonsmokers had lung hemorrhage. Intercurrent infection also appeared to be an important factor in relapse in many patients. Their therapeutic results from a combination of daily plasmapheresis and three agent immunosuppression (prednisone, azathioprine, and cyclophosphamide) continue to be impressive in patients whose treatment is initiated before onset of renal failure; 15 of 17 patients achieved long-term improvement. Conversely, only 1 of 24 patients presenting with a serum creatinine in excess of 7 mg/dl or in end-stage renal failure was improved. Lung hemorrhage was controlled in 29 of 33 patients. In most cases, 2 weeks of daily plasmapheresis was sufficient to reduce the anti-GBM titer almost to normal, and antibody rebound after discontinuation of plasmapheresis was rarely seen when this reduction had been achieved first. Immunosuppression was continued for a longer period. Late relapses have been uncommon, and the long-term outlook appears to be good.

Systemic Vasculitis

Uncertainty has persisted concerning the immunopathogenesis of Wegener's granulomatosis. Because typical granular immune deposits have been seen in the glomeruli of some patients with this condition, it has generally been thought to be mediated by circulating immune complexes. But the glomerular deposits are inconsistent from patient to patient, and immune deposits have rarely been found in other involved tissues. Two papers (159,160) this year report for the first time the presence of typical immune complex deposits in lung and sinus tissue, primarily associated with small vessels. Circulating immune complexes were detected in two patients tested for them. These findings strengthen the hypothesis that Wegener's granulomatosis is mediated by immune complexes. Another study (161) reports on the vascular lesions that may be seen in the kidney in this condition. The acute vascular lesions are sparse, focal, and mainly confined to the interlobular arteries. The lesions are characterized by the presence of platelets and fibrinoid material; immune complexes are usually absent. Detection of these lesions on biopsy is more specific for Wegener's granulomatosis than the very nonspecific glomerulonephritis and may help in establishing the diagnosis. Cohen and Meltzer (162) call our attention to "strawberry gums," a gingival lesion highly suggestive of Wegener's granulomatosis that is readily recognized by dentists but frequently overlooked by physicians. Recognition of this fairly common physical finding may assist in early diagnosis. Though Wegener's granulomatosis usually responds well to cyclophosphamide therapy, occasional patients have rapidly progressive courses leading to acute renal failure. Dabbagh et al. (163) report on one such patient who required dialysis for 7 weeks, after which he regained a GFR of 35 ml/min. He was still well 1 year later. Apparently even prolonged renal failure in this syndrome may resolve to a substantial degree. Those patients who progress to permanent renal failure have no further evidences of recurrent disease on dialysis; recurrent disease has not appeared after transplantation (164).

When Herreman et al. (165) found one patient with Behçet's syndrome and glomerulonephritis, they undertook a systemic evaluation, including renal biopsy, of 10 other patients. Although none of the patients had any symptoms of renal disease, proteinuria was found in five and leukocyturia in two. Eight patients had mesangial and extramembranous glomerular capillary deposits and 10 had subendothelial and medial arteriolar deposits. Immunofluorescence showed the glomerular and arteriolar deposits to contain C3. Circulating immune complexes were found in six of seven of these patients. The occurrence of circulating immune complexes, glomerular and arteriolar immune deposits, and clinical evidences of glomerular injury suggest that Behçet's disease may be another example of an immune complex mediated disease.

The circulating cryoglobulins in essential mixed cryoglobulinemia appear to be immune complexes containing IgM rheumatoid factor. It is thought that they deposit in the glomeruli and thereby initiate glomerular inflammation and damage. Maggiore et al. (166) have shown that glomerular immune deposits in some patients with this condition do indeed contain rheumatoid factor activity, always in association with IgM deposits. Patients with glomerular deposits of rheumatoid factor have more severe glomerular disease, supporting the hypotheses that cryoglobulins deposited in the glomerulus are pathogenic.

Hypocomplementemia is frequently associated with vasculitis and glomerulonephritis. When these three abnormalities are accompanied by urticaria, low molecular weight (7S) precipitins of C1q are often found in the circulation, the constellation then being called the *hypocomplementemic vasculitis-urticaria syndrome* (HVUS). However, Schultz et al. (167) describe two patients with the same clinical picture of urticaria, vasculitis, glomerulonephritis, and hypocomplementemia who were found to have high molecular weight circulating immune complexes more suggestive of systemic lupus erythematosus. One had circulating antibodies to Sm protein. These authors conclude that HVUS may result from several different disease processes. Minta and associates (168) have reported a new inherited complement deficiency, complete absence of C1q, associated with vasculitis and glomerulonephritis. While the association of different complement deficiencies with vasculitides may suggest a pathogenetic relationship, this may simply represent an ascertainment bias, since complement assays are most frequently ordered in patients with one form or another of vasculitis.

Ridolfi and Bell (169) have written this year a major review of thrombotic thrombocytopenic purpura (TTP), analyzing 25 new patients together with 250 patients previously reported in the medical literature since 1964. Their findings are in close agreement with what has been written previously about TTP, the greatest interest centering on the improved prognosis of patients seen since 1965 and on the authors' summary of the results of the various therapies used in this condition. Whereas only 10% of the patients seen prior to 1965 survived their illness, almost half of the patients in this series survived. No one therapy was associated with a dramatically better survival than the others, with "favorable" therapies associated with survival rates ranging from about 55% to 70%. Patients treated with some form of plasma exchange therapy seem to have the best chance of surviving. Because TTP is thought to result from endothelial damage or primary activation of platelets, antiplatelet therapy is frequently prescribed. Rosove et al. (170) have retrospectively reviewed the results of antiplatelet therapy in 19 patients seen at their institution. They found no evidence of benefit from these agents; instead the risk of serious bleeding episodes appeared to be substantially increased. They recommend that they not be used. Since the etiology of TTP remains unknown, it is pertinent to note that it can recur following transplant in the new kidney (171). It appears that the cause of the renal vascular lesions is a circulating factor and not a primary defect of the vascular endothelium.

The pathology of hemolytic-uremic syndrome (HUS) closely resembles that of TTP, but it is not at all certain that these two conditions have the same etiology or pathogenesis. Bergstein et al. (172) have sought and found evidence in patients with HUS of a circulating low molecular weight inhibitor of fibrinolysis, similar to that found in the experimental Schwartzman phenomenon. The inhibitor was found in the sera of all 17 patients with HUS and was absent in all control subjects. It could be detected only during periods of active disease and disappeared as the disease remitted. They suggest that this factor may be important in the persistence of glomerular fibrin deposition in HUS, contributing both to the hemolytic state and the glomerular damage.

MISCELLANEOUS GLOMERULAR DISEASES

Familial Nephritis and Benign Familial Hematuria

The term *familial nephritis* is used to designate a group of diseases, most inherited as autosomal dominant traits, that are characterized by hematuria and proteinuria, and that tend to progress to end-stage renal failure. When familial nephritis is associated with nerve deafness, the condition is known as Alport's syndrome. *Benign familial hematuria* (BFH) is a term used to designate a condition also apparently inherited as an autosomal dominant trait and characterized by hematuria in which proteinuria does not occur and which is nonprogressive. There are no characteristic histopathological abnormalities by light or immunofluorescence microscopy early in the course of familial nephritis, and abnormalities by light or immunofluorescence microscopy never develop in BFH. Therefore, when children present with hematuria in the absence of a well-established family history, it can be difficult to distinguish between these two conditions with very different courses, or in fact to differentiate them from the sporadic forms of recurrent hematuria associated with minimal focal glomerular abnormalities. Over the past years several papers have asserted that these conditions could be distinguished by electron microscopy. The characteristic picture of familial nephritis is said to be an irregular thickening of the basement membrane with replication of the lamina densa, forming a "basket-weave" pattern enclosing electron-lucent spaces in which small dense particles are frequently found. Conversely, BFH is said to be characterized by a diffuse thinning of the GBM, especially of the lamina densa. However, several authors have questioned the specificity of these findings for these hereditary glomerulopathies, and there remains doubt as to whether the benign and progressive forms of familial glomerulopathy are really distinct conditions. Several papers this year have addressed themselves to these questions.

Yoshikawa et al. (173) reviewed electron micrographs of 366 renal biopsy specimens from children with various forms of renal disease to determine the specificity of the "basket-weave" abnormality for familial nephritis. They found the abnormality in 24 of 27 patients with well-documented familial nephritis. The abnormality was widespread in most, involving more than 50% of the capillary loops in 17 of the cases. Conversely, the abnormality was seen in only 19 of 283 other biopsy specimens. In two cases, the abnormality was widespread and the children had nerve deafness. These two patients were considered to be new mutant cases of Alport's syndrome. In no other case were the changes seen in more than a few capillary loops. In five children with BFH the "basket-weave" abnormality was not seen at all. These authors concluded that though the "basket-weave" lesions was not unique to familial nephritis, it was diagnostic when it was widely distributed. Another paper from this group (174) reported on the clinical and histological characteristics of 38 patients with familial hematuria. Twenty of these patients had Alport's syndrome, 11 had familial nephritis without deafness in the patient or the family, and seven had BFH. The "basket-weave" pattern was seen with equal frequency in the groups with Alport's syndrome and with familial nephritis without deafness. These two conditions were considered to be variants of the same disease, though the prognosis for patients with Alport's syndrome appeared to be worse. The only abnormality seen in the biopsy specimens of the seven patients with BFH was diffuse thinning of the lamina densa of the GBM. Because these patients had nonprogressive disease, BFH was considered to be distinct from familial nephritis. Tina et al. (175) reported on electron microscopic findings in 10 children with BFH and nine with sporadic hematuria. They found that measurement of the thickness of the GBM or the lamina densa distinguished reliably between those patients with and without a family history of hematuria. On the other hand, Piel et al. (176) found no sharp distinctions between biopsy findings from patients with familial nephritis, BFH, and sporadic hematuria. Both GBM thinning and reduplication were seen with essentially equal frequency in the three conditions, and patients from each category had progressed to chronic renal failure. They believe that these three conditions belong to a single spectrum of diseases.

The relationship between the various forms of familial glomerulopathies may be clarified as a result of the recent observation that the GBMs of some patients with familial nephritis lack the antigen responsible for Goodpasture's syndrome. McCoy et al. (177) have recently confirmed this finding in a very careful study of six patients from five families with Alport's syndrome. Biopsy specimens from each of these patients failed to stain with anti-GBM antibodies eluted from the kidneys of six other patients with Goodpasture's syndrome. The staining was absent even in patients with very early disease, but was present even in advanced forms of other glomerular diseases, so that it is unlikely to be the consequence of glomerular injury alone. The absence of this antigen is not found in all families with Alport's syndrome or familial nephritis, implying that there may be more than one genetic basis for the condition. Interestingly, if a patient with Alport's syndrome is transplanted, anti-GBM antibodies may appear in the graft or in the circulation (178). The outcome for these grafts, however, appears to be quite good.

Glomerular Lesions in Renal Allografts

Glomerular lesions of various etiologies can be seen in the biopsy specimens of transplanted kidneys. Glomerulonephritis may represent recurrence in the transplanted kidney of disease originally present in the recipient's own kidneys, may represent de novo disease, or, rarely, may be transplanted with the donor kidney. Transplant glomerulopathy may occur as a component of chronic rejection. In most cases, this injury is not associated with evidence of glomerular immune deposits, but when such deposits are found, the lesion is called *rejection glomerulonephritis*. This subject has been summarized this year by Briner (179), who has published an analysis of the glomerular lesions in 328 consecutive transplant biopsy and nephrectomy specimens, together with a detailed review of the literature on this topic. Glomerular lesions were present in about half of these specimens. The most common lesion was transplant glomerulopathy, present in 67 of the specimens. This lesion was most frequently seen with chronic graft rejection, was often associated with heavy proteinuria, and portended a poor outcome. Rejection glomerulonephritis was seen in another 49 specimens, and was associated with acute as well as chronic rejection. The outlook was similarly poor for these grafts. Nine patients developed recurrent glomerulonephritis of various types, which led to graft loss in seven. De novo glomerulonephritis was seen in 20 specimens (eight with MPGN), five with membranous nephropathy, and seven with pure mesangial proliferative disease). Those with de novo membranous nephropathy had rapid progression of their disease, but the patients with MPGN and mesangial proliferation had better preservation of function.

Morzycka et al. (180) reviewed the clinical outcome and biopsy material of 204 consecutive patients with tissue available both from their native and transplanted kidneys, in order to determine the frequency and type of recurrent glomerulonephritis. Of the 204 patients, 117 had had some form of chronic glomerulonephritis; a specific morphological type could be diagnosed in 61 patients. Nineteen of these 61 patients had recurrent glomerulonephritis in their grafts (Table 2). Recurrent glomerulonephritis appeared to be more frequent in related grafts than in cadaveric grafts. Two papers have reported specifically on the recurrence of focal segmental glomerulosclerosis in transplanted kidneys (181,182). The incidence of recurrent disease was similar in the two series (27% and 33%), and in both series about half of the patients with recurrent disease lost their kidneys as a result. Both groups found a strong correlation between the presence of mesangial proliferation in the native kidneys and recurrence in the transplanted kidneys. Finally, Cosyns et al. (183) have reported on nine patients with de novo membranous nephropathy in transplanted

Table 2. Incidence of Recurrent Glomerulonephritis

Host Disease	Total Patients	Patients with Recurrent Glomerulonephritis Number	%
Idiopathic membranous glomerulonephritis	7	4	57
IgA nephropathy	5	1	20
Focal glomerular sclerosis	20	3[a]	15
Antiglomerular basement membrane disease	2	2	100
Membranoproliferative glomerulonephritis, type I	16	6[a]	38
Membranoproliferative glomerulonephritis, type II	2	2	100
Crescentic proliferative glomerulonephritis	4	1	25
Proliferative glomerulonephritis	5	0	0
Total	61	19	31

SOURCE: Morzycka M et al: *Am J Med* 72:588–598, 1982. Reprinted with permission.
[a] One each of these patients had recurrent disease in two consecutive transplants.

kidneys. They found a high frequency of graft loss (5 of the 9) associated with this complication, which is in agreement with other studies (179). (For further discussion, see Chapter 3.)

PROTEINURIA AND THE NEPHROTIC SYNDROME

The Significance of Proteinuria

Proteinuria remains the most constant finding indicative of glomerular disease. Since urine analysis can detect proteinuria with good reliability, and since it is one of the most widely used screening tests, a significant number of patients are seen in whom proteinuria is the sole indicator of glomerular disease. Much attention has been paid over the years to the significance of isolated proteinuria in such patients. Robinson (184) has again reviewed this issue, emphasizing the importance of separating such patients into groups defined by the persistence of the proteinuria and the influence of posture on its appearance. Patients with postural proteinuria are substantially less likely to have significant glomerular lesions on biopsy than patients with persistent proteinuria in all positions. Patients with isolated proteinuria of any type appear to do well at least over the first 10 years following diagnosis. Lim et al. (185) have compared the biopsy findings of 90 patients with asymptomatic proteinuria in excess of 1.0 g per day with those of 83 patients with proteinuria of lesser degree. A high percentage of both groups (77%) had mesangial deposits of IgA, and there was no correlation between the degree of hematuria and the extent of glomerular damage. But patients with the higher degrees of proteinuria were significantly more likely to have areas of glomerular sclerosis (68%) than those with the lesser degree (19%). It is suggested that the degree of proteinuria may be the best predictor of outcome in these patients.

Complications of Nephrotic Syndrome

Proteinuria of nephrotic grade is associated with a number of complications such as infection, thrombosis, hyperlipidemia, and endocrine abnormalities that continue to attract the attention of investigators. This year progress has been made in each of these areas.

Krensky et al. (186) have studied the problem of peritonitis in children with idiopathic nephrosis. Nineteen of 351 patients seen at their institution over a 10-year period had at least one episode of peritonitis, and five of their patients had more than one episode. *Streptococcus pneumoniae* remains the most common agent (50%) and *Escherichia coli* the next most common (25%). Four patients (16%) were culture negative. Signs of peritoneal irritation were present in all patients irrespective of steroid therapy. No one morphological type of glomerular lesion appeared to be particularly associated with peritonitis, but substantially depressed levels of IgG appeared to be an important factor. Ballow et al. (187) have suggested that reduced levels of factor D of the alternative complement pathway may also contribute to the nephrotic patients' susceptibility to infection. Twenty-one of 27 patients in relapse had significantly reduced levels of this protein, whereas the levels of patients in remission were normal. Serum factor D levels were significantly correlated with serum levels of albumin, and it was postulated that this low molecular weight protein is lost in the urine similarly to albumin. Since nephrotic children are particularly susceptible to infection with *S. pneumoniae* (186), two groups have studied the responsiveness of these children to pneumococcal vaccine (188,189). Children with steroid responsive nephrotic syndrome have excellent responses to the vaccine. Those not currently on steroids appear to have better responses (188), but children on alternate-day steroids appear to have significant responses also (189). Children with steroid-resistant nephrotic syndrome have significantly lower levels of antipneumococcal antibody before immunization and unfortunately respond less well to the vaccine (188). The vaccine appears to be protective, since none of the children has had pneumococcal peritonitis over a period of 3 years (189).

The basis for the increased frequency of thrombosis in nephrotic syndrome is still not well understood. Two groups have reported this year that patients with nephrotic syndrome have increased plasma levels of factor VIII related antigen and factor VIII coagulant activity (190,191), which correlates inversely with plasma albumin level but less well with proteinuria. This abnormality was not associated with any particular histological type of glomerular lesion, and was not correlated with the patients' clinical courses or with the frequency of thrombotic disorders. The two groups concluded that the changes in factor VIII levels were probably epiphenomenal. Boneu et al. (192) have studied levels of three thrombin inhibitors, antithrombin III, α_1-antitrypsin, and α_2-macroglobulin in nephrotic children. Levels of antithrombin III and α_1-antitrypsin, two proteins with molecular weight close to that of albumin, were dramatically reduced in nephrotic patients. However, marked elevations of α_2-macroglobulin compensated for these reductions, accounting for the increased progressive antithrombin activity seen in all the children. Thus, it appears that the thrombotic diathesis is not, in most cases, attributable to reduced levels of antithrombins. Tomura et al. (193) have suggested that activation of platelets may be important in the susceptibility to thrombosis in nephrotics. They noted that nephrotic patients had significantly smaller platelet volume and higher plasma levels of β-thromboglobulin—evidences of platelet aggregation and release reaction—than normals or other patients with glomerulonephritis. One of the major manifestations of the thrombotic tendency of nephrotic patients is their susceptibility to renal vein thrombosis. This topic has been reviewed by Harrington and Kassirer (194).

It is now generally agreed, on the basis of animal experiments, that hyperlipoproteinemia in nephrotic patients is principally due to increased hepatic synthesis of lipoproteins. That this is true in humans as well is suggested by a study of Michaeli et al. (195), who found a generalized increase in all plasma lipoproteins, including high density lipoproteins, and enrichment of their lipid content, in 10 patients with moderate proteinuria. The finding of a parallel increase of HDLs in their patients suggested that the hyperlipoproteinemia might not be associated with increased atherogenesis. The increased hepatic synthesis of lipids appears to be part of a generalized hypertrophy of the liver and increase in protein synthesis in response to hypoalbuminemia (196), but it has been suggested that decreased renal clearance of mevalonate, a stimulator of cholesterol synthesis, may be a contributing factor (197). Finally, Chan et al. (198), using clearance studies of infused lipids, have confirmed that hyperlipoproteinemia is due principally to increased hepatic synthesis, but they have also found evidence for some decrease in the clearance rate in severely nephrotic patients. This may be due to urinary losses of HDLs.

Loss of hormone binding proteins in nephrotic syndrome may or may not be associated with a significant endocrine disturbance. It has been known for some time that total serum thyroxin is reduced in many nephrotics, but the mechanisms and significance of this reduction have not been thoroughly studied. Feinstein et al. (199) obtained thyroid function studies in 15 nondiabetic nephrotics with normal GFR. They confirmed low plasma levels of total thyroxin and triiodothyronine in about half of the patients, sometimes in association with low levels of thyroxin-binding globulin, but the levels of free thyroxin and triiodothyronine were normal in all patients. In addition, both basal and stimulated levels of thyroid-stimulating hormone were normal. They concluded that the abnormalities in thyroid function studies were the consequence of decreased levels of serum carrier proteins. On the other hand, more severe nephrotic syndrome may result in clinically significant abnormalities in thyroid function. McLean et al. (200) found that four of five infants with congenital nephrotic syndrome had not only low levels of thyroxine, but also elevated levels of thyroid-stimulating hormone suggesting true hypothyroidism. These patients all responded to thyroxine replacement. Serum levels of metabolites of vitamin D are also reduced in nephrotic patients. Sato et al. (201) have confirmed an increased urinary excretion of 25-OH-vitamin D in nephrotic patients, presumably the result of increased filtration of vitamin D binding globulin, a protein with a size and charge similar to those of albumin. Other vitamin D metabolites are also reduced in nephrotic syndrome, presumably by the same mechanism. This may lead to a metabolically significant defect in nephrotics that can be corrected by oral vitamin D therapy.

Treatment of Nephrotic Syndrome

Although there have been no major breakthroughs in the treatment of nephrotic syndrome, a new approach may improve the aesthetics of treatment. Two groups have reported on the effects of water immersion on sodium and water clearance in nephrotic patients (202,203). As has been seen with normal subjects and cirrhotics, immersion of nephrotic patients up to the neck in 1.3 meters of water at 34°C. for 4 hours is associated with a brisk diuresis, natriuresis, and kaliuresis, due to redistribution of plasma volume into the thorax. There is an associated reduction in plasma renin and aldosterone levels. These changes are directly correlated with the patients' estimated total plasma volumes. Some additional salt and water is lost in sweat. The advantages of this approach in the treatment of refractory nephrotic syndrome have not been established, but it seems likely that compliance would be higher to this therapy than to severe sodium restriction. The main risks of therapy seem to be drowning related to syncope or drowsiness induced by the warm water, and injury resulting from slipping on the edge of the deep bath (202).

REFERENCES

1. Cameron JS: Glomerulonephritis: Current problems and understanding. *J Lab Clin Med* 99:755–787, 1982.

2. Neale JT, Wilson CB: Glomerular antigens in Heymann's nephritis: Reactivity of eluted and circulating antibody. *J Immunol* 128:323–330, 1982.
3. Neale JT, Couser WG, Salant DJ, et al: Specific uptake of Heymann's nephritic kidney eluate by rat kidney: Studies in vivo and in isolated perfused kidneys. *Lab Invest* 46:450–453, 1982.
4. Cattran DC, Chodirker WB: Experimental membranous glomerulonephritis: The relationship between circulating free antibody and immune complexes to subsequent pathology. *Nephron* 31:260–265, 1982.
5. Border WA, Ward HJ, Kamil ES, et al: Induction of membranous nephropathy in rabbits by administration of an exogenous cationic antigen: Demonstration of a pathogenic role for electrical charge. *J Clin Invest* 69:450–461, 1982.
6. Vogt A, Rohrback R, Shimizu F, et al: Interaction of cationized antigen with rat glomerular basement membrane: In situ immune complex formation. *Kidney Int* 22:27–35, 1982.
7. Isaacs KL, Miller F: Role of antigen size and charge in immune complex glomerulonephritis: I. Active induction of disease with dextran and its derivatives. *Lab Invest* 47:198–205, 1982.
8. Haakenstad AO, Striker GE, Mannik M: The disappearance kinetics and glomerular deposition of small latticed soluble immune complexes. *Immunology* 47:407–414, 1982.
9. Steward MW, Collins MJ, Stanley C, et al: Chronic antigen-antibody-complex glomerulonephritis in mice. *Br J Exp Path* 62:614–622, 1981.
10. Raij L, Sibley RK, Keane WF: Mononuclear phagocytic system stimulation: Protective role from glomerular immune complex deposition. *J Lab Clin Med* 98:558–567, 1981.
11. Camussi G, Tetta C, Deregibus MC, et al: Platelet-activating factor (PAF) in experimentally induced rabbit acute serum sickness: Role of basophil-derived PAF in immune complex deposition. *J Immunol* 128:86–94, 1982.
12. Sharon Z, Schwartz MM, Pauli BU, et al: Impairment of glomerular clearance of macroaggregates in immune complex glomerulonephritis. *Kidney Int* 22:8–12, 1982.
13. Abrahamson DR, Caulfield JP: Proteinuria and structural alterations in rat glomerular basement membranes induced by intravenously injected anti-laminin immunoglobulin G. *J Exp Med* 156:128–145, 1982.
14. Salant DJ, Madaio MP, Adler S, et al: Altered glomerular permeability induced by F(ab')$_2$ and Fab' antibodies to rat renal tubular epithelial antigen. *Kidney Int* 21:36–43, 1981.
15. Biesecker G, Katz S, Koffler D: Renal localization of the membrane attack complex in systemic lupus erythematosus nephritis. *J Exp Med* 154:1779–1794, 1981.
16. Sterzel RB, Pabst R: The temporal relationship between glomerular cell proliferation and monocyte infiltration in experimental glomerulonephritis. *Virchows Archiv B (Cell Pathol)* 38:337–350, 1982.
17. Cattell V, Arlidge S: The origin of proliferating cells in the glomerulus and Bowman's capsule in nephrotoxic serum nephritis: Effects of unilateral renal irradiation. *Br J Exp Path* 62:669–675, 1981.
18. Nagle RB, Dong S, Janacek LL, et al: Glomerular accumulation of monocytes and macrophages in experimental glomerulonephritis associated with Trypanosoma rhodesiense infection. *Lab Invest* 46:365–376, 1982.
19. Schreiner GF, Kiely JM, Cotran RS, et al: Characterization of resident glomerular cells in the rat expressing Ia determinants and manifesting genetically restricted interactions with lymphocytes. *J Clin Invest* 68:920–931, 1981.
20. Kusuyama Y, Nishihara T, Saito K: Nephrotoxic nephritis in nude mice. *Clin Exp Immunol* 46:20–26, 1981.

21. Okada K, Oite T, Kihara I, et al: Masugi nephritis in the nude mice and their normal littermates. *Acta Pathol Jpn* 32:1–11, 1982.
22. Vehaskari VM, Root ER, Germuth FG, et al: Glomerular charge and urinary protein excretion: Effects of systemic and intrarenal polycation infusion in the rat. *Kidney Int* 22:127–135, 1982.
23. Bertani T, Poggi A, Pozzoni R, et al: Adriamycin-induced nephrotic syndrome in rats: Sequence of pathologic events. *Lab Invest* 46:16–23, 1982.
24. Bakker WW, Vos JTWM, Hoedemaeker PJ: Corticosteroid-sensitive peripheral blood cells are able to affect glomerular polyanion (GPA) in vitro. *Immunol Lett* 5:11–14, 1982.
25. Bakker WW, van der Laan SM, Vos JTWM, et al: The glomerular polyanion (GPA) of the rat kidney: I. Concanavalin-A-activated cells affect the glomerular polyanion in vitro. *Nephron* 31:68–74, 1982.
26. Melnick GA, LaDoulis CT, Cavallo T: Decreased anionic groups and increased permeability precedes deposition of immune complexes in the glomerular capillary wall. *Am J Pathol* 105:114–120, 1981.
27. Brenner BM, Meyer TW, Hostetter TH: Dietary protein intake and the progressive nature of kidney disease: The role of hemodynamically mediated glomerular injury in the pathogenesis of progressive glomerular sclerosis in aging, renal ablation, and intrinsic renal disease. *N Engl J Med* 307:642–649, 1982.
28. Hostetter TH, Rennke HG, Brenner BM: Compensatory renal hemodynamic injury: A final common pathway of residual nephron destruction. *Am J Kidney Dis* 1:310–314, 1982.
29. Baldwin DS: Chronic glomerulonephritis: Nonimmunologic mechanisms of progressive glomerular damage. *Kidney Int* 21:109–120, 1982.
30. Olson JL, Hostetter TH, Rennke HG, et al: Altered glomerular permselectivity and progressive sclerosis following extreme ablation of renal mass. *Kidney Int* 22:112–126, 1982.
31. Neugarten J, Feiner HD, Schacht RG, et al: Aggravation of experimental glomerulonephritis by superimposed clip hypertension. *Kidney Int* 22:257–263, 1982.
32. McLeish KR, Gohara AF, Gunning WT: Suppression of antibody synthesis by prostaglandin E as a mechanism for preventing murine immune complex glomerulonephritis. *Lab Invest* 47:147–152, 1982.
33. Kunkel SL, Zanetti M, Sapin C: Suppression of nephrotoxic serum nephritis in rats by prostaglandin E_1. *Am J Pathol* 108:240–245, 1982.
34. Fassett RG, Horgan BA, Mathew TH: Detection of glomerular bleeding by phase-contrast microscopy. *Lancet* 1:1432–1434, 1982.
35. Fairley KF, Birch DF: Hematuria: A simple method for identifying glomerular bleeding. *Kidney Int* 21:105–108, 1982.
36. Hauglustaine D, Bollens W, Michielsen P: Detection of glomerular bleeding using a simple staining method for light microscopy. *Lancet* 2:761, 1982.
37. Wickre CG, Golper TA: Complications of percutaneous needle biopsy of the kidney. *Am J Nephrol* 2:173–178, 1982.
38. Danovitch GM, Nissenson AR: The role of renal biopsy in determining therapy and prognosis in renal disease. *Am J Nephrol* 2:179–184, 1982.
39. Cairns SA, London AR, Mallick NP: Circulating immune complexes in idiopathic glomerular disease. *Kidney Int* 21:507–512, 1982.
40. Solling J: Molecular weight of circulating immune complexes in patients with glomerulonephritis. *Nephron* 30:137–142, 1982.
41. Schmitt E, Seyfarth M, Werner H, et al: Cellular immunity in glomerulonephritis. *Clin Nephrol* 18:271–276, 1982.

42. Tani Y, Kida H, Abe T, et al: B lymphocyte subset patterns and their significance in idiopathic glomerulonephritis. *Clin Exp Immunol* 48:201–204, 1982.
43. Heslan JM, Lautie JP, Intrator L, et al: Impaired IgG synthesis in patients with the nephrotic syndrome. *Clin Nephrol* 18:144–147, 1982.
44. Chapman S, Taube D, Brown Z, et al: Impaired lymphocyte transformation in minimal change nephropathy in remission. *Clin Nephrol* 18:34–38, 1982.
45. Sasdelli M, Cognoli L, Candi P, et al: Cell-mediated immunity in idiopathic glomerulonephritis. *Clin Exp Immunol* 46:27–34, 1981.
46. Fodor P, Saitua MT, Rodriguez E, et al: T-cell dysfunction in minimal change nephrotic syndrome of childhood. *Am J Dis Child* 136:713–717, 1982.
47. Wu MJ, Moorthy V: Suppressor cell function in patients with primary glomerular disease. *Clin Immunol Immunopathol* 22:442–447, 1981.
48. Matsumoto K, Osakabe K, Katayama H, et al: Concanavalin-A-induced suppressor cell activity in idiopathic membranous nephropathy. *Int Arch Allergy Appl Immunol* 69:26–29, 1982.
49. Matsumoto K, Osakabe K, Katayama H, et al: Concanavalin-A-induced suppressor cell activity in focal glomerular sclerosis. *Nephron* 31:27–30, 1982.
50. Zech P, Colon S, Pointet P, et al: The nephrotic syndrome in adults aged over 60: Etiology, evolution, and treatment of 76 cases. *Clin Nephrol* 18:232–236, 1982.
51. Depner TA: Nephrotic syndrome secondary to lithium therapy. *Nephron* 30:286–289, 1982.
52. Chatterjee GP: Nephrotic syndrome induced by tolmetin. *JAMA* 246:1589, 1981.
53. Finkelstein A, Fraley DS, Stachura I, et al: Fenoprofen nephropathy: Lipoid nephrosis and interstitial nephritis: A possible T-lymphocyte disorder. *Am J Med* 72:81–87, 1982.
54. International Study of Kidney Disease in Children: Primary nephrotic syndrome in children: Clinical significance of histopathologic variants of minimal change and of diffuse mesangial hypercellularity. *Kidney Int* 20:765–771, 1981.
55. Allen WR, Travis LB, Cavallo T, et al: Immune deposits and mesangial hypercellularity in minimal change nephrotic syndrome: Clinical relevance. *J Pediatr* 100:188–191, 1982.
56. Helin H. Mustonen J, Pasternack A, et al: IgM-associated glomerulonephritis. *Nephron* 31:11–16, 1982.
57. Vilches AR, Turner DR, Cameron JS, et al: Significance of mesangial IgM deposition in "minimal change" nephrotic syndrome. *Lab Invest* 46:10–15, 1982.
58. Kobayashi Y, Shigematsu H, Tateno S, et al: Nephrotic syndrome with diffuse mesangial IgM deposits. *Acta Pathol Jpn* 32:307–317, 1982.
59. Mampaso F, Gonzalo A, Teruel J, et al: Mesangial deposits of IgM in patients with the nephrotic syndrome. *Clin Nephrol* 16:230–234, 1981.
60. Editorial. Atopy and steroid-responsive childhood nephrotic syndrome. *Lancet* 2:964–965, 1981.
61. Pirotzky E, Hieblot C, Benveniste J, et al: Basophil sensitisation in idiopathic nephrotic syndrome. *Lancet* 1:358–361, 1982.
62. Kiprov DD, Colvin RB, McCluskey RT: Focal and segmental glomerulosclerosis and proteinuria associated with unilateral renal agenesis. *Lab Invest* 46:275–281, 1982.
63. Douglas MFS, Rabideau DP, Schwartz MM, et al: Evidence of autologous immune complex nephritis. *N Engl J Med* 305:1326–1329, 1981.
64. Taylor RG, Fisher C, Hoffbrand BI: Sarcoidosis and membranous glomerulonephritis: A significant association. *Br Med J* 284:1297–1298, 1982.
65. Tubbs RR, Gephardt GN, McMahon JT, et al: Membranous glomerulonephritis associated with industrial mercury exposure: Study of pathogenetic mechanisms. *Am J Clin Pathol* 77:409–413, 1982.

66. Lesavre PH, Digeon M, Back JF: Analysis of circulating IgA and detection of immune complexes in primary IgA nephropathy. *Clin Exp Immunol* 48:61–69, 1982.
67. Sancho J, Egido J, Sanchez-Crespo M, et al: Detection of monomeric and polymeric IgA containing immune complexes in serum and kidney from patients with alcoholic liver disease. *Clin Exp Immunol* 47:327–335, 1981.
68. Bene MC, Faure G, Duheille J: IgA nephropathy: Characterization of the polymeric nature of mesangial deposits by in vitro binding of free secretory component. *Clin Exp Immunol* 47:527–534, 1982.
69. Tomino Y, Sakai H, Miura M, et al: Detection of polymeric IgA in glomeruli from patients with IgA nephropathy. *Clin Exp Immunol* 49:419–425, 1982.
70. Tomino Y, Endoh M, Nomoto Y, et al: Specificity of eluted antibody from renal tissues of patients with IgA nephropathy. *Am J Kidney Dis* 1:276–280, 1982.
71. Egido J, Blasco R, Sancho J, et al: Increased rates of polymeric IgA synthesis by circulating lymphoid cells in IgA mesangial glomerulonephritis. *Clin Exp Immunol* 47:309–316, 1982.
72. Cosio FG, Lam S, Folami AO, et al: Immune regulation of immunoglobulin production in IgA-nephropathy. *Clin Immunol Immunopathol* 23:430–436, 1982.
73. Frasca GM, Vangelista A, Biagini G, et al: Immunological tubulo-interstitial deposits in IgA nephropathy. *Kidney Int* 22:184–191, 1982.
74. D'Amico G, Ferrario F, Colasanti G, et al: IgA-mesangial nephropathy (Berger's disease) with rapid decline in renal function. *Clin Nephrol* 16:251–257, 1981.
75. Yoshikawa N, White RHR, Cameron AH: Prognostic significance of the glomerular changes in Henoch-Schoenlein nephritis. *Clin Nephrol* 16:223–229, 1981.
76. Potter EV, Lipschultz SA, Abidh S, et al: Twelve to seventeen-year follow-up of patients with poststreptococcal acute glomerulonephritis in Trinidad. *N Engl J Med* 307:725–729, 1982.
77. Drachman R, Aladjem M, Vardy PA: Natural history of an acute glomerulonephritis epidemic in children: An 11-to 12-year follow-up. *Israel J Med Sci* 18:603–607, 1982.
78. Singhal PC, Malik GH, Narayan G, et al: Prognosis of post-streptococcal glomerulonephritis: Chandigarh study. *Ann Acad Med Singapore* 11:36–41, 1982.
79. Strife CF, McAdams AJ, West CD: Membranoproliferative glomerulonephritis characterized by focal, segmental proliferative lesions. *Clin Nephrol* 18:9–16, 1982.
80. Abreo K, Moorthy V: Type 3 membranoproliferative glomerulonephritis: Clinicopathologic correlations and long-term follow-up in nine patients. *Arch Pathol Lab Med* 106:413–417, 1982.
81. Fox A: Light microscopy of membranoproliferative glomerulonephritis type II (MPGN with homologous extraglomerular lesions). *Am J Clin Pathol* 76:644–651, 1981.
82. Couser WG: Idiopathic rapidly progressive glomerulonephritis. *Am J Nephrol* 2:57–69, 1982.
83. Magil AB, Wadsworth LD: Monocyte involvement in glomerular crescents: A histochemical and ultrastructural study. *Lab Invest* 47:160–166, 1982.
84. Arbeitsgemeinschaft fur Padiatrische Nephrologie: Effect of cytotoxic drugs in frequently relapsing nephrotic syndrome with and without steroid dependence. *N Engl J Med* 306:451–454, 1982.
85. Cameron JS: Membranous nephropathy: The treatment dilemma. *Am J Kidney Dis* 1:371–375, 1982.
86. D'Achiardi-Ray R, Pollak VE: Membranous glomerulonephropathy: There is no significant effect of treatment with corticosteroids. *Am J Kidney Dis* 1:386–391, 1982.
87. Glassock RJ: Corticosteroid therapy is beneficial in adults with idiopathic membranous glomerulopathy. *Am J Kidney Dis* 1:376–385, 1982.

88. Kobayashi Y, Tateno S, Shigematsu H, et al: Prednisone treatment in non-nephrotic patients with idiopathic membranous nephropathy: A prospective study. *Nephron* 30:210–219, 1982.
89. Ishikawa H, Honjo A, Hayashi M, et al: Effects of dipyridamole on proteinuria in chronic glomerulonephritis and the nephrotic syndrome. *Arzneim Forsch/Drug Res* 32:301–309, 1982.
90. Rose GM, Cole BR, Robson AM: The treatment of severe glomerulopathies in children using high dose intravenous methylprednisolone pulses. *Am J Kidney Dis* 1:148–156, 1981.
91. Thysell H, Bygren P, Bengtsson U, et al: Immunosuppression and the additive effect of plasma exchange in treatment of rapidly progressive glomerulonephritis. *Acta Med Scand* 212:107–114, 1982.
92. Hayslett JP, Hardin JA (eds): Proceedings of symposium: Advances in systemic lupus erythematosus. *Am J Kidney Dis* 2:97–236, 1982.
93. Koffler D (ed): Current perspectives in the immunology of systemic lupus erythematosus. *Arthritis Rheum* 25:721–897, 1982.
94. Winchester RJ, Nuñez-Roldan A: Some genetic aspects of systemic lupus erythematosus. *Arthritis Rheum* 25:833–837, 1982.
95. Ahearn JM, Provost TT, Dorsch CA, et al: Interrelationships of HLA-DR, MB, and MT phenotypes, autoantibody expression, and clinical features in systemic lupus erythematosus. *Arthritis Rheum* 25:1031–1040, 1982.
96. Schur PH: Complement and lupus erythematosus. *Arthritis Rheum* 25:793–798, 1982.
97. Sano Y, Nichimukai H, Kitamura H, et al: Hereditary deficiency of the third component of complement in two sisters with systemic lupus erythematosus-like symptoms. *Arthritis Rheum* 24:1255–1260, 1981.
98. Steinberg AD, Smith HR, Laskin CA, et al: Studies of immune abnormalities in systemic lupus erythematosus. *Am J Kidney Dis* 2:101–110, 1982.
99. Steinberg AD, Raveche ES, Laskin CA, et al: Genetic environmental, and cellular factors in the pathogenesis of systemic lupus erythematosus. *Arthritis Rheum* 25:734–743, 1982.
100. Sharp GC: Subsets of SLE and mixed connective tissue disease. *Am J Kidney Dis* 2:201–205, 1982.
101. Barada FA, Andrews BS, Davis JS, et al: Antibodies to Sm in patients with systemic lupus erythematosus. *Arthritis Rheum* 24:1236–1244, 1981.
102. Ballou SP, Kushner I: Lupus patients who lack detectable anti-DNA: Clinical features and survival. *Arthritis Rheum* 25:1126–1129, 1982.
103. Morrow WJW, Isenberg DA, Todd-Pokropek A, et al: Useful laboratory measurements in the management of systemic lupus erythematosus. *Q J Med* LI(202):125–138, 1982.
104. Agnello V, Mitamura T: Evidence for detection of low molecular weight DNA—anti-DNA complexes in systemic lupus erythematosus. *Arthritis Rheum* 25:788–792, 1982.
105. Tron F, Letarte J, Barreira MCR-A, et al: Specific detection of circulating DNA:anti-DNA immune complexes in human systemic lupus erythematosus sera using murine monoclonal anti-DNA antibody. *Clin Exp Immunol* 49:481–487, 1982.
106. Sano H, Morimoto C: DNA isolated from DNA/anti-DNA antibody immune complexes in systemic lupus erythematosus is rich in guanine-cytosine content. *J Immunol* 128:1341–1345, 1982.
107. Losito A, Cecchini C, Pittavini L, et al: Stimulation of polymorphonuclear leukocyte chemotaxis by cold precipitable complexes containing DNA–anti-DNA in active nephritis of systemic lupus erythematosus. *Nephron* 30:324–327, 1982.
108. Emlen W, Mannik M: Clearance of circulating DNA–anti-DNA immune complexes in mice. *J Exp Med* 155:1210–1215, 1982.

109. Looi LM, Prathap K: Hepatitis B virus surface antigen in glomerular immune complex deposits of patients with systemic lupus erythematosus. *Histopathology* 6:141–147, 1982.
110. Couser WG, Salant DJ, Madaio MP, et al: Factors influencing glomerular and tubulointerstitial patterns of injury in SLE. *Am J Kidney Dis* 2:126–134, 1982.
111. Hamburger MI, Lawley TJ, Kimberly RP, et al: A serial study of splenic reticuloendothelial system Fc receptor functional activity in systemic lupus erythematosus. *Arthritis Rheum* 25:48–54, 1982.
112. Medof ME, Oger JJF: Competition for immune complexes by red cells in human blood. *J Clin Lab Immunol* 7:7–13, 1982.
113. Iida K, Mornaghi R, Nussenzweig V: Complement receptor (CR_1) deficiency in erythrocytes from patients with systemic lupus erythematosus. *J Exp Med* 155:1427–1438, 1982.
114. Kazatchkine MD, Fearon DT, Appay MD, et al: Immunohistochemical study of the human glomerular C3b receptor in normal kidney and in 75 cases of renal diseases: Loss of C3b receptor antigen in focal hyalinosis and in proliferative nephritis of systemic lupus erythematosus. *J Clin Invest* 69:900–912, 1982.
115. Aguado MT, Perrin LH, Miescher PA, et al: Decreased capacity to solubilize immune complexes in sera from patients with systemic lupus erythematosus. *Arthritis Rheum* 24:1225–1229, 1981.
116. Jothy S, Sawka RJ: Presence of monocytes in systemic lupus erythematosus-associated glomerulonephritis: Marker study and significance. *Arch Pathol Lab Med* 105:590–593, 1981.
117. Camussi G, Tetta C, Segoloni G, et al: Localization of neutrophil cationic proteins and loss of anionic charges in glomeruli of patients with systemic lupus erythematosus glomerulonephritis. *Clin Immunol Immunopathol* 24:299–314, 1982.
118. Knutson DW: Initial management of lupus glomerulonephritis. *Am J Kidney Dis* 2:229–236, 1982.
119. McCluskey RT: The value of the renal biopsy in lupus nephritis. *Arthritis Rheum* 25:867–875, 1982.
120. Grishman E, Gerber MA, Churg J: Patterns of renal injury of systemic lupus erythematosus: Light and immunofluorescence microscopic observations. *Am J Kidney Dis* 2:135–141, 1982.
121. Pirani CL, Olesnicky L: Role of electronmicroscopy in the classification of lupus nephritis. *Am J Kidney Dis* 2:150–163, 1982.
122. Kashgarian M: New approaches to clinical pathologic correlation in lupus nephritis. *Am J Kidney Dis* 2:164–169, 1982.
123. Grishman E, Churg J: Focal segmental lupus nephritis. *Clin Nephrol* 17:5–13, 1982.
124. Magil AB, Ballon HS, Rae A: Focal proliferative lupus nephritis: A clinicopathologic study using the W.H.O. classification. *Am J Med* 72:620–630.
125. Baldwin DS: Clinical usefulness of the morphological classification of lupus nephritis. *Am J Kidney Dis* 2:142–149, 1982.
126. Whiting-o'Keefe Q, Henke JE, Shearn MA, et al: The information content from renal biopsy in systemic lupus erythematosus: Stepwise linear regression analysis. *Ann Int Med* 96:718–723, 1982.
127. Whiting-O'Keefe Q, Riccardi PJ, Henke JE, et al: Recognition of information in renal biopsies of patients with lupus nephritis. *Ann Int Med* 96:723–727, 1982.
128. Leehey DJ, Katz AI, Azaran AH, et al: Silent diffuse lupus nephritis: Long-term follow-up. *Am J Kidney Dis* 2:188–196, 1982.
129. Bennett WM, Bardana EJ, Norman DJ, et al: Natural history of "silent" lupus nephritis. *Am J Kidney Dis* 1:359–363, 1982.

130. Kant KS, Pollak VE, Weiss MA, et al: Glomerular thrombosis in systemic lupus erythematosus: Prevalence and significance. *Medicine* 60:71–86, 1981.
131. Schwartz MM, Roberts JL, Lewis EJ: Subepithelial electron-dense deposits in proliferative glomerulonephritis of systemic lupus erythematosus. *Ultrastruct Pathol* 3:105–118, 1982.
132. Bhathena DB, Sobel BJ, Migdal SD: Noninflammatory renal microangiopathy of systemic lupus erythematosus (lupus vasculitis). *Am J Nephrol* 1:144–159, 1981.
133. Schwartz MM, Fennell JS, Lewis EJ: Pathologic changes in the renal tubule in systemic lupus erythematosus. *Human Pathol* 13:534–547, 1982.
134. Ginzler EM, Diamond HS, Weiner M, et al: A multicenter study of outcome in systemic lupus erythematosus: I. Entry variables as predictors of prognosis. *Arthritis Rheum* 25:601–611, 1982.
135. Rosner S, Ginzler EM, Diamond HS, et al: A multicenter study of outcome in systemic lupus erythematosus: II. Causes of death. *Arthritis Rheum* 25:612–617, 1982.
136. Wallace DJ, Podell TE, Weiner JM, et al: Lupus nephritis: Experience with 230 patients in a private practice from 1950 to 1980. *Am J Med* 72:209–220, 1982.
137. Platt JL, Burke BA, Fish AJ, et al: Systemic lupus erythematosus in the first two decades of life. *Am J Kidney Dis* 2:212–222, 1982.
138. Morris MC, Cameron JS, Chantler C, et al: Systemic lupus erythematosus with nephritis. *Arch Dis Child* 56:779–783, 1981.
139. Ballou SP, Khan MA, Kushner I: Clinical features of systemic lupus erythematosus: Differences realted to race and age of onset. *Arthritis Rheum* 25:55–60, 1982.
140. Hayslett JP: Effect of pregnancy in patients with SLE. *Am J Kidney Dis* 2:223–228, 1982.
141. Jungers P, Dougados M, Pelissier C, et al: Lupus nephropathy and pregnancy: Report of 104 cases in 36 patients. *Arch Intern Med* 142:771–776, 1982.
142. Decker JL: The management of systemic lupus erythematosus. *Arthritis Rheum* 25:891–894, 1982.
143. Pollak VE, Dosekun AK: Evaluation of treatment in lupus nephritis: Effects of prednisone. *Am J Kidney Dis* 2:170–177, 1982.
144. Dinant HJ, Decker JL, Klippel JH, et al: Alternative modes of cyclophosphamide and azathioprine therapy in lupus nephritis. *Ann Int Med* 96:728–736, 1982.
145. Donadio JV, Holley KE, Ilstrup DM: Cytotoxic drug treatment of lupus nephritis. *Am J Kidney Dis* 2:178–181, 1982.
146. Elliott RW, Essenhigh DM, Morley AR: Cyclophosphamide treatment of systemic lupus erythematosus: Risk of bladder cancer exceeds benefit. *Br Med J* 284:1160–1161, 1982.
147. Ponticelli C, Zucchelli P, Banfi G, et al: Treatment of diffuse proliferative lupus nephritis by intravenous high-dose methylprednisolone. *Q J Med* LI(201):16–24, 1982.
148. Barron KS, Person DA, Brewer EJ, et al: Pulse methylprednisolone therapy in diffuse proliferative lupus nephritis. *J Pediatr* 101:137–141, 1982.
149. Sharon Z, Roberts JL, Fennel JS, et al: Plasmapheresis in lupus nephritis. *Plasma Ther Transfus Technol* 3:163–169, 1982.
150. Pollak VE, Glueck HI, Weiss MA, et al: Defibrination with ancrod in glomerulonephritis: Effects on clinical and histologic findings and on blood coagulation. *Am J Nephrol* 2:195–207, 1982.
151. Hunt JS, Macdonald PR, McGiven AR: Characterisation of human glomerular basement membrane antigenic fractions isolated by affinity chromatography utilising anti-glomerular basement membrane autoantibodies. *Biochem Biophys Res Comm* 104:1025–1032, 1982.
152. Sisson S, Dysart NK, Fish AJ, et al: Localization of the Goodpasture antigen by immunoelectron microscopy. *Clin Immunol Immunopathol* 23:414–429, 1982.

153. Jennette JC, Lamanna RW, Burnette JP, et al: Concurrent antiglomerular basement membrane antibody and immune complex-mediated glomerulonephritis. *Am J Clin Pathol* 78:381–386, 1982.
154. Leatherman JW, Sibley RK, Davies SF: Diffuse intrapulmonary hemorrhage and glomerulonephritis unrelated to anti-glomerular basement membrane antibody. *Am J Med* 72:401–410, 1982.
155. Dunn TL, Manning SH, McKinney TD: Hypersensitivity pneumonitis and mesangiopathic glomerulonephritis: An unusual pulmonary-renal syndrome. *South Med J* 74:1403–1406, 1981.
156. Lam M, Krous HF, Llach F: Massive pulmonary hemorrhage and fulminant renal failure associated with immune complex glomerulonephritis. *South Med J* 74:1338–1342, 1981.
157. Fukuda Y, Yamanaka N, Ishizaki M, et al: Immune complex-mediated glomerulonephritis and interstitial pneumonia simulating Goodpasture's syndrome. *Acta Pathol Jpn* 32:361–370, 1982.
158. Peters DK Rees AJ, Lockwood CM, et al: Treatment and prognosis in antibasement membrane antibody-mediated nephritis. *Transplant Proc* 14:513–521, 1982.
159. Shasby DM, Schwarz MI, Forstot JZ, et al: Pulmonary immune complex deposition in Wegener's granulomatosis. *Chest* 81:338–340, 1982.
160. Hui AN, Ehresmann GR, Quismorio FP, et al: Wegener's granulomatosis: Electron microscopic and immunofluorescent studies. *Chest* 80:753–756, 1981.
161. Novak RF, Christiansen RG, Sorensen ET: The acute vasculitis of Wegener's granulomatosis in renal biopsies. *Am J Clin Pathol* 78:367–371, 1982.
162. Cohen PS, Meltzer JA: Strawberry gums: A sign of Wegener's granulomatosis. *JAMA* 246:2610–2611, 1981.
163. Dabbagh S, Chevalier RL, Sturgill BC: Prolonged anuria and aortic insufficiency in a child with Wegener's granulomatosis. *Clin Nephrol* 17:155–159, 1982.
164. Kuross S, Davin T, Kjellstrand CM: Wegener's granulomatosis with severe renal failure: Clinical course and results of dialysis and transplantation. *Clin Nephrol* 16:172–180, 1981.
165. Herreman G, Beaufils H, Godeau P, et al: Behçet's syndrome and renal involvement: A histological and immunofluorescent study of eleven renal biopsies. *Am J Med Sci* 284:10–17, 1982.
166. Maggiore Q, Bartolomeo F, L'Abbate A, et al: Glomerular localization of circulating antiglobulin activity in essential mixed cryoglobulinemia with glomerulonephritis. *Kidney Int* 21:387–394, 1982.
167. Schultz DR, Perez GO, Volanakis JE, et al: Glomerular disease in two patients with urticaria-cutaneous vasculitis and hypocomplementemia. *Am J Kidney Dis* 1:157–165, 1981.
168. Minta JO, Winkler CJ, Biggar WD, et al: A selective and complete absence of C1q in a patient with vasculitis and nephritis. *Clin Immunol Immunopathol* 22:225–237, 1982.
169. Ridolfi RL, Bell WR: Thrombotic thrombocytopenic purpura: Report of 25 cases and review of the literature. *Medicine* 60:413–428, 1981.
170. Rosove MH, Ho WG, Goldfinger D: Ineffectiveness of aspirin and dipyridamole in the treatment of thrombotic thrombocytopenic purpura. *Ann Int Med* 96:27–33, 1982.
171. Stevenson JA, Dumke A, Glassock RJ, et al: Thrombotic microangiopathy: Recurrence following renal transplant and response to plasma infusion. *Am J Nephrol* 2:227–231, 1982.
172. Bergstein JM, Kuederli U, Bank NU: Plasma inhibitor of glomerular fibrinolysis in the hemolytic-uremic syndrome. *Am J Med* 73:322–327, 1982.

173. Yoshikawa N, Cameron AH, White RHR: The glomerular basal lamina in hereditary nephritis. *J Pathol* 135:199–209, 1981.
174. Yoshikawa N, White RHR, Cameron AH: Familial hematuria: Clinico-pathological correlations. *Clin Nephrol* 17:172–182, 1982.
175. Tina L, Jenis E, Jose P, et al: The glomerular basement membrane in benign familial hematuria. *Clin Nephrol* 17:1–4, 1982.
176. Piel CF, Biava CG, Goodman JR: Glomerular basement membrane attenuation in familial nephritis an "benign" hematuria. *J Pediatr* 101:358–365, 1982.
177. McCoy RC, Johnson HK, Stone WJ, et al: Absence of nephritogenic GBM antigen(s) in some patients with hereditary nephritis. *Kidney Int* 21:642–652, 1982.
178. Milliner DS, Pierides, AM, Holley KE: Renal transplantation in Alport's syndrome: Anti-glomerular basement membrane glomerulonephritis in the allograft. *Mayo Clin Proc* 57:35–43, 1982.
179. Briner J: Glomerular lesions in renal allografts. *Ergeb Inn Med Kinderheilkd* 49:1–76, 1982.
180. Morzycka M, Croker BP, Seigler HF, et al: Evaluation of recurrent glomerulonephritis in kidney allografts. *Am J Med* 72:588–598, 1982.
181. Maizel SE, Sibley RK, Horstman JP, et al: Incidence and significance of recurrent focal segmental glomerulosclerosis in renal allograft recipients. *Transplant* 32:512–516, 1981.
182. Habib R, Hebert D, Gagnadoux MF, et al: Transplantation in idiopathic nephrosis. *Transplant Proc* 14:489–495, 1982.
183. Cosyns J-P, Pirson Y, Squifflet J-P, et al: De novo membranous nephropathy in human renal allografts: Report of nine patients. *Kidney Int* 22:177–183, 1982.
184. Robinson RR: Isolated proteinuria. *Contrib Nephrol* 24:53–62, 1981.
185. Lim Ch, Woo KT, Chiang GS: Correlation of proteinuria with histopathology in asymptomatic glomerulonephritis. *Ann Acad Med Singapore* 11:9–14, 1982.
186. Krensky AM, Ingelfinger JR, Grupe WE: Peritonitis in childhood nephrotic syndrome: 1970–1980. *Am J Dis Child* 136:732–736, 1982.
187. Ballow M, Kennedy TL, Gaudio KM, et al: Serum hemolytic factor D values in children with steroid-responsive idiopathic nephrotic syndrome. *J Pediatr* 100:192–196, 1982.
188. Spika JS, Halsey NA, Fish AJ, et al: Serum antibody response to pneumococcal vaccine in children with nephrotic syndrome. *Pediatrics* 69:219–223, 1982.
189. Wilkes JC, Nelson JD, Worthen HG, et al: Response to pneumococcal vaccination in children with nephrotic syndrome. *Am J Kidney Dis* 2:43–46, 1982.
190. Coppola R, Guerra L, Ruggeri ZM, et al: Factor VIII/von Willebrand factor in glomerular nephropathies. *Clin Nephrol* 16:217–222, 1981.
191. Previato G, Loschiavo C, Lupo A, et al: Clinical significance of plasma factor VIII levels in renal disease. *Clin Nephrol* 16:200–206, 1981.
192. Boneu B, Bouissou F, Abbal M, et al: Comparison of progressive antithrombin activity and the concentration of three thrombin inhibitors in nephrotic syndrome. *Thromb Haemostasis* 46:623–625, 1981.
193. Tomura S, Ida T, Kuriyama R, et al: Activation of platelets in patients with chronic proliferative glomerulonephritis and the nephrotic syndrome. *Clin Nephrol* 17:24–30, 1982.
194. Harrington JT, Kassirer JP: Renal vein thrombosis. *Ann Rev Med* 33:255–262, 1982.
195. Michaeli J, Bar-on H, Shafrir E: Lipoprotein profiles in a heterogeneous group of patients with nephrotic syndrome. *Israel J Med Sci* 17:1001–1008, 1981.
196. Goldberg ACRK, Oliveira HCF, Quintao ECR, et al: Increased hepatic cholesterol production due to liver hypertrophy in rat experimental nephrosis. *Biochim et Biophys Acta* 710:71–75, 1982.

197. Golper TA, Swartz SH: Impaired renal mevalonate metabolism in nephrotic syndrome: A stimulus for increased hepatic cholesterogenesis independent of GFR and hypoalbuminemia. *Metabolism* 31:471–476, 1982.
198. Chan MK, Persaud JW, Ramdial L, et al: Hyperlipidaemia in untreated nephrotic syndrome, increased production or decreased removal? *Clin Chim Acta* 117:317–323, 1981.
199. Feinstein EI, Kaptein EM, Nicoloff JT, et al: Thyroid function in patients with nephrotic syndrome and normal renal function. *Am J Nephrol* 2:70–76, 1982.
200. McLean RH, Kennedy TL, Rosoulpour M, et al: Hypothyroidism in the congenital nephrotic syndrome. *J Pediatr* 101:72–75, 1982.
201. Sato KA, Gray RW, Lemann J: Urinary excretion of 25-hydroxyvitamin D in health and the nephrotic syndrome. *J Lab Clin Med* 99:325–330, 1982.
202. Berlyne GM, Sutton J, Brown C, et al: Renal salt and water handling in water immersion in the nephrotic syndrome. *Clin Sci* 61:605–610, 1981.
203. Krishna GG, Danovitch GM: Effects of water immersion on renal function in the nephrotic syndrome. *Kidney Int* 21:395–401, 1982.

ACKNOWLEDGMENT

We wish to thank Ms. Marge Landuyt for her assistance in the preparation of this manuscript.

CHAPTER 7

Urinary Tract Infections

John Z. Montgomerie

In the past two years there have been a number of excellent reviews of aspects of urinary tract infections. Hanson et al. (1) reviewed the pathogenesis of urinary tract infections, and the virulence factors in *E. coli* and the host defenses. It reviews much of the work carried out by this group in Goteborg, Sweden, in recent years. Other areas that have been reviewed include treatment (2–5), vesicoureteric reflux (6), the urethral syndrome (7), and infection stones (8).

MICROORGANISMS IN URINARY TRACT INFECTIONS

In the past few years, the number of species of microorganisms considered to be pathogens in the urinary tract has increased considerably (Table 1). The recognition of these organisms as pathogens has been the result of the more frequent use of suprapubic aspiration to obtain urine for culture. Ability to culture microorganisms from suprapubic urine has usually been considered sufficient to identify an organism as a pathogen. However, the presence of microorganisms in the bladder urine may not necessarily establish pathogenicity. For example, *Staphylococcus saprophyticus* is not a new bacterium, but a new name for an old bacterium (*Micrococcus*), not infrequently seen in community-acquired urinary tract infection. These strains were probably previously recognized as *S. epidermidis* or coagulase negative staphylococci (9,10). *S. saprophyticus* has been established as a pathogen because of the large number of patients from which this microorganism has been isolated. *S. saprophyticus* injected into the pelvis of the kidney resulted in pyelonephritis in monkeys (11). Although one of the early studies found *S. saprophyticus* in 42% of women in Sweden

Table 1. Newly Recognized Potential Pathogens in Urinary Tract Infection

Staphylococcus saprophyticus	Anaerobic bacteria?
Gardnerella vaginalis?	Chlamydia trachomatis?
Lactobacillus sp. ?	Ureaplasma urealyticum?

with bacteriuria (12), in more recent studies of urinary tract infection in young women in different countries, the incidence of this organism has been approximately 7% (13,14); since the organism was found to be part of the urethral flora in only 2% of healthy women, the source of the S. saprophyticus is still unclear. Marrie et al. also found that resistance of the organism to a 5 µg novobiocin disc had a 93% positive predictive accuracy as a presumptive test for S. saprophyticus (14).

The isolation of Chlamydia trachomatis has been associated with nonspecific urethritis in men and pelvic inflammatory disease in women. Recently it has been linked to the urethral syndrome or dysuria and frequency syndrome and the presence of white cells in the urine (15). Renal infection with this microorganism has not been described. The isolation of anaerobic organisms from pregnant women with bacteriuria (16) has been difficult to evaluate. The presence of positive antibody coating in some of these patients might suggest the involvement of deep tissues or the kidney (17). The isolation of Ureaplasma urealyticum from renal transplant recipients and patients with chronic pyelonephritis and vesicoureteric reflux was described by Birch et al. (18,19). The urine was obtained by suprapubic aspiration to avoid urethral contamination. Because U. urealyticum is part of the normal urethral flora, it may not be possible to regard it as pathogenic simply because it has been isolated from the urine. Others have isolated Gardnerella vaginalis and Lactobacillus species from urine obtained by suprapubic aspiration (20–22). Brumfitt et al. (21) isolated Lactobacillus species from the urine but did not consider them to be pathogens. The problem of deciding whether these microorganisms are pathogens or "accidentals" in the urinary tract was discussed by Kunin (23). He suggested that bacteria may enter and leave the bladder urine intermittently without persisting in the urine or invading the bladder wall. Documentation of pathogenicity should include some evidence of host–parasite interaction—the presence of inflammatory cells in the urine, histologic evidence of tissue invasion, antibody response, or evidence of renal infection. Repeated positive cultures of the pathogen in the urine over a significant period of time would imply multiplication in the urine and potential pathogenicity.

Single cases of pyelonephritis with Haemophilus parainfluenzae (24) and Legionella pneumophila (25) have been reported. Urinary tract infection with H. influenzae has been reported in at least 16 cases, but H. parainfluenzae had not been reported previously (24).

FACTORS PREDISPOSING TO INFECTION

Vesicoureteric Reflux

Smellie and co-workers were among the first to demonstrate the significance of vesicoureteric reflux (VUR) in children. They advocated prophylaxis with antibacterial agents to prevent further infections (26). They have continued to treat many children with urinary tract infection and VUR and have since provided us with the results of the studies over two decades (27,28). Between 1955 and 1975 they treated 744 children, 179 boys and 565 girls from less than 1 year to 12 years old who had urinary tract infection. These children were investigated by intravenous pyelogram and micturating cystogram. All children received 7–10 days of an appropriate antibiotic, and 570 of them received at least 6 months of low dose prophylaxis, the majority being treated with sulfafurazole, nitrofurantoin, or cotrimoxazole. In addition, children were encouraged to void regularly, frequently, and completely, and to void twice at bed time if VUR was present.

One-third of the patients had VUR. There was no difference in the sex or age between the patients with and those without VUR. Fever was more often a presenting symptom in those patients with VUR. They only two fresh scars observed developed after infection in boys with moderate to severe reflux. Hypertension developed only in children with renal damage. Twenty children had a sustained rise in blood pressure, and in all but two, reflux and renal scarring were also found. In the second study this group of workers investigated renal growth for periods ranging from 2 to 22 years in 70 children who presented between 2 weeks and 12 years of age with urinary tract infection and who were found to have VUR (28). They were managed on a conservative regimen of continuous prophylaxis and regular complete voiding. Recurrence of urinary tract infection was not entirely prevented by the medical program and this allowed a comparison of the effect of sterile reflux with reflux associated with urinary tract infection. One of the main points of the study was to observe the effect of sterile VUR in the unobstructed urinary tract on renal growth, since renal growth without scarring may be used as an indicator of normality. It was clear that while VUR persisted, normal growth occurred in unscarred, uninfected kidneys, whatever the severity; this was also true in most kidneys with moderate scarring. In kidneys that were severely scarred and had little normal parenchyma remaining, growth was invariably impaired. These kidneys were generally drained by a dilated ureter with continuing gross VUR. Reinfection was also more likely to occur in these kidneys.

This study showed an association of reflux and impaired renal growth with infection. Ten of the 11 kidneys with growth impairment were reinfected during follow-up. Infection also preceded the development of

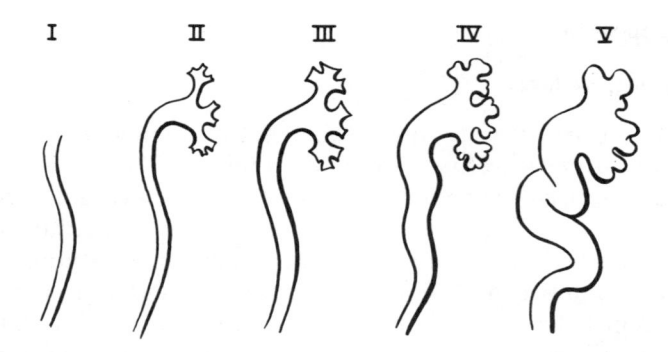

Figure 1. Grades of reflux (International Classification): I. ureter only; II. ureter, pelvis and calyces; no dilation, normal calyceal fornices; III. mild or moderate dilation and/or tortuosity of the ureter, and mild or moderate dilation of renal pelvis *but*—*no* or *slight* blunting of the fornices; IV. moderate dilation and/or tortuosity of ureter and moderate dilation of renal pelvis and calyces; complete obliteration of sharp angle of fornices *but* maintenance of papillary impressions in majority of calyces; V. gross dilation and tortuosity of ureter; gross dilation of renal pelvis and calyces; papillary impressions are no longer visable in majority of calyces. (Levitt SB: *Pediatrics* 67:396, 1981. Copyright 1981, American Academy of Pediatrics. Used with permission.)

two fresh scars, whereas no scarring developed in any uninfected refluxing urinary tract.

A review of VUR outlines the present attitudes towards medical and surgical therapy (6). Most causes of VUR not associated with dilatation of the upper urinary tract will disappear with time. However, spontaneous resolution is less likely when dilatation of the pelvis is present. In a study of 75 children followed for 9–15 years, VUR disappeared from more than 80% of undilated ureters and from 41% of dilated ureters (29). Medical management is indicated for these children if the urine can be kept sterile. The international study is designed to test (*1*) whether sterile major VUR is harmful in itself and (*2*) whether a difference exists between early successful surgery and medical management in preventing the possibly deleterious effect of VUR on renal growth rate, development of new scars, and progression of established scars. The study is also comparing the incidence of recurrent urinary tract infections and hypertension in surgically treated and medically treated patients. Patients with grade IV as VUR, as well as patients with grade III VUR beyond infancy, are included in the study (Fig. 1).

The international reflux study committee regards VUR as a congenital condition. It has not discussed the possible role of infection in the development or persistence of VUR, or of glomerulosclerosis, which may also be associated with VUR (30).

HOST–PARASITE INTERACTION

Bacterial Virulence

A considerable number of studies have correlated the ability of *Escherichia coli* to adhere to cells of the urinary tract and its ability to cause infection of the urinary tract. Hanson et al. (1) reviewed this evidence and the bacterial factors that influence adhesion. The adhesion of E. coli to epithelial cells depends on bacterial surface factors (adhesins), which have receptors in the epithelial cell surface. Attachment to epithelial cells has been classified according to the ability of the bacteria to bind to other cells, particularly erythrocytes. Two main groups of adhesins have been found on *E. coli* causing urinary tract infections. One group agglutinates erythrocytes and its action is reversed in the presence of D-mannose. There is some evidence that *E. coli* strains carrying only these adhesins attach poorly to human epithelial cells from the urinary tract but do bind to urinary slime. A second group of adhesins induces agglutination of erythrocytes and is resistant to D-mannose. *E. coli* with these adhesins attach to epithelial cells from the urinary tract and have been found in patients with acute pyelonephritis but rarely in normal fecal isolates. Most work has centered on the possibility that the adhesins are pili or fimbriae, but the existence of nonfimbriate adhesins has been suggested.

Globoseries glycolipids, related to the human P blood group, may be receptors for *E. coli* attaching to human urinary epithelial cells (31,32). Not all studies have shown a correlation of adherence to epithelial cells with urinary tract infection. Harber et al. studied freshly isolated pathogens from patients who had urinary tract infections (33). These organisms were tested for adhesion to normal buccal cells and epithelial cells from the urinary tract. All but one of the fresh isolates were nonfimbriate and all but one were nonadherent to each test system. However, after subculture in broth, 14 of 20 strains developed fimbriae and 17 became adherent to buccal cells. These observations suggest that adherence was not a factor in virulence once the organisms had entered the urinary tract. There were no differences in adherence between symptom-producing strains and non-symptom-producing strains. Fowler and Stamey had also been unable to find a correlation between bacterial adhesion and uropathogenecity (34). There have also been contradictory data on the significance of adherence to bladder epithelial cells in experimental animals (35).

Host Defenses

Many host factors, such as the shortness of the female urethra, bladder emptying, intact vesicoureteric valve, and the hypertonicity of the medulla, are considered to influence the infection of the urinary tract. The role of the immune system and polymorphonuclear leukocytes (PMNs) is unclear. PMNs in the urine have been an indicator of bacterial infection.

Suzuki et al. examined the opsonic effect of urine from normal adults and patients with acute cystitis (36). The urine contained an opsonic factor that increased phagocytosis of yeast or *E. coli*. The urine of patients with acute cystitis exhibited a more marked opsonic effect than normal urine. Several previous studies have suggested that PMNs in the urine may play a role in infection. Chernew and associates showed that PMNs carried out active phagocytosis in urine with a low osmotic pressure (37), and Bryant and associates demonstrated phagocytosis of *Staphylococcus* by PMns in urine (38). In both reports the PMNs were studied in serum derived from blood. In the present studies the addition of normal serum to urine at 1% markedly increased phagocytosis of yeast and *E. coli*. The authors believed that serum components found in the patient's urine may play an important role in opsonization. Heat inactivation of the test urine had no effect on the opsonic acitivity, suggesting that complement was not working in the system.

DIAGNOSIS

Since the studies of Kass, 10^5 bacteria/ml of urine has been considered to be a significant level of bacteriuria, indicating infection in the urinary tract (39). Stamm et al. studied 187 women who were referred for evaluation of dysuria and frequency to a student health center (15). Urine obtained by suprapubic aspiration was compared with midstream urine. The criterion of $>10^5$ bacteria/ml of midstream urine identified only 51% of women whose bladder urine contained coliforms. In these symptomatic young women, the best diagnostic criterion was $>10^2$ bacteria/ml. They noted that the isolation of $<10^5$ coliforms /ml of midstream urine has had a low predictive value in previous studies of asymptomatic women. It is not clear to what extent these results apply to other groups of patients with urinary tract infection. Additional studies will be necessary before we use $>10^2$ bacteria/ml in midstream urine as indicating infection.

The value of intravenous pyelography (excretory urography) in the investigation of women with uncomplicated urinary tract infection has frequently been questioned. Fowler and Pulaski examined the use of excretory urography, cystography, and cystoscopy in the evaluation of women with urinary tract infection (40). The majority of the women in this study had had two or more episodes before the study and none had bacteriologic evidence of persistent urinary tract infection. Among 75 cystograms and 74 cystoscopies, the only abnormalities that altered treatment of the infections were three instances of urethral diverticula. No abnormalities influencing treatment were found among 104 excretory urograms. Incidental findings, which the authors considered to be unrelated to urinary tract infection but necessitating therapeutic intervention, included a renal cell carcinoma (diagnosed on IVP) and a transitional cell

Table 2. Clinical Features of 26 Reported Cases of Eosinophilic Cystitis (15 Males, 11 Females; Mean Age 27.7 Years; Age Range 5 Days to 75 Years)

	Present No. (%)	Absent No. (%)	Not stated No. (%)
Hematuria	16 (61.5%)	5 (19.2%)	5 (19.2%)
Proteinuria	14 (53.8%)	1 (3.8%)	11 (42.3%)
Pyuria	15 (57.7%)	7 (26.9%)	4 (15.4%)
Peripheral eosinophilia	22 (84.6%)	2 (7.7%)	2 (7.7%)
Positive urine culture	8 (30.8%)	14 (53.8%)	4 (15.4%)
Irritative bladder symptoms	22 (84.6%)	4 (15.4%)	0 (0%)
Suprapubic pain or tenderness	14 (53.8%)	3 (11.5%)	9 (34.6%)
Palpable suprapubic mass	7 (26.9%)	3 (11.5%)	16 (61.5%)
History of allergy	7 (26.9%)	10 (38.5%)	9 (34.6%)

SOURCE: Tauscher JW, Shaw DC: *Clin Pediatr* 20:742, 1981. Used with permission.

carcinoma of the bladder (discovered at cystoscopy). Radiographic and cystoscopic examination of the urinary system rarely uncovers abnormalities that are important in the treatment of this group of patients. Another study confirmed the low diagnostic yield of IVP in women with uncomplicated urinary tract infections (41). The IVP was valuable in only 2.89% of 242 women with documented urinary tract infections with symptoms of lower urinary tract irritability.

June et al. (42) and others (43–45) have described the use of contrast-enhanced renal computed tomography (CT) (General Electric CT-8800) in 14 patients with pyelonephritis. Abnormal findings included linear and patchy areas of decreased density in the renal parenchyma, loss of corticomedullary delineation, and absence of normal renal separation from perirenal tissue (42). Intrarenal abscesses may also be detected. Further studies will be necessary to evaluate the usefulness of this technique in diagnosing acute nonobstructive urinary tract infection.

Eosinophilic Cystitis

Eosinophilic cystitis is an uncommon disease of the urinary bladder. Tauscher and Shaw reviewed 25 cases of eosinophilic cystitis that had been reported in the English literature (46). Symptoms of frequency, urgency, dysuria, and suprapubic abdominal pain were seen in 85% of cases. Gross or microscopic hematuria was seen in 62% (Table 2). Urine cultures were usually sterile, but proteinuria and pyuria were seen in more than half of the cases. Eosinophils were usually found in the submucosal and muscle layer of the urinary bladder. Peripheral eosinophilia was found in 85% of the cases. A number of authors have suggested that the etiologic agent may be a parasitic infection of the bladder. Only one reported case, however, seems to have been related to *Toxocara cati*. Others have suggested that eosinophilic cystitis is caused by allergy of the urinary tract (47). There are also reports of the association of eosinophilic gastroenteritis with eosinophilic cystitis (48,49). At the present time the cause of eosinophilic cystitis is unclear.

TREATMENT

The use of single dose antimicrobial treatment of uncomplicated urinary tract infections in women is now a well-accepted practice (5). Souney and Polk suggest that amoxicillin (2.9 g), sulfasoxazole (1.0 g), and trimethoprim-sulfamethoxazole (160/800 mg) are effective single dose regimens in this setting (5). However, the results should not be extrapolated to other populations, such as pregnant women, children, the elderly, or to the use of other antimicrobial agents. Lacey et al. compared single dose trimethoprim with a 5-day course for the treatment of urinary tract infections in the elderly (50). Single dose therapy was significantly less effective than the 5-day course. The study included both men and women, but there was no indication of the incidence of renal involvement or prostatitis. There have been few studies with cephalosporins. The authors suggest that cephalosporins may be less effective than the regimens recommended. McCracken et al. found that a 1-day regimen of cefadroxil was not as effective as a 10-day regimen for children with lower urinary tract infection (51). C-reactive protein concentrations were less than 28 µg/ml. These authors noted that one dose antibiotic therapy in children has been used successfully (52,53), but the number of children studied in a prospective randomized fashion is too small to allow meaningful conclusions.

Treatment of Acute Urethral Syndrome

Only 50% of women with symptoms of lower urinary tract infection have significant bacteriuria ($>10^5$/ml) in midstream urine. Patients with symptoms and significant bacteriuria may be considered to have cystitis. The terms *acute urethral syndrome* or *frequency-dysuria syndrome* have been reserved for women with symptoms similar to lower urinary tract infection in the absence of significant bacteriuria. Stamm et al. have found that many patients with acute urethral syndrome have counts of *E. coli* less than 10^5/ml and some of them are infected with *Chlamydia trochomatis* (15). For these patients, who require treatment for dysuria, single dose therapy with amoxicillin, sulfamethoxazole, or trimethorprim-sulfamethoxazole seems to be warranted until the results of cultures are available. The treatment of chlamydial infection producing this syndrome is not established. There is little place for surgical treatment (e.g., urethral dilatation, internal urethrotomy, etc.), and high fluid intake, frequent emptying of the bladder after sexual intercourse, and so on, are of questionable value. Failure of these patients to respond to amoxicillin or sulfonamides may be an indication to use tetracycline to treat a possible chlamydial infection. Stam outlined a clinical approach to treating women with acute dysuria and urinary frequency and discussed antimicrobial prophylaxis for recurrent urinary tract infection (4).

Drug concentrations in the urine have been used as the main criteria for the effectiveness of antimicrobial agents in the treatment of urinary tract infection (54–56). It is now becoming clear that the concentrations of aminoglycosides in the serum and urine are sometimes poor indicators of both intrarenal distribution of the drug and outcome of pyelonephritis in urinary tract infection in animals (57–59). The reason for this microbial persistence is unclear. It has been suggested that aminoglycosides are ineffective because they are incapable of reaching bacteria sequestered within the infected renal parenchyma. The relevance of these observations to human disease is unclear. Aminoglycosides have been very effective in the treatment of urinary tract infections and are widely used for severe urinary tract infections. There are some clinical studies that suggest that aminoglycosides may cause problems in certain groups of patients, and that antibacterial activity of aminoglycosides may be inhibited by factors in the urine (60). Aminoglycosides were not as effective as the third generation cephalosporins in the treatment of urinary tract infections in patients with spinal cord injury and neurogenic bladder (61).

Mayrer and Andriole reviewed the use of urinary tract antiseptics. They examined the antimicrobial spectrum, pharmacokinetics, and side effects of these frequently used agents (3). Nitrofurantoin seemed to be the most versatile agent. It is effective against acute uncomplicated symptomatic bacteriuria and has a low incidence of associated resistance when used as a long-term suppressive agent in children and pregnant women (Table 3). The authors point out that methenamine mandalate or hippurate contain only 480 mg of methenamine and 520 mg of mandelic or hippuric acid. These combinations contain an amount of acid that is unlikely to contribute significantly to the antibacterial activity in the urine. There is also little evidence that these acid forms contribute to the antibacterial activity of the methenamine. Urine acidification with ascorbic acid is widely used as a means of preventing bacteriuria. It now seems clear that neither oral nor intravenously administered ascorbic acid significantly alters the urine pH (62,63).

Antiseptic Agents in Urinary Drainage Bags

There are now several papers (64,65) that claim the frequency of urinary tract infection in catheterized patients can be reduced by placing an

Table 3. Urinary Tract Antiseptics

Agent	Dose	Use
Nalidixic acid	Adults 1 g q.i.d. for 1–2 wk; thereafter, if needed, 0.5 g q.i.d. for periods longer than 2 wk. Children: 55 mg/kg day in 4 divided doses for 1–2 wk; thereafter, if needed, 33 mg/kg/day for periods longer than 2 wk.	Acute and recurrent uncomplicated urinary tract infections due to susceptible organisms; or long-term suppressive therapy for frequently recurrent bacteriuria (single daily dose of 1 g). Do not use in infants < 3 months or patients with renal carbuncle, perinephric abscess, or pyelonephritis.
Oxolinic acid	Adults: 750 mg b.i.d. for 2 wk. Children: Not recommended.	Acute and recurrent uncomplicated urinary tract infections due to susceptible organisms. Do not use in patients with renal insufficiency, renal carbuncle, perinephric abscess, pyelonephritis, or in infants or nursing mothers.
Nitrofurantoin	Adults: 50 or 100 mg q.i.d. for 1–2 wk. Children: 1.25–0.75 mg/kg q.i.d. for 1–2 wk.	Acute and recurrent uncomplicated urinary tract infections due to susceptible organisms; or long-term suppressive therapy for frequently recurrent bacteriuria (single doses of 50–100 mg in adults, or 1 mg/kg b.i.d. in children). Do not use in patients with renal insufficiency, renal carbuncle, perinephric abscess or in infants.
Methenamine	Adults 0.5–2g (usually 1 g) q.i.d. or b.i.d. Children: 15 mg/kg q.i.d.	Chronic suppressive treatment of urinary tract infections when urine pH is 5.5 or less. Not a primary drug for acute urinary tract infection.
Methenamine mandelate	Adults: 1 g q.i.d. Children: 15 mg/kg q.i.d.	Chronic suppressive treatment of urinary tract infections when urine pH is 5.5 or less. Not a primary drug for acute urinary tract infections.[a]
Methenamine hippurate	Adults: 1 g b.i.d. Children age 6–12: 0.5–1 g b.i.d.	Chronic suppressive treatment of urinary tract infections when urine pH is 5.5 or less. Not a primary drug for acute urinary tract infections.[a]

SOURCE: Mayrer AR, Andriole VT: *Med Clin North Am* 66:199–208, 1982. Used with permission.

[a] One gram of methenamine mandelate or hippurate contains only 480 mg of methenamine and 520 mg of mandelic or hippurate acid. These combinations contain an amount of acid that is unlikely to contribute significant antibacterial activity to the urine. Also, there is little evidence that these acid forms contribute to the antibacterial activity of methenamine.

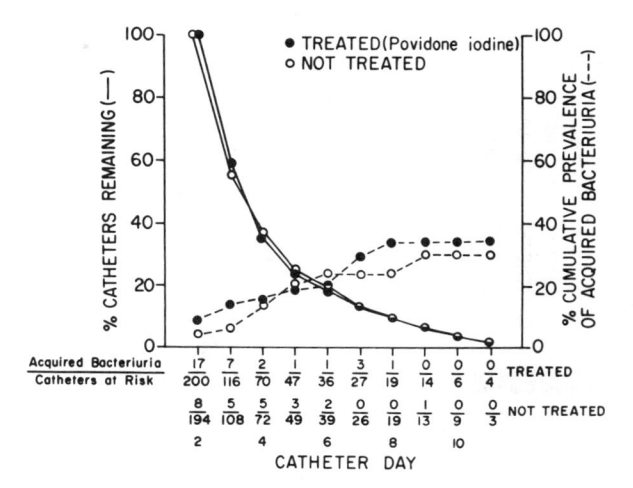

Figure 2. Povidone-iodine study. Prevalence of indwelling catheters and cumulative prevalence of acquired bacteriuria during the first 11 days of catheterization. (Burke JP et al: *Am J Med* 70:656, 1981. Used with permisstion.)

antiseptic solution such as chlorhexidine, povidone iodine, or hydrogen peroxide into the drainage bag. These studies suggest that sterilization of the bag by these methods may reduce cross-infection and that infection arises from the drainage bag. Such infection may occur at times but is probably rare (66,67). The major pathway for bladder infections appears to be entry of bacteria colonizing the periurethral zone. Topical agents applied to the meatus, however, do not prevent infection (68). Burke et al. attempted to prevent catheter-associated urinary tract infections by daily meatal cleaning with povidone iodine solution or soap (68). Neither was beneficial (Figs. 2 and 3). Indeed, the rates of bacteriuria were higher in the treated groups than in the untreated groups. Thus, the usually recommended approach at the present time appears to be unwarranted.

Immunosuppressive Agents

Miller et al. showed that immunosuppression during pyelonephritis enhanced the clearing of renal bacteriuria and did not increase the pathologic changes (76). However, Roberts et al. treated experimental pyelonephritis in monkeys with immunosuppressants and found that this prolonged bacteriuria and increased kidney pathology (77). Treatment with cyclophosphamide did not result in more efficient clearance of bacteria from the kidney. Indeed, cyclophosphamide- or azathioprim-treated monkeys were bacteriuric longer than controls.

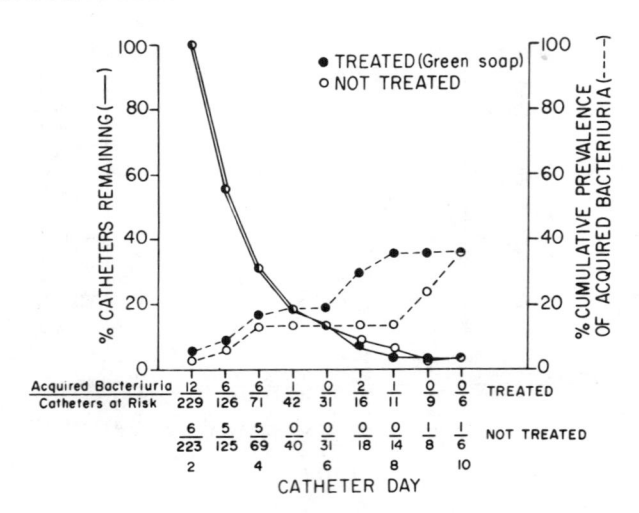

Figure 3. Green soap study. Prevalence of indwelling catheters and cumulative prevalence of acquired bacteriuria during the first 10 days of catheterization. Four patients in the untreated group had durations of catheterization longer than 10 days but did not acquire bacteriuria. (Burke JP et al: *Am J Med* 70:657, 1981. Used with permission.)

INFECTION STONES

The management of infection stones was reviewed by Resnick (8). Infection stones account for approximately 15–20% of all urinary calculi. Recent reports on the use of urease inhibitors such as acetohydroxamic acid and hydroxy urea have indicated that these agents may be of some value in the management of patients with infection stones, if used with antimicrobial therapy (69,70). Acetohydroxamic acid has low toxicity and has been shown to inhibit urinary alkalinization and precipitation of magnesium ammonium phosphate and carbonate apatite in the presence of *Proteus* infection in vitro (71). Studies of patients with infection stones in urea-splitting bacterial infections have demonstrated that the administration of this agent reduces urinary alkalinity and ammonia concentration and is well tolerated (72). The size of some stones is reduced, but these agents may be more useful in inhibiting the growth of residual stones when complete surgical removal is not possible and in preventing formation of new stones in patients with intractable urinary tract infections. The options for surgery include nephrectomy and pyelolithotomy. The objectives of renal surgery for infected calculi, usually of a staghorn configuration, are to remove all calculi and repair of the kidney. Without operation, patient mortality ranges from 28–50% within 10 years; in addition, approximately 50% of these patients will eventually lose the kidney because of the persistent infection and stones. Infusion and irrigation with acid solution (hemiacidrin) may dissolve struvite stones (73). Irrigation by way of urethral catheters is of limited value because the patient must remain at bed rest since repositioning of the catheter is frequently necessary. Only small amounts of the solution can be infused and at a slow rate, thereby prolonging the time required for stone dissolution. Placement of a nephrostomy following surgical exposure of the kidneys has also been effective, but primarily as a means of dissolving residual stones following an open surgical procedure.

Dretler and associates reported the results of hemiacidrin irrigation by way of percutaneous nephrostomy (74). Complete stone dissolution occurred in six of the eight kidneys treated in this way. These techniques are new and promising. Resnick, however, stressed that there were considerable risks associated with this technique (8). Following surgery, residual stone rates range from 5% to 26% (8). In approximately 60–80% of patients, the urinary tract infection will be eradicated following stone removal and treatment with appropriate antibiotics. The stone recurrence rate is approximately 30% in 6 years (75), with the recurrence rate in males being higher than that in females.

REFERENCES

1. Hanson LA, Fasth A, Jodal U, et al: Biology and pathology of urinary tract infections. *J Clin Pathol* 34:695–700, 1981.
2. Andriole VT: Advances in the treatment of urinary infections. *J Antimicrob Chemother* 9(Suppl A):163–172, 1982.
3. Mayrer AR, Andriole VT: Urinary tract antiseptics. *Med Clin North Am* 66:199–208, 1982.
4. Stamm WE: Recent developments in the diagnosis and treatment of urinary tract infections—University of Washington (Specialty Conference). *West J Med* 137:213–220, 1982.
5. Souney P, Polk BF: Single-dose antimicrobial therapy for urinary tract infections in women. *Rev Infect Dis* 4:29–34, 1982.
6. Report of the International Reflux Study Committee. Medical versus surgical treatment of primary vesicoureteral reflux. *Pediatrics* 67:392–400, 1981.
7. Turck M: New concepts in genitourinary tract infections. *JAMA* 246:2019–2023, 1981.
8. Resnick MI: Evaluation and management of infection stones. *Urol Clin North Am* 8:265–276, 1981.
9. Pereira AT: Coagulase-negative strains of staphylococcus possessing antigen 51 as agents of urinary infection. *J Clin Pathol* 15:252–253, 1962.
10. Mitchell RG: Classification of *Staphylococcus albus* strains isolated from the urinary tract. *J Clin Pathol* 21:93–96, 1968.
11. Mardh P, Hovelius B, Melsen F, et al: Experimental acute pyelonephritis in grivet monkeys provoked by *Staphylococcus saprophyticus*. *Acta Pathol Microbiol Scand* [Section B] 88:225–230, 1980.
12. Wallmark G, Arremark I, Telander B: *Staphylococcus saprophyticus*. A frequent cause of urinary tract infection among female outpatients. *J Infect Dis* 138:791–797, 1978.

13. Anderson JD, Clarke AM, Anderson ME, et al: Urinary tract infections due to *Staphylococcus saprophyticus* biotype 3. *Can Med Assoc J* 124:415–418, 1981.
14. Marrie TJ, Kwan C, Noble MA, et al: *Staphylococcus saprophyticus* as a cause of urinary tract infections. *J Clin Microbiol* 16:427–431, 1982.
15. Stamm WE, Counts GW, Running KR, et al: Diagnosis of coliform infection in acutely dysuric women. *N Engl J Med* 307:463–468, 1982.
16. Dankert J, Mansink WFA, Aarnoudse JG, et al: The prevalence of anaerobic bacteria in suprapubic bladder aspirates obtained from pregnant women. *Z Entrabl Bacteriol Hyg* 244:260–267, 1979.
17. Meijer-Severs GJ, Aarnoudse JG, Mensink WFA: The presence of antibody coated anaerobic bacteria in asymptomatic bacteriuria during pregnancy. *J Infect Dis* 140:653–658, 1979.
18. Birch DF, Fairley KF, Pavillard RE: Unconventional bacteria in urinary tract disease: *Ureaplasma urealyticum*. *Kidney Int* 19:58–64, 1981.
19. Birch DF, D'Apice AJF, Fairley KF: *Ureaplasma urealyticum* in the upper urinary tracts of renal allograft recipients. *J Infect Dis* 144:123–127, 1981.
20. Maskell R, Pead L, Allen J: The puzzle of "urethral syndrome": a possible answer? *Lancet* 1:1058–1059, 1979.
21. Brumfitt W, Ludlam H, Hamilton-Miller JMT, et al: Lactobacilli do not cause frequency and dysuria syndrome. *Lancet* 2:393–395, 1981.
22. McDowall DRM, Buchanan JD, Fairley KF, et al.: Anaerobic and other fastidious microorganisms in asymptomatic bacteriuria in pregnant women. *J Infect Dis* 144:114–122, 1981.
23. Kunin CM: In defense of the bladder. *West J Med* 137:237–239, 1982 (editorial).
24. Back E, Carlsson B, Hylander B: Urinary tract infection from *Haemophilus parainfluenzae*. *Nephron*, 29:117–118, 1981.
25. Dorman SA, Hardin NJ, Winn WC Jr: Pyelonephritis associated with *Legionella pneumophilia* serogroup 4. *Ann Intern Med* 93:835–837, 1980.
26. Normand ICS, Smellie JM: Prolonged maintenance chemotherapy in the management of urinary infection in childhood. *Br Med J* 1:1023–1026, 1965.
27. Smellie JM, Normand ICS, Katz G: Children with urinary infection: A comparison of those with and those without vesicoureteric reflux. *Kidney Int* 20:717–722, 1981.
28. Smellie JM, Edwards D, Normand ICS, et al. The effect of vesicoureteric reflux on renal growth in children with urinary tract infection. *Arch Dis Child* 56:593–600, 1981.
29. Normand C, Smellie J: Vesicoureteral reflux: The case of conservative management, in Hodson J, Kincaid-Smith P (eds.): *Reflux Nephropathy*. New York, Masson Publishing Co, 1979.
30. Montgomerie JZ, Meares EM Jr: Urinary tract infections, in Gonick HC, (ed): *Current Nephrology*, vol 5. New York, John Wiley & Sons, 1982, pp 169–188.
31. Vaisanen V, Elo J, Tallgren LG, et al: Mannose-resistant hemagglutination and P-antigen recognition are characteristic of *Escherichia coli* causing primary pyelonephritis. *Lancet* 2:1366–1369, 1981.
32. Korhonen TK, Vaisanen V, Saxen H, et al: P-antigen-recognizing fimbriae from human uropathogenic *Eschericha coli* strain. *Infect Immunol* 37:286–291, 1982.
33. Harber MJ, Chick S, MacKenzie R, et al: Lack of adherence to epithelial cells by freshly isolated urinary pathogens. *Lancet* 1:586–588, 1982.
34. Fowler JE, Stamey TA: Studies of introital colonization in women with recurrent urinary infection. X. Adhesive properties of *Escherichia coli* and *Proteus mirabilis*: Lack of correlation with urinary pathogenicity. *J Urol* 120:315–318, 1978.

35. Montgomerie JZ, Turkel S, Kalmanson GM, et al: *E. Coli* adherence to bladder epithelial cells of mice. *Urol Res* 8:163–165, 1980.
36. Suzuki Y, Fukushi Y, Orikasa S, et al: Opsonic effect of normal and infected human urine on phagocytosis of *Escherichia coli* and yeasts by neutrophils. *J Urol* 127:356–360, 1982.
37. Chernew I, Braude AI: Depression of phagocytosis by solutes in concentrations found in the kidney and urine. *J Clin Invest* 41:1945–1953, 1962.
38. Bryant RE, Sutcliffe MC, McGee ZA: Human polymorphonuclear leukocyte function in urine. *Yale J Biol Med* 46:113–124, 1973.
39. Kass EH: Asymptomatic infections of the urinary tract. *Trans Assoc Am Phys* 69:56–63, 1956.
40. Fowler JE, Pulaski ET: Excretory urography, cystography, and cystoscopy in the evaluation of women with urinary tract infection. *N Engl J Med* 304:462–465, 1981.
41. Lieberman E, Macchai RJ: Excretory urography in women with urinary tract infection. *J Urol* 127:263–264, 1982.
42. June CH, Browning MD, Pyatt RS: Renal computed tomography is abnormal in pyelonephritis. *Lancet* 2:93–94, 1982 (letter).
43. Hoffman EP, Mindelzun RE, Anderson RU: Computed tomography in pyelonephritis associated with diabetes. *Radiology* 135:691–695, 1980.
44. Rosenfield AT, Glickman MG, Taylor KJW, et al: Acute focal bacterial nephritis (acute lobar nephronia). *Radiology* 132:533–562, 1979.
45. Lee JKT, McClennan BL, Melson GL, et al: Acute focal bacterial nephritis. *AJR* 135:87–92, 1980.
46. Tauscher JW, Shaw DC: Eosinophlic cystitis. *Clin Pediatr* 20:741–743, 1981.
47. Goldstein M: Eosinophilic cystitis. *J Urol* 160:854–857, 1971.
48. Palubinskas AJ: Eosinophilic cystitis: Case report of eosinophilic infiltration of the urinary bladder. *Radiology* 75:589–591, 1960.
49. Rebhun J: Systemic eosinophilic infiltrative disease (SEIDI). *Ann Allergy* 32:86–93, 1974.
50. Lacey RW, Simpson MHC, Lord VL, et al: Comparison of single-dose trimethoprim with a five-day course for the treatment of urinary tract infections in the elderly. *Age and Aging* 10:179–185, 1981.
51. McCracken GH, Ginsburg CM, Namasonthi V, et al: Evaluation of short-term antibiotic therapy in children with uncomplicated urinary tract infections. *Pediatrics* 67:796–801, 1981.
52. Bailey, RR, Abbott GD: Treatment of urinary tract infection with a single dose of amoxicillin. *Nephron* 18:316–320, 1977.
53. Bailey RR, Abbott GD: Treatment of urinary tract infection with a single dose of trimethoprim-sulfamethoxazole. *Can Med Assoc J* 118:551–552. 1978.
54. Stamey TA, Govan DE, Palmer JM: The localization and treatment of urinary tract infection: The role of bactericidal urine levels as opposed to serum levels. *Medicine* (Baltimore) 44:1–36, 1965.
55. Stamey TA, Fair WR, Timothy MM, et al: Serum versus urinary antimicrobial concentrations in cure of urinary tract infections. *N Engl J Med* 291:1159–1163, 1974.
56. McCabe WR, Jackson GG: Treatment of pyelonephritis. Bacterial, drug and host factors in success or failure among 252 patients. *N Engl J Med* 272:1037–1044, 1965.
57. Bergeron MG, Bastille A, Lessard C, et al: Significance of intrarenal concentrations of gentamicin for the outcome of experimental pyelonephritis in rats. *J Infect Dis* 146:91–96, 1982.
58. Miller T, Phillips S, North D: Pharacokinetics of gentamicin in the treatment of renal infection: A therapeutic anomaly explained. *Kidney Int* 15:160–166, 1979.

59. Glauser MP, Lyons JM, Braude AI: Prevention of pyelonephritis due to *Escherichia coli* in rats with gentamicin stored in kidney tissue. *J Infect Dis* 139:172–177, 1979.
60. Minuth JN, Musher DM, Thorsteinsson SB: Inhibition of antibacterial activity of gentamicin by urine. *J Infect Dis* 133:14–21, 1976.
61. Montgomerie JZ, Morrow JW, Canawati HN, et al: Ceftizoxime in the treatment of urinary tract infection in spinal cord injury patients: Comparison with tobramycin. *J Antimicrob Chemother* 10(Suppl):247–252, 1982.
62. Barton CH, Sterling ML, Thomas, R, et al: Ineffectiveness of intravenous ascorbic acid as an acidifying agent in man. *Arch Intern Med* 141:211–212, 1981.
63. Nahata MC, Shimp L, Lampman T, et al: Effect of ascorbic acid on urine pH in man. *Am J Hosp Pharmacol* 34:1234–1237, 1977.
64. Maizels M, Schaeffer AJ: Decreased incidence of bacteriuria associated with periodic instillations of hydrogen peroxide into the urethral catheter drainage bag. *J Urol* 123:841–845, 1980.
65. Southhampton Infection Control Team. Evaluation of aseptic techniques and chlorhexadine on the rate of catheter-associated urinary tract infection. *Lancet* 1:89–91, 1982.
66. Kunin CM: Chlorhexidine and urinary drainage bags. *Lancet* 1:626, 1982.
67. Kunin CM, McCormack RC: Prevention of catheter-induced urinary tract infections by sterile closed drainage. *N Engl J Med* 274:1155–1162, 1966.
68. Burke JP, Garibaldi RA, Britt MR, et al: Prevention of catheter-associated urinary tract infections. Efficacy of daily meatal care regimens. *Am J Med* 70:655–658, 1981.
69. Griffith DP, Musher DM: Acetohydroxamic acid: Potential use in urinary infection caused by urea splitting bacteria. *Urology* 5:299–302.
70. Griffith DP, Gibson JR, Clinton CW, et al: Acetohydroxamic acid: Clinical studies of a urease inhibitor in patients with staghorn renal calculi. *J Urol* 119:9–15, 1978.
71. Griffith DP, Muscher DM, Itin C: Urease: The primary cause of infection-induced urinary stones. *Invest Urol* 13:346–350, 1976.
72. Martelli A, Buli P, Cortecchia V: Acetohydroxamic acid therapy in infected renal stones. *Urology* 17:320–322, 1981.
73. Nemoy NJ, Stamey TA: Use of hemiacidrin in management of infection stones. *J Urol* 116:693–695, 1976.
74. Dretler SP, Pfister RC, Newhouse JH: Renal stone dissolution via percutaneous nephrostomy. *N Engl J Med* 300:341–343, 1979.
75. Griffith DP: Infection-induced stones, in Coe FL (ed.): *Nephrolithiasis, Pathogenesis and Treatment.* Chicago, Year Book Medical Publishers, 1978 pp. 203–228.
76. Miller TE, Burnham S, North JDK: Immunological enhancement of the pathogenesis of pyelonephritis. *Clin Exp Immunol* 24:336–345, 1976.
77. Roberts JA, Domingue GJ, Martin LN, et al: Immunology of pyelonephritis in the primate model. II. Effect of immunosuppression. *Invest Urol* 19:148–153, 1981.

CHAPTER 8

Hypertension

Vito M. Campese
James Sowers
Michael Golub
Matthew Conolly

This year, the review on hypertension will deal primarily with the role of the sympathoadrenal system in hypertension and with the hypertension in the elderly. The adrenergic nervous system plays an important role in the regulation of blood pressure and in the pathogenesis of various forms of experimental and human hypertension. Recent evidence suggesting that sodium ingestion and obesity are important factors in the genesis of hypertension and that abnormalities of the sympathetic nervous system activity are present in salt-sensitive and in obese patients will be reviewed. The most recent diagnostic approach to the diagnosis of pheochromocytoma will also be discussed. Recently, hypertension in the elderly has been generating increased attention; knowledge of the pathophysiology and treatment of this form of hypertension will be reviewed.

THE ADRENERGIC NERVOUS SYSTEM IN ESSENTIAL HYPERTENSION

Anatomy and Biochemistry of the Sympathoadrenal System

This subject has been reviewed more extensively elsewhere (1). The sympathoadrenal system comprises a central and a peripheral component. The nucleus tractus solitarius is probably the most important integrative center modulating the autonomic control of the cardiovascular system.

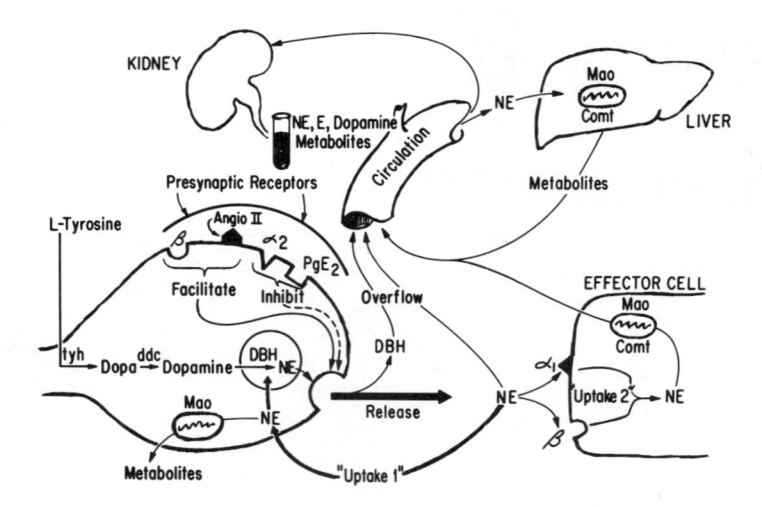

Figure 1. Metabolic pathways of catecholamines. NE, norepinephrine; E, epinephrine; TYH, tyrosine-hydroxylase; ddc, dopadecarboxylase; DβH, dopamine-beta-hydroxylase; MAO, monoamine oxidase; COMT, catechol-O-methyltransfere; Angio II, receptors for angiotensin II. (Campese VM: *Am J Nephrol* 3:128–138, 1983. Used with permission.)

The peripheral component is composed of the thoracolumbar system, with cell bodies of the preganglionic myelinated fibers arising in the intermediolateral gray portion of the spinal cord and being distributed via the anterior roots of the spinal nerves to the sympathetic ganglia and to the adrenal medulla.

The major known neurotransmitters of the sympathoadrenal system are norepinephrine (NE), epinephrine, and dopamine. NE is the main neurotransmitter of the sympathetic nerves and acts locally on effector cells. Epinephrine is synthesized mainly in the adrenal medulla and is released in the circulation to act as a hormone on distant target organs. Dopamine is an important neurotransmitter in the central nervous system (CNS) and also acts as a precursor of norepinephrine.

The biosynthesis of these amines occurs in the postganglionic sympathetic fibers, in the CNS, and in the chromaffin cells of the adrenal medulla. The amino acid precursor of these amines is L-tyrosine which is converted to L-dihydroxy-phenylalanine (L-dopa) by the enzyme tyrosine-hydroxylase (Fig. 1). L-Dopa is subsequently converted to 3,4-dihydroxyphenylethylamine (dopamine) through the catalytic action of the enzyme dopadecarboxylase. Dopamine is converted to NE by the enzyme dopamine-β-hydroxylase (DβH). In the adrenal medulla, most of the NE is converted to epinephrine by the enzyme 4-phenylethanolamine-N-methyltransferase. In the peripheral sympathetic nerves, 80–90% of NE is stored within the vesicles and the remainder is stored in the cytosol in equilibrium with the vesicles. The concentration of NE in the cytosol regulates synthesis through feedback inhibition of the enzyme tyrosine-hydroxylase.

Upon depolarization of the sympathetic neurons, storage vesicles fuse with the axonal membrane and, by exocytosis, release NE, DβH, and other contents of the vesicles in the synaptic cleft. The amount of neurotransmitter released depends upon the frequency and duration of excitatory impulses and it is modulated by a system of presynaptic receptors (Fig. 1). Following release, catecholamines exert their actions by binding to specific postsynaptic receptors. The action of NE is rapidly terminated primarily by active reuptake into the sympathetic nerve terminals. Approximately 75–80% of this amine is, in fact, disposed by active transport from the extracellular space across the axonal membrane into the free pool in the cytosol. Subsequently, NE is actively taken up into the storage vesicles to reestablish the equilibrium between the free and bound pools. Excessive amounts of NE in the cytosol are metabolized by the enzyme monoamine oxidase. This process of reuptake is called uptake 1 and is to be distinguished from uptake 2, which occurs in extraneuronal peripheral tissues.

Part of the catecholamines, released from the sympathetic nerve endings, overflows into the circulation where, in conjunction with the catecholamines released from the adrenal medulla, they constitute the measurable pool in the blood. The amount of NE that overflows into the circulation depends not only on the rate of release from the sympathetic nerve endings but also on the density, distribution, and width of the neuroeffector junction. At narrow junctions, the action of NE is terminated mainly by reuptake into the neurons, whereas at wider junctions, a greater amount of neurotransmitter will diffuse into the circulation. Smooth muscles in the walls of arteries and veins seem to have wider neuroeffector junctions than the vas deferens and, therefore, may be the most important source of plasma NE. Circulating catecholamines are rapidly metabolized, mainly in the liver, by the enzymes monoamine oxidase and catechol-0-methyltransferase. The half-life of intravenously infused NE is approximately 2 minutes.

Since normally only approximately 29% of total plasma NE and epinephrine and less than 1% of total dopamine are free in the blood, with the rest being conjugated, it has been suggested that conjugation is an important pathway of inactivation of catecholamines. Catecholamines in man are predominantly sulfoconjugated by the enzyme phenolsulfotransferase.

The main metabolites of NE and epinephrine detectable in the urine are vanillylmandelic acid (VMA) and 4-hydroxy-3-methoxyphenylglycol (MHPG). Normetanephrine and metanephrine are excreted in the urine in smaller amounts, but they reflect more closely the amount of NE and epinephrine released by the peripheral sympathetic nerves. The main metabolites of dopamine found in the urine are homovanillic acid (HVA) and methoxytyramine. Only small quantities of catecholamines appear unchanged in the urine: 1–5% of NE and approximately 1% of epinephrine.

Pathogenetic Links Between Increased Sympathetic Activity and Hypertension

Increased activity of the sympathetic nervous system may lead to a sustained rise in arterial blood pressure through a variety of mechanisms. First, it can cause an increase in cardiac output via the direct inotropic and chronotropic action on the heart, and via increased venous return due to venous constriction. The increase in cardiac output, in the long run, may stimulate autoregulatory vasoconstriction and/or arteriolar hypertrophy, ultimately leading to an increase in vascular resistance. Second, the increased sympathetic drive may directly stimulate α_1-adrenergic receptors of the arteriolar vessels and result in vasoconstriction. Third, increased sympathetic neuronal activity may cause sodium retention via a direct action on the renal tubules or via enhanced release of renin. Finally, the sympathetic tone may increase vascular resistance by stimulating the synthesis of contractile protein in vascular smooth muscle cells (2) and by triggering membrane abnormalities in vascular muscle, which leads to exaggerated vasoconstrictor response and hypertension (3).

Increased contractile response to NE has been shown in various experimental forms of hypertension as well as in human essential hypertension. Dietz et al. have presented evidence that early structural changes of the resistance vessels occur in spontaneously hypertensive rats (SHR) at a time when blood pressure is only moderately elevated. These early vascular changes may exert an important pathogenetic role in the development of hypertension (4). Philipp et al. have demonstrated an inverse correlation between plasma levels of NE during physical exercise and reactivity to exogenous NE in normal subjects (5). This relationship was invariably disturbed in age-matched patients with essential hypertension, so that pressor responses to NE at any given basal NE level was increased in these patients. A highly significant correlation existed between the combination of plasma levels of NE and vascular reactivity to infused NE and the height of mean arterial pressure, suggesting that the interrelation between these two factors forms an important determinant of the blood pressure levels in these patients.

Evidence for Neurogenic Factors in Human Essential Hypertension

Since the discovery that the sympathoadrenal system plays a central role in the regulation of blood pressure, a large number of studies have attempted to investigate whether essential hypertension in humans is related to hyperactivity of this system. The evidence available to substantiate this hypothesis is, for the large part, indirect. Wallin et al. have shown that a rise in arterial pressure results in suppression of electrical activity in hypertensive humans (6).

Arterial baroreceptors have higher threshold and reduced sensitivity to increases in arterial pressure in patients with essential hypertension (7). The decreased sensitivity of the arterial baroreceptor may increase the sympathetic drive and cause hypertension. A significant resetting of baroreceptors has been identified in the early stages of labile hypertension. suggesting that it might have a causative role in the initiation of hypertension. However, the resetting of baroreceptors may occur within hours after elevation of arterial pressure (8), which raises the provocative question of whether this abnormality is causative or secondary.

Since the introduction of sensitive techniques for measuring plasma levels of catecholamines and with the demonstration that the NE levels correlate with sympathetic neural activity in various physiologic and pathologic states, these measurements have been extensively used to search for evidence of increased sympathetic neuron activity in essential hypertension.

A review of 32 studies comparing plasma NE concentrations in hypertensive and normotensive groups indicated higher levels of NE in hypertensive patients in 88% of these studies (9). It is interesting to note that mean levels of NE in the hypertensive groups in these various studies were largely comparable. However, what determined the presence or absence of differences in plasma levels of NE was primarily the great variability of levels in normal subjects among the various studies. This raises serious questions about the criteria used by various investigators in the selection of the control population. In earlier studies, for example, elevated levels of catecholamines were demonstrated in a greater proportion than in later studies (10,11). This difference can now be attributed to the fact that in the older studies the hypertensives and normal subjects were not age-matched and the latter usually consisted of younger individuals selected from the personnel working in those laboratories (12).

Among 24 studies involving orthostatic stress, the increments in NE with standing were similar for hypertensives and normotensives. In contrast, the increments in plasma concentrations of NE during isotonic or isometric exercise is usually greater in hypertensives than in normotensives (13). Franco-Morselli et al. have described greater levels of epinephrine but not NE in patients with essential hypertension (14). These findings, however, have not been confirmed by others. A significant positive correlation between plasma NE and blood pressure has also been demonstrated in some studies (15,16) not not in others (17).

Pharmacologic studies with antiadrenergic agents have also been put forward in support of the hypothesis for a role of the sympathetic nervous system in the genesis of essential hypertension. Louis et al. demonstrated a positive and significant correlation between the decrease in diastolic blood pressure and the decrease in plasma NE after the administration of pentolinium, a ganglionic blocking agent (16). We recently demonstrated a similar finding after the administration of clonidine, a central acting antiadrenergic agent (18).

Relationship between Sodium Intake and Plasma Catecholamines in Hypertension

Available evidence suggests that hypertension is related to sodium ingestion, both in man and animals (19–22). A number of epidemiologic studies have shown a direct relationship between sodium intake and the incidence of hypertension (21,23,24). It is also well known that sodium restriction reduces blood pressure in a great number of patients with essential hypertension (22,23). Kawasaki et al. identified two subgroups of patients with essential hypertension. There was an increase in blood pressure during sodium loading in one group ("salt-sensitive"), while blood pressure remained unchanged in the other group ("non-salt-sensitive") (25). Furthermore, certain strains of rats also demonstrate this phenomenon. The Dahl "S" (salt-sensitive) rats become hypertensive only when their intake of sodium is high; in contrast, the "R" (salt-resistant) rats remain normotensive irrespective of the amount of sodium in their diet (26). The mechanisms underlying the sensitivity to sodium intake have not been fully elucidated.

Kawasaki et al. (25) and Fujita et al. (27) have shown that salt-sensitive patients retain a greater amount of sodium than salt-resistant patients during high sodium intake. In contrast, we did not find any difference in renal sodium handling between salt-sensitive patients and normal subjects (28).

We have evidence, however, suggesting that an abnormal relationship between the activity of the sympathetic nervous system and the state of sodium volume balance may be responsible for the rise in blood pressure during sodium loading in patients with essential hypertension (28). The recumbent blood levels of NE, epinephrine, and dopamine in normal subjects are higher during ingestion of low sodium intake (10 mEq/day) than with higher sodium intake (Fig. 2). An inverse significant correlation is present between the blood levels of NE, epinephrine, and dopamine and urinary sodium excretion in normal subjects (29). The relationship between plasma levels of NE or epinephrine and sodium excretion is most evident when sodium intake and excretion are below 50 mEq/day. In contrast, an inverse relationship between urinary sodium excretion and plasma levels of dopamine is evident throughout the entire range of sodium excretion. No substantial changes in plasma NE levels are evident with sodium excretion between 50 and 300 mEq/day. However, extremely

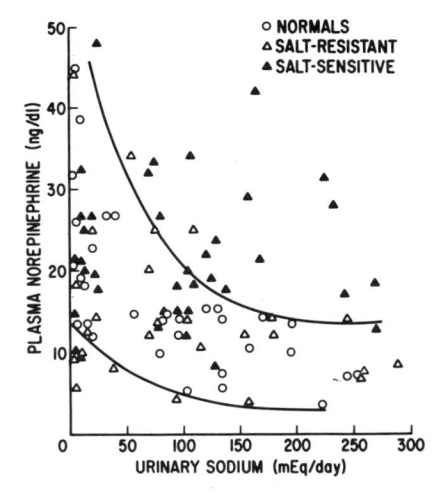

Figure 2. Relationship between plasma levels of NE and urinary excretion of sodium in normal subjects (open circles), salt-sensitive (solid triangles), and salt-resistant (open triangles) patients with essential hypertension. (Campese VM et al: *Kidney Int* 21:371–378, 1982. Used with permission.)

higher sodium intake, in the range of 800–1,500 mEq/day, can result in further suppression of plasma NE levels (30).

Urinary excretion rate of NE and epinephrine also increases during dietary sodium restriction. On the contrary, urinary excretion of dopamine increases with the ingestion of greater amounts of sodium (31). There is less consistency in the data on the effect of acute extracellular volume expansion with saline infusion on plasma catecholamines. A decrease or no change in plasma levels and in urinary excretion of NE and epinephrine and a rise in urinary excretion of dopamine have been observed (32). In patients with essential hypertension, there is no significant inverse relationship between plasma concentration of NE and urinary sodium excretion (28). When we attempted to correlate this finding with blood pressure response to high sodium intake, it became apparent that approximately 50% of hypertensive patients respond to salt loading with a rise in blood pressure greater than 10% (salt-sensitive), whereas in the remaining patients (salt-resistant) and in normal subjects, blood pressure does not change significantly (Fig. 3). Plasma NE levels were not significantly different between normal subjects and salt-sensitive or salt-resistant patients during low sodium intake. However, during high sodium intake, plasma NE concentration decreased significantly in normal subjects and in salt-resistant patients but not in salt-sensitive patients.

On the contrary, plasma NE levels increased instead of decreasing in the majority of salt-sensitive patients during high sodium intake. There was a significant and direct correlation ($r = 0.49$, $p < 0.01$) between the change in plasma NE and the change in mean blood pressure observed when these subjects modified their diet from low to high sodium intake. The increments in plasma NE after 5 minutes of upright posture were significantly greater in salt-sensitive patients than in salt-resistant patients and in normal subjects during both low or high sodium intake.

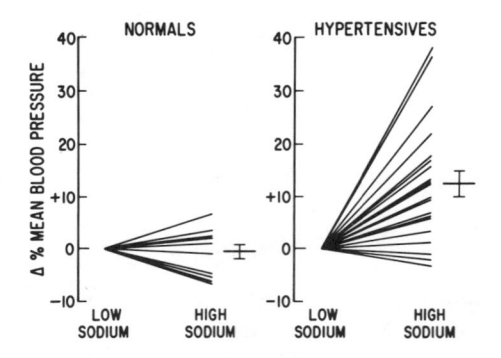

Figure 3. Percent change in the supine mean blood pressure in normal subjects and in patients with essential hypertension. Values obtained during high sodium intake (200 mEq/day) were compared with the values obtained during low sodium intake (10 mEq/day). (Campese VM et al: *Kidney Int* 21:371–378, 1982. Used with permission.)

These data indicate that a subset of patients with essential hypertension may have impaired suppressibility of plasma NE during high sodium intake, both in the supine and the upright position, which suggests hyperactivity of the sympathetic nervous system. These studies also indicate that any evaluation of sympathetic nervous system activity in hypertensive patients must take into account the state of sodium volume balance. Dietz et al. obtained similar findings in stroke-prone SHR (33). Consistent with this notion is the observation that sodium depletion may reduce blood pressure by inhibiting the sympathoadrenal drive (34–35).

The mechanisms responsible for the greater activation of the sympathetic nervous system during high sodium intake in rats and in humans with essential hypertension are not clear. Both central and peripheral mechanisms could be responsible. Winternitz et al. have put forward some findings substantiating the hypothesis that the exaggeration of hypertension following high sodium intake in SHR may result from an alteration in central noradrenergic activity. High sodium intake, in fact, produced significant increases in the NE content of the dorsomedial and anterior hypothalamic nuclei, which have been implicated in cardiovascular regulation (36).

Dietz et al. observed that high salt intake in stroke-prone SHR results in reduced reuptake of NE in the sympathetic end terminals, which points to a peripheral mechanism of activation of the sympathetic nervous system (33). High salt intake facilitates the release of the neurotransmitter, probably by reducing prejunctional α_2-receptors in SHR (37) as well as in Dahl salt-sensitive rats (38). Furthermore, it has been suggested that excessive sodium intake may suppress the Na^+-K^+ pump in the adrenergic terminal and facilitate the release of NE from nerve terminals (39). Finally, high sodium intake may potentiate neurogenic vasoconstriction by increasing vascular reactivity (40).

OBESITY AND HYPERTENSION

An association between hypertension and obesity has been documented by a number of clinical and epidemiological studies (41,42), and obesity

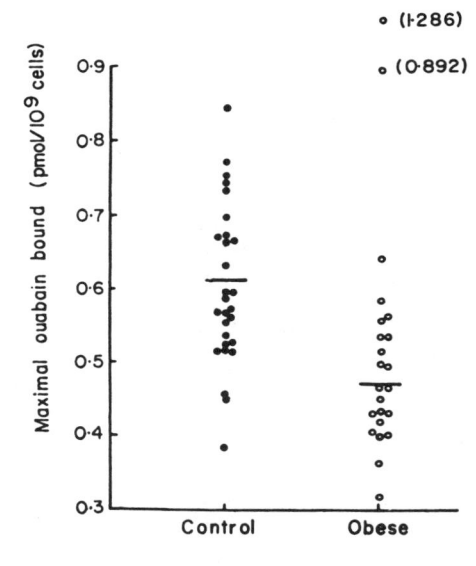

Figure 4. Individual values for maximal ouabain-binding capacity of erthyrocytes from obese subjects and controls. Horizontal lines denote the mean values for the controls (0.611 ± 0.020) and for the other 21 obese subjects (0.474 ± 0.018); the difference between these means is significant ($p < 0.001$). (De Luise M et al: *N Engl J Med* 303:1017–22, 1980. Used with permission.)

and/or weight gain during young adulthood are well-recognized risk factors for later development of hypertension (43,44). A relationship between increasing age and high blood pressure appears to be specific for Westernized populations in which there is an association of increasing body weight with age (45). In contrast, in rural or tribal nonaffluent populations, there is no relation between blood pressure and age in these nonobese individuals (46).

Despite the considerable epidemiological evidence, pathogenetic mechanisms of the relationship between hypertension and obesity remain poorly understood. Increased total blood volume and cardiac output in the presence of normal peripheral vascular resistance are observed in obese hypertensive patients (47). However, when these measurements were carefully corrected for body surface area, no differences could be found between obese and nonobese hypertensive patients (48). Increased salt intake associated with excessive caloric intake has been suggested to be an important factor explaining the high blood pressure associated with obesity. Salt restriction rather than caloric reduction has been suggested as being responsible for the fall in blood pressure associated with weight reduction. However, recent studies have shown that weight loss reduces blood pressure independent of salt intake (49,50).

Obese individuals have been reported to have increased erythrocyte intracellular sodium levels and reduced numbers of sodium-potassium adenosine triphosphatase (ATPase) units (Fig. 4) (51,52). Reductions in sodium transport and higher intracellular sodium content have also been described in the liver and muscle of obese (ob/ob) mice (53). In a recently reported study (52), erythrocyte Na^+, K^+-ATPase activity, and rubidium-

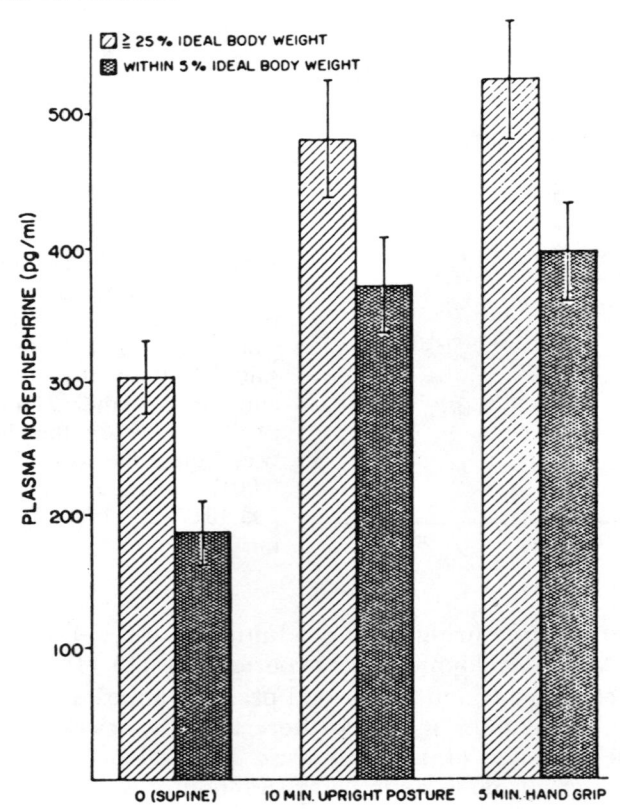

Figure 5. Mean (± SEM) plasma NE responses to 10 minutes of upright posture and 5 minutes of isometric handgrip exercise in 10 obese subjects and 12 age-, sex-, and race-matched nonobese subjects. (Sowers JR et al: *J Clin Endocrinol Metabol* 54:1181–1186, 1982. Used with permission.)

86 (^{86}Rb) uptake were observed to be low while intracellular sodium was high in obese patients. In obese individuals undergoing 12 weeks of weight loss, erythrocyte Na$^+$, K$^+$-ATPase activity, and ^{86}Rb uptake did increase and intracellular sodium decreased moderately, they never returned to levels observed in nonobese subjects (52). The authors suggested that the defects in sodium transport are not secondary to the obese state but may have contributed to the development of obesity. However, no relationship was observed between erythrocyte pump activity and blood pressure before onset of weight loss. Thus, these observations did not support a relationship between abnormalities in sodium pump activity and blood pressure in obese individuals. Recently conducted studies (54) have demonstrated that hypertensive obese patients have elevated plasma NE (Fig. 5) and that reductions in blood pressure associated with caloric restriction and the accompanying weight loss were related to reductions in plasma NE.

Reduction in plasma renin activity was also observed in these obese patients undergoing weight loss (54). Since the reductions in renin activity were not observed until plasma catecholamines were significantly lowered, it was suggested that a reduction in sympathetic nervous system activity and circulating catecholamines was, at least in part, responsible for the depression in renin activity. The investigators concluded from these studies that enhanced sympathetic nervous system activity may play a role in the maintenance of elevated blood pressure associated with obesity.

During the early days after onset of fasting or of a hypocaloric diet, there is a very prominent natriuresis which may account for some of the early reductions in blood pressure (55). This early natriuresis has been suggested to result from accompanying hyperketonemia, relative hypoinsulinemia, relative hyperglucagonemia, and mineralcorticosteroid resistance. However, the natriuresis associated with fasting and hypocaloric diets may also result from changes in the influence of catecholamines on renal sodium excretion (56). Dopamine influences the regulation of renal sodium excretion causing increased excretion of sodium (56). Circulating plasma NE and epinephrine as well as renal sympathetic nerve impulses result in increased renal tubular reabsorption of the sodium ion. Recent observations that plasma dopamine does not decline in the presence of dropping plasma levels of NE and epinephrine during early caloric deprivation suggest that these changing catecholaminergic influences on the renal tubule may account for the observed natriuresis.

Thus, studies reported in the past year provide evidence for derangements in several systems involved in blood pressure regulation which could account for hypertension associated with obesity. These derangements include increased intracellular sodium levels, high levels of plasma NE, and renin activity. Weight loss associated with caloric reduction in obese individuals is accompanied by a reduction in blood pressure as well as correction of some of the above-mentioned derangements.

Pheochromocytoma

Hormone deficiency and excess syndromes have been very important in our understanding of basic endocrinology. It is interesting to speculate what we would know of the actions of glucocorticoids without the clinical descriptions of Cushing and Addison, or what we would know of growth hormone without the existence of acromegaly and pituitary dwarfism. In the field of hypertension, such "experiments of nature" are a fundamental aspect of our study of the mechanisms that control blood pressure. Every syndrome that is associated with hypertension may yield a clue to the etiologies of essential hypertension. Thus, an adrenal adenoma producing aldosterone and certain patients with congenital adrenal hyperplasia represent a volume expansion model of hypertension. The rare renin-secreting tumors and renovascular hypertension illustrate the potential role of the renin-angiotensin system in hypertension. Pheochromocytomas, on the other hand, represent a natural model of hypertension induced by activation of the sympathoadrenal system. It is debatable how much the endocrinology of this tumor resembles essential hypertension, but the study of this tumor has definitely enhanced our understanding of the pathophysiology of the sympathetic system.

Although this tumor is fairly rare (estimated at 0.1% of the hypertensive population) (57), it is a very important clinical entity, and it should be surgically removed.

The classic clinical presentation of pheochromocytoma is well known. Few patients, however, present with classic symptoms, and the spectrum of presenting symptoms is far greater than is generally recognized. It is very rare, however, for a patient to be totally symptom-free, and non-functioning tumors are even rarer. Most series have reported an approximately equal occurrence of paroxysmal and sustained hypertension. The presenting symptoms are similar, although they are less pronounced in sustained hypertension. Paroxysms occur from once every few months to 25 times daily, but a weekly attack is common in 75% of patients (58). The attacks last less than 1 hour in 80% of patients and less than 15 minutes in 50% (58). Certain foods, anxiety, exercise, anesthesia, tight clothing, abdominal massage, bladder distention, and micturition may precipitate an attack. The most frequently mentioned symptom is headache, often throbbing, bilateral, and severe, but occasionally it is mild and indistinguishable from tension headache. Sweating, often perfuse and involving most of the body, occurs in the majority of patients. This is paradoxical because the major control of sweat glands not associated with hair follicles is cholinergic. The mechanism by which catecholamines activate this process remains unclear. It is of interest that patients with sustained tumor secretion may have continuous sweating as well as persistent hypertension. Palpitations are the third most common symptom. It is likely that this symptom is due to epinephrine, since infusions of this catecholamine will reproduce the cardiac symptoms and NE infusions rarely cause palpitations (59). Anxiety, nausea, vomiting, faintness, chest, and abdominal pain are frequent symptoms. It should be kept in mind that there is an increased incidence of cholelithiasis in pheochromocytoma patients. Following an attack, a sense of weakness and fatigue often occurs for a variable length of time. Some weight loss occurs, particularly in patients with sustained secretion. Obese patients with the tumor who do not lose weight are very uncommon (60). The hypermetabolism of this condition is occasionally associated with a sensation of warmth and heat intolerance.

Dyspnea may be a consequence of hypertensive heart disease, but this can be complicated by a catecholamine myocarditis (61). Visual disturbances are more frequently reported in patients with sustained secretion and chronic hypertensive retinopathy. Constipation may accompany chronically elevated catecholamine levels and can help to differentiate the hypermetabolic patient thought to have hyperthyroidism where hyperdefecation is the rule. Paresthesias are more characteristic of those patients with paroxysmal hypertension, probably due to acute vasoconstriction.

The physical findings in pheochromocytoma are even less specific than the symptoms. Hypertension, of course, is the most frequent finding. As previously stated, approximately 50% of patients have sustained hypertension while 40–50% have intermittent elevations. Nonfunctioning or predominantly epinephrine-secreting tumors may not cause hypertension at all. Transition from intermittent to sustained hypertension and sudden onset of sustained hypertension have been documented in patients with the disease. Significant severe fluctuations of blood pressure is seen frequently, even in those with sustained hypertension. Orthostatic fall in blood pressure is a common finding; both decreased blood volume and decreased sympathetic responsiveness may be responsible for this phenomenon (62), which is seen more commonly in the patient with sustained hypertension. This finding in a patient who is not currently taking antihypertensive drugs should alert the clinician to the possibility of pheochromocytoma. Interestingly, the blood pressure fall is usually accompanied by an increase in heart rate, demonstrating the intactness of the baroreceptor reflexes.

The presence of diaphoresis in a cool room in a hypertensive subject should also be a "red flag." Tachycardia and premature contractions are seen frequently, but sudden hypertension can result in reflex bradycardia. Pallor during an attack is common, presumably related to cutaneous vasoconstriction. Sometimes flushing occurs with the fall in pressure and some patients manifest only flushing, though this is rare. The retinopathy of this disorder is the same as that of essential hypertension, although grades III and IV lesions are probably seen more frequently. Lacrimation and papillary dilation often occur during attacks. A fine tremor, similar to that of hyperthyroidism, can be seen during attacks or, less frequently, in sustained hypertensives. Unexplained low grade fever has been reported in a majority of patients upon careful examination (63). A thorough skin examination for neurofibromatosis, cafe-au-lait spots, and axillary freckling should be performed. Neurofibromatosis is seen in about 5% of patients with pheochromocytoma, but less than 1% of all patients with von Recklinghausen's disease have pheochromocytoma. Nevertheless, hypertensives with this disorder should be screened. According to one report, axillary freckling is almost always present, and large, multiple cafe-au-lait spots are very suggestive (64). In several series, about 10% of patients had palpable abdominal masses.

The etiology of pheochromocytoma is unknown, but it is interesting to note that the tumor is seen in several domestic animals. A spontaneous tumor rate of 80% occurs in a Wistar strain of rats over 25 months of age. In humans, up to 10% of tumors are familial. Ten percent of tumors are bilateral and half of these are contributed by familial cases where bilaterality approaches 50%. In sporadic cases, the right adrenal is more often involved, but when the patient has neurofibromatosis, the left predominates. In familial cases, the inheritance is dominant. The peak incidence is in the fourth and fifth decades; slightly more than half the cases occur in women. Nearly 90% of tumors are in the adrenal and 99% are intraabdominal. The most common extraadrenal site is the organ of Zuckerkandl. The tumors vary considerably in size but average approximately 100 g.

Although normal adrenal tissue produces a predominance of epinephrine, most adrenal pheochromocytomas produce a predominance of norepinephrine. However, if some epinephrine is produced, it is highly likely that the tumor is located in the adrenal. The reason that extraadrenal pheochromocytomas rarely produce epinephrine has been attributed to the fact that the methyltransferase enzyme that converts NE to epinephrine is induced by high concentrations of glucocorticoids, concentrations attainable only within the adrenal (65). Nonetheless, extraadrenal production of epinephrine has been documented several times, so elevated epinephrine secretion does not totally rule out an extraadrenal site. Pheochromocytoma tissue often has a very large synthetic capacity relative to normal adrenal medulla, but the mechanisms that trigger release of these catecholamines is not known.

Nervous innervation has not been demonstrated. Small and large tumors tend to behave differently in terms of their metabolism and secretion. Small tumors have rapid turnover rates and release unmetabolized catecholamines, whereas large tumors have low turnover rates and release mainly metabolites as demonstrated by a high metabolite-to-catecholamine ratio in the urine (66). What then is responsible for the intermittent paroxysms seen in some patients? One interesting postulate is that the excessive NE is taken up by sympathetic nervous tissue and released as a large bolus with sympathetic stimulation (67). In other words, the paroxysms are due to sympathetic activity and not to tumor release. As we shall see, more recent studies suggest an important role for the sympathetic nervous system in blood pressure control in patients with pheochromocytomas.

In the 1960s and 1970s, a great deal of interest has developed in the identification of familial clusters of multiple endocrine tumors. Two such syndromes, both autosomal dominant, have as a component a high incidence of pheochromocytoma. In 1961, Sipple (68) described a very high incidence of thyroid carcinoma in patients with pheochromocytoma. This concurrence became identified as Sipple's syndrome. Further reports indicated that bilateral pheochromocytomas were very frequent in these patients, that the tumor of the thyroid was frequently a medullary carcinoma, and that familial cases also had an increased incidence of hyperparathyroidism. This familial pattern is generally referred to as multiple endocrine neoplasia, type II. Another rarer familial constellation of pheochromocytoma (often bilateral), medullary thyroid carcinoma, and multiple mucosal neuromas is multiple endocrine neoplasia, type IIb or type III. In these families, a Marfanoid appearance is also a feature. Interestingly, these families do not appear to have an increased incidence of hyperparathyroidism. Other features include thickened corneal nerves, a characteristic facial appearance with thickened lips and an "acromegalic" aspect, muscular wasting, and gastrointestinal tract abnormalities including megacolon and diffuse intestinal ganglioneuromatosis. In both of these familial conditions, the questions of family monitoring and early case finding are important. Clearly a good family history, measurement of serum calcium, and careful thyroid palpation should be part of the evaluation of any new case with pheochromocytoma. In identified families, the frequency of investigation and the means of studying asymptomatic relatives is highly controversial. The medullary tumor is multicentric and may be proceeded by hyperplasia of the C cells of the thyroid. Since calcitonin is produced by the tumor, it has been used as a marker of the disease. However, stimulation tests (pentagastrin, calcium, or glucagon) may be necessary to show an abnormality (69). These same investigators have detected unsuspected cases of medullary thyroid tumors in sporadic cases of pheochromocytomas. Thus, these investigators are aggressive in performing stimulatory tests in all new cases and in relatives of familial cases. The pheochromocytomas in these patients, although frequently bilateral, are almost always intraadrenal. Sustained hypertension is less frequent in these patients. As the tumors are in the adrenal, they produce some epinephrine, and one investigation in a large kindred identified urinary epinephrine excretion as the most sensitive test in finding new tumors (70).

The concept that epinephrine might be the most sensitive test for early tumors may also apply to small tumors not associated with the familial syndromes. As mentioned previously, small tumors might not elevate metabolites to the extent large tumors do, so urinary catecholamine elevations may precede metabolic product elevations. Brown and co-workers (71) recently pointed out that only 2% of the circulating NE is derived from adrenal secretion, whereas all of the epinephrine is from this source. Therefore, the secretion of NE from a tumor in the adrenal has to be 50 times the normal amount to double blood concentrations (assuming unchanged clearance), but a doubling of epinephrine secretion increases the blood concentration proportionately. In their series of 18 patients with the disease, the plasma epinephrine was the most sensitive discriminator of disease in the eight patients with small tumors.

Other investigators have emphasized the utility of plasma concentrations of catecholamines in making the diagnosis of pheochromocytoma. Bravo and co-workers evaluated 24 patients with the tumor and 40 control subjects who were suspect for the disease but who were subsequently found to be tumor-free (72). In this series, the urinary metabolites were disappointing in helping to discriminate the two groups of patients. Eleven of 22 patients had VMA levels overlapping with the nontumor subjects, and five of 22 had metanephrine excretion similar to control subjects. In three patients, both values were in the same range as those of the control group. With regard to the metanephrine determination, much of the overlap appeared to be due to a rather high range (up to 2 mg/24 hr) of excretion in the control group, although two patients had values below 1 mg/24 hr. With the VAM, the values of all the control subjects were below 10 mg/day, but so were the values of 11 patients with tumor. These results are certainly poorer than previous series, and it is unclear if the tumors are being identified earlier than previously and if the smaller tumors produce fewer metabolites. Unfortunately, this study did not analyze urinary catecholamines to see if this determination was more sensitive in detecting patients with the disease. The authors did find, however, that plasma total catecholamines was a very good test for detecting patients with pheochromocytoma. Only one patient had a value overlapping that of the control group (Fig. 6). On another occasion, this patient had an elevated value and responded to a glucagon challenge with a blood pressure response and marked elevation of catecholamine levels. The study also emphasized that catecholamine levels correlated poorly with blood pressure. Although the total catecholamines proved very useful, it is conceivable that fractionated levels (NE and epinephrine values) might be even more discriminatory. Only 10 subjects had these levels performed, and in all both values were elevated, including those of the five patients with normal blood pressure at the time of study. It would have been interesting to see if the three patients with normal VAM and metanephrine values had a greater elevation of epinephrine than NE as in the English series previously cited, but fractionated values were not reported.

This report requires further confirmation, since there may be some potential problems in using plasma levels of catecholamines in the diagnosis of pheochromocytoma. Plasma catecholamines fluctuate rapidly, and stress and venipuncture can elevate the levels. Therefore, careful technique in drawing blood at least 30 minutes after venipuncture with the patient relaxed and supine is important to avoid many false positives. Secondly, the assay itself requires careful technique and quality control, and variability in the values remains a critical problem. Finally, the question of whether this series is representative of most patients is critically important. Only five of 24 patients were normotensive at the time of the study. It has been a long held concept that patients with sustained hypertension have continuous secretion while those with intermittent hypertension may not. In Manger and Gifford's series, all but one of 20 patients with sustained hypertension had elevated catecholamine levels on several occasions (57). In six of 16 patients without hypertension at the time of the study, plasma catecholamines were normal. Thus, plasma catechola-

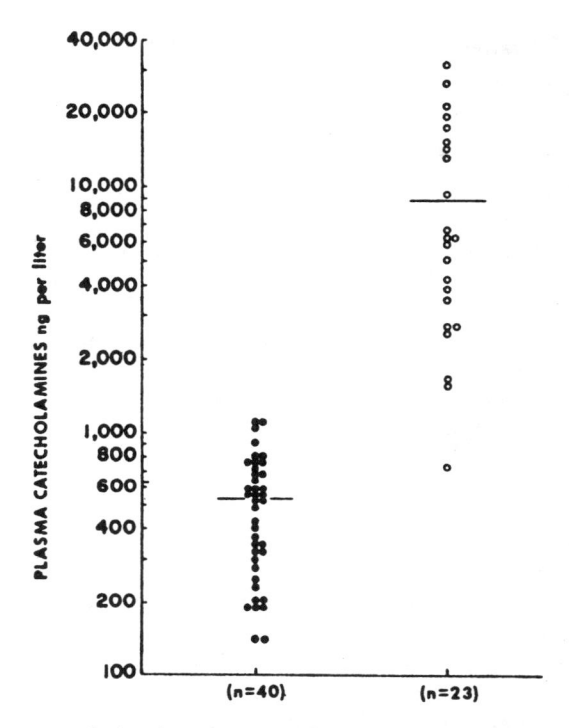

Figure 6. Plasma catecholamines measured at rest in patients with (open circles) and without (solid circles) evidence of pheochromocytoma. All but one of the 23 patients with pheochromocytoma had plasma catecholamine values greater than the highest values in patients without pheochromocytoma. (Bravo EL et al: *N Engl J Med* 301:682–686, 1979. Used with permission.)

mine levels, particularly if fractionated, have great diagnostic promise in those patients with sustained hypertension, but a proportion of those with paroxysmal hypertension may not be identified by this assay.

A further diagnostic approach to this question may help to eliminate false-positive elevations of plasma catecholamines. One of the major difficulties in diagnosing pheochromocytoma has been the lack of an appropriate suppression test. Several stimulatory tests have been used throughout the years, all having the significant danger of precipitating a major hypertensive crisis. The two groups mentioned above have utilized their plasma catecholamine assays to devise suppression tests. The principle of each test is that normal adrenal secretion is controlled by nervous innervation. Decreasing the nervous stimulation of the gland should decrease catecholamine release, whereas the noninnervated pheochromocytoma secretion would be unaffected. In the study of Brown et al. (71), the innervation of the adrenal was interrupted by the short-acting ganglion blocker, pentolinium 2.5 mg intravenously, and blood was obtained before

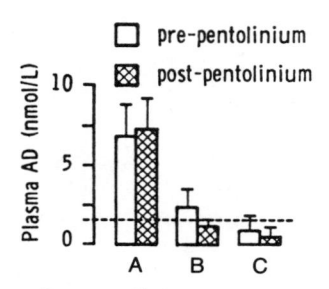

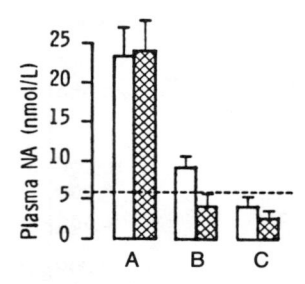

Figure 7. Pentolinium-suppression test. Plasma noradrenaline and adrenaline levels are shown before and after 2.5 mg pentolinium IV. Group A was pheochromocytoma patients. Group B was nontumor patients who underwent venous sampling but in whome no tumor was found. Group C was 12 patients who had intermittently elevated levels of NA or AD and did not undergo venous sampling. The columns represent the mean ± SE for each group. (Brown MJ et al: *Lancet* 1:174–177, 1981. Used with permission.)

and 10 minutes after the injection. The tumor patients showed little change in plasma catecholamines with no drop exceeding 8%. Each control group (one group of suspect patients who underwent intensive evaluation and another group who had some features suggestive of the disease) showed significant decreases in both epinephrine and NE levels (Fig. 7).

Bravo et al. (73) reported a second suppressive maneuver utilizing clonidine, a centrally acting sympathetic suppressant. In this study, the plasma levels of epinephrine and NE were measured before and 3 hours after the oral administration of 0.3 mg clonidine. The 10 patients and the 15 controls were clearly distinguished by plasma NE level responses, with all the controls suppressing into or below the normal range and all the patients' values remaining elevated. In this series, there was more overlap of baseline NE levels than their previous series using catecholamine levels. Also, in contrast with the series of Brown et al. (71), plasma epinephrine response was not as good a predictor of the diagnosis, and basal epinephrine levels were normal in two patients. The question in each of these series is whether a basal elevation is necessary to show a lack of suppressibility. If a pheochromocytoma patient has normal catecholamine levels, is the source the normal adrenal or the tumor? This basic question in "intermittent secretors" is yet to be resolved. A very interesting observation in this study was that both pheochromocytoma patients and control subjects had similar blood pressure decreases despite very dissimilar NE responses. This suggests that the sympathetic nervous system is more important in blood pressure regulation in pheochromocytoma than is the tumor secretion.

Another approach to identifying patients with pheochromocytoma by elevated catecholamine plasma levels was reported by Zweifler and Julius (74). In their series, elevated platelet catecholamine concentrations were

HYPERTENSION   285

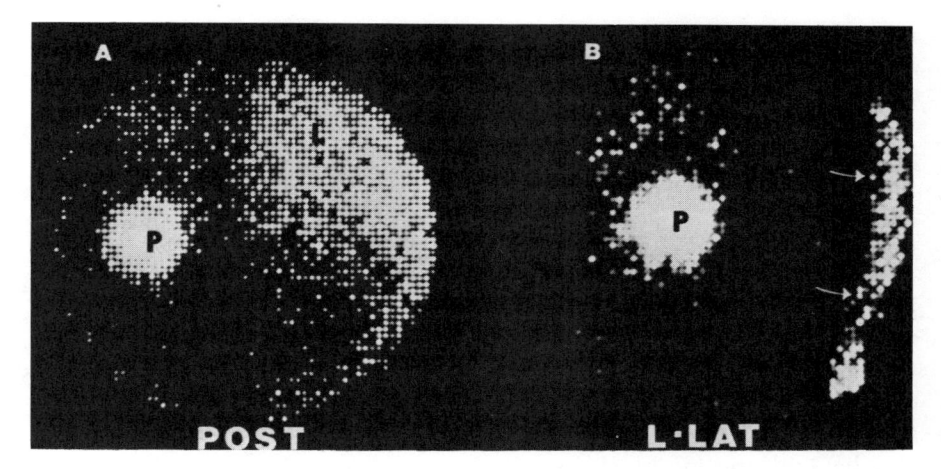

Figure 8. Scintigrams made one day after injection of [^{131}I] MIBG in one patient who had a 24 g tumor in the left adrenal gland. The pheochromocytoma (P) is readily identified in (*a*) (Post, posterior view) and (*b*) (L-lat, left lateral view). The liver (L) is seen in (*a*). Arrows in (*b*) point to a radioactive marker on the patient's back. (Sisson JC et al: *N Engl J Med* 305:12–17, 1981. Used with permission.)

found in 10 patients with the tumor while normal platelet concentrations of catecholamines were found in six subjects with elevated plasma levels and no tumor and in 22 normal control subjects. Since the platelet concentrations fell more slowly than plasma levels after tumor removal, it suggests that platelets store circulating catecholamines and their level is an integration of circulating levels over time.

Major advances in nuclear medicine and radiology are having a major impact in diagnosing and localizing pheochromocytoma tissue. A new radiopharmaceutical, ^{131}I-metaiodobenzylguanidine (MIBG) has been studied in Ann Arbor. This material is taken up by adrenergic tissue and incorporated into storage vesicles. In a series of patients with multiple endocrine neoplasia, types II and III, the agent was studied to see if early pheochromocytomas could be detected with this scanning material (75). Images were obtained 24–48 hours after scanning. In two subjects without symptoms and with normal laboratory findings, no adrenal image was seen. In four other subjects who had some abnormal urinary or plasma catecholamines, the imaging technique showed adrenal uptake. One patient had surgery, and tumor tissue was found in the predicted locations. In another series of eight patients with pheochromocytoma, it was shown that nuclear imaging was possible in intra- and extraadrenal locations, in malignant and benign tumors, and in tumors as small as 0.2 g (76) (Fig 8). Four of these patients had uptake in tissue that was not localized by computerized tomography (CT). The sensitivity and specificity of this procedure is still not determined, but the noninvasive and functional nature of the study makes it very attractive for localization and follow-up. The limited availability of this isotope, however, currently restricts its use. Angiography is still extensively used to localize pheochromocytomas. However, hypertensive crises may ensue during these procedures. High resolution CT offers a noninvasive, less hazardous alternative for identifying these tumors. However, it is not clear how often small lesions within or outside the adrenal can be missed with this procedure. False-positive findings in the adrenal are also seen more frequently with this procedure.

Once diagnosis and localization have been established, surgical removal is the accepted treatment. However, proper preoperative management is highly debatable (57), and experienced physicians have very good results with several approaches, including (1) long-term phenoxybenzamine up to the time of surgery, (2) phenoxybenzamine up to 72–48 hours prior to surgery, (3) no alpha-adrenergic blockade at all, and (4) combined alpha- and beta-adrenergic blockage. The most important aspect of successful surgery is careful preparation and teamwork of endocrinologist, anesthesiologist, surgeon, and nursing staff.

CURRENT CONCEPTS IN GERIATRIC HYPERTENSION

The elderly represent the fastest growing population in our country. There are now approximately 25 million Americans aged 65 years or older, and it is estimated that by 1990 there will be 29 million. In the United States, approximately 40% of whites and more than 50% of blacks aged 65–74 years have hypertension (defined as systolic above 160 mmHg and diastolic above 95 mmHg) or isolated systolic hypertension (systolic blood pressure below 160 mmHg and diastolic below 95 mmHg), and 30% have borderline hypertension (systolic blood pressure 140–159 mmHg and diastolic pressure 90–94 mmHg (77). Diastolic blood pressure rises to a maximum around 50–59 years of age, while systolic pressure continues to rise with age.

Both the Veterans Administration Study (78) and the Framingham Study (79) clearly demonstrated that hypertension in the elderly is a major risk factor for stroke, congestive heart failure, and coronary artery disease. Furthermore, other studies have shown that elevated systolic blood pressure is a major determinant of increased cardiovascular mortality and morbidity, particularly strokes, in the elderly population (80). Age-related rises in systolic pressure reflect a loss of elasticity within the aorta and other large vessels. Thus, when the cardiac output is ejected into a less distensible aorta, the systolic pressure rises at a steeper slope. It is still controversial whether the increased cardiovascular morbidity and mortality associated with systolic hypertension reflects the atherosclerotic process that caused the development of systolic hypertension or the elevated systolic blood pressure itself. Kannel et al. (80) addressed this issue in a study using the disappearance of the dicrotic notch of vasculogram-recorded pulse waves as a measure of aortic rigidity. Although there was a relationship between systolic blood pressure and loss of the dicrotic notch, stroke incidence correlated better with systolic blood pressure than with diastolic blood pressure or disappearance of the dicrotic notch. These observations have been interpreted as suggesting that it is the systolic blood pressure per se and not the atherosclerotic process that accounts for the increased cardiovascular morbidity and mortality.

Etiology of Hypertension in the Elderly

Relatively little attention has been devoted to the study of the etiology of hypertension in the elderly. There is some evidence that the tendency for blood pressure to increase with age may be related to a genetically determined decreased ability of the aging kidney to excrete sodium (81). This finding may be particularly important in the United States, where there is high sodium consumption. Increased rigidity of the aortic and carotid walls results in impairment of baroreceptor function with aging (82), leading to decreased ability to buffer swings in arterial pressure. This reduction in baroreceptor sensitivity may play a role in the pathogenesis of elevated blood pressure as well as in the high incidence of orthostatic hypotension in the elderly. Reduction in baroreceptor sensitivity may, in part, explain the greater variability in systolic pressure in elderly compared to younger hypertensive individuals (83).

There is a physiological age-related increase in plasma NE levels. This age-related increase has been reported to be greater at night (84) and with upright posture (85) than in the supine position in the morning hours. With aging, there is a loss in the number of functional beta-adrenergic receptor sites (86) (Fig. 9). This may reflect a process of desensitization associated with exposure to high levels of catecholamines (87). However, no age-related desensitization of alpha-adrenergic receptors has been demonstrated. Thus, with increasing levels of plasma NE associated with aging, diminished beta-adrenergic mediated effects such as vasodilatation could leave unopposed alpha-adrenergic vasoconstrictor responses. The sympathetic nervous system plays a role in regulating renin secretion, and beta-adrenergic receptors appear to be involved in mediating renal renin release in association with renal nerve stimulation and circulating catecholamines. Despite having increased plasma levels of NE, both basal plasma renin activity (PRA) and renin responses to various stimuli decrease with age, particularly in elderly hypertensive patients (88). One factor that may play a role in the decreased PRA responses with aging is decreased beta-adrenergic activity mediating renal renin release, although this remains to be studied. The expected age-related fall in plasma aldosterone has been reported not to occur when aldosterone levels were measured in patients assuming an upright posture (88). Thus,

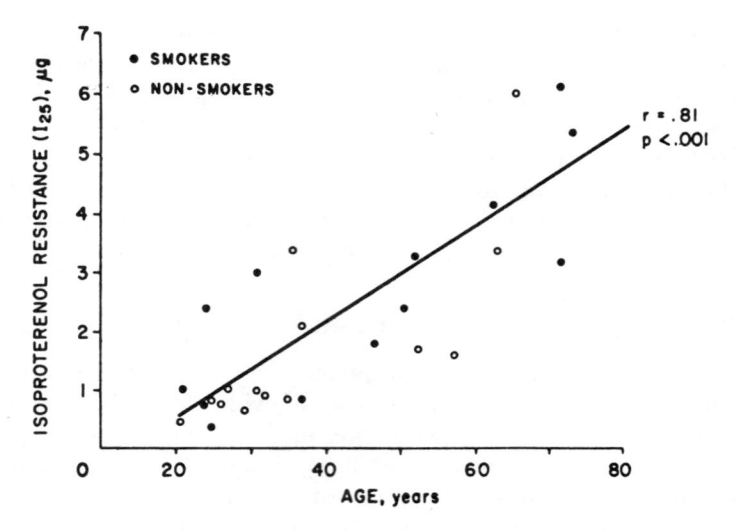

Figure 9. Relationship between isoproterenol resistance and age. (Vestal RE et al: *Clin Pharmacol Ther* 26:181–186, 1979. Used with permission.)

plasma aldosterone may be inappropriately elevated, considering the marked suppression of PRA levels, and may contribute to increased sodium retention and hypertension in the elderly. Adipose tissue constitutes a greater proportion of body mass in elderly than in younger individuals (89). Thus, it is likely that the increased incidence of hypertension with increasing age may be related, in part, to an increased incidence of obesity with advancing age. The relationship between obesity and hypertension has been discussed in a previous section of this chapter.

Evaluation and Treatment

Before beginning antihypertensive therapy in the elderly, it is imperative to determine if there is sustained elevation of diastolic, systolic, or both diastolic and systolic pressures. As previously noted, there is marked variability in systolic blood pressure readings in the elderly (83). Thus, the approach advocated by Gifford seems reasonable. He advocates taking three measurements on each of at least three office visits over a period of weeks before deciding to begin therapy. It has been suggested that "pseudohypertension" in the elderly may occur due to rigid sclerotic vessels that cannot be adequately occluded with a sphygmomanometer cuff. However, available limited studies indicate that indirect blood pressure measurement is misleading in only a small number of elderly patients.

An extensive workup for secondary causes of hypertension is seldom indicated in the elderly. However, it is indicated if diastolic hypertension appears after age 55 or if the hypertension is resistant to medical management. If the blood pressure is found to be very high in an elderly person or if there is an abrupt exacerbation of stable hypertension, then a secondary factor, particularly renovascular disease, should be sought.

Both the European Working Party on High Blood Pressure in the Elderly (EWPHE) (89) and the Hypertension Detection and Follow-Up Program (HDFP) (90) have demonstrated that elderly patients benefit from the treatment of diastolic-systolic hypertension and that they tolerate antihypertensive drug therapy if it is carefully administered. However, data from prospective, well-controlled studies designed to determine if control of isolated systolic hypertension improves prognosis is lacking. A cooperative trial on the treatment of predominantly systolic hypertension has begun in the United States, but final results will probably not be available before 1990. The goal in treatment of diastolic blood pressure in the elderly is generally accepted as similar to that for younger hypertensive patients, that is, reduction of diastolic pressures to below 90 mmHg (77,88,89). Although there is controversy as to what the goal should be in the treatment of systolic hypertension, it has been suggested that a gradual reduction in systolic blood pressure to the 140–160 mmHg range should be attempted (77).

In many elderly patients, moderate restriction of salt and caloric intake is adequate to control either diastolic-systolic or isolated systolic hypertension (77). This is particularly true if the patient is obese or is a heavy salt user. If drug therapy is necessary, most recommend initial therapy with a diuretic (77,88,89). The EWPHE employs hydrochlorothiazide with triamterene as step 1 and methyldopa as step 2 therapy. The HDFP study employed chlorthalidone as step 1 and either reserpine or methyldopa as step 2 therapy. Thus, a small dose of a diuretic of intermediate duration of action such as 12.5 or 25 mg of hydrochlorothiazide each morning would appear to be a reasonable initiating therapy in treating elderly patients with hypertension. Careful attention must be directed to diuretic-induced potassium deficits in elderly hypertensive patients. The elderly often consume diets very low in potassium and may be more susceptible to cardiac complications secondary to hypokalemia. Some recommend a beta-blocker as the initial treatment (91), but there is increasing evidence that the elderly do not respond as well to beta-blockers given alone (86). Furthermore, beta-blockers are contraindicated in obstructive lung disease, peripheral vascular disease, and heart failure, all of which are relatively common in the elderly. In the absence of adequate blood pressure reduction with a thiazide diuretic, employment of a central acting sympathetic inhibitor such as clonidine or methyldopa appears to be the best choices as step 2 drugs (77,89,90). Although the EWPHE study is not complete, an interim report indicated that only in a minority of patients (15%) was it necessary to add the second line of therapy (methyldopa) to the thiazide/triamterene regimen. When given at a low dosage and then gradually increased, clonidine and aldomet seldom cause central nervous system depression and symptomatic orthostatic hypotension. The fact that clonidine does not impair renal sodium excretion (18) may constitute a distinct advantage over aldomet (92) in treating elderly hypertensives. Though the evidence for their effectiveness and safety is limited, direct acting vasodilators such as hydralazine and calcium ion influx inhibitors (nifedepine, verapamil and diltiazem) may be used as second or third step drugs, since therapy with such drugs would not be expected to cause significant reflex tachycardia in the elderly with sluggish baroreceptor reflexes. Verapamil has been successfully used as step 1 treatment in older patients with hypertension (93). Indeed, because of their potent vasodilatory effects and the fact that they do not cause reflex tachycardia and fluid retention, both verapamil and diltiazem may prove to be the ideal drugs for treating hypertension in the elderly (94,95).

DRUG TREATMENT OF HYPERTENSION

The Problem of "Mild" Hypertension

Physicians faced with a hypertensive patient must always consider not only which drugs to use, but, even more fundamentally, whether a given patient merits life-long drug therapy. The hazards of such a course of action, which is far from benign, were reviewed in volume 4 of this series. Nevertheless, given the results of the earlier VA studies, which clearly indicated the benefits of treating hypertension when the diastolic pressure was greater than 109 mmHg, and the Framingham studies, which have indicated the continuous nature of the relationship between blood pressure level and risk of developing cardiovascular disease, the temptation to treat milder hypertensives has grown as the side effects of the drugs available have become less severe. The dilemma is one of enormous magnitude. If one were to accept the recommendation of the Joint National Committee on Detection, Evaluation, and Treatment of High Blood Pressure that the aim should be to reduce every patient's diastolic blood pressure to less than 90 mm Hg, then between 20 and 40 million extra patients would require treatment. The price of this would be as high as $20 billion. In "Pentagonal" spending units, this is equivalent to the cost of 100 B-1 bombers or 10 nuclear-powered aircraft carriers. Of course, if it could be shown that such treatment would decrease the risk of cardiovascular disease, we would have no choice but to shoulder this burden. The question is, can it?

Three studies that address this problem have been recently reported, one from the United States (96), one from Australia (97), and one from Norway (98). (A fourth study, by the Medical Research Council in England, has yet to be completed). At first sight, these three reports appear to indicate that mild hypertension should indeed be treated, but within the past year, two critical reviews of the data (99,100) have suggested an opposite conclusion. Briefly reviewed, their arguments are as follows:

The Hypertension Detection and Follow-Up Program study in this country (96) was seriously flawed in that there was no true control group. Instead, one group of patients was given free detailed medical care, including, but not confined to, antihypertensive treatment, while the other patients merely continued with the best treatment they could either find or afford. Not surprisingly, mortality from causes other than cardiovascular disease was reduced in the "treatment" group. The frequency with which the "control" group was seen was sufficiently low that deterioration in hypertension could have gone undetected for many months, thereby making the "treatment" group *seem* even better. In the subset of the "control" group where care was given as intensively as in the "treatment" group, there was no difference between the two.

The Norwegian study from Oslo (97) used a more conventional trial design, but despite an average blood pressure reduction of 17/10 mmHg, no convincing benefit emerged, perhaps because at least a half of the placebo group showed a spontaneous fall in blood pressure. Only in those patients whose diastolic pressure (untreated) remained above 100 mmHg was the incidence of cardiovascular disease reduced (7.6% versus 16.4%).

At the present time, it still is not possible to make a blanket recommendation based on blood pressure alone. It is appropriate in all patients to seek associated risk factors, such as cigarette smoking, hypercholesterolemia, glucose intolerance, and evidence of end organ damage. Patients with multiple risk factors especially merit attention and treatment. In our present state of knowledge, Kaplan's (99) recommendations seem a reasonable compromise. They are as follows:

1. Patients with diastolic pressures above 110 mmHg or, if other risk factors are present, above 100 mmHg, should receive drug treatment.
2. Patients with diastolic pressures below 110 mmHg should be followed for approximately 6 months while common sense measures such as weight reduction, exercise, and reduced salt intake are instituted.
3. If the diastolic blood pressure falls below 100 mmHg, these patients should be followed up and checked at least twice a year.
4. If the diastolic blood pressure stays above 100 mmHg or if in spite of the above measures it goes above 100 mmHg, drug treatment should be instituted.

The Problem of Hypokalemia

American physicians, more often than European physicians, begin treatment especially in milder hypertension with a diuretic, since this has been regarded as a very safe form of therapy. Increasingly, however, this view is being challenged. Holland et al. (101) showed that in a group of 21 patients with mild essential hypertension, the administration of hydrochlorothiazide (50 mg bid) was associated with a fall in plasma potassium (<3.5 mEq/liter). Seven patients developed multifocal preventricular contractions (PVCs), while in four, multiple ectopics, ventricular couplets, and/or ventricular tachycardia was seen. Despite data of this type, in a provocative editorial, Harrington et al. (102) have again challenged the routine administration of potassium supplements to any patients with the exception of those already on digitalis. It seems that those on each side of this issue base their views on the problems they most often encounter. Naturally, nephrologists are very concerned about hyperkalemia. Conversely, cardiologists concern themselves with situations they regard as arrhythmogenic. Until the issue is resolved to everyone's satisfaction, physicians should measure the potassium regularly if using diuretics, and consider the possibility that in many patients beta-blocking drugs may make a better first-line drug.

New in '82

Two drugs mentioned in earlier editions of this volume have finally cleared all the FDA hurdles and have appeared in the therapeutic arena.

Pindolol

This is a relatively water soluble nonselective beta-blocker whose outstanding feature is a marked degree of intrinsic sympathomimetic activity (ISA). The paradox of a blocking drug having agonist activity is not too surprising when one recalls that structurally all beta-blocking drugs are recognizable derivatives of isoproterenol. Drugs are to receptors as keys are to keyholes. An agonist fits the keyhole and turns the lock. An antagonist fits the keyhole (and thereby denies access to the agonist), but cannot turn the lock. An antagonist with intrinsic activity fits the lock and so excludes the agonist, but also retains at least some ability to turn the lock. It has been claimed that because of its high level of ISA, pindolol does not reduce resting cardiac output or muscle blood flow (103). Numerous double-blind trials conducted in this country have shown that in doses up to 60 mg/day, it is as effective an antihypertensive agent as propranolol, methyldopa, and diuretics (104). Early studies gave rise to speculation that ISA might prevent some of the complications that limit the usefulness of beta-blockers, such as exacerbation of peripheral vascular disease and Raynaud's phenomenon, and provocation of bronchial asthma. In the clinical setting, it does not seem that these hopes will be borne out (105,106). However, ISA may be useful in those patients where the usefulness of beta-blockade is limited by the development of marked bradycardia, especially during sleep (107).

Guanabenz

Guanabenz, a centrally acting alpha agonist, resembles clonidine and alpha methyl norepinephrine (the active metabolite of alpha methyldopa). In its quality of control and lack of orthostasis, it closely resembles clonidine, although its longer half-life permits once-daily therapy (108), and may be the basis for the reported lesser incidence of withdrawal symptoms such as are sometimes seen with abrupt clonidine withdrawal (109–111). Given the fact that it acts via the same central mechanisms, it is not surprising that side effects, notably sedation and dry mouth, are similar to those seen with clonidine. One other possible advantage over clonidine is that it has greater selectivity for the α_2 receptor (112). Clonidine in higher doses acts also on the α_1 receptors, so that intravenous injections produce an initial pressor response, and high oral doses lead to a paradoxical increase in blood pressure. Guanabenz is less active on the vascular (α_1) receptors and may prove to be a more flexible agent than clonidine in that respect.

REFERENCES

1. DeQuattro V, Campese VM: Functional components of the sympathetic nervous system. Regulation of organ systems, in DeGroot: *Endocrinology*. New York, Grune & Stratton, 1977, pp 1261–1278.
2. Bevan RD: Effect of sympathetic denervation on smooth muscle cell proliferation in the grown rabbit ear artery. *Circ Res* 37:14, 1975.
3. Abel PW, Hermsmeyer K: Sympathetic cross-innervation of SHR and genetic controls suggest a trophic influence on vascular muscle membranes *Cir Res* 49:1311, 1981.
4. Dietz R, Schmig A, Haebara H, et al: STudies on the pathogenesis of spontaneous hypertension of rats. *Circ Res* 43(suppl I):98–106, 1978.
5. Phillip T, Distler A, Cordes U: Sympathetic nervous system and blood pressure control in essential hypertension. *Lancet* 1:959–963, 1980.
6. Wallin BG, Delius W, Hagbarth KE: Comparison of sympathetic activity in normo and hypertensive subjects. *Cir Res* 33:9–21, 1973.
7. Gribbin B, Pickering TC, Sleight P, et al: Effect of age and high blood pressure on baroreflex sensitivity in man. *Cir Res* 29:424, 1971.
8. Krieger EM: Time course of baroreceptor resetting in acute hypertension. *Am J Physiol* 218:486, 1976.
9. Goldstein DJ: Plasma norepinephrine in essential hypertension. A study of the studies. *Hypertension* 3:48–52, 1981.
10. Engelman K, Portnoy B, Sjoerdsma A: Plasma catecholamine concentrations in patients with hypertension. *Cir Res* 27(suppl):141–146, 1970.
11. DeQuattro V, Chan S: Raised plasma catecholamines in some patients with primary hypertension. *Lancet* 1:806–809, 1972.
12. Lake CR, Ziegler MG, Coleman MD, et al: Age-adjusted plasma norepinephrine levels are similar in normotensive and hypertensive subjects. *N Engl J Med* 296:208–209, 1977.
13. Goldstein DJ: Plasma norepinephrine during stress in essential hypertension. A study of the studies. *Hypertension* 3:551–556, 1981.

14. Franco-Morselli R, Elghozi JL, Joly E, et al: Increased plasma adrenaline concentrations in benign essential hypertension. *Br Med J* 2:1251–1254, 1977.
15. Campese VM, Mark R, Myers BS, et al: Neurogenic factors in low renin essential hypertension. *Am J Med* 69:83–91, 1980.
16. Louis WJ, Doyle AE, Anavekar S: Plasma norepinephrine levels in essential hypertension. *N Engl J Med* 288:599–601, 1973.
17. Pedersen EB, Christensen NJ: Catecholamines in plasma and urine in patients with essential hypertension determined by double-isotope derivative techniques. *Acta Med Scand* 198:373–377, 1975.
18. Campese VM, Romoff T, Telfer N, et al: Role of sympathetic nerve inhibition and body sodium volume state in the antihypertensive action of clonidine in essential hypertension. *Kidney Int* 18:351–357, 1980.
19. Tobian L: Interrelationship of electrolytes, juxtaglomerular cells and hypertension. *Physiol Rev* 40:280–312, 1960.
20. Dahl LK: Salt intake and salt need. *N Engl J Med* 258:1152–1156, 1958.
21. Freis ED: Salt, volume, and the prevention of hypertension. *Circulation* 53:589–595, 1976.
22. Haddy FJ: Mechanism, prevention and therapy of sodium-dependent hypertension. *Am J Med* 69:746–758, 1980.
23. Meneely GR, Battarbee HD: The high sodium-low potassium environment and hypertension. *Am J Cardiol* 38:768–786, 1976.
24. Page LB, Danion A, Moellering RC Jr: Antecedents of cardiovascular disease in six Soloman Islands societies. *Circulation* 49:1132–1146, 1974.
25. Kawasaki T, Delea CS, Bartter FC, et al: The effect of high-sodium and low-sodium intakes on blood pressure and other related variables in human subjects with idiopathic hypertension. *Am J Med* 64:193–198, 1978.
26. Dahl LK, Knudsen KD, Heine MA, et al: Effects of chronic excess salt ingestion. *Circ Res* 22:11–18, 1968.
27. Fujita T, Henry WL, Bartter FC, et al: Factors influencing blood pressure in salt-sensitive patients with hypertension. *Am J Med* 69:334–344, 1980.
28. Campese VM, Romoff MS, Levitan D, et al: Abnormal relationship between sodium intake and plasma norepinephrine in salt-sensitive patients with essential hypertension. *Kidney Int* 21:371–378, 1982.
29. Romoff MS, Keusch G, Campese VM, et al: Effect of sodium intake on plasma catecholamines in normal subjects. *J Clin Endocrinol Metab* 48:26–31, 1979.
30. Luft FC, Rankin LI, Henry DP, et al: Plasma and urinary norepinephrine values at extreme of sodium intake in normal man. *Hypertension* 1:261–266, 1979.
31. Alexander RW, Gill JR, Yamabe H, et al: Effects of dietary sodium and of acute saline infusion on the interrelationship between dopamine excretion and adrenergic activity in man. *J Clin Invest* 54:194–200, 1974.
32. Faucheux B, Buu NT, Kuchel O: Effects of saline and albumin on plasma and urinary catecholamines in dogs. *Am J Physiol* 232:F123–F129, 1977.
33. Dietz R, Schomig A, Rascher W, et al: Enhanced sympathetic activity caused by salt loading in spontaneously hypertensive rats. *Clin Sci* 59:171–173, 1980.
34. DeChamplain J, Krakoff L, Axelrod J: Interrelationship of sodium intake, hypertension, and norepinephrine storage in the rat. *Circ Res* 24/25(suppl I):I75–I92, 1969.
35. Brosnihan KB, Szilagyi JE, Ferrario CM: Effect of chronic sodium depletion on cerebrospinal fluid and plasma catecholamines. *Hypertension* 3:233, 1981.
36. Winternitz SR, Wyss JM, Meadows JR, et al: Influence of high sodium intake on blood pressure and norepinephrine content of hypothalamic nuclei in the spontaneously hypertensive rat. *Clin Res* 29:866A, 1981.

37. Collis MG, DeMey C, Vanhoutte PM: Renal vascular reactivity in the young spontaneously hypertensive rat. *Hypertension* 2:45, 1980.
38. Takeshita A, Mark AL: Neurogenic contribution to hindquarters vasoconstriction during high sodium intake in Dahl strain of genetically hypertensive rat. *Circ Res* 43(suppl I):86–91, 1978.
39. Nakazato Y, Okga A, Onoda Y: The effect of ouabain on noradrenaline output from peripheral adrenergic neurones of isolated guinea pig vas deferens. *J Physiol* 278:45–54, 1978.
40. Heistad DD, Abboud FM, Ballard DR: Relationship between plasma sodium concentration and vascular reactivity in man. *J Clin Invest* 50:2022–2032, 1971.
41. Kannel W, Brand N, Skinner J, et al: Relation of adiposity to blood pressure and development of hypertension: The Framingham Study. *Ann Intern Med* 67:48–59, 1967.
42. Chiang BN, Perlman LV, Epstein FH: Overweight and hypertension: A review. *Circulation* 39:403–421, 1969.
43. Paffenbarger RS Jr, Thorne MC, Wing AL: Chronic disease in farmer college students. VIII. Characteristics in youth predisposing to hypertension in later years. *Am J Epidemiol* 88:25–32, 1968.
44. Johnson AL, Cornoni JC, Cassel JC, et al: Influence of race, sex, and weight on blood pressure behavior in young adults. *Am J Cardiol* 35:523–530, 1975.
45. Stamler J, Rhomberg P, Schoenberger JA, et al: Multivariant analysis of the relationship of seven variables to blood pressure: Findings of the Chicago Heart Association Detection Project in Industry. *J Chron Dis* 28:527–548, 1975.
46. Severs PS, Gordon D, Peart WS, et al: Blood pressure and its correlates in urban and tribal Africa. *Lancet* 2:60–64, 1980.
47. Messerli FH, Christie B, DeCarvalho J, et al: Obesity and essential hypertension: Hemodynamics, intravascular volume, sodium excretion, and plasma renin activity. *Arch Intern Med* 141:81, 1981.
48. Dustan HP, Tarazi RC, Mujais S: A comparison of hemodynamic and volume characteristics of obese and nonobese hypertensive patients. *Int J Obes* 5(suppl 1):19–25, 1981.
49. Reisin E, Abel R, Modan M: Effect of weight loss without salt restriction in the reduction of blood pressure in overweight hypertensive patients. *N Engl J Med* 298:1, 1978.
50. Tuck ML, Sowers J, Dornfeld L, et al: The effect of weight reduction on blood pressure, plasma renin activity, and plasma aldosterone levels in obese patients. *N Engl J Med* 304:930–933, 1981.
51. DeLuise M, Blackburn GL, Flier JS: Reduced activity of the red-cell sodium-potassium pump in human obesity. *N Engl J Med* 303:1017–1032, 1980.
52. Sowers JR, Whitfield LA, Beck FWJ, et al: Role of enhanced sympathetic nervous system activity and reduced Na^+, K^+ dependent adenosine triphosphatase activity in maintenance of elevated blood pressure in obesity: Effects of weight loss. *Clin Sci* 63:121–124, 1982.
53. Lin MH, Romsos DR, Ukera T, et al: Functional correlates of Na^+, K^+-ATPase in lean and obese (ob/ob) mice. *Metabolism* 30:431–438, 1981.
54. Sowers JR, Whitfield LA, Catania RA, et al: Role of the sympathetic nervous system in blood pressure maintenance in obesity. *J Clin Endocrinol Metab* 54:1181, 1982.
55. Sowers JR, Nyby M, Stern N, Beck F, et al: Blood pressure and hormone changes associated with weight reduction in the obese. *Hypertension* 4:596, 1982.
56. Bello-Reuss E, Higashi Y, Kaneda Y: Dopamine decreased fluid reabsorption in straight portions of rabbit proximal tubules. *Am J Physiol* 242:634–640, 1982.
57. Manger WM, Gifford RW Jr: *Pheochromocytoma*. New York, Springer-Verlag, 1977.

58. Thomas JE, Rooke ED, and Kvale WF: The neurologist's experience with pheochromocytoma. A review of 100 cases. *JAMA* 197:754–758, 1966.
59. Barnett AJ, Blacket RB, DePoorter AE, et al: The action of noradrenaline in man and its relation to pheochromocytoma and hypertension. *Clin Sci* 9:151–179, 1950.
60. Gifford RW Jr, Kvale WF, Maher FT, et al: Clinical features diagnosis and treatment of pheochromocytoma: A review of 76 cases. *Mayo Clinic Proc* 39:281–302, 1964.
61. Van Vliet PD, Burchell HB, and Titus JL: Focal myocarditis associated with pheochromocytoma. *N Engl J Med* 274:1102–1108, 1966.
62. Eugleman F, Zelis R, Waldmann T, et al: Mechanism of orthostatic hypotension in pheochromocytoma. *Circulation* 38(suppl 6):VI–72, 1968.
63. Greer WER, Robertson CW, and Smithwick RH: Pheochromocytoma: Diagnosis, operative experience, and clinical results. *Am J Surg* 107:192–201, 1964.
64. Page LB, Copeland RB: Pheochromocytoma, in Dowling HF (ed): *Chicago Disease-a-Month*. Chicago, Year Book Medical Publishers, 1968.
65. Wurtman RJ, Axelrod J: Control of enzymatic synthesis of adrenaline in the adrenal medulla by adrenal cortical steroids. *J Biol Chem* 241:2301–2305, 1966.
66. Crout JR, Sjoerdsma A: Turnover and metabolism of catecholamines in patients with pheochromocytoma. *J Clin Invest* 43:94–102, 1964.
67. Winkler H, Smith AD: Catecholamines in pheochromocytoma: Normal storage but abnormal release? *Lancet* 1:793–795, 1968.
68. Sipple JH: The association of pheochromocytoma with carcinoma of the thyroid gland. *Am J Med* 31:163–166, 1961.
69. Sizemore GW, Go VLW: Stimulation tests for diagnosis of medullary thyroid carcinoma. *Mayo Clinic Proc* 50:53–56, 1975.
70. Hamilton BP, Lansberg L, Levine RJ: Measurement of urinary epinephrine in screening for pheochromocytoma in multiple endocrine neoplasia type II. *Am J Med* 65:1027–1032, 1978.
71. Brown MJ, Allison DJ, Jenner DA, et al: Increased sensitivity and accuracy of pheochromocytoma diagnosis achieved by use of plasma adrenaline estimations and a pentolinium suppression test. *Lancet* 1:174–177, 1981.
72. Bravo EL, Tarazi RC, Gifford RW, et al: Circulating and urinary catecholamines in pheochromocytoma. *N Engl J Med* 301:682–686, 1979.
73. Bravo EL, Tarazi RC, Fouad FM, et al: Clonidine-suppression test. A useful aid in the diagnosis of pheochromocytoma. *N Engl J Med* 305:623–626, 1981.
74. Zweifler AJ, Julius S: Increased platelet catecholamine content in pheochromocytoma. *N Engl J Med* 306:890–894, 1982.
75. Valk, TW, Frager MS, Gross MD, et al: Spectrum of pheochromocytoma in multiple endocrine neoplasia. *Ann Int Med* 94:762–767, 1981.
76. Sisson JC, Frager MS, Valk TW, et al: Scintigraphic localization of pheochromocytoma. *N Engl J Med* 305:12–17, 1981.
77. Gifford RW: Isolated systolic hypertension in the elderly: *JAMA* 247:781–785, 1982.
78. Veterans administration cooperative study group on antihypertensive agents. Effects of treatment on morbidity in hypertension III. Influence of age, diastolic pressure, and prior cardiovascular disease. Further analysis of side effects. *Circulation* 45:991–1004, 1972.
79. Kannel WB, Gordon T: Evaluation of the cardiovascular risk in the elderly: The Framingham study. *Bull NY Acad Med* 54:573–579, 1978.
80. Kannel WB, Wolf PA, McGee OL, et al: Systolic blood pressure, arterial rigidity, and risk of stroke: The Framingham study. *JAMA* 245:1225–1229, 1981.

81. Luft FC, Grim CE, Fineberg N, et al: Effects of volume expansion and contraction in normotensive whites, blacks, and subjects of different ages. *Circulation* 59:643–650, 1979.
82. Gribbon B, Pickering TG, Sleight P, et al: Effect of age and high blood pressure on baroreflex sensitivity in man. *Circ Res* 29:424–429, 1971.
83. Drayer JIM, Weber MA, DeYoung JL, et al: Circadian blood pressure patterns in ambulatory hypertensive patients: Effects of age. *Am J Med* 73:493–499, 1982.
84. Prinz PN, Halter J, Benedetti C, et al: Circadian variation of plasma catecholamines in young and old men: Relation to rapid eye movement and slow wave sleep. *J Clin Endocrinol Metab* 49:300–304, 1979.
85. Young JB, Rowe JW, Pallotta JA, et al: Enhanced plasma norepinephrine response to upright posture and oral glucose administration in elderly human subjects. *Metabolism* 29:532–539, 1980.
86. Vestal RE, Wood AJ, Shand DG: Reduced B-adrenoreceptor sensitivity in the elderly. *Clin Pharmacol Ther* 26:181–186, 1979.
87. Roth GS: Hormone receptor changes during adulthood and senescence: Significance for aging research. *Fed Proc* 38:1910, 1979.
88. Weidmann P, Beretta-Piccoli C, Ziegler WH, et al: Age versus urinary sodium for judging renin, aldosterone, and catecholamine levels: Studies in normal subjects and in patients with essential hypertension. *Kidney Int* 14:619–628, 1978.
89. Amery A, Berthaux P, Birkenhager W, et al: Antihypertensive therapy in patients above 60 years: Fourth interim report of the European Working Party on High Blood Pressure in the Elderly. *Clin Sci Mol Med* 55(suppl):263–270, 1978.
90. Five-year findings of the Hypertension Detection and Follow-Up Program: 1. Reduction in mortality of persons with high blood pressure including mild hypertension, Hypertension Detection and Follow-Up Program Cooperative Group. *JAMA* 242:2562–2571, 1979.
91. O'Malley K, O'Brian E: Management of hypertension in the elderly. *N Engl J Med* 302:1397–1401, 1980.
92. Grabie M, Nussbaum P, Goldfarb S, et al: Effects of methyldopa on renal hemodynamics and tubular function. *Clin Pharmacol Ther* 27:522–527, 1980.
93. Buhler FR, Hulthen L, Bolli P, et al: Verapamil's potent vasodilatory and antihypertensive effect, particularly in the older and low renin hypertensives opens up a new treatment concept. *Clin Sci* (Dec.).
94. Agabiti-Rosei E, Alicandri C, Beschi M, et al: Blood pressure, catecholamines, renin, and aldosterone during short- and long-term treatment of essential hypertension with verapamil. *Am J Cardiol* 49:912, 1982.
95. Bonrassa MG, Cato P, Theronx P, et al: Hemodynamics and coronary flow following diltiazem administration in unesthetized dogs and in humans. *Chest* 78:224–230, 1980.
96. Hypertension Detection and Follow-Up Program Cooperative Group. Five-year findings of the Hypertension Detection and Follow-Up Program. I. Reduction in mortality of persons with high blood pressure, including mild hypertension. *JAMA* 242:2562–2571, 1979.
92. Report by the Management Committee. The Australian Therapeutic Trial in Mild Hypertension. *Lancet* 1:1261–1269, 1980.
98. Helgeland A: Treatment of mild hypertension: A 5-year controlled trial. The Oslo Study. *Am J Med* 69:725–732, 1980.
99. Kaplan NM: Whom to treat: The dilemma of mild hypertension. *Am Heart* 101:867–870, 1982.
100. Fries ED: Should mild hypertension be treated? *N Engl J Med* 307:306–309, 1982.

101. Holland OB, Nixon JV, Kuhnert L: Diuretic-induced ventricular ectopic activity. *Am J Med* 70:762–768, 1981.
102. Harrington JT, Isner JM, Kassirer JP: Our national obsession with potassium. *Am J Med* 73:155–159, 1982.
103. Acllig WH: Clinical pharmacology of pindolol. *Am Heart J* 104:346–356, 1982.
104. Gonasun LM: Antihypertensive effects of pindolol. *Am Heart J* 104:374–387, 1982.
105. Louis WJ, McNeil JJ: Beta adrenoceptor blocking drugs: The relevance of intrinsic sympathomimetic activity. *Br J Clin Pharmacol* 13:317S–320S, 1982.
106. Rufin RE, McIntyre ELM, Latimer KM, et al: Assessment of beta adrenoceptor antagonists in asthmatic patients. *Br J Clin Pharmacol* 13:325S–335S, 1982.
107. Sleight P: Clinical use of beta blockers in hypertension. *Aviat Space Environ Med* 52:S2–S8, 1981.
108. Walker BR, Hare LE, Deitch MW: Comparative antihypertensive effects of guanabenz and clonidine. *J Int Med Res* 10:6–14, 1982.
109. Deitch MW, Walker BR, Schneider BE, et al: Multicenter comparison of guanabenz and clonidine in hypertension. *Clin Pharmacol Ther* 31:215–216, 1982.
110. Franklin SS, Conolly ME, Tuck M: Hypertension, Gonick H (ed): *Current Nephrology*, vol. 3. Boston, Houghton Mifflin, 1979, pp 225–294.
111. Winer N, Carter CM: Effects of abrupt discontinuation of guanabenz and clonidine in hypertension patients. *Clin Pharmacol Ther* 31:282–283, 1982.
112. Unnerstall JR, Kopajtic TA, Deitch MW, et al: Specificity and potency of guanabenz at the α_2 adrenergic receptor. *Fed Proc, Fed Am Soc Exp Biol* 41:1667, 1982.

ACKNOWLEDGMENT

We wish to thank Ms. Joann Little for her assistance in the preparation of this manuscript.

CHAPTER 9

Acid-Base Metabolism

Jose A. L. Arruda
Robert Gold
Richard Wheeler
Shiva Rastogi

This review describes new clinical aspects of acid-base physiology and pathophysiology. We have attempted to review most of the new information available while emphasizing areas in which significant developments have occurred. Most of the papers reviewed deal directly with clinical acid-base physiology, but we also include material dealing with basic aspects of acid-base physiology thought to be essential to the understanding of the clinical disorders.

CALCIUM AND URINARY ACIDIFICATION

Background

The role of calcium in urinary acidification has been described in Volumes 5 and 6 of *Current Nephrology* (1,2). This segment of the chapter is intended to provide an update on the effect of hypercalcemia, vitamin D, and parathyroid hormone on renal and extrarenal acid base homeostasis. As we pointed out in our last review, the interaction of calcium and acid-base homeostasis at the level of the kidney has been difficult to evaluate because hypercalcemia directly causes hemodynamic effects on the kidney and decreases the GFR and renal plasma flow. These alterations can, by themselves, decrease net acid excretion. If calcium chloride is given orally, it can react with $NaHCO_3$ in the bowel according to the following reaction:

$NaHCO_3 + CaCl_2 \rightarrow CaCO_3 + HCl + NaCl$. It is obvious from this reaction that administration of $CaCl_2$ will result in an acid load to the body, and this will increase acid excretion by the kidney. Oral administration of $CaCl_2$ has been utilized as a test of urinary acidification in subjects who cannot tolerate oral ingestion of NH_4Cl (3). Calcium given in the form of $CaCO_3$ results in a high alkaline load to the organism, and this per se can alter urinary acidification. From the above considerations, it becomes apparent that the effect of oral administration of calcium on urinary acidification is critically dependent on the anion accompanying the calcium (Table 1). The administration of intravenous calcium is complicated not only by hemodynamic effects but, in addition, by changes in parathyroid hormone (PTH) (4). PTH inhibits urinary acidification; a decrease in its secretion brought about by hypercalcemia can lead to the enhancement of urinary acidification, not because of a direct effect of calcium itself on urinary acidification, but rather because of the removal of the inhibitory effect of PTH on acid excretion by the kidney (4,5).

It has been recognized for many years that patients with hypercalcemia associated with malignancy may present with metabolic alkalosis (6). The mechanism of the metabolic alkalosis was not studied in detail, but it was proposed to be mediated by enhanced mobilization of CO_3 from the bone and by increased acid excretion by the kidney. The mechanism, whereby chronic hypercalcemia alters acid-base homeostasis, has recently been reinvestigated in detail and these new studies (6–9) provide a better understanding of the overall effect of hypercalcemia on acid-base physiology. It should be emphasized that clinical hypercalcemia usually arises either from enhanced bone resorption or increased gastrointestinal absorption of calcium. The kidney only plays a role in the maintenance of hypercalcemia by reducing calcium excretion. The kidney by itself, in the absence of enhanced bone resorption or increased gastrointestinal absorption of calcium, is incapable of producing hypercalcemia. Stimulation of calcium absorption by the kidney should raise plasma calcium and the increase in plasma calcium would supress PTH, which then decreases bone resorption and normalizes serum calcium. Thus, studies dealing with the effect of experimental hypercalcemia on acid-base homeostasis should use a model that closely resembles most of the clinical conditions that cause hypercalcemia; that is, it should be associated with enhanced bone resorption. Hypercalcemia caused by enhanced bone resorption may be associated with increased mobilization of buffer from bone, and therefore its effects on acid-base homeostasis may differ from those caused by the intravenous or oral administration of calcium.

Hypercalcemia, Vitamin D, and Acid-Base Homeostasis

Two recent studies examine the effect of chronic hypercalcemia on acid-base homeostasis in the dog and in the rat (7,8). Hulter et al. (7), examined

Table 1. Acid-Base Homeostasis Associated with Alterations in PTH, Calcium, Phosphate, and Vitamin D

Agent or Condition	Renal Acidification	Extrarenal Buffer Mobilization	Experimental Model	Clinical Disorder
Parathyroid hormone	Proximal acidification ↑ Distal acidification normal or ↑	↑	Metabolic alkalosis	*Hyperparathyroidism* Proximal RTA
			No change	*Hypoparathyroidism* Metabolic alkalosis
Calcium	Proximal acidification ↑ Distal acidification ↑ or ↓	Endogenous hypercalcemia ↑ Exogenous hypercalcemia ↑	Metabolic alkalosis	*Hypercalcemia* Metabolic alkalosis Distal RTA
			—	*Hypocalcemia* Metabolic alkalosis
Vitamin D	Proximal acidification ↑ Distal acidification ↓ by vitamin D deficiency	↑	Distal acidification defect	*Vitamin D deficiency* Proximal RTA
			Metabolic alkalosis	*Vitamin D excess* Metabolic alkalosis
Phosphate depletion	Proximal acidification normal or ↓ Distal acidification ↑	↑	Distal or proximal acidification defect	*Phosphate depletion* Proximal or distal RTA

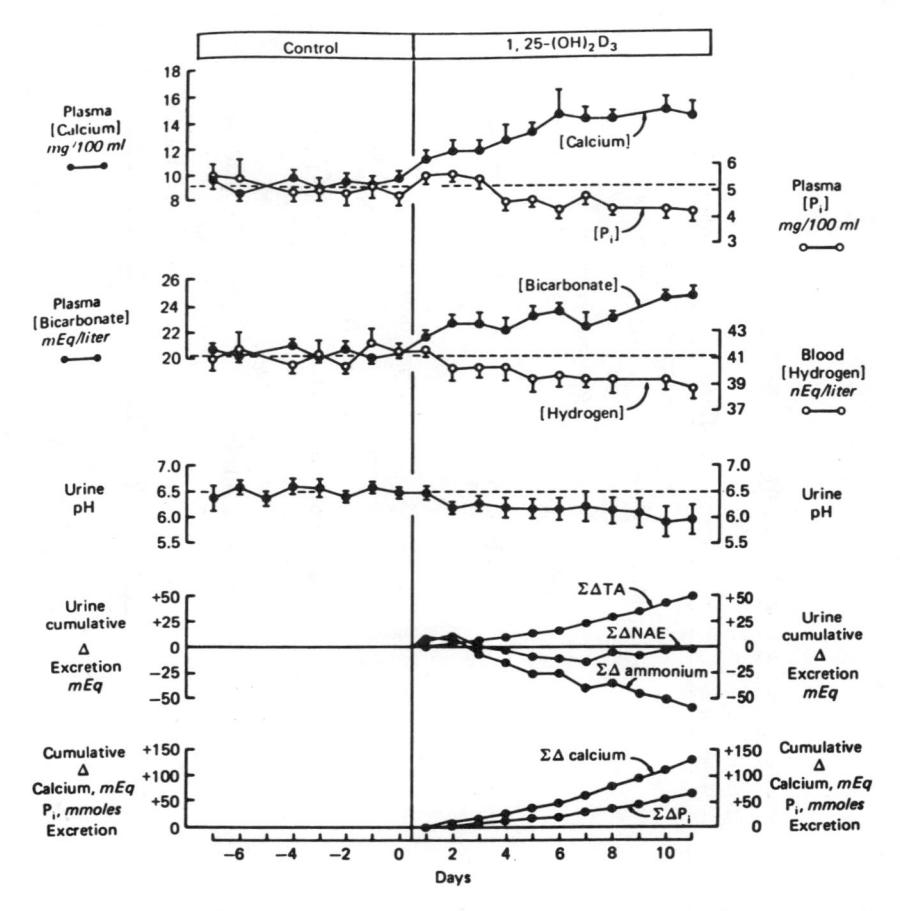

Figure 1. Effect of 1,25-(OH)₂-D₃ on plasma and urinary acid-base and electrolyte composition in TPTX dogs ingesting a high calcium diet. NAE, net acid excretion; Pi, inorganic phosphate; TA, titratable acid excretion. (Hulter HN et al: *Kidney Int* 21:445–448, 1982. Reproduced by permission.)

the effect of chronic hypercalcemia induced by 1,25-dihydroxycholecalciferol in thyroparathyroidectomized dogs maintained on a diet high in calcium in the form of $CaCO_3$. Administration of 1,25 vitamin D_3 caused hypercalcemia, and paralleling the increase in plasma calcium was a concomitant increase in plasma HCO_3 (Fig. 1). Urine pH decreased, but net acid excretion did not change because the increase in titratable acid excretion was paralleled by a decrease in ammonia excretion, leaving net acid excretion unchanged. The increase in titratable acid excretion was due to the increase in phosphate excretion elicited by the hypercalcemia. The decrease in ammonia excretion was attributed to a direct effect of calcium on ammonia production, but the latter parameter was not measured. Thus, the metabolic alkalosis observed with vitamin D administration was from extrarenal origin because net acid excretion remained constant, indicating that the kidney did not play a role in the generation of the metabolic alkalosis. The authors argued that the kidney played a role in the maintenance of the metabolic alkalosis because of the fact that net acid excretion should have decreased in response to the increase in plasma HCO_3 and to the decrease in blood H+ concentration. The latter contention, however, is difficult to accept without reservation. It is unclear whether mild elevations in plasma HCO_3 of 2–3 mEq/liter, especially in the face of a decrease in body weight (probably reflecting volume contraction), are associated with a supression of net acid excretion by the kidney.

To evaluate further the role of the kidney in the metabolic alkalosis induced by vitamin D, Hulter and co-workers examined the effect of this hormone on acid excretion by the kidney in the presence of phosphate restriction. Phosphate restriction of short duration minimized the phosphaturia induced by vitamin D and obviated the increase in titratable acid excretion. In these dogs, net acid excretion decreased because of the decrease in ammonia excretion. Despite the decrease in net acid excretion, plasma HCO_3 increased, thus clearly indicating that the kidney is not required either for the generation or for the maintenance of metabolic alkalosis induced by pharmacologic doses of vitamin D. Further evidence against an important role of the kidney on the metabolic alkalosis induced by 1,25-vitamin D_3 is the fact that when the hormone was given to animals ingesting a high phosphate diet, there was a significant increase in net acid excretion; however, the observed increase in plasma HCO_3 was not greater than that observed in animals in which net acid excretion did not change or actually decreased.

Metnick and co-workers (8) studied the effect of chronic administration of 1,25-vitamin D_3 for 2 weeks to intact rats. The animals developed hypercalcemia, hypercalciuria, and hyperphosphaturia. Plasma HCO_3 increased slightly by about 2 mEq/liter, and blood pH did not change because of the presence of high P_{CO_2}. Although the results were complicated by the presence of hypercapnia, there was a modest increase in plasma HCO_3. As compared to control rats, vitamin D-treated rats showed a lower urine pH and a greater net acid excretion. The increase in net acid excretion could be totally accounted for by the increase in titratable acid excretion, which was probably due to the increase in absolute phosphate excretion caused by the hyperphosphatemia.

Thus the data obtained in dogs and in rats are similar, suggesting that chronic administration of vitamin D is associated with an increase in plasma HCO_3 that is independent of the presence of the parathyroid gland, since it was observed in thyroparathyroidectomized (TPTX) animals. The role of the kidney in the generation or maintenance of metabolic alkalosis is questionable. Although there was an increase in titratable acid excretion, this increase was not necessary for the elevation in plasma HCO_3, since plasma HCO_3 rose regardless of whether or not there was a change in net acid excretion. Furthermore, ingestion of a high phosphate diet increases titratable acid and net acid excretion without causing an increase in plasma HCO_3. This finding supports the contention that an increase in titratable acid excretion need not necessarily increase plasma HCO_3.

Inasmuch as an increase in net acid excretion does not seem necessary for the increase in plasma HCO_3 induced by vitamin D, the metabolic alkalosis induced by this hormone could either be mediated by increased gastrointestinal absorption of alkali or by increased mobilization of alkali from the bone. The role of the gastrointestinal tract in the generation of metabolic alkalosis induced by vitamin D has not been investigated, but the gastrointestinal tract may have played a role in the studies of Hulter and colleagues; since some of the animals were given a high alkali load. The role of the gastrointestinal tract and dietary intake in acid-base homeostasis is discussed below.

Bone Resorption and Acid-Base Homeostasis

The role of increased bone resorption and mobilization of alkali in the generation of metabolic alkalosis induced by vitamin D was investigated by Hulter et al. (7) and by Arruda et al. (9). Hulter et al. (7) pretreated dogs with the diphosphonate (dichloromethanediphosphonate—Cl_2DM) before and during vitamin D administration. This diphosphonate is a potent inhibitor of bone resorption that has been shown to decrease bone resorption effectively. In the presence of the diphosphonate pretreatment, 1,25-dihydroxy vitamin D caused only a modest, nonsignificant increase in plasma calcium, indicating that bone resorption was effectively blocked by the drug. The increase in plasma HCO_3 in the latter group was of smaller magnitude than in the group not treated with diphosphonate, suggesting that bone resorption played a significant role in the generation of metabolic alkalosis. It remains unknown whether bone resorption had been totally blocked by diphosphonate treatment; if this was the case, then the observed increase in plasma HCO_3 would be due to a mechanism not dependent on bone (renal or gastrointestinal). Alternatively, it is possible that diphosphonate pretreatment may not have totally inhibited the bone resorption induced by vitamin D or that vitamin D mobilizes calcium and buffer by different mechanisms. The possible ability of vitamin D to mobilize buffer from bone needs to be studied in greater detail.

Arruda et al. (9) studied the effect of chronic administration of vitamin D (calciferol 200,000 units/day for 3 days) on the buffering of an acute acid load. After 3 days of treatment with vitamin D, the rats were mildly hypercalcemic, but baseline blood pH and plasma bicarbonate were not different from controls. The animals were bilaterally nephrectomized and infused with 0.1N hydrochloric acid at a rate of 5 mEq/kg/hour for 90

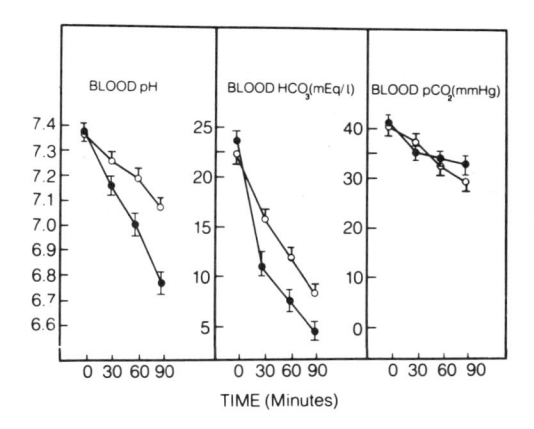

Figure 2. Effect of vitamin D treatment on the buffering of an acute acid load. Control rats (closed circle) and vitamin D-treated rats (open circle) (calciferol 200,000 units/day for 3 days) were bilaterally nephrectomized and then infused with HCl 5 mEg/kg/hr. (Arruda JAL et al: *Min Elect Met* 8:36–43, 1982. Reproduced by permission.)

minutes. Figure 2 compares the blood pH, HCO_3, and P_{CO_2} in vitamin-D-treated rats and in control rats during infusion of HCl. Vitamin-D-treated rats had a significantly smaller decrease in plasma HCO_3 and blood pH than did control rats. The site where vitamin D enhances the buffering of an acid load was not elucidated by this study, and it is possible that either bone or muscle could have played a role. We feel that chronic vitamin D administration acted at the level of the bone, but the issue clearly needs additional studies.

The above studies clearly demonstrate that chronic vitamin D administration increases plasma HCO_3 and also increases the capacity of the nephrectomized animals to buffer an acute acid load. This effect seems at least in part to be mediated by increased bone resorption and buffer mobilization, since the increase in plasma HCO_3 can be blocked by diphosphonate pretreatment. The increase in bone resorption induced by vitamin D seems to be independent of PTH, but the presence of parathyroid glands may enhance the degree of buffer mobilization and the magnitude of the metabolic alkalosis.

As we discussed in Volume 6 of *Current Nephrology* (2), phosphate deprivation or depletion, a condition associated with enhanced bone resorption, is also associated with increased capacity to buffer an acid load (Table 1), suggesting increased mobilization of bone buffer (10–12). Arruda et al. (9) have further evaluated the role of phosphate deprivation and parathyroid glands in the buffering of an acute acid load. They showed that the enhanced buffering capacity of phosphate deprivation is present with or without parathyroid glands, which suggests that PTH is not necessary for this effect. They further demonstrated that exogenous PTH can increase the buffering capacity of phosphate-deprived rats to buffer an acute acid load. Taken together, the observations strongly suggest that enhanced bone resorption, regardless of how accomplished, is associated with increased mobilization of buffer and protection against metabolic acidosis. PTH is not necessary for this effect, but it can greatly increase the buffer mobilization. The important message to the clinician is that conditions associated with increased bone resorption are likely to be associated with a tendency to metabolic alkalosis. There is also an enhanced capacity to buffer an acid load, which protects or minimizes the degree of metabolic acidosis of any cause in these patients.

The role of decreased bone resorption in acid-base homeostasis has only been partially studied (9). Chronic administration of diphosphonate does not seem to alter baseline acid-base homeostasis (9). In addition, experimental chronic hypoparathyroidism (Table 1) does not cause any acid-base abnormality (14). These observations tend to suggest that inhibition of bone resorption, either by diphosphonate or by lack of PTH, does not cause metabolic acidosis. The implication of this finding is that mobilization of bone buffers does not play a role in the day to day regulation of acid-base homeostasis. Arruda and colleagues (9) studied the effect of agents capable of inhibiting bone resorption on the buffering of an acute acid load. Chronic administration of diphosphonate to rats did not change the buffering of an acute acid load. However the mortality rate in diphosphonate-treated rat during the infusion of HCl (5 mEq/kg/hour) was 88%, as compared to 10% in the controls. The authors speculated that the increased mortality rate in the diphosphonate-treated rats might reflect the impaired buffering capacity of these animals; however, it is difficult to exclude other causes responsible for the high mortality rate, for example, hemodynamic alterations. To further evaluate the role of bone resorption, these workers evaluated the effect of thyrocalcitonin administration to intact and TPTX rats. The rats were infused with HCl (5 mEq/kg/hour). In intact rats, but not in TPTX rats, thyrocalcitonin decreased the ability of the animals to buffer an acid load. The ability of TPTX and calcitonin to impair buffering of an acute acid load were not additive, suggesting that TPTX blocks the effect of PTH to mobilize buffer and calcium from bone. These observations suggest that bone resorption may play a role in acid-base homeostasis only when there is a need to buffer an excess acid load. Under normal conditions chronic inhibition of bone resorption may not alter acid-base homeostasis. The contention that inhibition of bone resorption plays a role in acid-base homeostasis only when there is an excess acid load to be buffered is supported by the studies of Goulding and Broom (15). The authors evaluated the effect of diphosphonate or colchicine administration on intact and nephrectomized animals. The drugs were given for 2 days. In intact rats, diphosphonate or colchicine did not alter blood pH or bicarbonate. In animals with bilateral nephrectomy, diphosphonate or colchicine caused a significant decrease in blood pH and bicarbonate as compared to animals with bilateral nephrectomy not treated with these drugs. Intracellular pH of the muscle was also decreased in nephrectomized rats receiving diphosphonate. The results are compatible with the interpretation that in the presence of a high acid load (created by the nephrectomy), the bone plays a significant role in acid buffering. Inhibition of bone resorption by colchicine or diphosphonate increases the severity of metabolic acidosis.

Parathyroid Hormone, Hypercalcemia, and Acid-Base Homeostasis

The role of PTH in acid-base homeostasis continues to be investigated. As discussed in Volume 6 of *Current Nephrology,* Fraley and Adler (16) demonstrated that infusion of pharmacologic does of PTH significantly increased the buffering of an acute high acid load. Arruda et al. (7) expanded these initial observations and showed that PTH excess either from exogenous or endogenous source (stimulated by EDTA or colchicine administration) significantly increased the buffering of an acute acid load. Madias and co-workers (18) reinvestigated the role of endogenous PTH by administering an acid load to intact and TPTX rats. They clearly demonstrated that under experimental conditions, endogenous PTH was not necessary for the buffering of an acute acid load. They correctly pointed out that the studies of Fraley and Adler and of Arruda et al. did not show a difference in plasma HCO_3 between control and TPTX rats infused with HCl and that both studies showed only an increased mortality rate in TPTX rats as compared to controls. Madias et al. attributed the increased mortality rate of TPTX animals in the previous studies to the "unstable" hemodynamic condition of the thyroparathyroidectomized animals. The reason for the difference is difficult to determine, but it is possible that the dose of acid, rate of administration, and the level of plasma HCO_3 required for the effect of PTH to become apparent may have been different among the three studies. Fraley and Adler (19) have recently reinvestigated the role of PTH on the buffering of an acute acid load. They demonstrated that 2–5 mEq of HCl per kg given in 30 minutes was buffered equally in control and TPTX rats. The authors suggested that a critical level of plasma HCO_3 must be reached (plasma $HCO_3 < 11$ mEq/liter) before the effect of endogenous PTH can be disclosed. These conflicting results are difficult to reconcile at present and further studies are needed to determine whether normal amounts of endogenous PTH are needed to buffer an acute acid. Although this issue is unresolved, the results are clear as regards the effect of excess PTH. Acute excess of PTH, of either exogenous or endogenous origin, clearly enhanced the buffering of acute acid load (17).

The effect of chronic excess of PTH on acid-base homeostasis was investigated in dogs and in rats. Hulter et al. (7) studied the effect of chronic administration of bovine PTH to dogs (10–15 units/kg daily for 1 week). As shown in Figure 3, PTH administration resulted in hypercalcemia, hyperphosphatemia, and hypercarbonatemia. The urine pH did not change but net acid excretion increased significantly. Pretreatment of the dogs with diphosphonate prevented the increase in serum calcium

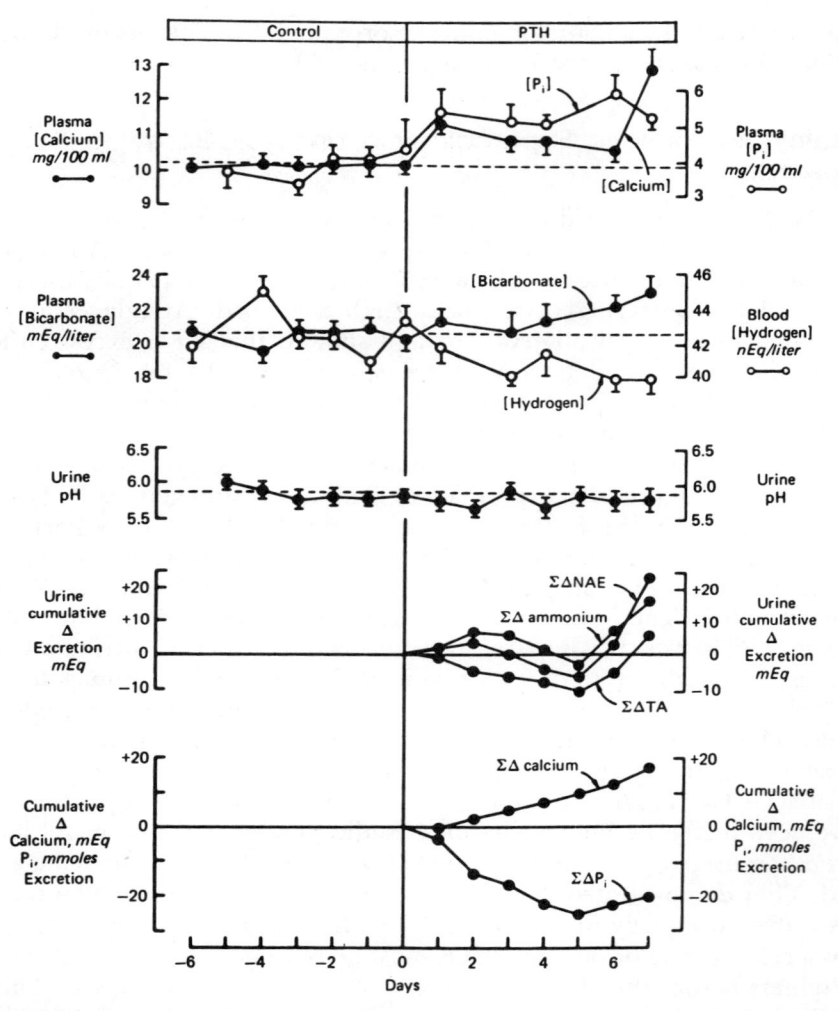

Figure 3. Effect of PTH administration on plasma and urinary acid-base and electrolyte composition in intact dogs. NAE, net acid excretion; P$_i$, inorganic phosphate; by TA, titratable acid excretion. (Hulter HN et al. *Kidney Int* 21:445–448, 1982. Reproduced by permission.)

and plasma bicarbonate, suggesting that enhanced bone resorption played a significant role in the elevation of plasma HCO$_3$. Further evidence that bone resorption was involved in the generation of the alkalosis was the presence of hyperphosphatemia. Licht and Vicker (20) reported results very similar to those of Hulter et al., in that PTH administration to dogs resulted in metabolic alkalosis that was thought to result from renal and nonrenal mechanisms.

Metnick et al. (8) used an ingenious approach to evaluate the effects of PTH on acid-base homeostasis. Rats were made hyperparathyroid by implanting several parathyroid glands in the lower limb musculature. The aminals developed hypercalcemia, hypophosphatemia, and an increase in plasma HCO_3 of 3–4 mEq/liter. The increase in plasma HCO_3 correlated well with the increase in plasma calcium. Net acid excretion was greater in hyperparathyroid rats than in controls, but the increase in net acid excretion was mainly due to an increase in phosphate excretion. Although the authors postulated that increased net acid excretion played a role in the generation of metabolic alkalosis, the same question raised earlier could be asked: Is the increase in net acid excretion necessary for the development of metabolic alkalosis? On the basis of Hulter's studies, it would appear that inhibition of bone resorption abolishes the effect of PTH to induce metabolic alkalosis. The results obtained with PTH are thus similar to those obtained with vitamin D and strongly suggest that enhanced bone resorption is associated not only with hypercalcemia but also with release of alkali and metabolic alkalosis. These studies provide support for our contention that PTH excess of endogenous origin (elicited by EDTA or colchicine) is capable of mobilizing extrarenal buffer. These observations would suggest that chronic endogenous PTH excess should be associated with the development of metabolic alkalosis.

Effect of pH on Bone Resorption In Vitro

In vivo animal studies showing an effect of PTH on buffer mobilization from bone must be compared with in vitro studies analyzing the effect of PTH to mobilize calcium from bone in the face of different pH. Dominguez and Raisz (21) analyzed the effect that variations in pH (induced by changing the HCO_3 and the P_{CO_2}) had on bone resorption in vitro. They utilized rat fetal bone labeled with ^{45}Ca and cultured in 2%, 5%, or 10% CO_2. They then measured the release of ^{45}Ca from devitalized bone (non-cell-mediated ^{45}Ca release) and from live bone (cell-mediated ^{45}Ca release). The tissue was cultured with or without PTH and/or 1,25-$(OH)_2$-vitamin D_3. The authors observed that calcium release from devitalized bone was linearly related to H+ concentration and the same response was observed regardless of whether H+ concentration was altered by varying the HCO_3 concentration or the P_{CO_2}. This finding indicates that calcium release from devitalized bone is a function of H+ concentration regardless whether these changes are induced by metabolic or respiratory acidosis. This loss of calcium from dead bone presumably consisted of both exchange and mineral dissolution, but most of the calcium release was apparently mediated by bone dissolution. The authors did not study the release of bone buffers, but based on other studies, there is reason to believe that hydroxyapatite and $CaCO_3$ were released from bone during acidosis.

Opposite to the effect of pH on calcium from dead bone, Dominguez and Raisz observed that cell-mediated bone resorption was not influenced by pH over a wide range (6.9–7.5). The effect of PTH or 1,25-(OH)$_2$-vitamin D$_3$ to mobilize ^{45}Ca was also not altered over a wide pH range; although an inhibition of the ability of PTH to mobilize calcium was observed at very low (< 6.9) or very high (> 7.6) pH. These in vitro studies therefore do not support the two contentions that (1) in vivo metabolic acidosis directly enhances osteoclastic bone resorption and (2) metabolic acidosis enhances the effect of PTH on bone. The reason for these discrepancies is unclear, but it is possible that other factors present in vivo might influence the effects of acidosis and PTH. The effect of PTH to mobilize buffer is not elucidated by this study. One would expect buffer to be mobilized with calcium; the lack of effect of pH on PTH-induced calcium mobilization suggests that bone buffer mobilization is not enhanced by PTH during acidosis. It is possible, however, that buffer is mobilized independently of calcium. Careful studies measuring bone buffer release in vivo and in vitro in response to PTH are needed to verify the contention that PTH is capable of altering acid-base homeostasis by controlling bone buffer release.

Effect of Intravenous Calcium Infusion on Acid-Base Homeostasis

All the above studies have concentrated on hypercalcemia produced by enhanced bone resorption and its effects on acid-base homeostasis. Hulter and co-workers (7) also evaluated the effect of intravenous calcium in the form of calcium chloride or calcium thiosulfate in TPTX dogs. During the control period, the animals were infused with the sodium salt, and during the experimental period, the calcium salt was infused. Administration of the calcium salt resulted in hypercalcemia associated with a significant decrease in blood pH and plasma HCO$_3$ (Table 1). The metabolic acidosis caused a significant decrease in urine pH and an increase in net acid excretion. The authors postulate that administration of calcium to TPTX animals results in the consumption of base, which is deposited along with calcium in bone or soft tissue, and thus results in metabolic acidosis. Thus hypercalcemia can be associated with metabolic alkalosis or metabolic acidosis depending on the mechanism of generation of hypercalcemia. Endogenous hypercalcemia is usually associated with metabolic alkalosis, whereas exogenous hypercalcemia is associated with metabolic acidosis (Table 1).

Effect of Hypercalcemia-Producing Agents on Renal Acidification

The finding of metabolic alkalosis with hypercalcemia induced by vitamin D or PTH suggests that enhanced bone resorption, regardless of how induced, tends to cause metabolic alkalosis. It should be pointed out that this effect may be enhanced or decreased by the effect of these hormones on the kidney. PTH suppresses proximal HCO_3 reabsorption (22). In the distal nephron, PTH either does not alter acidification or may actually increase acidification (22,23) (Table 1). The effect of vitamin D on the kidney has only been partially studied. Vitamin D deficiency may inhibit urinary acidification (2), whereas vitamin D excess may increase bicarbonate reabsorption (24–26). As discussed earlier, clearance studies in dogs have suggested that acute hypercalcemia enhances bicarbonate reabsorption in the presence and absence of PTH (5). It was suggested that hypercalcemia directly stimulates bicarbonate reabsorption, but because of hemodynamic alterations caused by the hypercalcemia, it could not be excluded that the changes observed represented a hemodynamic effect rather than a direct effect of calcium on bicarbonate reabsorption.

McKinney and Myers (27) examined the effect of various concentrations of calcium on bicarbonate absorption by the isolated proximal convoluted and straight tubules of rabbit in vitro. They showed that in the proximal convoluted tubule, but not in the proximal straight tubule, elevation of calcium concentration in the perfusate in the bath to 5 mM resulted in an increase in bicarbonate absorption. Removal of calcium from the perfusate inhibited bicarbonate absorption. These studies reveal a modest increase in bicarbonate absorption; however, in order to see this modest increase in HCO_3 absorption, it was necessary to increase ionized calcium from 0.9 mM to 2.5 mM in the bath, which corresponds to an increase in total plasma calcium from 2 mM to 5 mM (20 mg/dl). Therefore, the clinical significance of these observations is questionable, since at these high calcium concentrations, the hemodynamic effects of calcium would predominate. The experiments dealing with the effect of calcium removal from the bath are difficult to interpret because removal of calcium may alter membrane permeability nonspecifically and therefore may alter bicarbonate absorption. In summary these studies somewhat support the notion that very high levels of calcium may enhance bicarbonate absorption, but they do not clarify the role of mild changes in cytosolic calcium on urinary acidification.

Role of Cytosolic Calcium on Urinary Acidification

In Volume 5 of *Current Nephrology*, the studies by Arruda et al. (28) of the effect of alterations in cytosolic calcium on urinary acidification in the turtle bladder were partially discussed. The turtle bladder is an analog of the mammalian distal nephron, capable of acidification in vitro, and is thus an ideal model to examine the effect of calcium on acidification independent of hemodynamic changes.

The concentration of calcium in the cytosol is regulated by several mechanisms that maintain the concentration of calcium in this compartment at 10^{-6} M, as compared to the extracellular fluid concentration of

10^{-3} M. The concentration of calcium is kept low not only because the permeability of the plasma membrane to calcium is very low, but also because various intracellular organelles are capable of taking up calcium. In addition, calcium is extruded from the cell very effectively by a sodium–calcium exchange system and by a calcium-stimulated ATPase. All these mechanisms act to maintain the concentration of calcium in the cytosol at very low levels; thus, the presence of a high extracellular calcium concentration need not be accompanied by corresponding changes in intracellular calcium (28). As discussed earlier, an increase in cytosolic calcium by the ionophore A23187 or by the cholinergic agent carbachol resulted in an inhibition of urinary acidification by the turtle bladder. Quinidine, an agent that liberates calcium from intracellular organelles, also caused a significant inhibition of H+ secretion by the turtle bladder that was independent of extracellular calcium concentration (29–32).

More recently, the possible role of the sodium–calcium exchange system in the regulation of cytosolic calcium was examined (33). Removal of serosal sodium (substituted by sucrose) resulted in a significant increase in calcium uptake (33). In the absence of serosal sodium, the increase in calcium uptake is explained by the fact that the outward movement of sodium (due to a favorable concentration gradient) leads to an increase in calcium uptake. When sodium is present in the serosal solution, the energy generated by passive entry of sodium into the cell extrudes calcium. This increase in calcium uptake, elicited by removal of serosal sodium, could be prevented by pretreatment with lanthanum chloride. Removal of serosal sodium was associated with a significant inhibition of H+ secretion that could be prevented, at least in part, by pretreatment with lanthanum. The observation that lanthanum prevents the effect of sodium removal on calcium uptake and on H+ secretion strongly suggests that two phenomena (i.e., the increase in calcium uptake and the inhibition of transport) are causally related. Interestingly, removal of mucosal Na failed to inhibit H+ secretion; thus, the sodium–calcium exchange system may operate only at the serosal membrane.

These observations suggest that maneuvers that increase intracellular calcium by different mechanisms (i.e., increase in the permeability of the plasma membrane to calcium with ionophore A23187, release of calcium from intracellular organelles with quinidine, and increase in calcium uptake by removing serosal sodium) result in inhibition of H+ secretion. The fact that prevention of calcium uptake prevents or minimizes the inhibition of H+ secretion strengthens the contention that two phenomena are causally related. In all the above studies inference about cytosolic calcium was obtained with the use of radioactive calcium uptake and efflux. These studies should be expanded by direct measurement of the concentration of calcium in the cytosol. This would determine whether the alterations in cytosolic calcium precede the inhibition of urinary acidification.

Intracellular calcium seems to inhibit urinary acidification not by impairing the force of the H+ pump, but, rather, by decreasing the active conductance of protons through the pump. In vivo, calcium may inhibit distal acidification both by affection H+ secretion directly and by interferring with sodium transport. Thus, calcium decreases the favorable electric gradient for H+ secretion. The mechanism(s) whereby changes in intracellular calcium affect urinary acidification by the turtle bladder remains unexplored. Calcium is capable of producing several alterations in cell metabolism. A systematic analysis of these alterations as possible mechanisms of the inhibition of acidification needs to be undertaken. The effect of calcium to inhibit urinary acidification does not seem to be related to changes in intracellular pH. Arruda et al. (34) measured intracellular pH before and after addition of ionophore A23183 or carbachol, or replacement of serosal sodium by sucrose. These maneuvers are thought to increase cytosolic calcium and did result in a decrease in intracellular pH. It was postulated that the increase in cytosolic calcium resulted in calcium uptake by the mitochondria. Studies performed in isolated mitochondria have established that an increase in calcium uptake is associated with ejection of protons from the mitochondria into the medium (cytosol) and a decrease in intracellular pH. Thus, the inhibition of urinary acidification by high levels of intracellular calcium cannot be attributed to an increase in intracellular pH. The inhibition of urinary acidification also does not seem to result from metabolic alterations based on the fact that ATP, ADP, and the ATP:ADP ratio remained normal (33).

It is interesting to consider the possibility that the effects of calcium on urinary acidification may depend on the nephron segment. The studies of McKinney and Myers (27) and clearance studies (5) suggest that calcium stimulates acidification in the proximal convoluted tubule but does not alter acidification in the straight tubule, whereas studies in the turtle bladder suggest that calcium inhibits distal acidification. Other agents, such as PTH, inhibit proximal HCO_3 reabsorption but stimulate distal acidification (23). In addition, calcium may be deposited in the medulla, causing nephrocalcinosis associated with impaired distal acidification (4). In summary, it seems clear from the above consideration, that calcium has important effects on acid-base homeostasis (Table 1). The effects of calcium depend on degree and duration of hypercalcemia and the mechanism whereby the hypercalcemia is generated. In addition, the overall effect of calcium is the result of a complex interplay of bone mobilization of alkali, enhanced gastrointestinal absorption of alkali, and its effect on the kidney, which may be associated with an enhancement of proximal acidification and inhibition of distal acidification.

Metabolic Acidosis, Bone Disease, and Vitamin D

The relationship between chronic metabolic acidosis and bone disease continues to be of interest to clinicians and renal physiologists. Cunningham et al. (35) studied two patients with chronic metabolic acidosis, secondary to urinary diversion, who developed osteomalacia proven by bone biopsy. One patient had a normal glomerular filtration rate (GFR) and the other patient had a GFR decreased to 30% of normal value. Plasma 25-OH-vitamin D_3 and 1,25-dihydroxy-vitamin D_3 were normal in one patient and low in the second patient. Administration of alkali, without vitamin D, resulted in clinical and histologic improvement of the osteomalacia. In the patient with low levels of plasma 25- and 1,25-vitamin D_3, the levels of these metabolites increased to normal ranges during alkali treatment. Thus, significant osteomalacia can develop in the presence of chronic acidosis and correction of acidosis alone can lead to significant improvement of the bone disease.

Various mechanisms may contribute to the osteomalacia induced by chronic acidosis, including a direct effect of acidosis on bone, enhancement of the effect of PTH to promote bone resorption, alterations of the effect of PTH on the kidney that lead to hypophosphatemia, and the impairment of vitamin D metabolism by acidosis (36–38). Let us briefly consider the effects of metabolic acidosis on vitamin D metabolism. Metabolic acidosis has been associated with a decrease in the activity of the enzyme 1α-hydroxylase, the enzyme that mediates the conversion of 25- to 1,25-vitamin D_3 (36). Metabolic acidosis decreases the effect of PTH in the kidney by inhibiting the effect of PTH-sensitive adenylate cyclase. Since PTH is an important stimulator of the 1α-hydroxylase activity in the kidney, the effect of metabolic acidosis to inhibit this enzyme could be mediated by inhibition of the PTH-sensitive adenylate cyclase. There are two 1α-hydroxylase systems in the rat kidney: one is located in the proximal convoluted tubule and is regulated by the PTH-cyclic AMP system; the other is found in the proximal straight tubule and it is regulated by calcitonin. Kawashima et al. (39) studied the two 1α-hydroxylase systems in kidneys from rats with vitamin D deficiency in the presence and in the absence of metabolic acidosis. The acitivity of 1α-hydroxylase systems was assayed in microdissected proximal convoluted and straight tubules. Metabolic acidosis of 3 days duration caused a significant decrease in 1α-hydroxylase activity in the proximal convoluted tubule. Metabolic acidosis of shorter duration or lowering the pH of the incubation medium failed to reduce the enzyme's activity. In the proximal straight tubule, the activity of 1α-hydroxylase was unaltered in both control and acidotic rats. To elucidate the mechanism of the decrease in 1α-hydroxylase, the authors studied the effect of PTH, cyclic AMP, and calcitonin administration to rats with chronic metabolic acidosis. PTH failed to stimulate the suppressed 1α-hydroxylase activity of rats with metabolic acidosis, whereas cyclic AMP administration restored the activity of the enzyme to the levels found in control rats. Calcitonin stimulated the 1α-hydroxylase activity equally in control and in acidotic rats. The results convincingly demonstrate that metabolic acidosis selectively decreases the activity of 1α-hydroxylase in

Table 2. Radiographic Evidence of Skeletal Abnormalities in Patients with Different Types of Renal Tubular Acidosis

	Renal Tubular Acidosis (%)		
Skeletal Abnormality	Distal (type I)	Proximal (type II)	Hyperkalemic (type IV)
Overall prevalence	2	67	12
Nonazotemic patients	0	47	0
Azotemic patients	2	20	12

SOURCE: Modified after Brenner RJ et al: *N Engl J Med* 307:217–221, 1982.

the proximal convoluted tubule, probably by inhibiting PTH-stimulated adenylate cyclase. The normal response of rats with metabolic acidosis to cyclic AMP indicates that metabolic acidosis does not affect the intracellular process necessary for the stimulation of 1α-hydroxylase beyond the generation of cyclic AMP.

The clinical significance of these observations at the present moment remains unclear. The levels of 1,25-$(OH)_2$-D_3 in metabolic acidosis have not been studied in detail: one study showed increased levels of 1,25-$(OH)_2$-D_3 in response to metabolic acidosis in vitamin-D repleted rats. This increase was thought to result from a decrease in plasma phosphate. Others have shown that metabolic acidosis causes a marked decrease of 1,25-$(OH)_2$-D_3 levels in vitamin-D repleted rats fed a low calcium diet supplemented with phosphate to prevent decrease in plasma phosphate (37–40). The effect of metabolic acidosis on 1,25-$(OH)_2$-D_3 clearly requires more study. One can speculate that the effects of metabolic acidosis may well depend on the degree and duration of acidosis, on possible changes in serum phosphate and serum calcium, and on preexisting vitamin D stores.

Renal Tubular Acidosis and Bone Disease

Distal renal tubular acidosis (RTA) (type I) of the idiopathic type is thought to be commonly associated with nephrocalcinosis and osteomalacia (41). More prevalent in children, osteomalacia leads to failure of growth. Proximal RTA is not thought to be associated with significant bone disease because hypercalciuria is not common. In distal RTA there would be continous hypercalciuria, whereas in proximal RTA the presence of large amounts of bicarbonate in the distal nephron stimulates calcium absorption, thus preventing hypercalciuria.

Brenner reviewed radiographs of bones and kidneys in 92 patients with RTA (42). Tables 2 and 3 show that 48% of the patients had distal RTA, 20% had proximal RTA, and 32% had type IV RTA. The last type is a variant of distal RTA characterized by (*1*) the ability to lower the urine pH maximally during acidosis, (*2*) a fractional bicarbonate excretion of

Table 3. Frequency (%) of Various Types of Renal Tubular Acidosis and Percentage Prevalence of Renal Calcification within Each Group

Abnormality	Distal (type I) (48%)	Proximal (type II) (20%)	Hyperkalemic (type IV) (32%)
GFR > 60 ml/min	98	67	80
Nephrocalcinosis and/or nephrolithiasis	63	0	0
Nephrocalcinosis alone	56	0	0
Nephrolithiasis alone	5	0	0
Nephrocalcinosis and nephrolithiasis	2	0	0

SOURCE: Modified after Brenner RJ et al: *N Engl J Med* 307:217–221, 1982.

less than 10% when plasma HCO$_3$ is normal, (3) reduced ammonia excretion, (4) hyperkalemia, and (5) reduced potassium excretion in the urine. Distal RTA (Type I) was the most common type in adults, accounting for 75% of the cases, whereas only 30% of children belonged to this category. In children the most common type was type IV followed by type I and type II. Radiographs of the bones (knee, hand, spine, and pelvis), available for 82 patients, were examined independently by two observers. The following terminology was used to describe the "bone disease": *osteopenia* was used to indicate generalized bone demineralization (thinning of the cortices); *rickets* was used when there was wide and irregular epiphyseal and metaphyseal junction or evidence of bone softening in the long bones of children; *osteomalacia* was used where there was evidence of incomplete cortical fracture (Looser's zones and pseudofractures) in the skeleton of the adults.

Bone disease occurred in 17% of all patients. Table 2 shows the prevalence of bone disease in each type of renal tubular acidosis. Bone disease was more frequent in the azotemic patients and in patients with proximal RTA. This study provides the only systematic and long-term radiologic evaluation of patients with RTA. In 21 patients with RTA previously reported by Courey and Pfister (44), osteopenia was twice as common as in the series described by Brenner et al., but Courey and Pfister did not divide the patients with RTA into various types, and it is thus impossible to determine whether the real prevalence of bone disease was higher. The present study negates the contention that proximal RTA is not associated with bone disease and indicates that distal RTA is not the type most frequently associated with bone disease. The main problem associated with the study is the fact that bone biopsies were not done and thus it is impossible to determine whether the radiologic diagnoses were correct.

The presence of bone disease in patients with proximal RTA merits further discussion. In clinical states of vitamin D deficiency, a Fanconi-type syndrome may develop. The mechanism of the Fanconi syndrome has not been completely studied, but it is possible that vitamin D deficiency itself, PTH excess, phosphate depletion, and hypocalcemia may all depress proximal tubular reabsorption of bicarbonate, glucose, and amino acids, thus leading to a Fanconi syndrome. Administration of 1,25-(OH)$_2$ vitamin D corrects both the rickets and the Fanconi syndrome. Similarily, in patients with idiopathic Fanconi syndrome the administration of 1,25(OH)$_2$ vitamin D may lead to improvement of the rickets. The development of rickets in these patients may be related to impaired vitamin D metabolism. It is possible that injury of the proximal tubule may impair the conversion of 25(OH) to 1,25(OH)$_2$ vitamin D. Experimental studies in animals showing that administration of maleic acid, a poison that causes proximal RTA, results in impaired conversion of 25(OH) vitamin D to 1,25(OH)$_2$ vitamin D (44) support the hypothesis. It should be pointed out, however, that serum levels of 1,25(OH)$_2$ vitamin D$_3$ may not be low in certain patients with proximal RTA. Ishitsu et al. studied a patient with proximal RTA and osteomalacia (45). A child who had been treated with anticonvulsants and acetazolamide for many years because of seizures presented with hypocalcemia, hypophosphatemia, hyperchloremic acidosis, and rickets. PTH levels were elevated, 1,25(OH)$_2$ vitamin D$_3$ levels were normal, but 25(OH) vitamin D levels were reduced. Discontinuation of the acetazolamide corrected the metabolic acidosis and increased serum phosphate levels but did not alter serum calcium. Unfortunately, vitamin D levels were not measured after discontinuation of the drug. Administration of 1,25(OH)$_2$ vitamin D$_3$ failed to elevate the serum calcium and to improve the rickets, but administration of cholecalciferol normalized the serum calcium and the alkaline phosphatase and increased the levels of 25(OH) vitamin D to normal. The authors concluded that 1,25(OH)$_2$ vitamin D levels may not be decreased in metabolic acidosis. The failure of the patients to respond to 1,25(OH)$_2$ vitamin D and the presence of normal levels of 1,25(OH)$_2$ vitamin D, suggest the existence of tissue resistance to action of 1,25(OH)$_2$ vitamin D$_3$ in metabolic acidosis. The normalization of biochemical features and improvement of the rickets with 25(OH) vitamin D suggests that this metabolite plays an important role in bone formation. The interrelationship of vitamin D, metabolic acidosis, and Fanconi syndrome is of considerable interest and additional studies are necessary to unravel their complex interaction.

DIETARY INTAKE AND ACID EXCRETION BY THE KIDNEY

The role of the gut in acid-base homeostasis remains unclear because detailed studies dealing with the effect of both diet and acid-base status on gut absorption of base or acid are lacking. To define acid balance it is necessary to measure acid production and acid excretion under defined dietary intake (13). In normal subjects ingesting a chemically defined neutral liquid diet, acid production is the result of oxidation of neutral dietary sulfur (present in methionine and cysteine) to inorganic sulfate and the incomplete combusion of proteins, fat, and carbohydrates to organic acids. Acid production, taken as the sum of the excretion of urinary sulfate plus the sum of the excretion of urinary organic anions, equals net acid excretion, taken as the sum of the excretion of titratable acid plus ammonia minus bicarbonate (46). Since acid production equaled acid excretion, acid balance was zero, therefore, it was thought that the gut played no regulatory role in acid balance.

Under normal dietary conditions, when subjects ingest whole food, it becomes more complicated to estimate endogenous acid production. Food can be analyzed in terms of its potential alkalinity or acidity by measuring acidity or alkalinity of the ash that is present after removal of the organic matter by combustion. Foods containing an excess of inorganic cations (Na, K, Ca, Mg) as compared to inorganic anions (Cl, PO_4, sulfate) have alkaline ash. This difference is made by organic anions that are metabolized to bicarbonate when absorbed. In foods containing an excess of inorganic anions over inorganic cations, the organic cations are responsible for the difference. When absorbed, these organic cations are metabolized, yielding $H+$. The average American diet contains an excess of inorganic cations over inorganic anions. The difference consists of organic anions that are absorbed and metabolized to bicarbonate. The average ingestion of organic anions is about 75 mEq/day or approximately 1 mEq/kg of body weight. Of this amount, 35 mEq are found in the stool and thus, theoretically, 35 mEq of organic anions (potential bicarbonate) are absorbed daily (46). Lemman and Lennon have pointed out that these calculations are based on the assumption that phosphate has a valence of 1.8 in the diet and in the stool (46). Obviously the valence of phosphate used in these calculations has a profound impact on whether acid or base is liberated in the gastrointestinal tract and, hence, in the body fluids. In the stool, the mean valence of phosphate is unknown because of the heterogenous mixture of the material, with only 5% of phosphorus being dialyzable. The valence of phosphate has been estimated to be between 1.8 and 3.0.

Few studies have evaluated the changes in fecal anion composition during acid loading. During NH_4Cl induced acidosis, fecal organic anions decreased during induction of the acidosis and returned to normal levels as ammonia excretion increased (47,48). These data suggest that absorption of organic anions was increased during the induction of acidosis. Thus, one would be tempted to speculate that the gut contributed to the adaptation of the acid load. The contribution was transient however, and in quantitative terms, it was of small magnitude since it accounted for only 3% of the cumulative acid load. Although these data suggest that the gut may, under certain conditions, play a role in acid-base homeostasis, it remains unclear whether alterations in fecal excretion of potential base play a role in the day to day regulation of acid-base homeostasis in normal subjects.

It is possible, however, that constant and chronic changes in dietary intake may alter the pattern of the gut absorption of organic anions and thus influence acid-base homeostasis. Richardson and co-workers (49) studied this issue by examining rabbits and rats under different dietary intakes. Under normal dietary intake, rabbits excrete an alkaline urine and rats excrete an acid urine. Rabbits, under normal dietary intake, have decreased distal acidification as evidenced by their inability to raise urine Pco_2 in response to bicarbonate loading. These investigators examined the role of diet on acidification by rats and rabbits fed different diets. The diets contained an excess of inorganic cations over anions. Rats fed a rat diet excreted an acid urine, whereas rabbits fed the rat diet excreted an alkaline urine. Conversely, rabbits eating a rabbit diet excreted an alkaline urine, whereas rats fed the same rabbit diet excreted much less alkali in the urine than did the rabbit. The difference between the two species can only be explained by postulating a difference in the absorption of the organic anions (potential bicarbonate) from the diet. To verify this hypothesis, Richardson et al. (49) measured absorption of organic anions (potential bicarbonate in the rabbit and in the rat) under the same dietary intake. Rabbits absorbed twice as much potential bicarbonate from the diet as did the rats (61% as compared to 26%). In the rabbit, 76% of the potential bicarbonate absorbed was excreted in the urine as HCO_3 and 24% as organic anions. In contrast, the rat excreted 33% as HCO_3 and 67% as organic anions. Thus, the rabbit absorbs more potential HCO_3 from the diet and excretes more HCO_3 in the urine as compared to the rat.

These findings strongly suggest that the type of diet may influence the absorption of organic anions, which may directly or indirectly influence distal acidification. To evaluate the effect of diet on urinary acidification, the authors studied urinary acidification in rabbits fed a rat diet for 2 weeks and given NH_4Cl loading. Under these conditions, rabbits fed a rat diet were able to lower urine pH but were not capable of increasing ammonia excretion. Feeding the rabbits the rat diet plus NH_4Cl did not correct the inability to increase ammonia excretion. The authors concluded that low acid excretion present in the rabbits cannot be explained by the diet. It should be emphasized, however, that the change in the dietary intake was of short duration, and it is possible that a distal acidification apparatus that has been dormant for a long time may not adapt quickly to the change in dietary intake.

The role of the dietary intake on acid excretion by the kidney has been examined in detail in the rat and in the rabbit (49–51). Cruz-Soto et al. (50) fed rats a solution containing $NaHCO_3$ or $NaCl$ for 1 week. After 1 week, they measured the ability of these rats to raise urine P_{CO_2} in response to HCO_3 infusion. In rats fed $NaHCO_3$, urine P_{CO_2} was lower than that of control rats at comparable levels of urine HCO_3 concentration, indicating the presence of a distal acidification defect. Thus it would appear that feeding alkali to rats can turn off distal nephron H+ secretion. This defect is similar to that found in rabbits ingesting a normal diet (49), supporting the hypothesis that chronic high alkali dietary intake can modulate distal acidification. To test this hypothesis they examined distal acidification in rabbits under normal conditions, during acid dietary intake, and during metabolic acidosis. Under normal dietary intake, rabbits were incapable of raising urine P_{CO_2} in response to HCO_3 administration, confirming the data of Giammarco et al. (50). Infusion of $NaHCO_3$, however, greatly increased the blood pH, which could account, at least in part, for the inhibition of distal acidification. To examine this issue, P_{CO_2} was measured in urine made alkaline by infusion of acetazolamide. Administration of acetazolamide raised urine HCO_3 concentration and urine P_{CO_2} increased, albeit not to normal values. These data suggested a role for blood pH in the regulation of distal acidification in the rabbit.

The role of the dietary intake was also examined by measuring urine P_{CO_2} during $NaHCO_3$ loading to weanling rabbits. Weanling rabbits have never been exposed to a high dietary intake of alkali and should thus allow testing the hypothesis that the dietary intake plays a role in distal acidification. Weanling rabbits raised urine P_{CO_2} in response to $NaHCO_3$ infusion. The increase in urine P_{CO_2} was not of the same degree as that observed in normal rats but it should be remembered that $NaHCO_3$ infusion raised blood pH which, as discussed above, could partially inhibit distal acidification. it seems clear from these experiments that the dietary intake and the blood pH played a role in distal acidification. When the rabbits were fed an acid diet and blood pH was normal, the urine P_{CO_2} (measured during phosphate administration) was close to normal. When the rabbits were made acidotic and blood pH was kept in the acidotic range during the experiment, urine P_{CO_2} increased to the same level as that found in normal rats. In these experiments, urine P_{CO_2} was measured during phosphate and acetazolamide administration. This protocol allowed the investigators to measure urine P_{CO_2} when the urine had a pH close to the pK of phosphate while keeping the blood pH in the acidotic range. These data clearly demonstrated that the ability of rabbits to raise urine P_{CO_2}, is critically dependent on dietary intake and blood pH. Figure 4 shows urine–blood P_{CO_2} in the rabbits during various dietary and blood pH conditions. It is clear that the lower the blood pH the greater the capacity of the rabbits to raise urine P_{CO_2}. These data would support the concept that chronic dietary intake turns off the distal acidification apparatus in rabbits and in rats. When rabbits are given a high acid diet, they are able to lower urine pH maximally but are unable to increase ammonia excretion to normal values. The finding that dietary intake

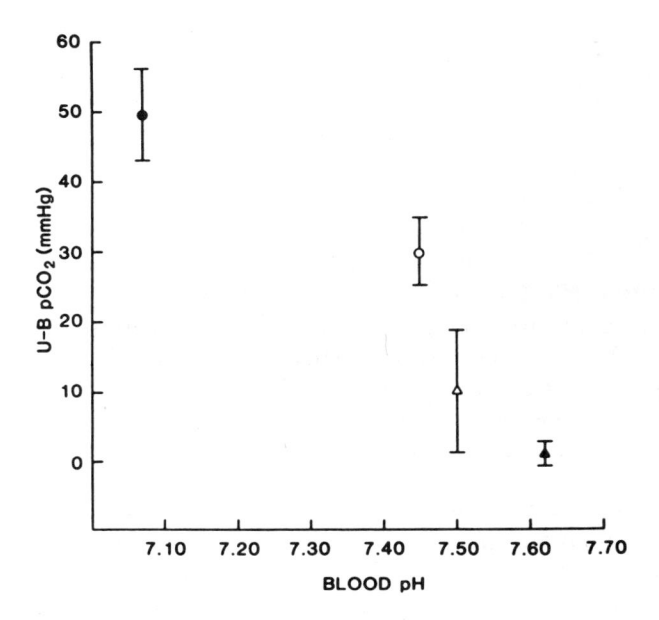

Figure 4. Urine minus blood (U-B) P_{CO_2} in rabbits at different blood pH levels. Closed triangle represents rabbits eating a regular diet, studied during alkalinization of urine. Remaining groups were studied during infusion of neutral sodium phosphate to rabbits chronically fed with cow's milk (open triangle) or ammonium chloride. Blood pH was kept within acidotic range by acetazolamide infusion (closed circle) or it was restored to normal by sodium bicarbonate infusion (open circle). (Cruz-Soto M. et al: *Am J Physiol* 243:371, 1982. Reproduced by permission.)

influences distal acidification is in agreement with the study described in Volume 6 of *Current Nephrology* showing that kidneys isolated from rats with a high alkali intake have a defect to lower urine pH when perfused in vitro, thus suggesting the kidney "remembers" the dietary intake from which it originated (52). These observations are of considerable interest from the clinical point of view because they strongly suggest that individuals with high dietary intake of potential HCO_3 will have a dormant distal acidification apparatus.

The effect of blood pH on acidification has been a subject of continued interest. In Volume 6 of *Current Nephrology* (2) we reviewed the data obtained in the turtle bladder showing that urinary acidification was a curvilinear function of serosal pH. Sasaki et al. (53) performed similar experiments in isolated proximal convoluted tubules of the rabbit. They showed that increasing the peritubular HCO_3 concentration, but not the mucosal HCO_3 concentration, inhibited HCO_3 absorption by 45%. The inhibitory effect of high peritubular HCO_3 on HCO_3 absorption was reversed by increasing bath P_{CO_2} and maintaining a high peritubular

HCO_3 concentration. This decrease in HCO_3 absorption could arise either because of increased HCO_3 permeability, which would allow HCO_3 to backleak into the lumen, or because of alterations in intracellular pH. The authors measured HCO_3 permeability and calculated that only a small fraction of the inhibition of HCO_3 absorption could be accounted for by increased passive loss of HCO_3 from peritubular fluid into the lumen. In contrast to the above findings, increasing luminal HCO_3 concentration led to an increase in HCO_3 absorption. These findings are similar to those observed in the turtle bladder and in the kidney in that an increase in mucosal HCO_3 concentration stimulates HCO_3 absorption, probably by reducing the H+ gradient against which the sodium–hydrogen ion antiporter operates. Increasing the peritubular concentration of HCO_3 reduces the electrochemical driving force for HCO_3 removal from the cell, leading to an increase in intracellular HCO_3 concentration and in intracellular pH, which in turn decreases the availability of protons for the sodium–hydrogen ion antiporter. The conclusion of this study is that HCO_3 absorption in the proximal tubule of the rabbit is a function of peritubular pH. These data would suggest that any maneuver that decreases HCO_3 removal from the cell should increase intracellular pH and decrease HCO_3 reabsorption. Recent measurements of intracellular pH in proximal tubule of the rabbit kidney showed an increase in intracellular pH with SITS, furosemide, and chloride removal from the bathing solution (54). Furosemide and chloride removal from the bath decreased HCO_3 removal from the cell, probably by inhibiting the Cl–HCO_3 exchange system. The disulfonic stilbene, SITS, directly inhibits the Cl–HCO_3 exchange system in red blood cells; the finding that this agent increases intracellular pH in the proximal tubule suggests that a Cl–HCO_3 exchange is also present in this system. Obviously, further studies are necessary to understand the mechanisms regulating intracellular pH in the proximal tubule since this factor seems to be important in the regulation of acidification not only in the distal but also in the proximal nephron.

RENAL TUBULAR ACIDOSIS

Nephrocalcinosis and Citrate Excretion

Brenner et al. studied the prevalence of nephrocalcinosis in the different types of RTA (42). The prevalence of nephrocalcinosis according to the localization and type of calcification in the kidney is shown in Table 3. The authors examined 82 radiographs of patients with RTA without prior knowledge of the type of RTA. The radiographs were examined for parenchymal (nephrocalcinosis) and for renal pelvicalyceal califications (nephrolithiasis). Nephrocalcinosis was present in 29% of all patients, and it occurred only in patients with distal RTA. When the group with distal

RTA was analyzed it was found that 56% of patients had nephrocalcinosis, 5% had nephrolithiasis, and 2% had both. The finding of nephrocalcinosis in distal RTA was more frequent in adults than in children (58% versus 10%). Thus the presence of nephrocalcinosis in a patient with RTA would be strong evidence of type I distal RTA.

The relationship between distal RTA and nephrocalcinosis is complex but of considerable interest. In some patients, the acidification defect is the consequence of nephrocalcinosis, whereas in others, the nephrocalcinosis is the consequence of the distal RTA. There is experimental and clinical evidence to suggest that certain conditions associated with chronic hypercalcemia or hypercalciuria can lead to a distal acidification defect. These conditions include hyperparathyroidism, hypercalcemia secondary to vitamin D intoxication, and medullary sponge kidney, to mention only a few (4). In some familial cases, the hypercalciuria also seems to lead to an acidification defect (55,56). In other patients, especially those with idiopathic distal RTA, the nephrocalcinosis seems to be the consequence of the distal acidification defect, since correction of metabolic acidosis leads to a decrease in the hypercalciuria and regression of the nephrocalcinosis (41).

To understand the mechanism whereby correction of distal RTA leads to regression of nephrocalcinosis, it is necessary to consider the mechanism whereby citrate excretion is altered in acid-base disturbances (57,58). Correction of the acidosis increases citrate excretion in patients with RTA. Although citrate excretion increases with acute metabolic alkalosis and with an increase in urine pH, citrate excretion is best correlated with intracellular pH of the kidney. An increase in intracellular pH increases citrate excretion and, conversely, a decrease in intracellular pH decreases citrate excretion. In the presence of RTA or chronic acetazolamide administration, citrate excretion decreases despite the presence of a high urine pH, presumably because the presence of metabolic acidosis leads to a decrease in intracellular pH, which in turn leads to a decrease in citrate excretion.

The mechanism whereby changes in intracellular pH alter citrate excretion has been partially studied. Metabolic alkalosis increases tissue citrate levels and could alter citrate excretion by impairing reabsorption of citrate from the proximal nephron because of the high level of citrate in the cell. Although this explanation is reasonable, other conditions capable of increasing tissue levels of citrate do not increase citrate excretion, suggesting that tissue citrate content does not regulate citrate reabsorption. The kidney is capable of taking up citrate both from the luminal and the basolateral membrane. When the plasma citrate levels are increased, citrate uptake across the basolateral membranes increases five times without an increase in citrate excretion. The citrate taken up by the tubule is either oxidized or transformed into glucose or other metabolic products. In the presence of a normal blood pH, plasma citrate levels are primarily regulated by uptake and metabolism. In metabolic acidosis, tissue citrate levels fall, and renal extraction of citrate increases. Conversely, in metabolic alkalosis citrate levels increase and the renal extraction of citrate decreases.

The effect of metabolic acidosis or alkalosis on citrate metabolism has been examined in tissue slices incubated at different pH (58). A decrease in pH increases the uptake, oxidation, and conversion of citrate to glucose. All these factors will decrease citrate levels. In vitro, an increase in pH of the medium decreases citrate oxidation, which increases citrate levels. Thus, the intracellular pH seems to alter citrate oxidation by modulating the rate of entry of citrate into the mitochondria. Studies performed with different buffers would appear to indicate that intracellular bicarbonate, and not other buffers, is the important regulator of citrate entry into the mitochondria. The effect of acidosis seems to be mediated by changes in intracellular bicarbonate concentration; this effect on citrate metabolism is present not only in the kidney but in other organs as well. In addition to pH, plasma calcium also seems to be an important regulator of citrate oxidation in the kidney, in that an increase in plasma calcium decreases citrate oxidation by the kidney. Thus, the conditions associated with hypercalcemia should be associated with an increased level of citrate in the tissue and enhanced excretion of citrate by the kidney.

In patients with proximal RTA, the increased excretion of amino acids and other organic anions would bind calcium and thereby prevent precipitation of calcium and nephrocalcinosis. In type I distal RTA, the decrease in citrate excretion prevents binding of calcium and leads to precipitation of calcium and nephrocalcinosis.

Hyperkalemic Renal Tubular Acidosis

The idiopathic forms of hyperkalemic RTA were reviewed in detail in Volume 6 of *Current Nephrology* (2). Sanjard et al. (59) studied a 13-year-old girl with severe hypertension, short stature, and hyperkalemic RTA. The hypertension was associated with expanded plasma volume and with suppressed plasma renin activity and plasma aldosterone. Dietary salt restriction or diuretic administration increased plasma renin activity and plasma aldosterone, which indicates that the supression of renin and of aldosterone was secondary to the expansion of the plasma volume. Administration of fludrocortisone led to a normal increase in potassium excretion and to a decrease in sodium excretion; thus, the distal nephron was responsive to aldosterone. This finding excludes the possibility of pseudohypoaldosteronism. The hyperkalemia was due to a defect in potassium excretion as assessed by the low levels of urine potassium for the degree of hyperkalemia. Administration of Na_2SO_4 in the presence of a low sodium diet increased potassium excretion to normal levels. The renal tubular acidosis was of the distal type, as assessed by the presence of low fractional HCO_3 excretion in the presence of acidosis. It is interesting that the patient was able to lower the urine pH maximally in the presence of acidosis but that net acid excretion was low mainly because of a decrease in ammonia excretion. Ingestion of a low salt diet corrected the hyperkalemia and increased net acid excretion by increasing ammonia excretion. In summary, all the abnormalities of this patient—hypertension, suppressed plasma renin activity and plasma aldosterone, hyperkalemia, and RTA—were corrected by a low salt diet or the administration of thiazide and furosemide. This case is very similar to that described by Schambelan et al. (60), which was reviewed in the last volume of *Current Nephrology* (2). Both patients behaved as if their tubules were avidly retaining sodium chloride, which leads to volume expansion, hypertension, and suppression of plasma renin activity and plasma aldosterone. The hyperkalemia and RTA can be explained by postulating the existence of abnormal permeability of the distal nephron to chloride. This chloride shunt would not allow the generation of a lumen negative potential difference and, hence, the lack of a favorable electric gradient for potassium and H+ secretion. When sodium delivery is increased with a nonreabsorbable anion, such as sulfate, the lumen negative voltage is established, which leads to normal potassium and H+ secretion.

The patient described by Sanjard et al. thus can be classified as having a chloride shunt, but the nature of the acidification defect of patients with a chloride shunt has not been completely studied. It is interesting that both patients reported in the literature were able to lower urine pH maximally in response to acidosis; their net acid excretion was low because of the decrease in ammonia excretion. Correction of the hyperkalemia increased net acid excretion, suggesting that suppression of ammonia production by the high level of potassium played a significant role in the inhibition of urinary acidification. It is unclear why these patients should be able to lower the pH maximally, since nullification of the distal nephron electric gradient by amiloride administration impairs the ability of experimental animals to lower urine pH maximally. It is possible that the low urine pH in these patients may reflect the low buffer capacity of this tubular fluid. Hyperkalemia could lead to a suppression of ammonia production that would lower urine ammonia concentration and urine buffer concentration. In the presence of decreased urine buffer concentration, the urine pH may be lowered maximally even though the function of the H+ pump is impaired by lack of a favorable electric gradient.

Distal Renal Tubular Acidosis in Systemic Disease

Distal RTA continues to be reported in association with systemic disease. Although the initial descriptions of distal RTA were of the idiopathic type, it is likely that in adults, distal RTA will frequently be associated with systemic disease. In multiple myeloma, proximal RTA is a well-recognized complication of the disease that may reflect the damage of the proximal tubule induced by light-chain proteins (61). More recently, cases of distal RTA have been described in patients with multiple myeloma. Lazar and Feinstein reported a patient with multiple myeloma and hyperchloremic acidosis who was unable to acidify urine (62). The patient had less than 5% fractional HCO_3 excretion in the urine at normal plasma HCO_3 levels, indicating the presence of distal RTA. It is interesting that the patient had normal serum potassium levels, but data for potassium excretion were not presented. The mechanism of distal RTA was not elucidated, but since the patient had a normal serum potassium level, the distal RTA was either a rate-dependent defect or an impairment of the proton pump (2). It is unknown whether the defect is the result of light-chain damage to the distal nephron. Experimental studies in animals should be undertaken to determine whether light-chain proteinuria can cause distal RTA.

The association of hyperthyroidism and distal RTA has been described in the literature. Bolonos et al. (63) described the association of distal RTA acidosis with hyperthyroidism and the presence of periodic paralysis without hypokalemia. The patient also had a defect in urine concentration. The patient was studied before and after treatment of hyperthyroidism. The defect in urine acidification and concentration did not correct, suggesting that either the association with hyperthyroidism was just coincidental or that the distal tubular damage caused by the hyperthyroidism was irreversible. The pathogenesis of the periodic paralysis in this patient was unclear but it was postulated to result from the hyperthyroidism and the mild potassium depletion present in the patient.

Allergia et al. described the presence of hypokalemic distal RTA in a patient with idiopathic hypergammaglobulinemia. Renal biopsy showed positive IgG and C_3 fluorescence in the interstitium and in the tubule. The patient had elevated levels of IgG and IgA and also had circulating immunocomplexes, and it is possible that the distal acidification defect was secondary to immunocomplex deposition in the tubule and the interstitium. These cases show that RTA may be found in association with a variety of systemic diseases; however, the mechanism responsible for the distal RTA has not been clarified.

Heparin-Induced Selective Hypoaldosteronism

Heparin sodium and heparinoids (polysulfonated mucopolysaccharides) have been confirmed as decreasing mineralocorticoid synthesis (65,66). This inhibition is thought to be located at the step at which corticosterone is converted to 18-hydroxycorticosterone. Heparin and heparinoid administration to normal subjects and to patients with primary and secondary hyperaldosteronism decreases aldosterone production and leads to potassium retention and sodium wastage. The sodium wastage increases plasma renin activity. Cortisol levels are normal indicating a selective inhibition of mineralocorticoid synthesis. Despite the well known inhibitory effect of these compounds on aldosterone synthesis, the syndrome of selective hypoaldosteronism has been found only infrequently in patients receiving heparin or heparinoids. Leehey et al. (67) reported the development of selective hypoaldosteronism presenting as hyperkalemic metabolic acidosis in a patient treated with heparin for 41 days. The patient had low levels of plasma aldosterone and high levels of plasma renin activity. Discontinuation of heparin therapy corrected the hyperkalemia and the metabolic acidosis and increased the levels of plasma aldosterone. Readministration of heparin led to reappearance of the hyperkalemic metabolic acidosis associated with a decrease in plasma levels of aldosterone. Thus, this study clearly establishes a link between the administration of heparin and the development of selective hypoaldosteronism. Review of the literature indicated the existence of only two case reports of heparin-induced hypoaldosteronism (68,69). One patient had received 20,000 units of heparin per day for 4 years and the second had received 20,000 units of heparin per day for 5 days. The reason for the rare occurrence of the syndrome of selective hypoaldosteronism in patients receiving these drugs is surprising since these compounds uniformly decrease aldosterone levels. It is possible that only patients who have other factors compromising potassium excretion, such as renal insufficiency, diabetes mellitus, and volume contraction, will develop the full blown syndrome. In subjects without these risk factors, heparin or heparinoid administration may decrease aldosterone, but hyperkalemia does not develop because the kidney is capable of maintaining potassium homeostasis if volume contraction or renal insufficiency is not present.

Renal Acidification Defect Induced by Lithium

The acidification defect induced by lithium was reviewed in detail in Volume 6 of *Current Nephrology* (2). Bank et al. (70) studied the effect of intraperitoneal injection of LiCl (4 mEq/kg/day for 3 days) to rats on urinary acidification. The animals developed metabolic acidosis and were unable to acidify urine, indicating the presence of a distal acidification defect. Micropuncture of the proximal tubule showed a small defect in proximal HCO_3 reabsorption leading to increased distal delivery of HCO_3. The inhibition of proximal HCO_3 reabsorption was attributed to inhibition of the sodium–hydrogen ion antiporter system by lithium. This hypothesis has recently been verified by studies of brush border membrane vesicles showing that lithium inhibits the sodium–hydrogen ion antiporter system (71). Micropuncture of the distal tubule showed normal rates of HCO_3 reabsorption, and the amount of HCO_3 present in the distal nephron of lithium treated rats was not different from that of controls. Lithium-treated rats, however, had significantly greater amounts of HCO_3 in the final urine than did control rats. The increased urine bicarbonate excretion of lithium-treated rats could result from either the defect in acidification in the collecting duct or a more profound effect of lithium on the deep nephrons. The authors also performed studies on the isolated turtle urinary bladder and confirmed the observations of Arruda et al. (72) that mucosal addition of lithium inhibited H+ secretion by the turtle bladder under open-circuited but not under short-circuited conditions. Furthermore, they confirmed that the acidification defect of lithium was voltage dependent, since restoration of the potential difference to baseline values returned H+ secretion to normal despite the continuing presence of lithium in the mucosal solution. In summary, these micropuncture studies confirm previous clearance and turtle bladder experiments showing that lithium administration induces a distal acidification defect that is voltage dependent. In addition, the study also shows that lithium induces a proximal defect in HCO_3 reabsorption attributed to an inhibition of the Na–H+ antiporter by lithium.

Renal Acidification in Elderly Subjects

Renal function of elderly subjects has recently been of interest to physiologists and nephrologists. A progressive decline in GFR and renal plasma flow with age has been described (73). There is also impaired capacity to concentrate and dilute the urine and to conserve sodium (73). It was reported that elderly patients have decreased acid excretion but this study was difficult to evaluate because the patients had a 50% decline in GFR as compared to young subjects (74).

Agarwal and Cabebe evaluated urinary acidification in subjects over 60 years old with the short ammonium chloride test and compared their response to results in younger subjects (73). Elderly subjects were able to lower the urine pH below 5.0. The increase in net acid excretion in the elderly subjects was significantly lower than that of control subjects. The decrease in net acid excretion was mainly due to a decrease in ammonia excretion. Although the elderly subjects had a slightly lower GFR than the controls (76 ml/min versus 92 ml/min), ammonia excretion corrected per GFR was still lower in the elderly subjects than in the controls. In addition, the control subjects increased ammonia excretion as the pH was lowered, whereas the elderly subjects failed to display the same response. For any given urine pH, ammonia excretion was lower in the elderly subjects than in controls. These findings suggest that ammonia production is decreased by the kidney of elderly subjects. The mechanism of the decrease in ammonia excretion in the elderly was not clarified by the present study. Since aldosterone secretion is known to decrease with age, it is possible that this hormone, which plays an important role in acid excretion, may be involved in the diminished capacity of the kidney to excrete acid. These findings indicate that elderly subjects have a decreased ability to increase acid excretion and thus may be more vulnerable to metabolic acidosis.

Proximal Renal Tubular Acidosis in Association with Renal Amyloidosis

The effect of multiple myeloma on electrolyte and acid-base homeostasis has been described above. Rochman et al. (75) described a patient with chronic lymphocytic leukemia and κ light-chain proteinuria. The patient developed hypokalemic hyperchloremic metabolic acidosis with hypophosphatemia and hypouricemia. The excretion of uric acid, glucose, and phosphate in urine was high, indicating the presence of a Fanconi syndrome. Autopsy showed the presence of amyloid fibrils in the tubular basement membrane, in the tubular lumen, and in the interstitium.

Fanconi syndrome has been described in association with light-chain proteinuria. It is thought to be caused by reabsorption of the light-chain protein, which causes damage of the proximal tubule, as shown by Pirani et al. (76). Their study suggests another mechanism for the development of Fanconi syndrome, that is, that amyloid infiltration of the proximal tubule may also be responsible for the tubular damage. It is impossible to state with certainty whether the light-chain proteinuria or the amyloidosis was responsible for the Fanconi syndrome. The presence of "amyloid" cast in the tubular lumen might suggest a role for the amyloid in the tubular damage. The message from this study is that the presence of Fanconi syndrome in patients with leukemia can be caused by the rare occurrence of light-chain proteinuria or the presence of amyloidosis. More common is the development of hypokalemia due to renal potassium wastage, which is thought to be the result of tubular cell injury by lysozymes liberated by the leukemic cells.

METABOLIC ACIDOSIS

Ketoacidosis

New approaches to the treatment of diabetic ketoacidosis continue to be sought. Patients with diabetic ketoacidosis usually have high serum phosphate levels but are actually phosphate depleted. The phosphate depletion is due to urinary phosphate losses induced by the glycosuria and probably also to the lack of dietary intake of phosphate. Administration of insulin to these patients causes a rapid decline in serum phosphate levels because of the rapid shift of phosphate into the cell. The decrease in serum phosphate may reach levels reported to cause many of the manifestations of the severe syndrome of profound hypophosphatemia, which includes rhabdomyolysis, cardiomyopathy, and alterations in the central nervous system. Initial studies suggested that phosphate replacement could be beneficial in treatment of diabetic ketoacidosis by reducing the time needed to correct the acidosis as well as decreasing the amount of insulin required to correct the acidosis.

Table 4. Serum Phosphate Levels During the Course of Diabetic Ketoacidosis Therapy

Group	Serum Phosphate Levels (mg/dl)				
	0 hr	4 hr	8 hr	16 hr	24 hr
1. n = 15; no phosphate	5.1 ± 2.3	3.9 ± 1.6	2.1 ± 0.8	1.8 ± 0.6	1.9 ± 0.6
2. n = 17; sodium phosphate, 15 mmol	4.9 ± 2.3	3.7 ± 2.0	2.8 ± 0.8	2.4 ± 0.8	2.0 ± 0.6
3. n = 12; sodium phosphate, 45 mmol	4.9 ± 1.3	4.2 ± 3.3	2.8 ± 1.4	2.5 ± 0.7	2.3 ± 0.9

SOURCE: Wilson HK et al: *Arch Intern Med* 142:517–520, 1982. Reproduced with permission.

Wilson and co-workers (77) evaluated the efficacy of phosphate replacement therapy in diabetic ketoacidosis. Forty-four patients with diabetic ketoacidosis were randomly assigned to three treatment groups: one group received no phosphate replacement; the second group received 15 mmol of sodium phosphate 4 hours after treatment was begun; the third group received 15 mmol of sodium phosphate at 2, 6, and 10 hours after beginning treatment. In all other aspects the treatment protocol was very similar. Table 4 shows the levels of serum phosphate in the three groups. The group that received only one dose of 15 mmol of phosphate had a decline in serum phosphate at 16 and 24 hours, whereas the third group had a serum phosphate level that was greater than that of controls, but there was a significant decrease in serum phosphate levels at 16–24 hours. The results of this study clearly indicate that phosphate replacement did not affect the duration of acidosis, the amount of insulin required to correct acidosis, muscle enzyme levels, or the rate of glucose disappearance. These studies, therefore, strongly suggest that routine phosphate replacement is not indicated in patients with diabetic ketoacidosis. It should be pointed out, however, that if the serum phosphate level is initially low, then phosphate replacement is indicated to prevent the serum phosphate from falling to dangerous levels of less than 1 mg/dl.

It could be argued that since phosphate replacement in the present study did not prevent the decline in the serum phosphate, aggressive phosphate replacement capable of preventing a decrease in serum phosphate could be beneficial. Figure 5 shows the amount of phosphate used in various studies of diabetic ketoacidosis. It is clear that doses ranging from 40–220 mmol are needed to maintain the serum phosphate within the normal range in diabetic ketoacidosis. High doses of phosphate may cause hypocalcemia, metastatic calcification, and acute renal failure. The obvious conclusion from this study is that only in patients that present initially with low serum phosphate levels should phosphate replacement

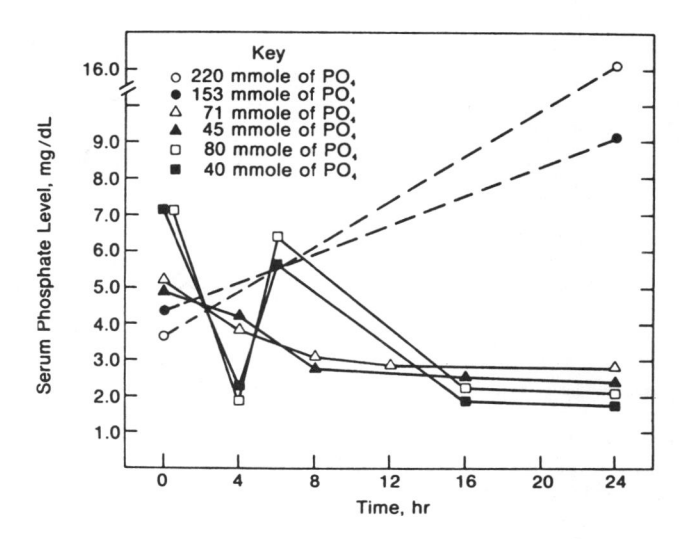

Figure 5. Changes in serum phosphate level during phosphate (PO$_4$ given as the sodium salt) replacement in diabetic ketoacidosis reported by various authors. (Wilson HK et al. *Arch Int Med* 142:517–520, 1982. Reproduced by permission.)

be used. Phosphate replacement could be either in the form of sodium or potassium phosphate. Since potassium requirements are invariably greater than phosphate requirements, phosphate replacement should be in the form of sodium phosphate while potassium is replaced as potassium chloride.

It has been generally accepted that in ketoacidosis, the increase in the ketoacids leads to an increase in the anion gap, which is accompanied by a symmetrical decrease in plasma HCO$_3$ (78–80). In several studies, it was observed that the mean increase in the anion gap was equal to the mean decrease in the plasma HCO$_3$. Although this contention has been widely accepted, it may not be entirely correct. Adrogue and co-workers (78) correctly pointed out that several factors may alter the 1:1 stoichiometry between the increase in anion gap and the decrease in plasma HCO$_3$. There are several buffers present in the extracellular fluid, all of which can accept protons from the ketoacids and a 1:1 relationship would be expected only if HCO$_3$ were the only buffer capable of accepting H+. Thus, the increase in plasma ketoacids should be equal to the combined decrease in plasma HCO$_3$ and other nonbicarbonate buffers. Furthermore, some of the ketoacids may be buffered inside the cell; the H+ entering the intracellular fluid is exchanged for sodium or potassium which leaves the cell to the extracellular fluid. Another mechanism capable of increasing the anion gap is volume contraction, which increases the concentration of plasma proteins and also impairs the excretion of the ketoacids. Gain of HCO$_3$ (either from vomiting or from parenteral administration) will also

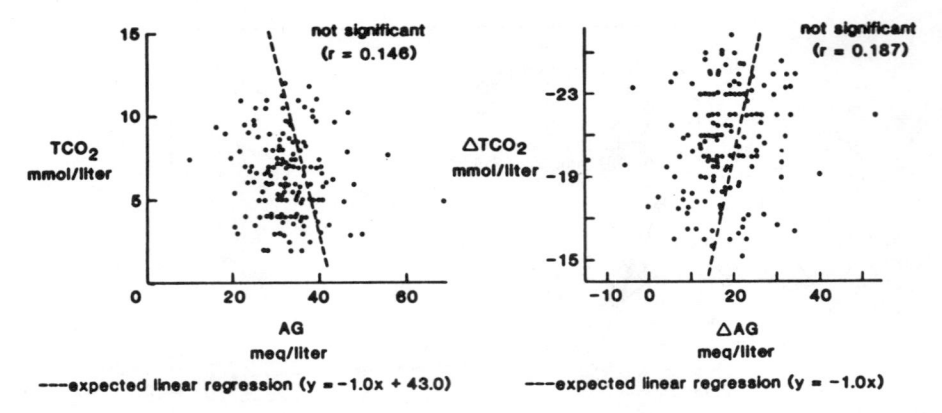

Figure 6. Relationship between the level of unmeasured anions in plasma and the severity of the metabolic acidosis for diabetic ketoacidosis. The left panel relates the values of plasma anion gap (AG) to serum total CO₂ content (TCO₂), and the right panel compares the excess anion (ΔAG) with the bicarbonate deficit (ΔTCO₂) on admission. No significant correlations were found in either of these relations. Each symbol represents an admission (n = 150). Broken lines represent the expected significant linear regressions between each set of values in pure anion-gap acidosis; the corresponding theoretical equations are presented at the bottom. (Adrogue HJ et al: *N Engl J Med* 307:1603–1610, 1982. Reproduced by permission.)

increase the plasma HCO₃ without correcting the anion gap. All these factors may influence the relationship between the increment in the anion gap and the decrement in the plasma HCO₃. Intrigued by these clinical physiologic considerations, Adrogue et al. studied acid-base patterns in 196 admissions for diabetic keoacidosis. The study was divided in three parts: 150 admissions were studied restrospectively, 42 admissions were studied prospectively, and a prospective balance study was done on four patients. Essentially the same results were obtained in the prospective and in the retrospective studies. Androgue et al. observed, as had previous investigators, that the mean decrease in plasma HCO₃ was equal to the mean increase in the anion gap. However, the correlation between total plasma HCO₃ or the total decrement in plasma HCO₃ and total increase (or Δ increment) in anion gap was poor and not significant. In other words, instead of a predicted slope of 1, a total lack of correlation between the increase in the anion gap and the decrease in plasma HCO₃ was observed. It is clear from Figure 6 that in many patients with ketoacidosis, the anion gap was normal or actually decreased.

If the anion gap is normal or decreased in the face of metabolic acidosis, then hyperchloremia must be present. Hyperchloremia is known to occur during the first 4–8 hours of recovery from ketoacidosis, but the study of Adrogue et al. clearly demonstrates that hyperchloremia is present at admission in many patients with diabetic ketoacidosis. In pure anion gap

ACID-BASE METABOLISM   **333**

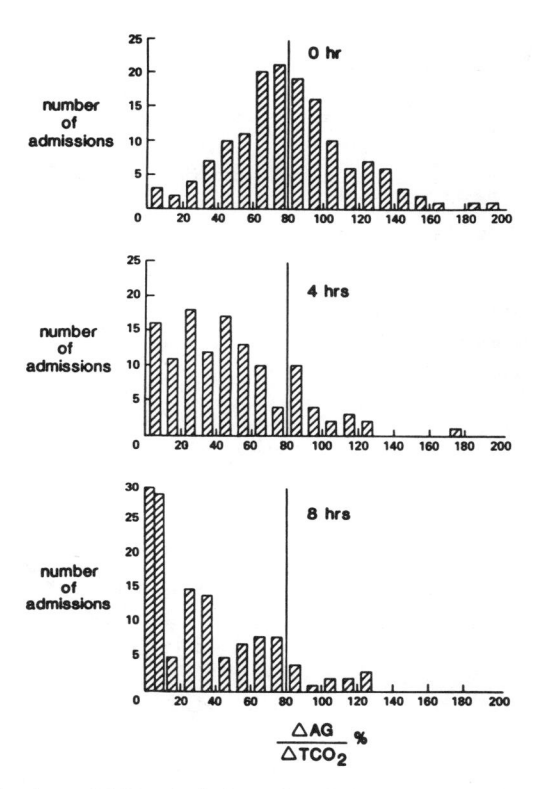

Figure 7. Distribution of 150 admissions for diabetic ketoacidosis according to the underlying mechanism of the metabolic acidosis, as evaluated from the acid-base and electrolyte composition of the plasma. Each panel shows the distribution according to the fraction of the bicarbonate deficit that is accounted for by the retention of anions ($\Delta AG/\Delta TOC_2\%$) on admission (0 hr) and 4 and 8 hours after the initiation of therapy, respectively. The vertical line drawn at 80% arbitrarily separates admissions of patients with mainly anion-gap acidosis. Although about half the patients had a component of hyperchloremic acidosis on admission, most of them (91%) had hyperchloremic acidosis 8 hours afterward. (Adrogue HS et al: *N Engl J Med* 307:1603–1610, 1982. Reproduced by permission.)

acidosis, the increase in plasma anion gap should account for 100% of the decrement in plasma HCO_3. In other words, the Δ increase in the anion gap divided by the Δ decrease in plasma HCO_3 (expressed as a percentage) should be 100%. If the increase in Δ anion gap is less than the decrease in plasma HCO_3 (i.e., the ratio is less than 100%), then a component of hyperchloremia must be present. Adrogue et al. arbitrarily chose the value of less than 80% to define the presence of a component of hyperchloremic acidosis. As can be seen from Figure 7, 52% of the patients had a component of hyperchloremic acidosis on admission (0 hours in Fig. 7).

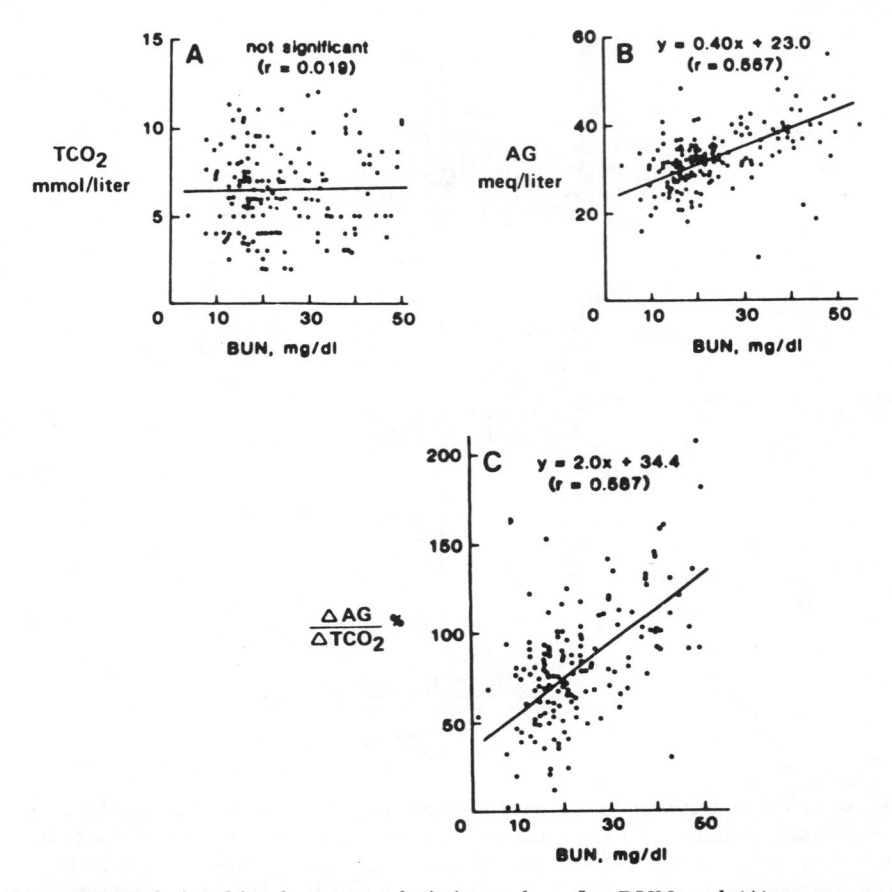

Figure 8. Relationships between admission values for BUN and (A) serum total CO_2 content (TCO_2), (B) the plasma anion gap (AG), and (C) the fraction of the bicarbonate deficit accounted for by the retention of anions ($\Delta AG/\Delta TCO_2 \%$). Each symbol represents an admission (n = 150). Although no significant correlation was found between BUN and TCO_2, significant correlations were found between BUN and the plasma anion gap and between BUN and the fraction of the bicarbonate deficit that is accounted for by the increase in plasma anion gap. (Adrogue HJ et al: *N Engl J Med* 307:1603–1610, 1982. Reproduced by permission.)

Volume contraction could influence the level of the anion gap. The authors studied the correlation between the level of the anion gap and blood urea nitrogen (BUN). The increase in BUN was thought to reflect the presence of volume contraction, and this was subsequently confirmed by showing normalization of BUN with volume replacement. Although plasma HCO_3 did not correlate with BUN, the anion gap was significantly correlated with BUN with a correlation coefficient of 0.557 (Fig. 8). They also found a correlation between the fraction of the HCO_3 deficit (accounted for by the increase in anion gap) and BUN. What is the reason for the correlation between the anion gap and BUN? The authors argue convincingly that the correlation between BUN and the increase in the anion gap is not the result of retention of phosphate and sulfate by the kidney. If this were the case, one would expect that the decrease in total HCO_3 should be correlated with BUN, which was not the case. They further pointed out that the slope of the relationship between the anion gap and BUN is five times greater than the slope expected in renal insufficiency. From these observations, the authors suggest that volume contraction increases the retention of the ketoacids, and this leads to high anion gap metabolic acidosis. In patients who are able to maintain a good salt and water intake, severe volume contraction does not develop. In these patients, the ketoacids which have titrated the plasma HCO_3 are excreted as sodium or potassium salts of the ketoacid. Acidosis develops and the kidney is stimulated to retain sodium. Sodium can be retained mainly as NaCl as or $NaHCO_3$. During the development of ketoacidosis, $NaHCO_3$ reabsorption is complete, and because of the fact that plasma HCO_3 is decreased, the only anion available to be reabsorbed with the sodium is chloride; thus, chloride is reabsorbed at a greater rate than normal, leading to hyperchloremic acidosis. This is the same mechanism, proposed many years ago, to explain the presence of hyperchloremic acidosis in renal insufficiency (81). Presence of hyperchloremic acidosis suggests the presence of moderate volume contraction. If volume contraction becomes more severe, the GFR decreases and organic acids are retained and a high anion gap develops. This hypothesis was confirmed by balance studies showing that chloride is retained in excess of sodium, leading to development of hyperchloremic metabolic acidosis during the recovery phase of diabetic ketoacidosis. The retention of chloride in excess of sodium is caused by the obligatory loss of sodium by the ketoacids. Thus, the proportion of sodium that is reabsorbed as a chloride salt is increased, which leads to hyperchloremia. Obviously, the loss of ketoacids in the urine represents the wastage of potential HCO_3. The presence of hyperchloremic metabolic acidosis should therefore be associated with delayed time to correct the metabolic acidosis. Indeed, Adrogue et al. found that in patients with hyperchloremic acidosis, recovery from metabolic acidosis was significantly slower than in patients with high anion gap metabolic acidosis.

The explanation proposed by Adrogue et al. for the development of hyperchloremic metabolic acidosis is somewhat different than that proposed by Oh et al. (80) who studied eight patients before and during recovery from diabetic ketoacidosis. They showed that during the recovery phase of diabetic ketoacidosis, sodium was retained and net acid excretion by the kidney was increased, indicating that the kidney was generating HCO_3. Although Oh and associates concluded that renal loss of ketoacids was the ultimate factor responsible for the development of hyperchloremic metabolic acidosis, they proposed that the lack of disparity between the increase in anion gap and the decrease in plasma HCO_3 was due to the fact that the volume of distribution of ketoacids was different than the volume of distribution of HCO_3. The organic acids would be confined to the extracellular space; once converted to HCO_3, they are distributed in the intracellular and extracellular compartments and thus the increase in extracellular HCO_3 is not paralleled by the symmetrical decrease in the anion gap. Although this is an interesting hypothesis, the volume of distribution of organic acids is not known with certainty. The mechanism proposed by Adrogue et al. is more appealing and is substantiated by the data presented. In summary, the finding of hyperchloremic metabolic acidosis in a patient with diabetic ketoacidosis or renal failure indicates the presence of moderate volume contraction. More severe volume contraction impairs the excretion of the acids and leads to high anion gap metabolic acidosis (81).

Metabolic Acidosis in Carcinoid Syndrome

In patients with carcinoid syndrome, persistent diarrhea, and metabolic acidosis, $NaHCO_3$ administration is the usual form of therapy. Feldman (82) reported the use of parachlorophenylalanine, an inhibitor of serotonin synthesis, in the treatment of diarrhea of patients with carcinoid syndrome. Approximately 10% of the patients in his series developed metabolic acidosis and/or hypokalemia. In some of the patients, serotonin antagonists failed to decrease the diarrhea and ameliorate the metabolic acidosis. Parachlorophenylalanine (an investigational drug) 250–500 mg every 6 hours decreased the amount of diarrhea and corrected the metabolic acidosis. Serum serotonin and urinary levels of 5-hydroxyindolacetic acid fell significantly with therapy. The mechanism of the diarrhea in the carcinoid syndrome was not elucidated, but experimental studies suggest that serotonin may stimulate electrolyte secretion in the bowel; therefore, inhibition of serotonin synthesis may prove beneficial in patients with carcinoid syndrome and life-threatening diarrhea.

LACTIC ACIDOSIS

Treatment of Experimental Lactic Acidosis

Lactic acidosis is one of the most common causes of metabolic acidosis in clinical practice. It is associated with a high mortality despite aggressive $NaHCO_3$ therapy (83–85). Recent studies (86) have even suggested a detrimental effect of bicarbonate therapy in certain forms of lactic acidosis. Therefore, interest has developed in new therapeutic approaches to lactic acidosis. Lactic acidosis is found in a variety of clinical settings: tissue hypoxia, diabetes mellitus, liver disease, malignancy, drug therapy including phenformin, and inborn errors of metabolism. The evaluation of the efficacy of therapy in lactic acidosis is hampered by the diversity of etiologies that generate lactic acidosis of variable prognoses. Hence the necessity of studying experimental models of lactic acidosis in which the variables capable of influencing the course of lactic acidosis can be monitored and the efficacy of different forms of therapy prospectively evaluated.

Arieff et al. (87,88) utilized the phenformin model of lactic acidosis to study the effect of $NaHCO_3$ therapy. Phenformin induces lactic acidosis both by increasing splanchnic bed lactate production and by decreasing hepatic uptake of lactate. Lactic acid levels of greater than 5 mmol were induced in diabetic dogs by phenformin administration and the effect of $NaHCO_3$ or NaCl therapy on the mortality of the lactic acidosis was evaluated. They found that mortality was similar in both $NaHCO_3$- and NaCl-treated animals. Of particular interest was the finding of a decrease in cardiac output and intracellular pH of the liver in dogs treated with $NaHCO_3$ but not with NaCl. In addition, $NaHCO_3$ treatment resulted in an increase in extrahepatic splanchnic lactate production, and despite continuous infusion of $NaHCO_3$, blood bicarbonate and pH were unchanged. Several mechanisms could account for the increase in lactate production with $NaHCO_3$ administration. Bicarbonate administration may cause tissue hypoxia secondary to the acute elevation of pH that impairs O_2 unloading into tissues by the Bohr effect, causing an acute shift of the oxygen–hemoglobin dissociation curve to the left. The decrease in cardiac output alone can cause tissue underperfusion and hypoxia. The reason for the greater fall in cardiac output in $NaHCO_3$-treated animals is unclear. The increased lactate production in animals treated with $NaHCO_3$ could be caused either by a direct effect of $NaHCO_3$ or by gut ischemia due to lowered cardiac output. The rise in blood lactate was not due to decreased hepatic extraction, as liver lactate uptake was the same in both NaCl- and $NaHCO_3$-treated animals.

The rise in lactate levels with $NaHCO_3$ therapy may not be unique to this experimental model. A similar increase in lactate production has been noted in a cancer patient with lactic acidosis (89,90). Fields et al. (90) described a patient with cancer of the colon metastatic to the liver and lactic acidosis with lactate levels of 15 mmol/L. Despite aggressive bicarbonate therapy there was no change in either plasma bicarbonate level or anion gap, suggesting continued lactate production. Urinary lactate excretion was high, again suggesting increased lactate production. An explanation of the increase in lactate production with $NaHCO_3$ therapy may be found in the increase in pyruvate production caused by the transient alkalemia. The transient increase in blood pH caused by $NaHCO_3$ administration activates the enzyme phosphofructokinase and as a result there is an increase in glycolysis. As the equilibrium constant for lactate dehydrogenase normally favors lactate production and the normal tissue concentration ratio of lactate to pyruvate is 10:1, is blood lactate levels increase.

The failure of NaHCO$_3$ to improve the lactic acidosis prompted these authors to investigate the efficacy of new therapeutic approaches on experimental lactic acidosis (91). Dichloroacetate (DCA) is a drug that lowers blood levels of lactate and pyruvate by inhibiting the regulatory enzyme pyruvate dehydrogenase kinase and activating pyruvate dehydrogenase (PDH) (91,92). The latter is the rate-limiting enzyme that regulates entry of pyruvate into the Krebs cycle; activation of PDH leads to oxidation of pyruvate to acetyl-CoA (12). There is thus a decrease in pyruvate and lactate levels. Arieff et al. (88) studied the effect of dichloroacetate on two experimental models of lactic acidosis; one model utilized diabetic dogs treated with phenformin and the second model was a functional hepatectomy produced by shunting the hepatic portal vein into the inferior vena cava and ligating the hepatic artery. The animals were then treated with DCA or NaHCO$_3$, and measured serially for bicarbonate, glucose, cardiac output, intracellular pH, lactate, and pyruvate in arterial, hepatic, and portal circulations. Significant lactic acidosis was induced in both models, as assessed by the fact that lactate levels rose to values greater than 8 mmol/liter. In the phenformin model, the 4-hour mortality was 22% in the DCA-treated animals as compared to 91% with NaHCO$_3$ treatment. Blood pH rose with DCA therapy but was unchanged with bicarbonate therapy. It is likely that larger doses of bicarbonate could have normalized the blood pH, but the enormous quantity of NaHCO$_3$ required to achieve a normal blood pH would have increased serum osmolality to fatal levels. As noted in the previous study described above (88), cardiac index declined with bicarbonate therapy and increased in the DCA-treated animals. Blood lactate increased after NaHCO$_3$ therapy while DCA treatment resulted in a fall in blood lactate levels. Of particular interest was the decrease in intracellular pH of the liver with NaHCO$_3$ while in the animals treated with DCA the intracellular pH rose and this was associated with increase hepatic lactate extraction. In summary, DCA treatment resulted in an increase in survival, cardiac index, serum bicarbonate, and blood pH, and a fall in blood lactate levels. In the "hepatectomy model" DCA treatment also increased blood pH and cardiac output, decreased lactate levels, and improved survival as compared to NaHCO$_3$-treated dogs.

What is the mechanism responsible for the beneficial effect of DCA in lactic acidosis? DCA increased hepatic lactate extraction from a negative value in phenformin-treated dogs to values similar to controls, whereas in NaHCO$_3$-treated dogs, lactate uptake was unchanged. These findings suggest that DCA improved lactic acidosis in part by increasing lactate removal by the liver. The authors, therefore, postulate that the increased hepatic uptake may be caused by the increase in pH of liver cells in the

DCA-treated animals, which results in increased glucose synthesis. The major rate-limiting enzyme for glucose synthesis is pyruvate carboxylase, which is a pH-sensitive enzyme whose activity falls when pH decreases below 6.9. Lactate is a major substrate for gluconeogenesis and inactivation of the enzyme pyruvate carboxylase at the low intracellular pH found in the control and NaHCO$_3$-treated animals may have been responsible for the decreased hepatic lactate extraction. It is unknown whether DCA caused an increase in cellular lactate uptake and proton consumption, thereby raising intracellular pH (pHi), or whether it had a direct action on intracellular pH. DCA pretreatment in the "hepatectomy" model also resulted in a decrement in blood lactate levels. Since a functioning liver was absent in this model, these results suggest that DCA may also cause a decrease in extrahepatic lactate production. The source of the extrahepatic lactate is undefined as the gut lactate production in DCA-treated animals was similar to that in controls. The mechanism for the decrease in extrahepatic lactate production is unclear. In addition to these biochemical effects, part of the effect of DCA to improve lactic acidosis may be hemodynamic. The improvement in cardiac output with DCA treatment may be due to the less severe acidosis and to the fact that DCA therapy may improve myocardial lactate extraction, thereby raising intracellular pH of the heart and thus improving cardiac contractility.

The finding of this study clearly shows that in two different experimental models of lactic acidosis, DCA treatment improves survival and various biochemical and physiological parameters. This study suggests that DCA therapy by activating PDH, may be useful in the treatment of lactic acidosis in the absence of hypoxia. It should be pointed out, however, that the clinical relevance of these experimental models of lactic acidosis is unclear. Phenformin is no longer available for clinical use in the USA; it is cardiotoxic, decreases cardiac output, and causes an underperfusion of the splanchic bed, thus increasing lactate production. Furthermore, the "hepatectomy model" may not have a similar clinical counterpart. Thus, although the findings of DCA treatment in experimental lactic acidois are provocative, the clinical applications of this drug are unclear at the present time and randomized studies comparing DCA to NaHCO$_3$ in certain types of clinical lactic acidosis are indicated.

As discussed above, new approaches to the treatment of lactic acidosis are being sought experimentally. These approaches in one way or another are based on enhanced utilization of the excess lactate through various metabolic pathways. These studies have mainly employed experimental models of lactic acidosis and the clinical evaluation of these approaches has yet to be performed. One such experimental treatment of lactic acidosis involves the use of pyridoxine α-ketoglutorate (PAK), which has been shown to reduce ketosis and lactate levels in experimental animals. Capetti et al. (93) evaluated the efficacy of PAK in lactic acidosis induced in the rat by biguanide administration. Metformin, a biguanide similar to phenformin was used because of its short half-life. Metformin administration to rats resulted in an increase of lactate to seven times above the baseline values and in a decrease in plasma glucose. Pretreatment of the animals with PAK or administration of PAK after administration of metformin significantly blunted the increase in plasma lactate and the decrease in blood glucose levels. The mortality rate was 83% in the control animals and 10% in the animals treated with PAK. It is unclear from the study whether the mortality was related to the lactic acidosis per se or to the severe hypoglycemia that developed in the animals treated with metformin alone. Metformin is thought to produce lactic acidosis by blocking gluconeogenesis and preventing conversion of lactate and pyruvate to glucose. The mechanism whereby PAK improves lactic acidosis was not clarified by the present study but it was postulated that PAK partially reverses the inhibitory effect of metformin on gluconeogenesis. Others have postulated that PAK promotes oxidation of the pyruvate by stimulating the entry of this metabolite into the Krebs cycle.

The possible clinical application of PAK to decrease lactate levels in patients was evaluated by Belvisi et al. (94) in 25 cirrhotic patients. Twenty patients received 2300 mg of PAK dissolved in 250 ml of saline by intravenous drip and 25 patients received a placebo. Both groups were treated for 10 days; lactate levels decreased from 22.7 mg/dl to 16 mg/dl and ammonia decreased from 110.6 μg/dl to 68 μg/dl. It was not determined whether larger doses of PAK would lead to a greater reduction in plasma lactate levels. Lactate and ammonia levels remained unchanged in patients receiving placebo. No apparent serious side effects were observed with this short-term administration but the long-term effects of PAK administration have yet not been evaluated. It remains unestablished whether PAK is effective in other forms of lactic acidosis, other than that induced by biguanide intoxication. The low incidence of side effects makes this compound an attractive drug to be evaluated in the treatment of certain types of lactic acidosis.

The optimal form of alkali therapy in lactic acidosis is unknown. Different etiologies may require different sources of bicarbonate. There are a number of congenital forms of lactic acidosis due to inborn errors of metabolism. These include enzyme deficiencies in the Embden-Meyerhof pathway, Krebs cycle, pruvate dehydrogenase complex, and the respiratory chain (Table 5). (For a complete discussion of congenital lactic acidosis see reference 95.) Hamat et al. (96) evaluated the effect of acetate therapy in a model of "lactic acidosis" caused by a defect in pyruvate oxidation. They postulated that acetate would function as an alternate subtrate for the Krebs cycle, bypassing pyruvate. The ATP and citrate thus generated would inhibit phosphofructokinase, thereby decreasing glycolysis and lactate accumulation. In their model, "lactic acidosis" was produced in a rat hemidiaphragm by inhibitors of pyruvate oxidation in the absence of hypoxia. Pyruvate metabolism requires entry into mito-

Table 5. Enzyme Deficiencies Associated with Congenital Lactic Acidosis

Glucose-6-phosphatase
Fructose bisphosphatase
Phosphoenolpyruvate carboxykinase
Pyruvate carboxylase
Pyruvate dehydrogenase
Cytochrome aa$_3$
Cytochrome b
NADH-CoQ Reductase

chondria either by diffusion or by a transport system. The authors used two compounds to produce "lactic acidosis." Cyanolhydroxycinnamate (CNCM) is a specific inhibitor of mitochondrial pyruvate transport and when added to the preparation caused almost a twofold increase in cytosol pyruvate concentration. Aminooxyacetate (AOA) causes cytoplasmic pyruvate levels to fall by inhibiting the main shuttle system of cytoplasmic reducing power (NADH) into mitochondria. The addition of AOA results in a rise in cytoplasmic NADH and fall in pyruvate levels, thus decreasing the rate of pyruvate diffusion into the mitochondria. The rise in cytoplasmic NADH shifts the equilibrium of the reaction catalyzed by lactate dehydrogenase towards lactate. With the addition of both AOA and CNCM, lactate production in the rat hemidiaphragm increased by 50%. The authors analyzed the effect of acetic acid and sodium acetate on lactate production. Lactate output was decreased by two-thirds with the addition of acetic acid. A similar but smaller decrement was found with the addition of sodium acetate. A small, but statistically significant, decrease in lactate production was observed with the addition of HCl to the medium, suggesting that the decrease in pH per se causes a fall in lactate levels, presumably by the inhibition of glycolysis secondary to the acidemia. The authors proposed that this model might be representative of the type of lactic acidosis due to a genetic defect in the enzyme pyruvate–dehydrogenase (PDH) (Table 5); therefore, acetate therapy may have theoretical advantages in patients with lactic acidosis due to a defect in PDH since it can bypass the metabolic block and thus improve the lactic acidosis. The efficacy of acetate therapy in this form of congenital lactic acidosis has not been evaluated and it should be compared to the efficacy of NaHCO$_3$ in the long-term treatment of this acidosis. The authors, however, raise the possible importance of individualizing the treatment on the basis of the etiology of the lactic acidosis.

D-Lactic Acidosis

High anion gap metabolic acidosis and D-lactic acidosis were reviewed in Volumes 4 and 5 of *Current Nephrology*. Acidosis caused by the D-sterioisomer of lactate has been recently recognized in humans (97). The syndrome of D-lactic acidosis is well known to veterinarians and occurs in ruminants overfed with grain (98). The bacterial fermentation of carbohydrate to D-lactic acid occurs in the digestive tract and it is subsequently absorbed into the blood, resulting in acidosis. Treatment of wheat-induced lactic acidosis in lambs has been studied by Muir et al. (98). They induced lactic acidosis in lambs by wheat feeding; fermentation of the carbohydrate by *Streptococcus bovis* was believed to be responsible for the D-lactate production. Survival was improved and lactic acidosis was prevented by a single dose of the antibiotic thiopeptin. In a human with this syndrome, both the L and D forms of lactate are produced but only the enzyme capable of metabolizing the L-form is present, allowing the D-form to accumulate.

The occurrence of anion gap acidosis in humans due to D-lactic acid was first reported by Oh et al. (97) in a patient with bowel resection and history of ingesting *Lactobacillus acidophillus* tablets. Recently there have been additional reports of patients who presented with neurologic symptoms and metabolic acidosis, which were subsequently proven to be due to D-lactic acidosis (98–100). Carr et al. (99) reported a 36-year-old patient who had jejunoileal bypass for morbid obesity at age 31. He presented with transient episodes of hypothalamic dysfunction consisting of hypersomnia, thirst, irritability, dysarthria, and ataxia associated with high anion gap metabolic acidosis. Urine was analyzed by gas chromatography and mass spectrometry to identify the nature of the unmeasured anions, and abnormal levels of lactic and phenolic acids were found. Serum lactate levels were normal upon routine laboratory assay to measure lactate. This assay uses the enzyme L-lactate dehydrogenase, which is sensitive only to the L form of lactate and thus does not detect D-lactate. The presence of D-lactate was suggested by gas chromatography, which, however, does not distinguish between the two isomeric forms of lactic acid. The presence of D-lactate was confirmed by analyzing the serum with D-lactate dehydrogenase, and levels of 1.8–3.3 mmol/liter of D-lactate were found. D-Lactate was also detected in the urine. The patient was treated with 2 g oral neomycin for 2 days and ampicillin 2 g daily for 10 days with complete chemical and clinical remission.

Stoleburg and his colleagues (100) described two patients with short bowel and D-lactic acidosis. One patient had extensive surgical resection of the small bowel for mesenteric infarction and the second patient had a jejunoileal bypass for morbid obesity. Both patients presented with neurologic symptoms of lethargy, dysarthia, and ataxia and an elevated anion gap metabolic acidosis. Both had elevated D-lactate levels. Oral vancomycin therapy resolved symptoms in both patients. In search of the bacteria responsible for production of D-lactate, stool samples from both patients and controls were cultured anaerobically. Lactate production was measured from each organism isolated, before and after therapy. The

Table 6. D-Lactic Acidosis

Clinical setting	Presence of small bowel bypass or resection, neurologic symptoms, and presence of high anion gap metabolic acidosis
Presumptive diagnosis	High lactate levels by gas chromatography or by proton nuclear magnetic resonance but normal levels by L-lactate dehydrogenase assay
Definitive diagnosis	Assay of lactate by D-lactate dehydrogenase assay
Treatment	Oral nonabsorbable antibiotic such as neomycin or vancomycin

stool flora before treatment showed a predominance of gram positive anaerobes and relative absence of *Bacteroides* species, which are normally the most common stool bacteria. The number of D-lactate-producing species seemed to be higher in the patients than in controls. With therapy, the number of the lactate-producing strains decreased in both patients.

It is speculated that multiple factors contribute to the D-lactic acidosis, but an abnormality of the intestine seems to be necessary for the development of the syndrome. The fact that the disease remitted with fasting in one patient supports the intestinal origin of D-lactate and requirement of a carbohydrate load. Normally, sterile digestion takes place in the small bowel. However, if small bowel anatomy is altered, intestinal carbohydrate may either be exposed to colonic flora or undigested carbohydrate may be shunted to colon where fermentation occurs. In addition, the patients frequently have abnormal gut flora with predominance of lactate producing strains. Normally, simple sugars are anerobically metabolized to pyruvate and then, depending on the bacteria species present, are metabolized to D- or L-lactate. Increased acid production further decreases gut pH and the resulting acid environment favors the selection of acid-tolerant bacterial species such as *Lactobacillus*. Then, depending on the bacterial species, either D- or L-lactate is produced and absorbed, and since only the enzyme to metabolize L-lactate is present in humans, D-lactate accumulates.

The clinical diagnosis of D-lactic acidosis (Table 6) should be suspected in patients who present with mild metabolic acidosis, history of abnormal small bowel anatomy, and neurologic symptoms. That these patients had more neurologic abnormalities than would be expected on the basis of the acidosis suggests a direct toxicity of the D-lactate or other products on the CNS. A systematic study of the effect of D-lactate on neurologic function in animals needs to be undertaken to determine whether it can account for the findings observed in these patients. The diagnosis can be confirmed using a specific enzymatic assay for D-lactate or by the finding of an elevated peak on gas-chromatography for lactic acid in the absence of an elevation of L-lactate. Recently, Traube and co-workers (101) utilized proton nuclear magnetic resonance (NMR) spectroscopy to identify the presence of lactic acid in a patient with jejunoileal bypass, neurologic symptoms, and metabolic acidosis. The proton NMR spectrum of the patient's serum indicated the presence of lactate at a concentration of 10 mEq/liter. Serum lactate levels measured with L-lactate dehydrogenase assay were normal, but when the serum was assayed for D-lactate, elevated levels of 7.5 mEq/liter were found. Proton NMR is a simple screening test to identify organic acids and it is useful in screening for D-lactic acidosis. The clinical utility of culturing stool for lactate-producing bacteria is probably limited to a research setting due to the wide variation in normal flora and the difficulty in using quantitative culture due to the vast number of bacterial species present. The treatment of D-lactic acidosis involves correction of abnormalities of the intestinal tract, if possible, and the use of oral nonabsorbable antibiotics such as neomycin and vancomycin.

Lactic Acidosis in McArdle's Syndrome: Use of Phosphorus-31 Nuclear Magnetic Resonance (^{31}P NMR)

Ross and co-workers (103) utilized ^{31}P NMR to diagnose McArdle's syndrome by measuring intracellular pH. McArdle's syndrome is an inherited deficiency of the enzyme glycogen phosphorylase in skeletal muscles. During ischemic exercise the muscle fails to convert glycogen to glucose and is unable to generate lactic acid. The patients have marked exercise intolerance with muscle weakness. In a normal individual, lactate is produced during exercise and intracellular pH of the muscle decreases. Patients with McArdle's syndrome fail to increase lactate and intracellular pH does not decrease. The authors demonstrated that in one patient with McArdle's syndrome, intracellular pH of the muscle did not fall during exercise. In contrast, the pH in normal subjects fell to 6.67 during ischemic exercise because of increased lactic acid production and accumulation (Fig. 9). This study represents the first clinical diagnostic application of NMR, which provides a noninvasive method to study in vivo pH changes associated with an enzyme deficiency (103).

NMR is a technique that in the past was used primarily by the physicochemists. Recent advances and new spectrometers have made it possible to apply NMR to the biologic sciences. NMR is based on the intrinsic physical properties of atomic nuclei; nuclei with an odd number of protons and neutrons function as a magnetic dipole and NMR spectroscopy takes advantage of this fact. The measurement requires two electromagnetic fields. The first causes the magnet dipoles to align themselves in the same direction, either with the field or against it; this requires a strong magnetic field. The second field uses low energy electromagnetic radiation in the radiofrequency portion of the spectrum. Usually the magnetic field is held constant and the radiofrequency is varied. For a given magnetic field there is a specific radiofrequency that

ACID-BASE METABOLISM **345**

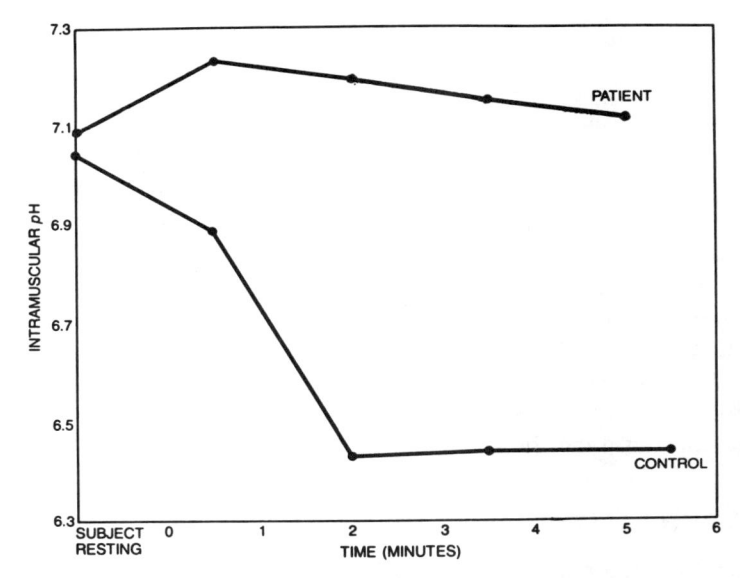

Figure 9. Intracellular pH of the muscle in a normal subject and in a patient with McArdle's syndrome. The diagnosis of disease by means of NMR spectroscopy has been reported by Ross et al. (103). McArlde's syndrome is characterized by fatigue following slight exertion and results from the deficiency of the enzyme glycogen phosphorylase, which takes part in making glucose in muscle tissue. The metabolites of glucose decrease the pH of cells, in NMR spectra. Therefore, the disease is revealed by a lack of change in pH, as is shown by the unchanging position of the inorganic phosphate peak in spectra of the patient's arm made as the patient exercised. The subjects of the measurement wore a cuff to keep fresh glucose from arriving in arterial blood. (Shulman RG: *Sci Am* 248:86:93, 1983. Reproduced by permission.)

will carry the correct amount of energy to change alignment of a certain nucleus, causing it to "flip." At this frequency, the nuclei will absorb the electromagnetic energy and resonate, and the absorption can then be analyzed by a computer. The nuclei commonly measured include hydrogen, ^{13}C, and ^{31}P. The frequency of the resonance is also dependent on the chemical environment of the nuclei. A carbon atom bound to two oxygen atoms ($COO-$) would have a spectrum different from a carbon bound to a hydrogen atom (CH). Since ^{13}C nuclei occur naturally in only 1.1% of all carbon atoms, NMR provides a technique to follow metabolic pathways. By labeling a compound in a particular position with ^{13}C at a higher concentration than naturally occurs, it is possible to follow that label as it changes positions in various molecules during metabolism and thus gain insight into metabolic pathways.

NMR spectroscopy with ^{31}P offers different advantages. Only ^{31}P occurs naturally, so no labeling of the tissue with phosphate is required. Phosphorus occurs in the cell in the form of inorganic phosphate, sugar phosphate, ATP, ADP, and phosphocreatine. Each of these phosphate compounds resonates at a certain position and can thus be identified by NMR (Fig. 10). The technique of phosporus NMR has been utilized to measure intracellular pH and to monitor ATP levels in several tissues, cells, and subcellular organelles (104,105). The advantage of this technique is that it allows rapid and noninvasive assessment of intracellular pH. Furthermore, it allows repeated measurements in the same sample. The principle by which phosphorus NMR can be used to measure intracellular pH is based on the fact that the resonance position (chemical shift) of inorganic phosphate (which exists in equilibrium between the forms $HPO_4 \rightleftharpoons H_2PO_4$ in the cell) is pH dependent (105). The resonance position of inorganic phosphorus is thus subject to changes in intracellular $H+$ concentration and can be used to calculate intracellular pH.

Other Causes of Lactic Acidosis

Lactic acidosis is a common finding in exertional heat stroke and is found in marathon runners, military recruits, and others after exhaustive exercise. In these conditions, very high levels of lactate may be found with strenuous exercise and they are usually well tolerated. In men with exertional heat stroke, the prognosis is good and no correlation has been found with blood lactate levels. These findings are significantly different from those found in patients with "classic heat stroke." In a recent paper, Hart et al. (106) compared the clinical features and acid-base status of patients presenting with classic heat stroke to those of patients with exertional heat stroke (Table 7). Classic heat stroke typically occurs in the elderly during heat waves and is often associated with a predisposing disease or use of medications. They reported a group of 28 patients, of which 20 survived with no sequelae, four had permanent neurologic deficits, and four died. The most common acid-base disorder was respiratory alkalosis, whereas in exertional heat stroke, lactic acidosis is more frequent. Mixed acid-base disorders were common, and only six patients had lactate levels greater than 5 mmol/liter, which correlated with a poor prognosis. Elevation of creatine phosphokinase levels was common, though no patient had clinically evident rhabdomyolysis. These findings suggest that lactate levels should be measured routinely in patients suspected of having classic heat stroke and the finding of elevated levels should alert the clinician to the possibility of a guarded prognosis.

Vaziri et al. (107) described a patient who developed severe lactic acidosis after ingestion of an overdose of papaverine. Papaverine is a peripheral vasodilator and a smooth-muscle relaxant. The authors suggested that lactic acidosis was due to inhibition of the mitochondrial respiratory chain at the step between the NADH dehydrogenase and coenzyme Q. Inter-

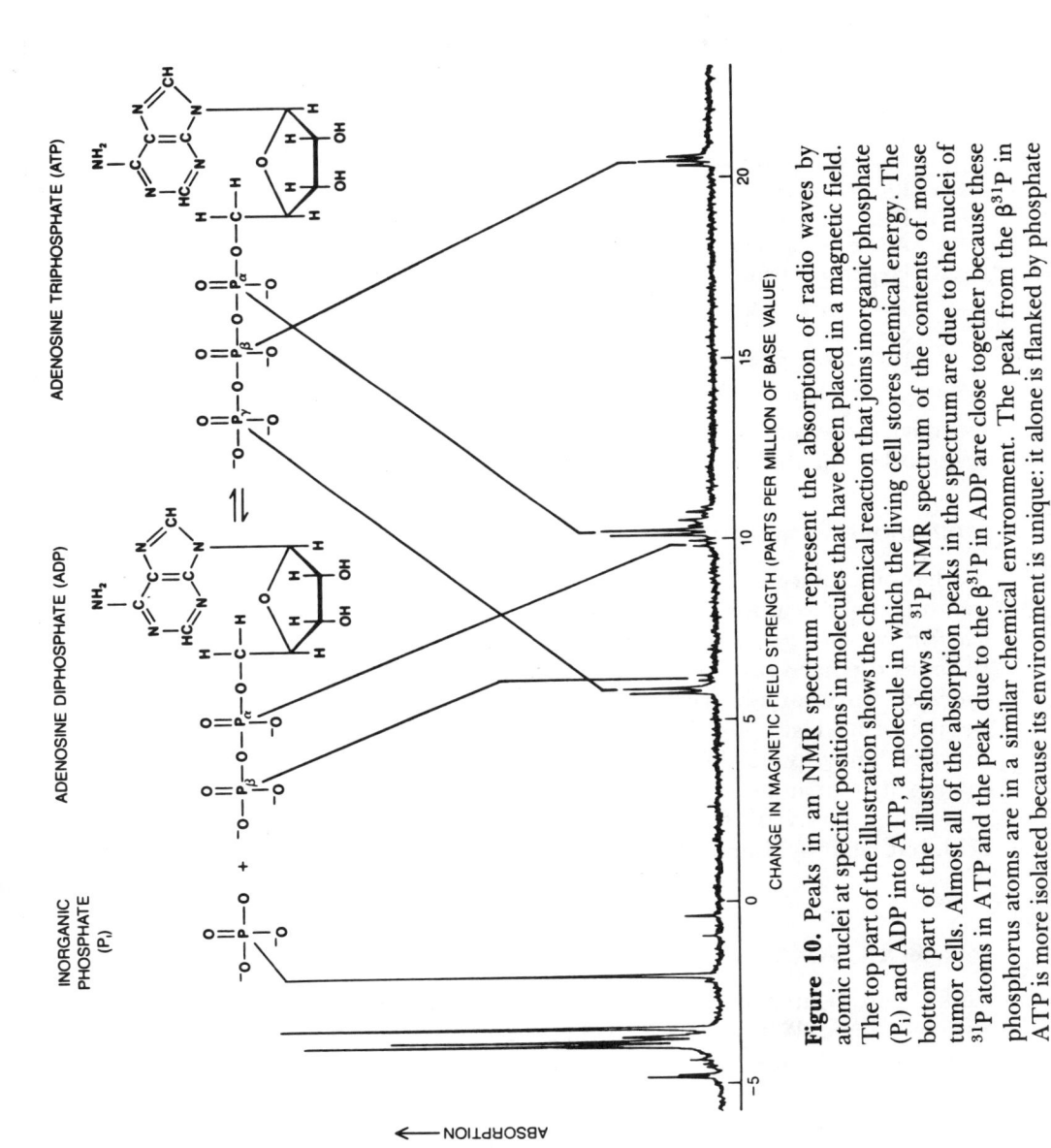

Figure 10. Peaks in an NMR spectrum represent the absorption of radio waves by atomic nuclei at specific positions in molecules that have been placed in a magnetic field. The top part of the illustration shows the chemical reaction that joins inorganic phosphate (P$_i$) and ADP into ATP, a molecule in which the living cell stores chemical energy. The bottom part of the illustration shows a ^{31}P NMR spectrum of the contents of mouse tumor cells. Almost all of the absorption peaks in the spectrum are due to the nuclei of ^{31}P atoms in ATP and the peak due to the β^{31}P in ADP are close together because these phosphorus atoms are in a similar chemical environment. The peak from the β^{31}P in ATP is more isolated because its environment is unique: it alone is flanked by phosphate groups. (Shulman RG: *Sci Am* 248:86–93, 1983. Reproduced by permission.)

Table 7. Clinical Characteristics of Two Forms of Heat Stroke

	Classic	Exertional
Age group affected	Older	Young
Occur in epidemics	Yes	No
Predisposing illnesses	Often	No
Prevailing weather	Prolonged heatwave	Variable
Sweating	Often absent	May be present
Acid base disturbance	Respiratory alkalosis	Lactic acidosis
Rhabdomyolysis	Rare	Common
DIC	Rare	Common
Acute renal failure	Rare	Common
Hyperuricemia	Mild	Marked

SOURCE: Hart GR et al: *Medicine* 61:189–197, 1982. Reproduced with permission.
DIC, disseminated intravascular coagulation.

estingly, there was also severe respiratory acidosis, but the mechanism responsible for the respiratory acidosis was not clarified.

Methanol Poisoning

Methanol intoxication is another well-recognized form of increased anion gap metabolic acidosis and has been discussed in detail in other issues of *Current Nephrology*. A recent review by Pappas and Silverman (108) emphasizes the need for early hemodialysis combined with ethanol and alkali therapy. Survival was related to the initial serum methanol level, the degree of acidosis, and the interval between ingestion and institution of therapy. They found the serum bicarbonate level was particularly discriminating in that none of the patients with bicarbonate levels less than 10 mmol/liter survived. The elevated anion gap is primarily due to formic acid, but lactic acid may also be present.

METABOLIC ALKALOSIS

Finkle and Dean (10) reported their experience in treating 21 patients with metabolic alkalosis with HCl. These patients were receiving parenteral amino acid solution and HCl was used in the hyperalimentation solution. The amount of HCl to be given to the patient was calculated from the following formula: (observed plasma bicarbonate − normal plasma HCO_3) × 0.5 × body weight in kilograms. This defines the excess of HCO_3 that needs to be buffered by the HCl. The HCl (12–13N solution) was diluted under sterile conditions to 2N solution and the amount required to correct the alkalosis was added to the amino acid solution. The final solution of HCl in the amino acid preparation should not be greater than 0.2N. A

```
                    ┌─────────────────┐          ┌─────────────────┐
                    │ ↓ Urinary Potassium │          │ ↑ Urinary Potassium │
                    │    (<30 mEq/L)      │          │    (>30 mEq/L)      │
                    └─────────────────┘          └─────────────────┘
                          Poor Intake
                          Diarrhea
```

```
        ┌─────────────────┐                    ┌─────────────────┐
        │ ↑ Urinary Chloride │                    │ ↓ Urinary Chloride │
        │    (>10 mEq/L)     │                    │    (<10 mEq/L)     │
        └─────────────────┘                    └─────────────────┘
                                                  Nasogastric Suction
   ┌──────────┐      ┌──────────┐                 Vomiting
   │Hypertension│      │Normotension│              Posthypercapneic State
   └──────────┘      └──────────┘
```

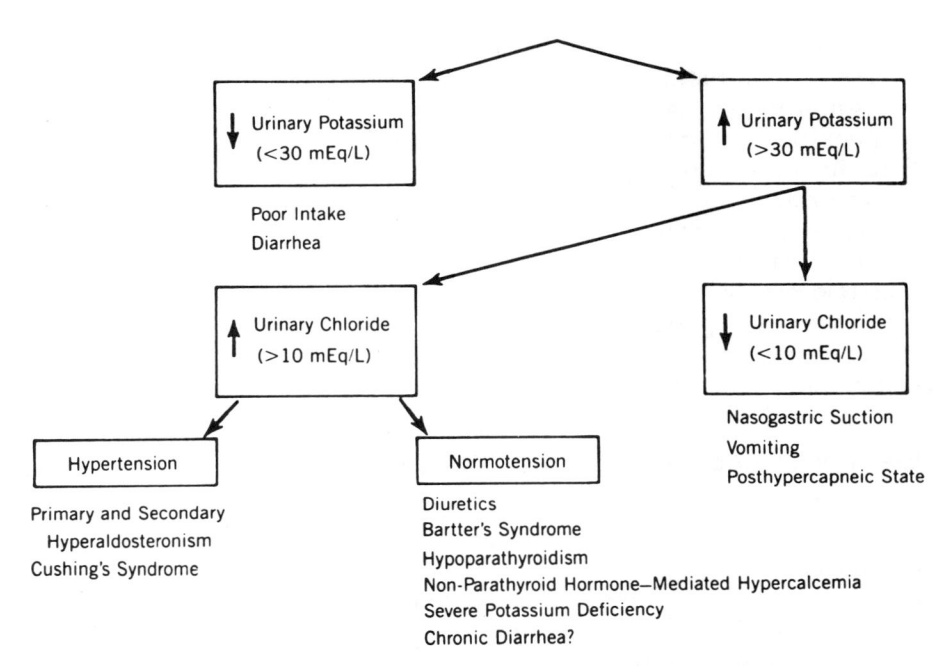

Primary and Secondary   Diuretics
   Hyperaldosteronism   Bartter's Syndrome
  Cushing's Syndrome   Hypoparathyroidism
                               Non-Parathyroid Hormone–Mediated Hypercalcemia
                               Severe Potassium Deficiency
                               Chronic Diarrhea?

Figure 11. Flow diagram of diagnosis of hypokalemia. (Parker MS et al: *Arch Intern Med* 140:1336–1337, 1980. Reproduced by permission.)

2N HCl solution contains 2000 mEq/liter. Thus, if one calculates that the patient needs 100 mEq/liter of HCl to correct the alkalosis, then 50 ml of 2N HCl solution should be added to 1000 ml of the amino acid solution. The advantage of adding HCl to the amino acid solution is the fact that the pH of this solution is higher than that of HCl added to saline. The same amount of HCl decreases pH to 1 when added in 0.9% saline and to 3–5 when added to 3.5% or 8.5% solution of amino acid. Thus, buffering of HCl increases the pH of the solution and prevents skin necrosis and thrombophlebitis. The treatment was effective in all patients and the amount of HCl infused ranged from 60 mEq to 2100 mEq in a period of 1–21 days. Buffered HCl should be considered in the treatment of patients with metabolic alkalosis in whom administration of saline and KCl is either dangerous or contraindicated, for example, in heart failure, hepatic failure, or severe edema.

Parker et al. (110) described the case of a patient with hypokalemic metabolic alkalosis. The metabolic alkalosis was persistent and did not correct with the administration of KCl. Urinary electrolytes showed a high urinary potassium and high urinary chloride, findings compatible with diuretic abuse, which was later confirmed. Figure 11 presents a practical flow diagram for differential diagnosis of hypokalemic metabolic alkalosis.

This diagram employs three essential parameters: the urinary potassium concentration, the urine chloride, and blood pressure. If the urine potassium is less than 30 mEq/liter it suggests extrarenal potassium loss or poor dietary intake. If urine potassium is greater than 30 mEq/liter then the urine chloride will provide a clue to the differential diagnosis. If the chloride is less than 10–20 mEq/liter, this suggests vomiting, posthypercapnic state, or volume contraction. If the chloride is greater than 10–20 mEq/liter and hypertension is present, then the syndrome of primary mineralocorticoid excess should be considered. In this group, patients with essential hypertension who abuse diuretics should also be included. If the blood pressure is normal and the urine chloride is high, the other conditions mentioned in Figure 11 should be considered.

Effect of Glucocorticoid on Acid-Base Homeostasis

Cushing's disease is associated with metabolic alkalosis and hypokalemia. These effects are related to the degree of cortisol excess and its mineralocorticoid effect of cortisol. The possible effect of glucocorticoid on acid-base homeostasis has now been subjected to systematic investigation and allows a better understanding of the role of this hormone in acid-base disorders. Administration of triamcinolone to rats has been known to increase plasma HCO_3 and increase ammonia production but the effect on net acid excretion was not reported. In dogs, triamcinolone administration in pharmacologic doses results in an increase in endogenous acid production paralleled by an increase in net acid excretion and thus plasma composition remained normal (111). It is difficult in this study to analyze the role of the glucocorticoid itself on acid excretion. The increase in acid production induced by the large doses of glucocorticoid could be the factor responsible for the increase in renal acid excretion without having to invoke any direct effect of the glucocorticoids per se on renal acidification. Hulter et al. evaluated the effect of small doses of dexamethasone (0.2 mg/day or 0.8 mg/day) on acid-base homeostasis in adrenalectomized dogs maintained on constant and fixed mineralocorticoid replacement (112). Administration of either dose of glucocorticoid to these dogs did not alter acid-base homeostasis, indicating that normal amounts of glucocorticoid do not play a role in the maintenance of acid-base homeostasis. Endogenous acid production, however, increased as the glucorticoid dose was increased from 0.2 mg/day to 0.8 mg/day. This increase in endogenous acid production was paralleled by an increase in net acid excretion and thus plasma composition remained constant. The authors then evaluated the effect of an acid load (HCl 5 mmol/kg/day) on acid-base composition in dogs maintained on 0.2 mg/day and 0.8 mg/day of dexamethasone. In response to HCl feeding, plasma HCO_3 decreased and net acid excretion increased in both groups of dogs: the decrease in plasma HCO_3 was smaller and increase in net acid excretion was greater in the dogs receiving

0.8 mg of dexamethosone than in the group receiving 0.2 mg. The increase in net acid excretion was mainly due to an increase in ammonia excretion. The authors concluded that glucocorticoid excess protects against metabolic acidosis induced by exogenous acids. They also concluded that glucocorticoid excess increases endogenous acid production, but this effect does not lead to metabolic acidosis because glucocorticoids also enhance net acid excretion and thus plasma composition is maintained at normal levels. These studies do not clarify the role of endogenous glucocorticoid on acid-base homeostasis.

To further define the role of glucocorticoids on urinary acidification, Frieberg et al. (113) studied the effect of glucocorticoid on sodium–hydrogen exchange in brush border membrane vesicles of the rat. This technique used renal cortical tissue; the plasma membranes of the tubular cells were separated into luminal and basolateral membranes. These membranes form vesicles which can then be used to study transport. This technique offers the advantage of allowing study of transport in the absence of metabolic factors. Adrenalectomized rats were divided in three groups; one group received injection of normal saline, the second group received dexamethasone (5 µg/100 g body weight), and the third group received the same dose of aldosterone. The dose of dexamethasone corresponds approximately to the high dose of dexamethasone (0.8 mg) given to the dogs by Hulter et al. (112), and it would be considered three times greater than the usual replacement dose of glucocorticoid required by adrenalectomized subjects. The authors prepared brush border membranes from the kidneys of these three groups of rats and used these membranes in vitro. In the proximal tubule, acidification is coupled to sodium through an electroneutral sodium–hydrogen antiporter which translocates H+ in response to a sodium gradient. The authors showed that sodium uptake and inferentially H+ secretion was greater in vesicles prepared from rats treated with dexamethasone than in vesicles from control rats. Amiloride blocked this effect, which suggests that the enhancement of sodium uptake was mediated by the sodium–hydrogen antiporter. The authors also evaluated the effect of dexamethasone on H+ efflux from the vesicles in response to sodium transport and showed that the rate of H+ efflux in vesicles from dexamethasone-treated rats was greater than that of control rats. Vesicles from aldosterone-treated rats did not show an enhancement of transport by sodium–hydrogen antiporter. These findings further substantiate the contention that glucocorticoid enhances the sodium–hydrogen antiporter. Vesicle studies provide information mainly about acidification from the proximal tubule since the vesicles are made from homogenates of the cortex from which brush border membranes are isolated. These studies would suggest that glucocorticoid enhances acidification by the proximal tubule and would thus enhance HCO_3 reabsorption by the proximal tubule. Glucocorticoid excess could then help maintain metabolic alkalosis generated by the distal nephron. The authors postulate that glucocorticoid induced a specific change in the activity of the sodium–hydrogen carrier since other transport functions also performed by the brush border membranes, such as glucose transport, were not altered by glucocorticoid.

In summary, these studies provide evidence that glucocorticoid in amounts slightly above the replacement dose can enhance proximal acidification and thus could play a role in urinary acidificiation, especially in the maintenance of metabolic alkalosis by the proximal tubule. The role of glucocorticoid on distal acidification has not been studied. Although glucocorticoid can interact with the mineralocorticoid receptor it is unlikely that the above observations resulted from a mineralocorticoid effect since administration of aldosterone failed to elicit the same response. Thus, these studies suggest that under certain defined experimental conditions, glucocorticoid may play a role in urinary acidification.

POTASSIUM, ALDOSTERONE, AND ACID-BASE HOMEOSTASIS
Effect of Chronic Dietary Potassium Depletion in Humans

In states of potassium depletion, there is commonly metabolic alkalosis (114). However, in most clinical situations where hypokalemia and metabolic alkalosis coexist, there is also associated mineralocorticoid excess, volume depletion, or chloride depletion, conditions that may cause metabolic alkalosis independently. Kassirer and Schwartz (115,116) demonstrated that gastric loss of hydrochloric acid in humans caused hypokalemia and metabolic alkalosis, yet metabolic alkalosis could be corrected by the infusion of saline alone, despite persistence of moderate potassium depletion. This suggests that moderate potassium depletion may not be essential for the maintenance of metabolic alkalosis. On the other hand, the effect of dietary deprivation of potassium on acid-base homeostasis in humans, rats, and dogs is controversial; no change, an increase, and a decrease in plasma bicarbonate concentration have been reported (117–120). Thus, the role of potassium depletion independent of other disorders in the acid-base balance in humans is not clear.

Jones and colleagues (121) studied the effects of uncomplicated potassium depletion on the acid-base homeostasis in normal subjects. Potassium depletion was induced in seven normal male volunteers by giving them an electrolyte-free synthetic diet to which 1.8 mmol of NaCl/kg body weight/day was added. During the control period, 1.5 mEq/kg body weight of potassium per day was provided as neutral phosphate. In the first 10 days of the experimental phase, potassium phosphate was substituted by sodium phosphate in equimolar amounts to keep the dietary anion content constant; thus the subjects received a potassium free diet during this phase. In the remaining 5 days of the study, one-tenth of dietary sodium

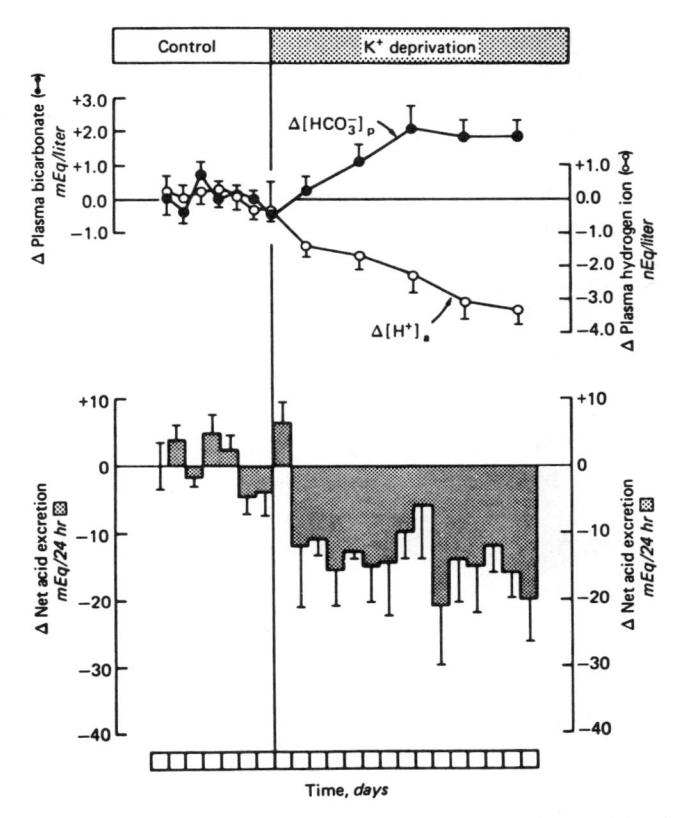

Figure 12. Effect of dietary potassium deprivation on plasma bicarbonate and hydrogen ion concentration and net acid excretion in normal subjects. The shaded bars depict the difference in mean daily net acid excretion from the mean control value. (Jones JW et al: *Kidney Int* 21:402–410, 1982. Reproduced by permission.)

phosphate was substituted by potassium phosphate to prevent further negative potassium balance and to achieve steady state potassium levels.

At the end of 2 weeks, serum potassium had decreased from a control value of 4 mEq/liter to 3 mEq/liter and a cumulative potassium deficit of 295 mEq occurred. Plasma HCO_3 increased by only 1.8 ± 0.3 mEq/liter H+ decreased by 3.1 ± 0.2 nmol/liter from control values (Fig. 12) and P_{CO_2} remained unchanged. This small but significant increase in plasma HCO_3 occurred despite a positive chloride balance, small but significant weight gain, increased creatinine clearance and a decrease in plasma aldosterone concentration. Although ammonia excretion increased, titratable acid excretion decreased and there was a cumulative decrease in net acid excretion of 169 mEq/liter. Thus it is not possible to attribute the generation of metabolic alkalosis to a renal mechanism since net acid excretion decreased. To invoke a renal mechanism in the generation of this alkalosis one would have to postulate that endogenous acid production decreased. Although the authors postulate this mechanism, they did not measure acid production, and therefore this hypothesis cannot be verified. It is not necessary, however, to invoke a renal mechanism in the generation of alkalosis, since the increase in plasma HCO_3 can be explained by an extrarenal mechanism: $K+$ moves out of the cell in exchange for extracellular $H+$ ion. Translocation of $H+$ into cells can explain both the decrease in net acid excretion and the increased plasma HCO_3. These studies demonstrate that uncomplicated potassium depletion in humans is associated with mild metabolic alkalosis that seems to be caused by a transcellular shift of $H+$ and is maintained, at least in part, by enhanced renal HCO_3 reabsorption. The maintenance of metabolic alkalosis can be explained by a renal mechanism since potassium depletion enhances proximal HCO_3 reabsorption (114) and thus can maintain the alkalosis regardless of how generated.

Effect of Hyperkalemia on Distal Acidification

Hyperkalemic disorders are commonly associated with metabolic acidosis. Hyperkalemia causes a decrease in extracellular pH by exchanging intracellular $H+$ for extracellular $K+$. In the kidney, hyperkalemia decreases urinary acidification. This effect is in part due to decreased proximal tubular bicarbonate reabsorption, which is thought to be caused by reduced availability of protons for secretion (114). This decrease of proximal HCO_3 reabsorption results in increased urinary excretion of HCO_3 and urine pH. The increase in urine pH decreases ammonia trapping, and thus net acid excretion decreases. Hyperkalemia also impairs the rate of synthesis of ammonia in the renal cortex, which contributes further to decrease net acid excretion. Renal mechanisms, therefore, can generate and sustain metabolic acidosis in hyperkalemia. On the other hand, hyperkalemia stimulates aldosterone secretion, which tends to increase renal acid excretion. Aldosterone stimulates sodium reabsorption in the distal nephron, thus creating a favorable electrical gradient for $K+$ and $H+$ secretion.

The effect of hyperkalemia on distal nephron $H+$ secretion is difficult to evaluate because measurement of net acid excretion reflects the contribution of the whole nephron rather than the selective contribution of the distal segment. Arruda et al. (122) and Pichette et al. (123) utilized the measurement of urine minus blood $(U - B)$ P_{CO_2} as an index of distal $H+$ ion secretion during normokalemia and hyperkalemia. Arruda et al. found no effect of $KHCO_3$ infusion on $U - B P_{CO_2}$ (i.e., distal nephron $H+$ was unchanged during $KHCO_3$ infusion). On the other hand, Pichette et al. observed a significant decrease in $U - B P_{CO_2}$ during $KHCO_3$ infusion in normovolemic dogs; $U - B P_{CO_2}$ was inversely related to the rate of potassium excretion. In hypervolemic dogs, however, $U - B P_{CO_2}$ was 50% lower than in the normovolemic dogs, and $KHCO_3$ infusion failed to depress U − BPco₂, suggesting that potassium infusion decreases distal acidification only in the normovolemic dogs. They suggested that a failure to observe a decrease in U − BPco₂ with KHCO₃ infusion in the studies of Arruda and co-workers was probably related to the fact that the dogs were volume expanded. During volume expansion, sodium transport in the distal nephron is inhibited, therefore, the favorable electric gradient for K+ or H+ ion secretion may not be present. Thus, hyperkalemia would seem to depress distal nephron H+ secretion only when this segment is avid for sodium reabsorption.

Aldosterone and the Renal Response to Sulfuric Acid Feeding in the Dog

Excretion of an acid load requires that filtered bicarbonate be completely reabsorbed and an additional bicarbonate be regenerated by the kidney and returned to the blood in order to minimize the degree of acidosis. The generation of new bicarbonate is mainly a function of the distal nephron, and H+ secretion in this segment depends to a large extent on the presence of a favorable electrical gradient. The favorable electrical gradient in the distal nephron is created by adequate delivery of sodium and enhanced sodium reabsorption by aldosterone, which increases proton secretion both by a direct effect on the proton pump as well as by its effect on sodium transport.

Chronic sulfuric acid feeding to dogs is characterized by a disparity in the rate at which administrated sulfate and H+ appear in the urine: administered sulfate is excreted rapidly, obligating the excretion of sodium and potassium while the excretion of H+ is delayed (125). Sodium deficits produced in this way stimulate aldosterone secretion and enhance acid excretion. Kraut et al. (125) examined the effect of sulfuric acid feeding on plasma renin activity, aldosterone production, and the role of aldosterone on renal excretion of acid in dogs fed sulfuric acid. They found that the plasma renin activity, the plasma aldosterone concentration, and the urinary aldosterone excretion increased significantly during sulfuric acid feeding, suggesting that aldosterone plays a role in acid excretion in this condition. To further evaluate the role of aldosterone on acid excretion, they studied intact dogs and adrenalectomized dogs replaced with glucocorticoid and maintained on subphysiologic doses of mineralcorticoid at two levels of sulfuric acid intake (7 mEq/kg and 3.5 mEq/kg per day) and adrenalectomized dogs receiving supraphysiologic doses of mineralocorticoid but receiving sulfuric acid at the higher dose (7 mEq/kg per day). They found that plasma bicarbonate decreased more in adrenalectomized dogs receiving subphysiologic replacement of mineralocorticoid than in either intact dogs or in the adrenalectomized dogs receiving supraphysiologic doses of mineralocorticoids (Fig. 13). In fact, the serum bicarbonate in intact and in adrenalectomized dogs receiving

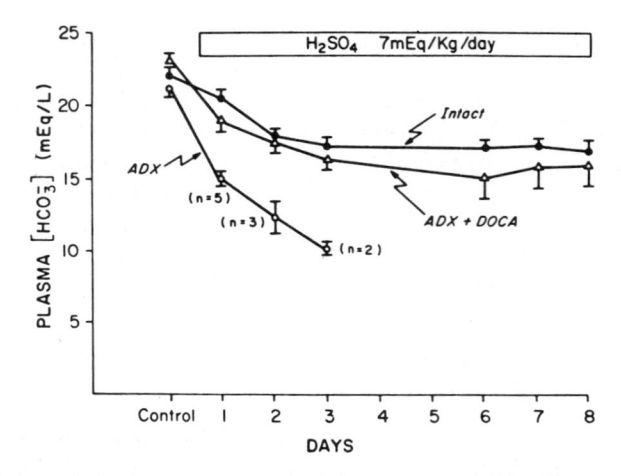

Figure 13. Effect of adrenalectomy on response of plasma bicarbonate concentration during daily feeding of H_2SO_4 (7 mEq/kg). Closed circles denote intact dogs; open circles, adrenalectomized dogs maintained on subphysiologic doses of mineralocorticoid; and open triangles, adrenalectomized dogs given supraphysiologic doses of deoxycorticosterone. (Kraut JA et al. *Am J Physiol* 243:F494–502, 1982. Reproduced by permission.)

supraphysiologic doses of mineralocorticoids were remarkably similar. They also observed that the cumulative increase in net acid excretion in adrenalectomized dogs, receiving glucocorticoid maintained on subphysiologic mineralocorticoid replacement and receiving high dose of sulfuric acid was 34% lower than that of intact dogs. The percent increment in net acid excretion in relation to sulfate excretion was also significantly less in the adrenalectomized dogs than in intact dogs at both dosage levels of sulfuric acid administration. Since the sulfate excretion was similar in all groups of dogs, sodium delivery to the distal nephron must have been comparable among the groups. The authors concluded that increased aldosterone secretion contributes in part to the increase in acid excretion observed with sulfuric acid feeding. The fact, however, that adrenalectomized dogs fed sulfuric acid were able to increase acid excretion indicates that factors other than aldosterone play an important role in the increase in acid excretion. Previous studies from the same laboratory provide further evidence for a role of factors other than aldosterone in the adaptation to sulfuric acid feeding. Kraut et al. (126) showed that dogs given pharmacologic doses of desoxycorticosterone acetate (DOCA) before and during the administration of sulfuric acid failed to increase acid excretion faster than normal dogs and therefore displayed a comparable decrease in plasma HCO_3. The authors suggest that the delay in the increase in acid excretion is not minimized by the existence of prior sodium avidity. This delay likely reflects the time necessary for ammonia production to increase and for distal H+ secretion rate to achieve a maximum. Thus, mineralocorticoids, either from endogenous or exogenous sources, play an important role in the adaptation to sulfuric acid feeding, but clearly this adaptation is the result of multiple factors.

AMMONIA METABOLISM

Ammonia accounts for about 50–60% of the acid excreted in the urine. In metabolic acidosis, the excretion of ammonia can increase five to 10 times. Ammonia is produced in the kidney according to need by the metabolism of glutamine to ammonia, and the pathways of ammoniagenesis are complex and involve multiple cytosolic and mitochondrial enzymes. The role of different pathways in the increased production of ammonia in metabolic acidosis continues to be investigated. We will briefly review the pathways involved in ammonia production before discussing new information on ammonia metabolism. The evidence for and against the relative importance of each of these pathways in ammoniagenesis has recently been reviewed extensively by Tannen (124) and will be only briefly discussed here (Fig. 14).

In the rat, the cytosolic pathway catalyzed by glutamine synthetase results in the amidation of glutamate to glutamine, thereby "using up" an ammonia. It is conceivable that slowing the rate of this reaction in acidosis might play a role in increasing the NH_3 available for secretion. This slowing is not felt to be important, however, because the enzyme is absent from the kidney of both dogs and humans, species able to enhance ammonia production in the presence of acidosis. (124). Two enzymes, glutamine ketoacid aminotransferase and Ω-amidase, make up the so-called glutaminase II pathway. These are also basically cytosolic enzymes and are found in human kidneys as well as in rat kidneys, but physiologic studies measuring enzyme activity and utilization of reactants suggest that they are not involved in the increased ammonia formation found in acidosis (127). Some confusion has arisen with regard to the enzyme "glutaminase I." It is now felt to be actually two enzymes. One of these is activated by phosphate, called *phosphate-dependent glutaminase,* and the other is activated by maleate, called *phosphate-independent glutaminase.* In the rat, the phosphate-independent glutaminase is felt to be γ-glutamyl transpeptidase. It is not known whether this is the case in the human kidney. Its role in the regulation of ammoniagenesis in acidosis is still being questioned, but Lemieux and co-workers (128) measured the enzyme and found no enhanced activity under conditions of acidosis, suggesting that it is at least not a major regulatory enzyme. On the other hand, phosphate-dependent glutaminase is felt to play a significant role in the regulation of ammoniagenesis (125). Phosphate-dependent glutaminase is located in the mitochondria. The most convincing evidence of its importance is the

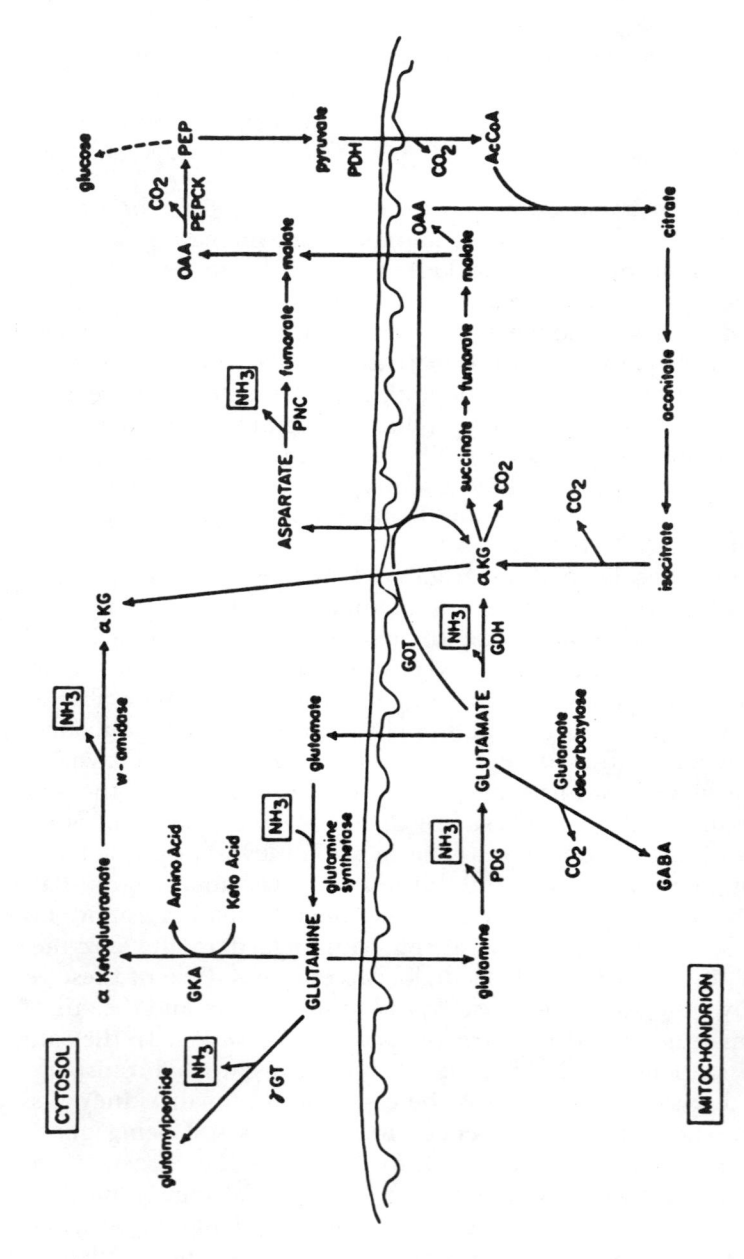

Figure 14. Pathways of renal ammoniagenesis. OAA, oxaloacetate; α-KG, α-ketoglutarate; AcCoA, acetyl-CoA; GKA; GDH and w-amidase, glutaminase II; PIC and γ-GT, phosphate-independent glutaminase; PDG, phosphate-dependent glutaminase; GDH, glutamate dehydrogenase; GOT, glutamate oxaloacetate transaminase; GABA, glutamate decarboxylase; PNC, purine nucleotide cycle. (Tannen RL: *Am J Physiol* 235:F265–F277, 1978. Reproduced by permission.)

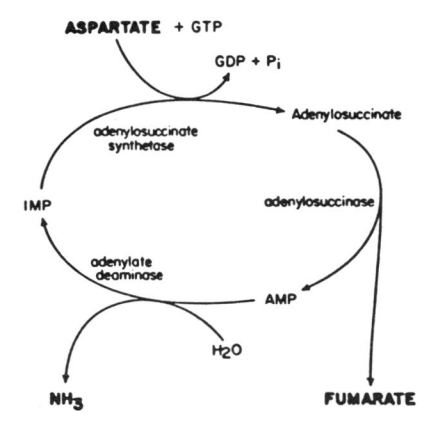

Figure 15. Purine nucleotide cycle. GTP, guanosine triphosphate; GDP, guanosine diphosphate; IMP, inosine monophosphate. Net reaction for one turn of the cycle is aspartate + GTP + H$_2$O → fumarate + GDP + P$_i$ + NH$_3$. (Tannen RL: *Am J Physiol* 235:F265–277, 1978. Reproduced by permission.)

fact that isolated mitochondrial preparations are capable of producing ammonia from glutamine. In fact, the capacity for ammoniagenesis by intact mitochondria is essentially the same as that by intact organs (129–131). While cytosolic pathways may be operative in ammoniagenesis, they are not of prime importance. Although phosphate-dependent glutaminase is felt to be important, it is unclear at this time whether or not it is the rate-limiting step in renal mitochondrial ammoniagenesis or whether the rate-limiting process is the entry of glutamine into the mitochondria. Utilizing ^{14}C glutamine, Simpson and Adam (129) have presented evidence that the entry of glutamine into the mitochondria is the rate-limiting step in ammonia production. They found ^{14}C glutamate but not ^{14}C glutamine in the mitochondria. This finding suggests that all the glutamine entering the mitochondria can be processed by phosphate-dependent glutaminase. This was true even when efforts were made to minimize the activity of the enzyme.

Another pathway considered important in ammoniagenesis is the purine nucleotide cycle (PNC) (Figs. 14 and 15). Unlike phosphate-dependent glutaminase, it is a cytosolic pathway. Its importance lies in the fact that it uses aspartate, which is a possible end-product of the phosphate-dependent glutaminase pathway. Its possible involvement in ammonia production was pointed out by Bogusky and co-workers and information concerning its role has recently been expanded by these investigators (132,133). They studied the activity of enzymes in the purine nucleotide cycle in rats made acidotic by feeding with NH$_4$Cl. They found that the activity of the rate-limiting enzyme in the cycle, adenylosuccinate synthetase, paralleled the rise in ammonia excretion. Discontinuation of NH$_4$Cl feeding and correction of the metabolic acidosis led to a decrease in ammonia excretion and to a decrease in the activity of this enzyme. In fact, the correlation between ammonia excretion and the activity of this enzyme was better than the correlation between ammonia excretion and the activity of phosphate-dependent glutaminase. While the study does not clarify the absolute contribution the purine nucleotide cycle makes to ammoniagenesis, it does seem to suggest that this pathway plays an important role in the adaptation to metabolic acidosis.

The involvement of PNC in the adaptation to metabolic acidosis illustrates an important concept in the regulation of ammoniagenesis. Since phosphate-dependent glutaminase has as its end product glutamate, the disposal of glutamate might function to "pull" through the reaction of glutamine to glutamate by way of phosphate-dependent glutaminase. The PNC can dispose of glutamate indirectly by using aspartate derived from glutamate through glutamine-oxaloacetate transaminase, but there are other enzyme systems that might function similarily. As the PNC increases its function, it would use glutamate as a substrate and hence lower the concentration of glutamate. This might make it easier for phosphate-dependent glutaminase to convert glutamine to glutamate and hence speed the reaction cycle. It therefore "pulls" through the reaction of glutamine to glutamate and this contributes to increased ammonia production.

This is not the only way to "pull" through this reaction. It is clear from Figure 14 that most of the metabolic pathways from glutamate go through α-ketoglutarate to phosphoenolpyruvate (PEP) and subsequently to glucose by the enzyme phosphoenolpyruvate carboxykinase (PEPCK). If PEPCK activity increases in acidosis, it leads to a decrease in the level of PEP and α-ketoglutarate; in this manner it "pulls" through the conversion of glutamine to glutamate. These considerations clearly indicate that there might be extensive interaction of various metabolic pathways in ammonia production, making it difficult to unravel the importance and contributions of each of these pathways.

While extensive work has been done on the biochemical pathways of ammonia synthesis, the sites where ammonia is produced and where it enters the nephron are less well defined. In the last volume of *Current Nephrology*, we reviewed evidence suggesting that ammonia may diffuse from the loop of Henle into the collecting duct. Additional studies suggest that most urinary ammonia is produced in the proximal tubule (134) and that addition of ammonia into the collecting duct occurs by diffusion of NH_3 from the loop of Henle into the collecting duct.

Buerkert and co-workers (135) recently addressed the question of ammonia handling in the various segments of the nephron by employing micropuncture of superficial and deep nephrons. They studied control and chronically acidotic rats. Plasma ammonia levels were higher in acidotic rats than in controls, indicating the need to correct the tubular values for the amount of ammonia filtered. Micropuncture samples were obtained from the proximal and distal tubules of superficial nephrons, from the bend in Henle's loop of selected deep nephrons, and from the collecting duct at the base and the tip of the papilla. The urinary ammonia excretion (absolute and fractional) was twice as great in the acidotic animals as compared to controls.

The amount of ammonia delivered to the end of the proximal tubule (superficial nephrons) in control rats was much greater than could be accounted for on the basis of filtration. In fact, expressed in fractional terms, the delivery of ammonia to the end of the proximal tubule was 853% of filtered load. This indicates that most of the ammonia found at the end of the proximal tubule was added by the proximal tubule. Samples obtained from the distal tubule revealed only about one-half of the ammonia found in the proximal tubule, indicating considerable loss of ammonia between the proximal and distal nephron. When similar studies were done in the acidotic rats, there was a greater increase (as compared to controls) in the delivery of ammonia to the end of the proximal tubule even when factored for the increase in filtered load. This would indicate that metabolic acidosis increases ammonia production by the proximal tubule. The amount of ammonia reaching the distal nephron, corrected for filtered load in the acidotic rats, was not different from that in control rats, indicating an even greater loss of ammonia (twice that observed in controls) between the proximal and distal nephrons in acidotic rats.

Samples obtained from the bend of Henle's loop (deep nephrons) in control rats revealed that the fractional delivery of ammonia to this site was significantly higher than that found in the end of the proximal nephron, indicating addition of ammonia between these two sites. This finding suggests that some structure (the pars recta and descending limb of loop of Henle) between the proximal tubule and the bend in Henle's loop continued to add ammonia to the luminal fluid. An alternative explanation is that the proximal tubules of deep nephrons make more ammonia than the proximal tubules of superficial nephrons. In the collecting ducts there was an increase in ammonia concentration between the base and the tip of the papilla, which could be accounted for by water extraction. There was considerably more ammonia at the base of the papilla than at the distal tubule, after correction fractional delivery. Therefore, ammonia was added to the tubule between the last accessible site of the distal tubule and the base of the papilla. In acidosis, the same findings were present but were magnified by a factor of two (Fig. 16).

This study provides strong evidence that the deep nephrons contribute significantly to the ammonia excretion as shown by the fact that ammonia delivered to the bend of Henle's loop was greater than that found at the end of the accessible proximal tubule. In metabolic acidosis, the contribution of the deep nephrons is greater, as evidenced by the larger amount of ammonia in the bend of Henle's loop than in the proximal tubule. Although the conclusion of this study seems reasonable, it should be remembered that one of the problems of the micropuncture technique is that samples are obtained only from limited sites and one must extrapolate what happens between those sites. In this case, fluid was sampled from

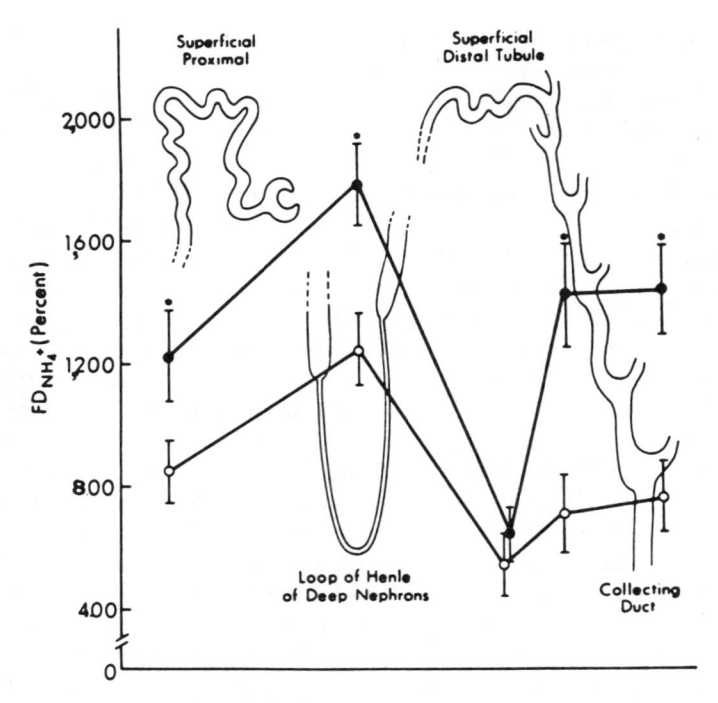

Figure 16. Profile of fractional delivery of ammonium to the micropuncture sites in controls (○) and after the chronic ingestion of an acid load (●). Asterisk denotes that the two values are significantly different. (Buerkert J et al: *J Clin Invest* 70:1–12, 1982. Reproduced by permission.)

the proximal tubule of superficial nephrons and from the bend of Henle's loop of deep nephrons. The assumption made is that the delivery to the end of the proximal tubule of superficial nephrons is the same as the ammonia delivery to the end of the proximal tubule of the deep nephrons, and this need not necessarily be correct.

It had been proposed that ammonia is generated in the proximal tubule and diffuses from the lumen of the bend of Henle's loop into the collecting structures (134). The physiologic explanation for this is that as the fluid proceeds down the Henle's loop, it becomes more alkaline. Therefore, more ammonia, in the nonionic form, can diffuse into the interstitium. It is then trapped in the collecting structures because of low pH. This concept is based on the fact that ammonia is transported as NH_3, which is a nonpolar species, and can easily pass through cell membranes (lipid layer) and therefore diffuse from cells into the tubular lumen. In contrast, it has been held that once the NH_3 is protonated to NH_4^+, it becomes a charged particle and loses its ability to cross lipid layers easily, becoming "trapped" in the lumen. Evidence is available to support the existence of

NH_4^+ transport in several species. This prompted Goldstein and coworkers (136) to further explore the exact nature of ammonia excretion. They examined the rate of gill ammonia excretion in isolated fish-head preparation. They studied the excretion of ammonia under two basic conditions. First, they held the concentration of total ammonia (NH_3 + NH_4^+) constant and varied the concentration of NH_3 in the perfusion fluid by varying its pH. In the second part of the experiment they held the concentration of NH_3 constant while increasing NH_4^+ concentration by varying the pH and the total ammonia concentration. They found that the rate of ammonia excretion was not significantly altered even after a twofold increase in the concentration of NH_3. However, there was a marked and significant increase in the excretion of ammonia when the NH_4^+ concentration was increased while holding the NH_3 concentration stable. Therefore, the increase in ammonia excretion actually appeared to be due to an increase in the NH_4^+ concentration rather than in the NH_3 concentration. This study suggests that the membrane is permeable to NH_4^+ and points out the need to reexamine the classic concepts of ammonia transport in the kidney and other acidifying epithelia.

REFERENCES

1. Narins RG, Bastl CP, Rudnick MP, et al: Acid base metabolism, in Gonick HC (ed): *Current Nephrology*, vol 5. New York, John Wiley & Sons, 1982, pp 79–130.
2. Arruda JAL, Wheeler RP: Disorders of acid base metabolism, in Gonick HC (ed): *Current Nephrology*, vol 6. New York, John Wiley & Sons, 1982, pp 237–282.
3. Oster JR, Hotchkiss JL, Carbon M, et al: A short duration renal acidification test using calcium chloride. *Nephron* 14:281–292, 1975.
4. Arruda JAL, Kurtzman NA: Hyperparathyroidism and metabolic acidosis: A complex interaction of multiple factors. *Nephron* 26:1–16, 1980.
5. Crumb CK, Martinez-Maldonado M, Eknoyan G, et al: Effects of volume expansion, purified parathyroid extract and calcium on renal bicarbonate absorption in the dog. *J Clin Invest* 54:1287–1293, 1974,
6. Heinemann HO: Metabolic alkalosis in patients with hypercalcemia. *Metabolism* 14:1137–1152, 1965.
7. Hulter HN, Sebastian A, Toto RD, et al: Renal and systemic acid base effects of chronic administration of hypercalcemia producing agents: Calcitriol, PTH and intravenous calcium. *Kidney Int* 21:445–448, 1982.
8. Metnick P, Greensburg A, Coffman T, et al: Effects of two models of hyperkalemia on renal acid base metabolism. *Kidney Int* 21:613–620, 1980.
9. Arruda JAL, Alla V, Rubenstein H, et al: Metabolic and hormonal factors influencing extrarenal buffering of an acute acid load. *Min Elect Met* 8:36–43, 1982.
10. Emmet M, Goldfarb S, Agus ZS, et al: The pathophysiology of acid base changes in chronically phosphate depleted rats: Bone-kidney interaction. *J Clin Invest* 59:291–298, 1977.
11. Arruda JAL, Julka NK, Rubinstein H, et al: Distal acidification defect induced by phosphate deprivation. *Metabolism* 29:826–836, 1980.

12. Baylink D, Wergedal J, Stauffer M: Formation, mineralization and resorption of bone in hypophosphatemic rats. *J Clin Invest* 50:2519–2530, 1971.
13. Lemann J, Lennon EJ, Goodman AD, et al. The net balance of acid in subjects given large loads of acid or alkali. *J Clin Invest* 44:507, 1961.
14. Hutler HN, Toto RD, Bonner EL, et al: Renal and systemic acid base effects of chronic hypoparathyroidism in dogs. *Am J Physiol* 10:F495–F501, 1981.
15. Goulding A, Broom MF: Effects of diphosphonate and colchicine administration upon acid base changes induced in rats by bilateral nephrectomy. *Clin Sci* 57:19–23, 1979.
16. Fraley DS, Adler S: An extrarenal role for parathyroid hormone in the disposal of acute acid loads in rats and dogs. *J Clin Invest* 63:985–997, 1979.
17. Arruda JAL, Venkateswararao A, Rubinstein H, et al: Parathyroid hormone and extrarenal acid buffering. *Am J Physiol* 239:F533–F538, 1980.
18. Madias NE, John CA, Homer SM: Independence of the acute acid buffering response from endogenous parathyroid hormone. *Am J Physiol* 243:141–149, 1982.
19. Fraley DS, Adler S: Effect of PTH on the buffering of an acute acid load. *Min Elect Met* (in press).
20. Licht JH, Vicker K: Parathyroid hormone induced metabolic alkalosis in dogs. *Min Elect Met* 8:78–91, 1982.
21. Dominguez JH, Raisz LG: Effects of changing on hydrogen ion carbonic acid and bicarbonate concentration on bone resorption in vitro. *Calcif Tissue Inter* 29:7–13, 1979.
22. Arruda JAL, Nascimento L, Kurtzman NA: Effect of parathyroid hormone on urinary acidification. *Am J Physiol* 232:F429–F433, 1977.
23. Bank N, Aynedjian HS: A micropuncture study of the effect of parathyroid hormone on renal bicarbonate reabsorption. *J Clin Invest* 58:336–344, 1976.
24. Booth BE, Tsai HC, Curtis-Morris R Jr: Metabolic acidosis in the vitamin D deficient chick. *Proc Am Soc Nephrol* 8:1, 1975, (abstract).
25. Siegfried D, Kumar R, Arruda JAL, et al: Influence of vitamin D on bicarbonate reabsorption. *Adv Exp Med Biol* 81:395–404, 1976.
26. Peraino R, Ghaffary E, Rouse D, et al: Effects of 25-hydroxy-vitamin D_3 on renal handling of sodium, calcium and phosphate during bicarbonate infusion. *Min Elect Met* 1:295–349, 1978.
27. McKinney TD, Myers P: Effect of calcium and phosphate on bicarbonate and fluid transport by proximal tubules in vitro. *Kidney Int* 21:433–438, 1982.
28. Arruda JAL: Effect of calcium on urinary acidification. *Min Elect Met* 7:1–7, 1982.
29. Arruda JAL: Calcium inhibits urinary acidification. Effect of ionophore A23178 in the turtle bladder. *Pflugers Arch* 381:107–111, 1979.
30. Arruda JAL, Dytko G, Mola R: Effect of calcium and magnesium on transport processes by the turtle bladder. *Arch Int Pharmacodyn Ther* 240:27–34, 1979.
31. Arruda JAL, Sabatini S: Effect of quinidine on Na, H+ and water transport by the turtle and toad bladders. *J Membr Biol* 55:141–147, 1980.
32. Arruda JAL, Sabatini S: Cholinergic inhibition of urinary acidification by the turtle bladder. *Kidney Int* 17:622–630, 1980.
33. Arruda JAL, Sabatini S, Westenfelder C: Serosal Na/Ca exchange and H+ and Na transport by the turtle and toad bladders. *J Memb Biol* 70:135–146, 1982.
34. Arruda JAL, Dytko G, Lubansky H, et al: Effect of calcium on intracellular pH. *Bioch Biophys Res Comm* 102:891–896, 1982.
35. Cunningham J, Frasher LJ, Clemens TL, et al: Chronic acidosis with metabolic bone disease. *Am J Med* 73:199–203, 1982.
36. Lee SW, Russel J, Avioli LV: 25-Hydroxycholicalciferol to 1-25 dihydroxycholicalciferol: Conversion impaired by systemic metabolic acidosis. *Science* 195:994–996, 1977.

37. Sawyer B, Gorabedian M, Fellot C, et al: The effect of induced metabolic acidosis on Vitamin D_3 metabolism in rachitic chicks. *Calcif Tissue Res* 23:121–124, 1981.
38. Beck N, Kim HP, Kim KS: Effect of metabolic acidosis on renal action of parathyroid hormone. *Am J Physiol* 228:1438–1488, 1975.
39. Kawashima H, Kraut JA, Kurokawa K: Metabolic acidosis supresses 25-hydroxy vitamin D_3 1-α-hydroxylase in the rat kidney. *J Clin Invest* 70:135–140, 1980.
40. Bushinsky DA, Favers MJ, Sen PK, et al: Effect of chronic metabolic acidosis on serum 1-25-dihyroxy vitamine D_3 levels in the rat. Proceeding of the American Society of Nephrology 14th Annual Meeting, 1981 (abstract).
41. Seldin DW, Wilson JD: Renal tubular acidosis, in Stanbury JB, Wyngaarden J, Frederickson DS (eds): *The Metabolic Basis of Inherited Diseases* (3d ed). New York, McGraw-Hill, 1971, pp 1548–1566.
42. Brenner RJ, Spung DB, Sebastian A, et al: Incidence of radiographic evident bone disease, nephrocalcinosis and nephrolithiasis in various types of renal tubular acidosis. *N Engl J Med* 307:217–221, 1982.
43. Courey WR, Pfister RC: The radiographic findings in renal tubular acidosis. *Radiology* 105:497–503, 1972.
44. Brewer ED, Tsai HC, Szeto KS, et al: Maleic acid induced impaired conversion of 25 (OH) D_3 to 1-25 $(OH)_2$ D_3: Implications for Fanconi's syndrome. *Kidney Int* 12:244–250, 1977.
45. Ishitsu T, Matsuda I, Suno Y, et al: Anticonvulsant induced rickets associated with renal tubular acidosis and normal levels of serum 1-25-dihydroxy vitamin D_3. *Am J Dis Child* 135:1140–1142, 1981.
46. Lemann J, Lennon E: Role of the diet, gastrointestinal tract and bone in acid base homeostasis. *Kidney Int* 1:275–279, 1972.
47. Camien MN, Gonick H: Relationship of renal "net acid" excretion to titrable ash acidity (Ash TA) in diet and feces. *Proc Soc Exp Biol Med* 126:45–51, 1967.
48. Lennon EJ, Lemann J Jr, Litzow JR: The effects of diet and stool composition on net external acid base balance of normal subjects. *J Clin Invest* 45:1610–1617, 1966.
49. Richardson RMA, Goldstein MB, Stinebaugh BJ, et al: Influence of diet and metabolism on urinary acid excretion in the rat and rabbit. *J Lab Clin Med* 94:510–518, 1979.
50. Giammarco RA, Goldstein MB, Halperin M, et al: Collecting duct hydrogen ion secretion in the rabbit: Role of potassium. *J Lab Clin Med* 91:948–959, 1978.
51. Cruz-Soto M, Battle D, Sabatini S, et al: Distal acidification in the rabbit: Role of diet and blood pH. *Am J Physiol* 243:F364–F371, 1982.
52. Terao N, Tanner RL: Characterization of acidification by distal nephron using the isolated perfused rat kidney: Evidence for adaptation to a high bicarbonate diet. *Kidney Int* 20:36–42, 1981.
53. Sasaki S, Berry CA, Rector FC Jr: Effect of luminal and peritubular HOC_3 concentration and Pco_2 on HCO_3 reabsorption in rabbit proximal convoluted tubules perfused in vitro. *J Clin Invest* 70:639–649, 1982.
54. Kleinman JG, Ware RA, Schwartz JH: Anion transport regulates intracellular pH in renal cortical tissue. *Biochem Biophys Acta* 648:87–92, 1981.
55. Buckalew, VM Jr, Purvis ML, Shulman MG, et al: Hereditary renal tubular acidosis. *Medicine* 53:229–54, 1974.
56. Hamed SA, Czerwinski AW, Coats B, et al: Familial absorptive hypercalciuria and renal tubular acidosis. *Am J Med* 67:385–391, 1979.
57. Cohen JJ, Kamm DE: Renal metabolism relation to renal function, in Brenner B, Rector FC Jr (eds): *The Kidney*, vol 1, ed 1. Philadelphia, WB Saunders, 1976, pp 126–201.

58. Simpson D: Regulation of renal citrate metabolism by bicarbonate ion and pH: Observations in tissue slices and mitochondria. *J Clin Invest* 46:225, 1967.
59. Sanjar SA, Mansour FM, Hernandez RH, et al: Severe hypertension, hyperkalemia and renal tubular acidosis responding to dietary sodium restriction. *Pediatrics* 69:317–324, 1982.
60. Schambelan M, Sebastian A, Rector FC: Mineralocorticoid-resistant renal hyperkalemia without salt wasting (type II pseudohypoaldosteronism): Role of increased renal chloride reabsorption. *Kidney Int* 19:716–727, 1981.
61. DeFronzo RA, Cooke CR, Wright JR, et al: Renal function in patients with multiple myeloma. *Medicine* 57:151–166, 1978.
62. Lazar GS, Feinstein DI: Distal renal tubular acidosis in multiple myeloma. *Arch Int Med* 141:655–657, 1981.
63. Bolanos F, Leon SP, Garcia G, et al: Hyperthyroidism associated with renal tubular acidosis, nephrocalcinosis, nephogenic diabetes insipidus and periodic paralysis. *Rev Invest Clin* 33:195–198, 1981.
64. Allegri L, Chizzolini C, Ciccone E, et al: Acidosi tubulare renale (ATR) con ipergammaglobulinemia idiopatica. (Studio immunopatologico di un caso.) *Minn Nephrol* 28:49–52, 1981.
65. Conn JW, Rovner DR, Cohen EL, et al: Inhibition by heparinoid of aldosterone biosynthesis in man. *J Clin Endocrinol Metab* 26:527–532, 1966.
66. Kloppenborg PWC, Casparie AF, Benraad JT, et al: Inhibition of adrenal function in man by heparin or heparinoid, RO1 8308. *Acta Med Scand* 197:99–108, 1975.
67. Leehey D, Gantt C, Lim V: Heparin induced hypoaldosteronism. *JAMA* 246:2189–2190, 1981.
68. Phelps KR, Oh MS, Carroll HJ: Heparin induced hyperkalemia: Report of a case. *Nephron* 25:254–258, 1980.
69. Wilson ID, Goetz FC: Selective hypoaldosteronism after prolonged heparin administration. *Am J Med* 36:635–640, 1964.
70. Bank N, Leif PD, Aynedjian HS, et al: Studies of urinary acidification defect induced by lithium. *Am J Physiol* 242:F23–29, 1982.
71. Warnock DG, Yee VJ, Ives HE: Cis and trans effect of Li on Na-H antiporter. *Kidney Int* 23:240, 1983 (abstract).
72. Arruda JAL, Dytko G, Mola R, et al: The mechanism of lithium induced renal tubular acidosis: Studies in the turtle bladder. *Kidney Int* 17:196–204, 1980.
73. Agarwal BJ, Cabebe FG: Renal acidification in elderly subjects. *Nephron* 26:291–295, 1980.
74. Adler S, Lindeman RD, Yiengst MJ: Effect of acute acid loading on urinary acid excretion by the aging human kidney. *J Lab Clin Med* 72:278–289, 1968.
75. Rochman J, Lichtig C, Ostenwell D, et al: Adult Fanconi's syndrome with renal tubular acidosis is associated with renal amyloidosis. *Arch Intern Med* 140:1361–1363, 1980.
76. Pirani C, Silver F, Appel G: Tubulointerstitial disease in multiple myeloma and other nonrenal neoplasia, in Cotran RS (ed): *Contemporary Issues in Nephrology*, vol 10. New York, Churchill Livingston, 1983, pp 287–334.
77. Wilson HK, Kewer SP, Leo S, et al: Phosphate therapy in diabetic ketoacidosis. *Arch Intern Med* 142:517–520, 1982.
78. Adrogue HJ, Wilson H, Boyd AE, et al: Plasma acid base patterns in diabetic ketoacidosis. *N Engl J Med* 307:1603–1610, 1982.
79. Oh MS, Carroll HJ, Goldstein DA, et al: Hyperchloremic acidosis during the recovery phase of diabetic ketosis. *Ann Intern Med* 89:925–927, 1978.

80. Oh MS, Banerji MA, Carroll HJ: The mechanism of hyperchloremic acidosis during the recovery phase of diabetic ketoacidosis. *Diabetes* 30:310–313, 1981.
81. Arruda JAL, Kurtzman NA: Metabolic acidosis and alkalosis. *Clin Nephrol* 7:201–225, 1977.
82. Feldman JM: Metabolic acidosis in patients with the carcinoid syndrome: Treatment with parachlorophenylalonine. *J Surg Oncol* 19:219–223, 1980.
83. Olivia P: Lactic acidosis. *Am J Med* 48:209–225, 1970.
84. Alberti KG, Nattrass M: Lactic acidosis. *Lancet* 2:25–29, 1977.
85. Kreisberg RA: Lactate homeostasis and lactic acidosis. *Ann Intern Med* 92:227–239, 1980.
86. Park R, Arieff AL: Lactic acidosis. *Adv Intern Med* 33:68, 1980.
87. Arieff AL, Park R, Leach WJ: Pathophysiology of experimental lactic acidosis in dog. *Am J Physiol* 239:F135, 1980.
88. Arieff AL, Park R, Lazarowitz VC, et al: Systemic effects of $NaHCO_3$ in experimental lactic acidosis in dogs. *Am J Physiol* 242:F586–F591, 1982.
89. Fraley DS, Adler S, Bruns FJ, et al: Stimulation of lactate production by administration of bicarbonate in a patient with a solid neoplasm and lactic acidosis. *N Engl J Med* 303:1100–1102, 1980.
90. Fields ALA, Wolman SL, Halperin ML: Chronic lactic acidosis in a patient with cancer. *Cancer* 47:2026–2029, 1981.
91. Park R, Arieff AL: Treatment of lactic acidosis with dichloroacetate in dogs. *J Clin Invest* 70:853–862, 1982.
92. Stacpoole PW, Moore GW, Kornhauser DM: Metabolic effects of dichloracetate in patients with diabetes mellitus and hyperlipoproteinemia. *N Engl J Med* 298:526–530, 1978.
93. Capetti L, Fici F, Coscelli C, et al: Pyridoxine-alpha-ketoglutarate in the treatment of experimental lactic acidosis. *Horm Metab Res* 13:472–473, 1981.
94. Belvisi A, Metergi M, Fici F: Treatment of hyperlactacidemia in cirrhotic patients with pyridoxine-alpha-ketoglutarate. *Int J Clin Pharmacol Therap Toxicol* 20:142–146, 1982.
95. Leonard JV: Problems in the congenital lactic acidosis. *Ciba Foundation Symposium* vol 87. Belmont, CA, Pitman, 1981, pp 340–356.
96. Hamat RB, Wolman SL, Fields ALA, et al: Evaluation of Na acetate as a source of alkali therapy in an experimental aerobic model of lactic acidosis due to decreased pyruvate oxidation. *Metabolism* 31:548, 1982.
97. Oh MS, Phelps KR, Traube M, et al: D-lactic acidosis in a man with short-bowel syndrome. *N Engl J Med* 301:249–252, 1979.
98. Muir LA, Rickes EL, Duquette PF, et al: Control of wheat-induced lactic acidosis in sheep by thiopeptin and related antibiotics. *Animal Science* 50:547–553, 1980.
99. Schoorel EP, Giesbert MAH, Blom W, et al: D-lactic acidosis in a boy with short bowel syndrome. *Arch Dis Child* 55:810–812, 1980.
100. Carr DB, Shih VE, Richter JM, et al: D-lactic acidosis simulating a hypothalamic syndrome after bowel bypass. *Neurology* 11:195–197, 1982.
101. Stolberg L, Rolfe R, Gitlin N, et al: D-lactic acidosis due to abnormal gut. *N Engl J Med* 306:1344–1348, 1982.
102. Traube M, Bock J, Boyer JL: D-Lactic acidosis after jejunoileal bypass: Identification of organic anion by nuclear magnetic resonance spectroscopy. *Ann Intern Med* 98:171–174, 1983.
103. Roos BD, Radda GK, Gadian PG, et al: Examination of a case of suspected McArdle's Syndrome by ^{31}P nuclear magnetic resonance. *N Engl J Med* 304:1338–1341, 1981.
104. Shulman RG: NMR spectroscopy of living cells. *Sci Am* 248:86–93, 1983.

105. Burt CT, Cohen SM, Barany M: Analysis of intact tissue by means of 31-P magnetic resonance. *Ann Rev Biophys Bioengin* 8:1–25, 1979.
106. Hart GR, Anderson RJ, Crumpler CP, et al: Epidemic classical heat stroke: Clinical characteristics and course of 28 patients. *Medicine* 61:189–197, 1982.
107. Vaziri ND, Stokes J, Treadwell TR: Lactic acidosis, a complication of papaverine overdose. *Clin Toxicol* 18:417–423, 1981.
108. Pappas S, Silverman M: Treatment of methanol poisoning with ethanol and hemodialysis. *Can Med Assoc J* 126:1391–1394, 1982.
109. Finkle DE, Dean RE: Buffered hydrochloric acid: A modern method of treating metabolic alkalosis. *Am Surg* 47:103–106, 1981.
110. Parker MS, Oster JR, Perez G, et al: Chronic hypokalemia and alkalosis: Approach to diagnosis. *Arch Intern Med* 140:1336–1337, 1980.
111. Hulter HN, Licht JH, Bonner ER, et al: Effects of glucocorticoids on renal and systemic acid base equilibrium. *Am J Physiol* 239:F30–43, 1980.
112. Hulter HN, Sigala JF, Sebastian A: Effect of dexamethasone on renal and systemic acid base metabolism. *Kidney Int* 20:43–49, 1981.
113. Freiberg JM, Kinsella J, Sacktor B: Glucocorticoids increase the Na-H exchange and decrease the Na gradient dependent phosphate uptake systems in renal brush border vesicles. *Proc Natl Acad Sci USA* 79:4932–4936, 1982.
114. Kurtzman NA, White MG, Rogers PW: The effect of potassium and extracellular volume on renal bicarbonate reabsorption. *Metabolism* 22:481–492, 1973.
115. Kassirer JP, Schwartz WB: The response of normal man to selective depletion of hydrochloric acid. Factors in the genesis of persistent gastric alkalosis. *Am J Med* 40:10–18, 1966.
116. Kassirer JP, Schwartz WB: Correction of metabolic alkalosis in man without repair of potassium deficiency. A re-evaluation of the role of potassium. *Am J Med* 40:19–26, 1966.
117. Burnell JM, Teubner EJ, Simpson DP: Metabolic acidosis accompanying potassium deprivation. *Am J Physiol* 227:329–333, 1974.
118. Hulter HN, Sebastian A, Sigala JF, et al: Pathogenesis of renal hyperchloremic acidosis resulting from dietary potassium restriction in the dog: Role of aldosterone. *Am J Physiol* 238:F79–F91, 1980.
119. Garella S, Chang B, Kahn SI: Alterations of hydrogen ion homeostasis in pure potassium depletion: Studies in rats and dogs during the recovery phase. *J Lab Clin Med* 93:321–331, 1979.
120. van Ypersele de Strihou C, Dieu J-P: Potassium deficiency acidosis in the dog: Effect of sodium and potassium balance on renal response to a chronic acid load. *Kidney Int* 11:335–347, 1977.
121. Jones JW, Sebastian A, Hulter HN, et al: Systemic and renal acid base effects of chronic dietary potassium depletion in humans. *Kidney Int* 21:402–410, 1982.
122. Arruda JAL, Nascimento L, Kumar SK, et al: Factors influencing the formation of urinary carbon dioxide tension. *Kidney Int* 11:307, 1977.
123. Pichette C, Tam SC, Chen CB, et al: Effect of potassium on distal nephron hydrogen ion secretion in the dog. *J Lab Clin Med* 100:374–384. 1982.
124. Tannen RL: Ammonia metabolism. *Am J Physiol* 235:F265–F277, 1978.
125. Kraut JA, Wish JB, Zoller KM, et al: Aldosterone and the renal response to sulfuric acid feeding in the dog. *Am J Physiol* 243:F494–502, 1982.
126. Kraut JA, Wish JB, Sweet SJ, et al: Failure of increased sodium avidity to facilitate renal acid excretion during H_2SO_4 feeding in the dog. *Kidney Int* 20:50–54, 1981.

127. Goldstein W: Pathways of glutamine deamination and their control in the rat kidney. *Am J Physiol* 213:983–989, 1967.
128. Lemieux G, Baverel G, Vinay P, et al: Glutamine synthetase and glutamyltransferase in the kidney of man, dog, and rat. *Am J Physiol* 231:1068–1073, 1976.
129. Simpson DP, Adam W: Glutamine transport and metabolism by mitochondria from dogs renal cortex. *J Biol Chem* 350:8148–8158, 1975.
130. Tannen RW, Kunin AS: Effect of pH on ammonia production by renal mitochondria. *Am J Physiol* 231:1631–1637, 1976.
131. Tannen RL, Kunin AS: Effect of potassium on ammoniagenesis by renal mitochondria. *Am J Physiol* 231:44–51, 1976.
132. Bogusky RT, Lowenstein WM, Lowenstein JM: The purine nucleotide cycle. A pathway for ammonia production in the rat kidney. *J Clin Invest* 58:326–335, 1976.
133. Bogusky RT, Stelle KA, Lowenstein LM: The purine nucleotide cycle in the regulation of ammoniagenesis during the induction and absorption of chronic acidosis in the rat kidney. *Biochem J* 196:323–326, 1981.
134. Sajo IM, Goldstein MB, Wilson DR, et al: Sites of ammonia addition to tubular fluid in rats with chronic metabolic acidosis. *Kidney Int* 20:353–358, 1981.
135. Buerkert J, Martin D, Trigg D: Ammonium handling by superficial and juxtamedullary nephrons in the rat. *J Clin Invest* 70:1–12, 1982.
136. Goldstein L, Clairborne JB, Evans DE: Ammonia excretion by the gills of two marine teleost fish: The importance of NH_4+ permeance. *J Exp Zoology* 219:395–397, 1982.

ACKNOWLEDGMENT

The original work cited in this paper was supported by the following grants: VA CO 7083, U.S. Public Health Service AM 20170, and Chicago Heart Association 7920. Dr. Robert Gold was Fellow of the National Kidney Foundation during part of this work. Nancy Leach of Merck-Sharp Dohme Co. provided invaluable help in the review of the literature.

CHAPTER 10

Disorders of Calcium, Phosphorus, and Magnesium

Nachman Brautbar
Helen Gruber
David B.N. Lee

DISORDERS OF CALCIUM ION METABOLISM

The last two years have witnessed major advances in our understanding of the regulation of calcium homeostasis by the parathyroid hormone and its role in metabolic bone disease.

Parathyroid Hormone

Biosynthesis

Parathyroid hormone (PTH) is a polypeptide of 84 amino acids and is synthesized from a larger precursor proparathyroid hormone which contains 115 amino acids (1). This large precursor is cleaved twice to finally produce the 84 amino acid PTH (Fig. 1). The first cleavage occurs at the rough endoplasmic reticulum (RER), and after removal of 25 amino acids, the preproparathyroid hormone is formed. The second step occurs at the Golgi complex, where six or more amino acids are removed to form the final PTH (2). The hormone is then released from the gland to the circulation, and a third cleavage occurs in the liver and kidney at position 34-35 to yield the metabolically active hormone (to be further discussed in peripheral metabolism of PTH).

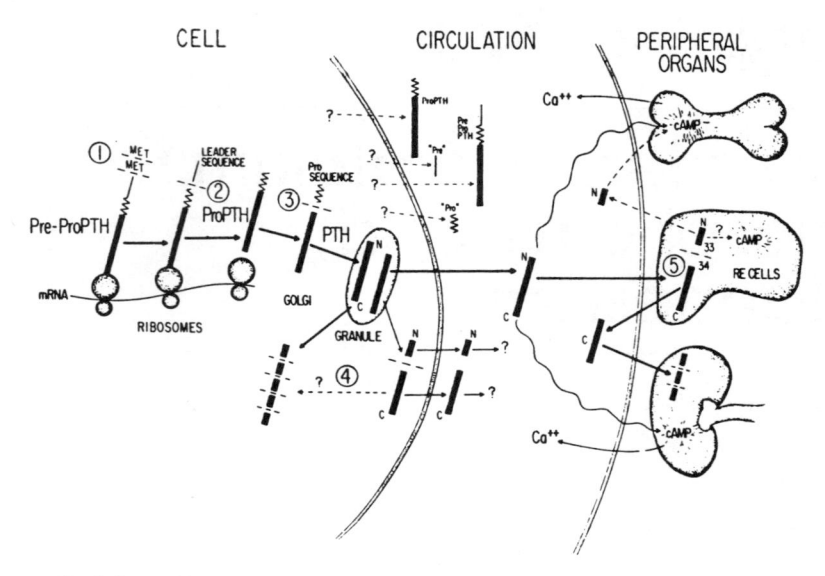

Figure 1. Schematic description of the biosynthesis, secretion, and peripheral metabolism of PTH. (Habener JF et al, in Hand AR, Oliver C (eds): *Methods in Cell Biology.* Academic Press, New York, 1981. Used with permission.)

Cellular Transport

The regulation and cellular pathway of preproPTH have been examined recently by Habener et al. (3). They have suggested a model whereby the initiation of the synthesis of preproPTH occurs on polyribosomes located within the cell matrix. When the growing polypeptide chain reaches a length of 20 to 30 amino acids, the NH_2 terminal emerges from the ribosome and the two NH_2-terminal methionines of preproPTH are removed by a putative amino peptidase.

As the chain continues to grow, the hydrophobic amino terminal sequence of preproPTH emerges and associates with the membrane of the endoplasmic reticulum (Fig. 2). Newly synthesized polypeptide chains are then transferred to the cisternal spaces of the sarcoplasmic reticulum (Figs. 2 and 3). This step is of major importance in the preservation of cellular proteins to be retained in the cell and those to be secreted via the cisternal step. The secretory proteins are then transferred within the membrane to the Golgi apparatus of the cell to be further incorporated into secretory granules and vesicles. In response to the appropriate stimulus the protein is either stored within the cell or released through the membrane by exocytosis. Habener et al. (3) performed experiments using very short pulse labeling periods and demonstrated newly synthesized preproPTH and proPTH as early as 30 seconds; furthermore, the labeled proPTH was found in association with the microsome of the PTH cell.

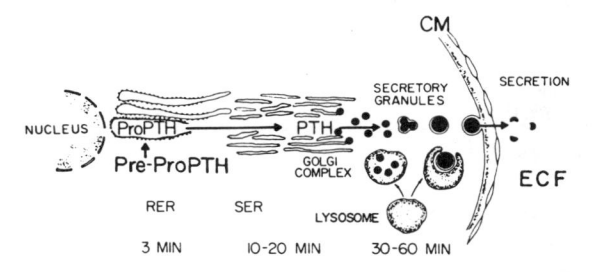

Figure 2. Schematic description of the intracellular biosynthesis of PTH from prepro-PTH to the secretion of the hormone. (Habener JF et al, in Hand AR, Oliver C (eds): *Methods in Cell Biology*. New York, Academic Press, 1981. Used with permission.)

Parathyroid Secretory Proteins

The parathyroid gland synthesizes and secretes two major proteins, PTH and parathyroid secretory protein (PSP), which is essentially a glycoprotein. PSP comprises 50–60% of the newly formed protein. The synthesis, cellular transport, and release of both proteins occurs together (2) and is regulated mainly by changes in extracellular calcium content (4). Majzoub et al. (5) examined the biosynthesis and cellular processing of PSP by analysis of the products of translation of PTH gland mRNA in cell-free systems supplemented with pancreatic microsomes and incubation of parathyroid gland slices in the presence of amino acids and sugars and measuring the PSP. The authors show that prePSP is converted to PSP by microsomal membranes during translocation of prePSP mRNA. Interestingly, the known heterogeneity of the cellular and secreted forms of PSP is the result of a modification of newly synthesized PSP by glycosylation, which takes place *after* completion of the synthesis and during the transport of the protein to the membrane. We suggest that the heterogeneity of the

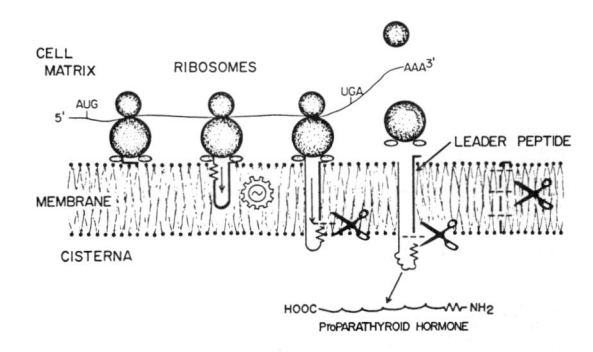

Figure 3. The secretory process of the hormone via the cisternal spaces and sarcoplasmic reticulum. (Habener JF et al, in Hand AR, Oliver C (eds): *Methods in Cell Biology*, New York, Academic Press, 1981. Used with permission.)

cellular and secreted forms of PSP and prePSP is an expression of several closely related genes. Whether PSP has any biologic activity once secreted into the circulation is not known. However, it is possible that excess secretion of the PSP in pathologic conditions may contribute to the various syndromes of excess PTH.

Regulation of Synthesis by Calcium
The regulation of cellular biosynthesis and cellular transport of PTH and PSP has been controversial. Raisz et al. (6) found a marked incorporation of radioactive amino acids in total cellular proteins of rat parathyroid glands at low rather than at high extracellular calcium concentrations and suggested a role for calcium in the regulation of PTH biosynthesis. Other investigators (7,8) who used bovine parathyroid slices found incorporation of labeled amino acids into peptides corresponding to bovine proPTH and intact PTH (1-84) that was higher at low than at high calcium concentrations in the incubation medium. These findings were not confirmed by others (9). Recent work by Moran et al. (10) has examined the incorporation of labeled amino acids into PSP, proPTH, and PTH (1-84) using dispersed bovine parathyroid cells incubated in vitro. The incorporation of the labeled amino acids was shown to be greater at low than at high calcium concentrations. This study for the first time presents evidence for calcium regulation of synthesis of prePTH, PTH, and PSP. These findings suggest that the calcium-regulated release of the hormone is accompanied, or possibly preceded, by a calcium-regulated synthetic pathway. At what step of cellular synthesis calcium exerts its regulatory role is not clear.

PTH Metabolism

Intravenous administration of intact 1-84 PTH is accompanied by a rapid appearance in the circulation of fragments of the hormone. The hormone is cleaved at positions 33-34 and 36-32, releasing fragments of the hormone that possess biologic activity (the first 34 amino acids possess biologic activity). It is possible that the step of peripheral metabolism is of major importance in activation of the hormone.

The peripheral clearance occurs in the liver and kidney. Administration of 1-84 PTH to partially hepatectomized animals has been shown to prolong the disappearance rate of the hormone. Several factors are involved in the regulation of hepatic metabolism of PTH.

Metabolism by the Liver
Studies performed in an isolated perfused liver preparation have shown that the concentration of calcium in the perfusate has a marked influence on the cleavage of the hormone: high calcium in the perfusate was associated with a slower rate of cleavage. This observation is compatible

with the notion that the amino terminal fragment is the metabolically active fragment in calcium homeostasis and that some kind of a feedback loop is regulating the production of this active fragment through the concentration of blood ionized calcium. Martin et al. (11) have shown that hepatic uptake is specific for the intact hormone and that the liver is the source of both the amino and carboxy terminal fragments.

Studies by D'Amour et al. (12) have localized the hepatic uptake cleavage and production of carboxy terminal PTH to the Kupffer cells. Other investigators have suggested a role for the hepatocyte in addition to the Kupffer cells.

The hepatic uptake of PTH has been shown to be impaired in uremia. Huruska et al. (13) have recently examined the effects of chronic renal failure on the peripheral metabolism of PTH by measuring plasma disappearance rate of intact PTH administered to awake dogs. The metabolic clearance rate of PTH was found to be very rapid, 21.6 ± 3.1 ml/min/kg; the liver accounted for 61%, while renal uptake accounted for 31% of the metabolic clearance rate. Interestingly, the metabolic clearance rate of intact PTH inactivated by oxidation was markedly reduced, demonstrating that the liver and renal sites responsible for the uptake are specific and recognize intact PTH. Chronic renal failure in these dogs reduced the metabolic clearance rate of the hormone largely due to impaired liver uptake. These data identify the liver as the major extrarenal site of PTH metabolism affected in chronic renal failure.

Segre et al. (14) examined the role of hepatectomy and nephrectomy on the peripheral metabolism of PTH. The rate of disappearance of ^{125}I-labeled and unlabeled bovine PTH from plasma and the appearance and disappearance and chemical and immunochemical characteristics of the fragments were evaluated in control and hepatectomized rats. After hepatectomy, the clearance rate of the intact hormone was significantly reduced. Injection of ^{125}I-labeled intact hormone in hepatectomized rats resulted in a marked reduction in the carboxy terminal fragment of the hormone. Carboxy terminal fragments having positions 34 and 37 of the intact hormone sequence were essentially absent in hepatectomized rats but abundant in control and uremic rats, further demonstrating the liver as the major organ for peripheral metabolism of PTH and the generation of most of the carboxy terminal fragments.

The role of the kidney in generating circulating fragments was also examined. It appears that the kidney has a lesser role in the quantitative generation of fragments. Plasma from nephrectomized rats contained twice the carboxy-terminal fragments than did controls, and the clearance rate of the fragments was significantly reduced. These results confirm the importance of renal clearance of both intact PTH and carboxy terminal fragments.

What is the cellular location and mechanism by which the liver accomplishes the peripheral metabolism of PTH? Segre et al. (15) examined this issue in isolated liver cells. The authors showed that Kupffer cells, rather than hepatocytes, contain enzymes that are responsible for proteolysis of PTH. The dominant PTH fragment recovered from the media of Kupffer cell incubations reacted in radioimmunassay to antibodies specific for the carboxy terminal portion of the hormone but not to antibodies specific for the aminoterminal. These studies also identified the properties of the enzymes responsible for PTH cleavage. The initial step is generation of both amino and carboxy terminal fragments by endopeptidases of the Kupffer cells. The amino terminal disappeared from the medium rapidly secondary to cleavage by exopeptidase. These in vitro results are consistent with the in vitro observation showing high concentration of carboxy terminal fragments but no amino terminal fragments.

Kidney Metabolism of PTH

The kidney has the capacity to metabolize intact PTH as well as to remove amino and carboxy terminal fragments. In chronic renal failure, the renal clearance of PTH is markedly reduced as a result of a reduction in renal plasma flow. The biologically active PTH (1-84) and the amino terminal fragment are removed by peritubular uptake and glomerular filtration, while the biologically inactive form (carboxy terminal) is removed exclusively by glomerular filtration and tubular reabsorption. This sequence of events has important chemical applications. The marked accumulation of carboxy terminal PTH in the plasma of rats with chronic renal failure is explained by the dependence of the renal clearance of the carboxy terminal fragment on the glomerular filtration rate. After successful renal transplantation, a marked reduction to normal levels of carboxy terminal PTH is noted.

The kidney has an important role in the production of PTH fragments. The metabolism of intact PTH to both carboxy and amino terminal PTH is accelerated in the presence of hypocalcemia and inhibited in the presence of hypercalcemia. Although the kidney and liver account for almost all the metabolic clearance of intact PTH, the kidney clears 45% of injected amino terminal fragment.

Bone Metabolism of PTH

Bone metabolism of PTH differs from that of liver and kidney by its ability to selectively uptake 1-34 PTH but not intact or carboxy terminal PTH. These observations correlate with the findings of biologic activity of 1-34 PTH on bone.

The effects of uremia on bone response to 1-34 PTH have recently been examined. An impaired calcemic response to PTH has been well documented in experimental animals and in patients with acute renal failure and various degrees of chronic renal failure. Olgaard et al. (16)

have evaluated the effects of acute renal failure on bone response to the administration of 1-34 PTH. The extraction of PTH and the stimulation of cyclic adenosine monophosphate (cAMP) were measured in isolated perfused bones. The extraction of 1-34 PTH by bone from uremic animals did not differ from the control group. However, despite a normal extraction of PTH, cAMP release by bone from uremic animals was markedly diminished. Interestingly, this was not observed in uremic animals who also underwent parathyroidectomy. The authors concluded that the high levels of endogenous PTH in the uremic animals desensitized the bone cAMP response, which was corrected in parathyroidectomized animals.

FACTORS REGULATING PARATHYROID HORMONE SECRETION (CELLULAR MECHANISMS)

Calcium

The concentration of ionized calcium in the blood and extracellular fluid is considered to be the major factor regulating the secretion of PTH from the gland. Little information is available about the mechanisms through which changes in extracellular calcium inhibit the secretory process.

Recent studies using dispersed PTH cells and bovine PTH slices have suggested that the rise of intracellular calcium concentration alters PTH secretion. Rothstein et al. (17) examined the role of Na–Ca exchange as a mediator of PTH secretion. Utilizing in vitro experiments with dispersed PTH cells the authors have shown that (1) ouabain affects PTH secretion by its action on Na–K ATPase and (2) a decrease in Na–Ca exchange by blocking the sodium pump increases intracellular calcium, which in turn inhibits PTH secretion. These observations suggest the existence of a Na–Ca exchanger in the parathyroid plasma cell membrane, and that this system participates in the regulation of cellular calcium concentration. Since an elevation in cellular sodium could raise cytosolic calcium, these data provide evidence for the mediatory role of cytosolic calcium concentration in regulation of PTH release. Further measurements of an increase in cytosolic calcium are needed to substantiate this hypothesis.

A direct effect of the calcium ions on the plasma membrane, rather than an intracellular increase in the concentration of the ion, has been suggested. Several types of endocrine cells are able to generate action potentials partly dependent on calcium, and these potentials play a key role in the stimulus–secretion coupling. Bruce et al. (18) have shown an increase in membrane potential in parathyroid glands at 1.5 mM as compared to 2.5 mM calcium. This hyperpolarization was abolished by an increase in extracellular potassium concentration. Membrane potential changes may play a role in stimulus-secretion coupling in PTH cells. Dempster et al. (19) examined the effects of raising extracellular potassium on PTH secretion and found a marked stimulation of PTH release. Whether these changes in PTH secretion are due to direct changes in the plasma membrane potential or are secondary to intracellular calcium is not clear from this study. Hove et al. (20) examined whether the changes in PTH are due to plasma membrane changes. The acute effects of various drugs on the release of PTH in goats was studied. The data were compatible with the notion that PTH cells possess voltage-sensitive potassium and calcium channels, and that exocytosis of stored PTH depends on influx of calcium. A suppressive effect of calcium ions on the permeability of the plasma membrane cell was postulated. Indeed, Wild et al. (21) reported quantitative changes of membranes in rat parathyroid cells related to variations in serum calcium. The results clearly demonstrate that stimulation and suppression of PTH through alteration in serum calcium caused quantitative changes in the Golgi complex and plasma membranes, suggesting recycling of membrane components. Support for an effect of calcium ions on the PTH cell membrane is taken from recent observations that calcium-mediated PTH secretion is associated with rapid membrane phospholipid turnover (22).

Mechanisms by Which Changes in Cytosolic Calcium May Mediate PTH Secretion

Cyclic AMP-Adenylate Cyclase System. Calcium has been shown to inhibit adenylate cyclase activity in PTH glands. A phosphodiesterase activated by calcium and calmodulin has been described in human (23) and in bovine PTH glands (24). Thus, inhibition of the synthesis or breakdown of cAMP in response to elevated intracellular calcium might mediate the secretory changes. Brown et al. (25) studied the effects of calcium on cellular cAMP and PTH release in dispersed PTH cells from patients with primary hyperparathyroidism. The results show considerable heterogeneity in the effects of calcium on cAMP accumulation and PTH secretion. These observations, and the report by Onties et al. (24) that adenylate cyclase from pathologic parathyroid tissue is resistant to the inhibitory effects of calcium, make the role of cAMP in the secretion of PTH questionable.

Calmodulin. Willgross et al. (26) have demonstrated the presence of a heat stable activator of calmodulin-stimulable phosphodiesterase in parathyroid adenomas. Recently, Oldham et al. (27) examined calmodulin in adenomas of patients with surgically diagnosed primary hyperparathyroidism. The authors found calmodulin activity in all adenomas. There was no correlation between the presurgical levels of PTH and the calmodulin concentration. Further studies in normal PTH cells are needed to find out whether calmodulin may play a role in the mediation of PTH secretion.

Increased Intracellular Degradation of PTH. Several investigators have reported increased intracellular PTH degradation in response to elevated calcium concentration. The regulating role of such a system is not clear.

Other Ions

The effects of magnesium on PTH secretion are comparable to those of calcium. Low magnesium stimulates and high magnesium suppresses PTH release. On a molar basis, magnesium is 2–3 times less effective in suppressing PTH release. On the other hand, severe magnesium depletion is known to inhibit PTH secretion.

Mahaffee et al. (28) examined the interaction of magnesium and calcium in PTH secretion and the role of the adenylate cyclase-cAMP system in parathyroid dispersed cells. Depletion of magnesium from the medium resulted in a marked decrease in PTH secretion at any given calcium concentration. At a constant calcium concentration of 1 mM, both PTH secretion and cAMP production rose to maximal rates as the magnesium concentration was increased from 0 to 2 mM. Adenylate cyclase sensitivity to calcium inhibition was dependent upon the magnesium concentration. The data suggest that magnesium may promote PTH secretion either by enhancing the activation of adneylate cyclase by endogenous guanine nucleotides or by competing with calcium for binding to a regulating enzyme.

Recently, lithium has been shown to affect PTH secretion. These studies were prompted by the clinical observations that manic depressive patients treated with lithium for a long period of time developed hypercalcemia in the face of elevated PTH hormone levels, a picture compatible with primary hyperparathyroidism. Brown et al. (29) examined the calcium-mediated PTH release in dispersed bovine PTH cells and the interaction with lithium. Preincubation with lithium for 4 hours caused a dose-dependent increase in the concentration of calcium required for half the maximal inhibition of PTH release (set point for calcium) A significant increase in the set point was observed following exposure to 1.25 mM lithium, a concentration within the therapeutic range for humans.

Other cations are known to exert changes in PTH secretion. Wallace et al. (30) examined recently the effects of lanthanum, manganese, strontium, barium, and magnesium on PTH secretion in vitro. All the ions suppressed low calcium-stimulated PTH release. La^{+3} and Mn^{+2} were about twice as effective as Ca^{+2} on a molar basis, Sr^{+2} was similar to Ca^{+2} while Mg^{+2} was about half as effective; Ba^{+2} had a minor effect.

Humoral Factors

A host of humoral factors have recently been thought to affect PTH secretion (Table 1). The relevance of these observations to in vivo day-to-day regulation of PTH secretion is not clear. The interested reader is referred to a recent monograph reviewing this topic (31).

Table 1. Humoral Factors Affecting PTH Secretion

Increased Secretion	Decreased Secretion
β-adrenergic catecholamines	α-Adrenergic catecholamines
Dopaminergic catecholamines	Parasympathomimetic agents
Histamine	Somatostatin
Calcitonin	PGE_1
Glucagon	PGE_2
Growth hormone	Vitamin D and metabolites
Prolactin	
PGE_2	
Cortisol	
Vitamin D and metabolites	

IN VIVO REGULATION OF PTH SECRETION

The major regulator of PTH secretion on a day-to-day basis is ionized calcium. Recent studies have examined the relationship between serum calcium and control of PTH secretion in normal and abnormal glands.

Early in vitro work by Habener et al. (32) has shown that the relationship between PTH release and serum calcium is sigmoidal. That this is the case in vivo has been shown by Mayer et al. (33), who infused calcium and measured PTH secretory rate. Segre et al. (34) examined the relationship between serum calcium and serum PTH secretory rates in humans and showed a curvilinear relationship.

Most of the studies examining the relationship between serum calcium and PTH secretion in vivo used hyper- or hypocalcemia induced by the intravenous infusion of calcium or calcium chelators (EDTA). The changes in serum calcium induced by these maneuvers was not sustained, making it difficult to interpret the data. Fox et al. (35) developed a new method for the study of PTH secretion in conscious dogs called the *calcium clamp*. In this method, intravenous administration of calcium or EDTA raises or lowers plasma calcium levels in 1–2 minutes. Rapid determination of plasma calcium concentration then permits feedback control of the infusion rates, to "clamp," or fix, the calcium concentrations for prolonged periods of time. The authors examined the effects of sustained hypocalcemia on PTH secretion and disappearance rate of PTH from plasma. When plasma calcium concentration was decreased acutely by 2 mg/dl, the secretion of PTH increased within 1 minute and plasma levels reached a peak within 4–10 minutes. The rapidity of the response to hypocalcemia contrasts with the in vitro studies, which reported a maximal secretory rate of 30–60 minutes. Moreover, despite persistent hypocalcemia the maximal secretory rates of PTH were not maintained, and there was an actual fall in the levels of PTH. When plasma calcium levels returned to normal, the secretion of PTH stopped and the hormone disappeared with a maximal $T_{\frac{1}{2}}$ of less than 4 minutes. These experiments demonstrate that during induced hypocalcemia, PTH secretory rates are not fixed and are immediately responsive to the restoration of serum calcium to normal levels. Furthermore, in a separate study, Fu et al. (36) examined the secretory rate of PTH under normocalcemic conditions, and demonstrated significant cycles of PTH secretion in the thyroid venous effluent plasma compatible with episodic secretion of the hormone and unrelated to detectable changes in serum calcium. These studies demonstrate the difficulty of clinical interpretation of one-time measurements of endogenous PTH levels.

Set Point of PTH in Normal and Abnormal Glands

The set point for calcium is defined as the concentration of calcium causing half of the maximal inhibition of PTH release. The set point for humans and experimental animals is fairly uniform. Recent human studies have shown this value to be 1 mM. Maximal inhibition of PTH secretion is achieved with serum calcium levels of 11–12 mg/dl. It is likely that the maximal suppressibility of PTH release by calcium may not be complete in some conditions or individuals and may be of major importance in patients with abnormal PTH secretory rate. Indeed, early work by Gittes et al. (37) showed that transplant of a large number of normal rat PTH glands to normal rats resulted in severe hypercalcemia with nonsuppressibility of PTH release. In vivo studies in cows (38) demonstrated persistent release of PTH despite high levels of serum calcium. These observations suggest that the set point for the release of PTH may be altered.

An increase in the set point of calcium has been recently described in PTH glands removed from patients with primary hyperparathyroidism (39). Dispersed cells were prepared from the adenoma and from a portion of the normal PTH glands. PTH release as a function of the concentration of calcium was determined by radioimmunoassay (C-terminal). Cells from the normal gland showed a lower set point for calcium than those from the adenoma. Moreover, both set point and maximal PTH release at low concentrations of calcium were significantly lower in normal glands from patients with adenoma than in patients with normal glands. These observations have important implications for the pathophysiology of PTH release. A decrease in the set point for calcium and maximal secretory rate for PTH would result in diminished release of PTH at any concentration of calcium. These studies provide an explanation for the transient postoperative hypocalcemia and hypoparathyroidism seen after removal of a parathyroid adenoma. The subsequent return to normocalcemia would be the result of normalization of the set point and maximal PTH secretion in the remaining normal glands.

Changes in set point are not limited to patients with parathyroid adenoma. Brown et al. (29) have recently described a shift in the set point in parathyroid glands from patients treated with lithium, which explains the hypercalcemia and elevated PTH levels seen in these patients. The concept of changes in the set point may be of great importance in the interpretation of PTH levels in various conditions. Brown et al. (40) have reported "normal" set points for calcium in some patients with primary parathyroid hyperplasia. This "normal" set point may be inappropriately high for the level of serum calcium. The majority of patients with primary hyperparathyroidism have a relative decrease in the sensitivity to the suppressive effects of extracellular calcium on PTH secretion.

Parathyroid hyperplasia is a well-known abnormality of chronic renal failure. Studies of parathyroid tissue in vitro suggested variable suppressibility of PTH release in uremia. In vivo studies during calcium infusion also suggest suppressibility. Brown et al. (41) have examined the regulation of PTH release using dispersed parathyroid gland cells obtained from patients undergoing parathyroidectomy for parathyroid bone disease in chronic renal failure. The authors demonstrated that in severe secondary hyperparathyroidism due to chronic renal failure there is frequently an increase in the set point for calcium without a change in the maximal secretory rate per cell. These observations suggest that the abnormalities in regulation of PTH secretion in chronic renal failure result both from an alteration in the set point for calcium and from an increase in the total number of cells and parathyroid gland mass.

OTHER CONDITIONS THAT ALTER PTH SECRETION

Acute Pancreatitis

Hypocalcemia is a known complication of acute pancreatitis. Low levels of PTH have been reported in three patients with acute pancreatitis and hypocalcemia (42). McMahon et al. (43) examined the renal handling of calcium, phosphate, serum PTH, and phosphorus levels in patients with acute pancreatitis. Hypocalcemia was found in six of 18 patients and was associated with hypocalciuria, hypophosphatemia, and decreased renal tubular reabsorption of phosphate; serum PTH levels were either normal or low. These findings indicated a discrepancy between the PTH levels and the renal findings, which are compatible with increased PTH activity. These data suggest that the hypocalcemia of acute pancreatitis is not solely the result of reduced PTH secretion but, in some cases, is a consequence of bone resistance to the calcemic effect of endogenous PTH.

Acute Rhabdomyolysis

Acute rhabdomyolysis-induced renal failure is commonly associated with marked hypocalcemia in the oliguric phase. Recent studies by Llach et al. (44) have examined the relationship between PTH levels, serum calcium, phosphorus, and 1,25 $(OH)_2D_3$ in the hypocalcemia of acute rhabdomyolysis. Elevated levels of both amino and carboxy terminal PTH have been found. A possible end organ (bone) resistance to the calcemic effect of PTH secondary to reduced 1,25 $(OH)_2D_3$ levels was suggested.

Familial Hypocalciuric Hypercalcemia

This is a familial autosomal dominant disorder associated with lifelong hypercalcemia and minimal signs and symptoms (i.e., nephrolithiasis and deterioration of renal function). The kidney shows avid tubular reabsorption of calcium. The circulatory levels of PTH are lower in familial hypocalciuric hypercalcemia than in typical primary hyperparathyroidism, suggesting that mechanisms other than PTH determine the renal handling of calcium. High levels of circulating PTH and an increased mass of the parathyroid glands in the face of hypercalcemia suggest an abnormal regulation of PTH secretion. A disturbance only in the proliferation of PTH cells does not adequately explain hypercalcemia in this syndrome, since hypercalcemia usually recurs after subtotal parathyroidectomy. The parathyroid gland may be insensitive to extracellular calcium, suggesting an altered set point in the suppression of PTH release by calcium in these patients (29).

Effects of Cimetidine

Various drugs have been evaluated for a possible effect on PTH secretion. Cimetidine has been reported to reduce intact PTH levels in chronic renal failure. Other investigators reported no change or an increase in endogenous PTH levels. Saxe et al. (45) examined the effects of cimetidine on PTH secretion in vitro using dispersed PTH cells and found no effects on the secretory rate of PTH. Mallett et al. (46) found no decrease in the levels of PTH in a patient with primary hyperparathyroidism who was treated with cimetidine. From the available data to date, it seems that cimetidine has no major effects on PTH secretory rate in patients with primary hyperparathyroidism or chronic renal failure. The conflicting reports may be the results of methodologic problems in the radioimmunoassay of PTH and its fragments.

PTH Levels in Cushing's Syndrome

Marked abnormalities in calcium metabolism have been described in Cushing's syndrome and in patients receiving chronic glucocorticoid administration. The role of PTH is not clear. Recent work has shown no difference in immunoreactive PTH in paired subjects during hyperglucocorticoid and euglucocorticoid states. Findling et al. (47) examined the role of PTH in patients with glucocorticoid excess. Serum PTH levels were normal during Cushing's syndrome but fell significantly after remission. These data suggest that cortisol excess may augment PTH secretion. Whether the changes in PTH levels represent decreased peripheral catabolism rather than increased secretion is not clear from these studies.

MEASUREMENT OF PTH AND ITS CLINICAL APPLICATION
Radioimmunoassay

Radioimmunoassay is now widely used for the determination of the intact hormone and its fragments. The interpretation of these measurements is complex and may not be useful in all clinical conditions since both carboxy terminal and amino terminal fragments circulate in the blood and may present difficulty with the different radioimmunoassays used. Several assays are available: (1) with antigenic determinant directed only to the amino terminal region of the intact PTH (N-terminal); (2) with antigenic determination only for the carboxy terminal region (C-terminal); (3) polyvalent antisera with both N- and C-terminals. Thus, an N-terminal assay will measure the intact hormone as well as the amino terminal fragment. The C-terminal assay will detect the intact hormone and the carboxy terminal fragment. Recent studies (48) have demonstrated that the C-terminal assay can distinguish patients with primary hyperparathyroidism from normals in 90–95% of the cases.

Bioassay

The inference of the functional state of the hormone from its immunochemical measurements in the circulation cannot be made unless the immunochemical activity can be attributed to biologic activity. Thus, a measurement of the biologic activity of the hormone is needed for clinical applications. Several PTH bioassays have been described in the past, including a bioassay that measures the production of hypercalcemia or stimulation of adenylate cyclase. These bioassays are not sensitive enough to quantitate PTH in human serum. Recently, Nissenson et al. (49) developed a bioassay to determine biologically active human PTH. This method is based on the augmented activation of canine renal cortical adenylate cyclase known to occur in the presence of a GTP analog. The authors correlated the values of intact and carboxy terminal PTH radioimmunoassay with the bioassay in parathyroid venous effluent from eight patients with primary hyperparathyroidism. There was a high correlation between the bioassay (biologically active PTH) and PTH measured using radioimmunoassay methods. Absolute concentrations of biologically active PTH were generally greater than those of intact PTH, but consistently

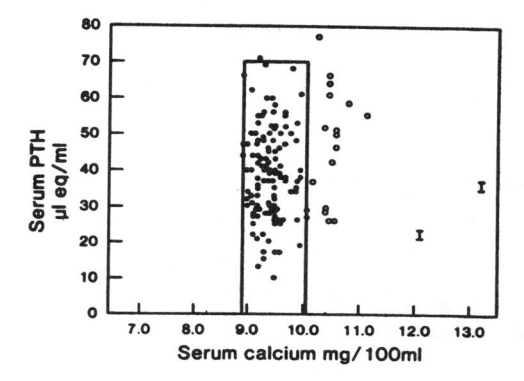

Figure 4. Serum PTH and calcium concentrations of normal subjects (closed circles), subjects on thiazide diuretics (opened circles), and patients immobilized by injury (I). (Kao PCK: *Mayo Clin Proc* 57:596–598, 1982. Used with permission.)

less than C-region I-PTH. The authors also correlated the bioassay and the radioimmunoassay of PTH in blood from patients with chronic renal failure. Most of the C-IPTH was found to be biologically inactive. In contrast, the values of intact PTH correlated highly with the biologically active PTH determined on bioassay.

With the development of monoclonal antibodies (50), the possibility of creating specific antibodies for the various fragments will allow their quantitation in different pathologic conditions.

PTH Assay in the Differential Diagnosis of Hypercalcemia

Of all PTH assays tested, only the radioimmunoassay developed by Reiss et al. (51) made it possible to differentiate between normal subjects and patients with primary hyperparathyroidism without overlap. Most of the other PTH assays showed some degree of overlap between normals, patients with primary hyperparathyroidism, and patients with hypercalcemia caused by malignancy. Recently, Kao et al. (52) have developed an antiserum that recognizes intact whole PTH and C-terminal fragments of 44-68 and 53-84 amino acid sequences but does not recognize the N-terminal 1-34 amino acid sequence. In a recent publication, the authors demonstrated an ability to differentiate clearly between normal subjects and patients with primary hyperparathyroidism, hypoparathyroidism, and chronic renal failure (Fig. 4). Patients with parathyroid carcinoma and hypernephroma who have ectopic secretion of PTH may also have highly elevated PTH and calcium levels (Fig. 5).

The differential diagnosis of hypercalcemia and the use of PTH blood levels should always take into account the clinical setting and serum calcium and phosphate levels. The reader is referred to a recent monograph for an extensive review of this issue (53).

PTH TOXICITY

In the last 2 years, several laboratories have reported the adverse effects of PTH on various organ systems. These adverse effects were reversible

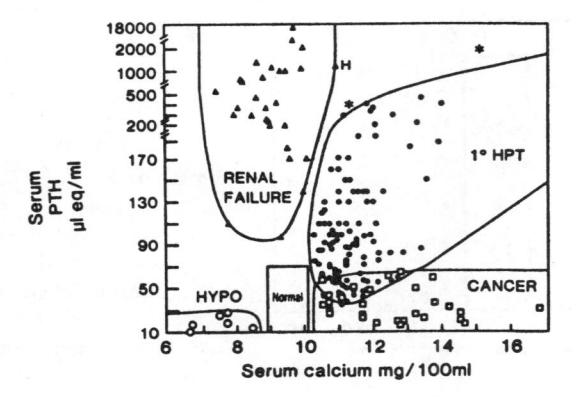

Figure 5. Serum PTH and calcium concentrations of patients with primary hyperparathyroidism (closed circles), cancer (open squares), hypoparathyroidism (Hypo, open circles), chronic renal failure (open triangles), parathyroid carcinoma (*), and hypernephroma (closed triangles). (Kao PCK: *Mayo Clin Proc* 57:596–598, 1982. Used with permission.)

upon removal of PTH from the system. These observations, linked with the knowledge that a major hormonal imbalance in chronic renal failure is elevation of PTH, suggest that various components of the uremic syndrome may result from excess PTH secretion.

Effect of PTH on the Nervous System

Several studies from our laboratory have demonstrated adverse effects of PTH on the central and peripheral nervous system. Acute uremia was associated with EEG abnormalities, which reversed after parathyroidectomy (54). Parathyroidectomy prior to induction of acute uremia prevented the EEG abnormalities in intact uremic dogs (55). The EEG abnormalities were correlated with an increased brain content of calcium. Data from patient studies support this notion; parathyroidectomy in chronic uremic patients was accompanied by reversal of EEG abnormalities. Recently, Akmal et al. (56) examined the role of PTH overactivity and EEG abnormalities in dogs with chronic renal failure. EEG abnormalities were associated with elevation of endogenous PTH levels. Parathyroidectomy prevented these changes. Interestingly, the EEG abnormalities in chronic uremia were abolished by parathyroidectomy, but brain calcium content remained elevated, suggesting a direct effect of the hormone on the brain.

Effects of PTH on the Hematopoietic System

Patients with chronic renal failure almost always have marked anemia. Decreased production and short survival of red blood cells have been implicated. Early studies have shown an inhibitory effect of uremic sera on erythropoiesis and suggest the presence of humoral inhibitors. Meytes et al. (57) examined the effects of intact PTH and some of its fragments on erythroid colony formation in human peripheral blood and mouse bone marrow. Intact (1-84 PTH) in concentrations comparable to those found in blood of uremic patients produced marked inhibition of mouse bone marrow erythroid colony forming units. Inactivation of the hormone abolished its effects on erythropoiesis. Increasing the concentration of erythropoietin in the medium overcame the inhibitory effects of PTH. The N-terminal fragment 1-34 bPTH and 53-84 hPTH had no effect. These data suggest that intact PTH and its carboxyterminal fragment exert an inhibitory effect on erythropoiesis, and that this inhibitory effect can be overcome with increased erythropoietin levels. These observations are complemented by the observations of Zevin et al. (58), who reported that PTH extract inhibits RNA and heme synthesis. These observations may be relevant to patients with chronic renal failure (59) as the anemia of uremia has been shown to improve after parathyroidectomy.

The interaction of PTH and erythropoietin is of major interest and suggests that if more erythropoietin were available to uremic patients, the adverse effects of PTH on erythropoiesis would be blunted. Indeed, an "experiment of nature" is available: patients with chronic renal failure due to polycystic kidney disease have been shown to have high erythropoietin levels and sometimes no anemia or even polycythemia.

Since erythrocyte survival has been implicated in the anemia of chronic renal failure, and since patients with chronic renal failure show reduced survival of red blood cells not corrected by dialysis, a role for a humoral factor was suggested. Bogin et al. (60) examined the effects of PTH on osmotic fragility of human erythrocytes. 1-34 bPTH and 1-84 bPTH were shown to produce hemolysis of red blood cells. This effect was dose related, required calcium, and was mimicked by calcium ionophore A23187. These data suggest that excess PTH may participate in the shortened life span of red blood cells in uremia.

Effects of PTH on the Heart

Patients with chronic renal failure often have a myocardiopathy. Early pathologic laboratory studies have shown that cardiac lesions of uremia in rats were prevented by parathyroidectomy and that administration of PTH enhanced the progression of the lesions. The observation that uremia is associated with an increase in the calcium content of the myocardium, and that these changes are due to excess PTH, suggests a role for PTH in the myocardiopathy of uremia.

Bogin et al. (61) examined the effects of both amino terminal 1-34 PTH and intact 1-84 PTH on an in vitro preparation of cultural isolated heart cells. Both the amino terminal and the intact hormone caused an immediate and sustained significant rise in beats per minute, and the cells died earlier than control cells. There was a dose response relationship between both moieties of PTH, but the effect of the intact hormone was greater than that of the amino terminal fragment. These effects of PTH required calcium, were mimicked by calcium ionophore, and were prevented by verapamil. Sera from uremic parathyroidectomized rats did not affect heart rate, but serum from intact uremic rats had effects similar to those of PTH. These data show an adverse effect of PTH on cells of the heart beating, and that this effect is mediated through an increase in intracellular calcium content or fluxes. These experimental data are complimentary to the observations by Drueke et al. (62), who reported a marked improvement in left ventricular function in 22 dialysis patients after parathyroidectomy.

The cellular mechanism by which PTH may mediate its adverse effects on the myocardium have recently been examined by Baczynski et al. (63). The authors evaluated myocardial cellular energetics (production, transport, and utilization) and tissue content of ash and radioactive calcium in rats injected with 1-84 PTH. A marked reduction in oxygen consumption, energy transport, and utilization by the myofibrils was associated with increased cellular calcium content and increased uptake of radioactive calcium. Bogin et al. (64) have reported inhibition of oxidative phosphorrylation by PTH using isolated myocardiol mitochondria in vitro.

Effects of PTH on Skeletal Muscle

Primary hyperparathyroidism and stages of secondary hyperparathyroidism are associated with skeletal myopathy. The observation that the myopathy is reversible after parathyroidectomy suggested a role of excess PTH. Recent studies by Brautbar et al. (65) examined the effects of excess PTH administration to experimental rats. All steps of cellular muscle energetics were impaired in PTH-treated rats. Interestingly, the tissue content of calcium was not elevated, suggesting a direct effect of the hormone on skeletal energetics.

Effects of PTH on Platelets and White Blood Cells

Several inhibitors of platelet functions have been described in blood from uremic patients. Recent studies by Remuzzi et al. (66) have examined the role of PTH excess in uremia and its effects on platelets. PTH inhibited aggregation of human platelets. This action of PTH mimicked the action of agents that stimulate cAMP. Secretion of intraplatelet serotonin induced by collagen was also prevented, in a concentration-dependent manner, by PTH. These effects of PTH on normal human platelets suggest that the elevated plasma levels of this hormone in uremia might contribute to the bleeding tendency in this disorder.

A high incidence of infections and impaired cellular immunity are known to occur in chronic uremia. Abnormalities in white blood cell random migration have been described in patients with primary hyperparathyroidism. A possible effect of excess PTH in chronic renal failure on white blood cells has been described recently by Massry et al. (67). A marked stimulation of random migration occurs initially when white blood cells are exposed to PTH. A reduction of random migration occurs after prolonged exposure. These effects were not blocked by verapamil and occurred in the absence of calcium in the incubation media. These preliminary studies suggest that excess PTH may have direct adverse effects on white blood cells.

Role of PTH in Muscular Dystrophy

Excessive calcium accumulation in muscle, which occurs in genetic, nutritional, and drug-induced muscular dystrophy, has been thought to play a major role in the generation of the dystrophic process. PTH increases the fluxes of calcium into the cytosol of cells, both directly by altering plasma membrane permeability, and indirectly, by increasing intracellular cAMP, which in turn stimulates the flux of calcium from mitochondria into the cytosol. Palmieri et al. (68) examined the effects of PTH ablation on muscle calcium, magnesium, protein synthesis, and histology as well as on plasma creatinine phosphokinase (CPK) in normal and in dystrophic hamsters. In intact dystrophic hamsters the calcium content in the heart was 20 times higher than in normal animals, but it was reduced by half in thyroparathyroidectomized (TPTX) dystrophic hamsters. The concentration of CPK in plasma from dystrophic hamsters was elevated but was abnormal in the PTH-ablated ones. Microscopic examination of the heart showed an amelioration of the dystrophic findings with PTH ablation. These changes were independent of plasma calcium levels. The authors concluded that PTH enhances the dystrophic process, probably by elevating the already increased calcium flux into the muscle, and that even normal levels of PTH in the presence of impaired membrane function may have deleterious effects. Thus, PTH may be a toxic substance in a disease with normal PTH levels but altered membrane permeability.

Effects of PTH on Renal Function and Nephrotic Syndrome in Experimental Nephritis

Recent studies have demonstrated that dietary restriction of phosphorus decreases the histologic damage and prevents renal function deterioration in immunologic and nonimmunologic forms of experimental renal disease. It was suggested that this protective effect is mediating by reducing the parenchymal calcification, possibly by reducing the calcium × phosphate product. The possibility that suppression of PTH occurred secondary to dietary phosphorus restriction has been suggested. Tomford et al. (69) examined the effects of dietary phosphate restriction and parathyroidectomy on the development of renal insufficiency and nephrotic syndrome in experimental nephritis. The authors found that TPTX protects renal function and markedly decreases the proteinuria and renal calcification, whereas parathyroidectomy (PTX) alone has no protective effects. The authors concluded that the protective effects of dietary phosphate restriction are not mediated primarily by PTH suppression or prevention of early renal parenchymal calcification. Borle et al. (70) examined the effects of high phosphate diet on the calcium metabolism of kidney cells in intact and PTX rats. In the control rats the high phosphate diet significantly increased kidney and mitochondrial calcium, the cytosolic and mitochondrial exchangeable calcium pools, and all calcium fluxes. In these controls, serum phosphate levels were normal, but plasma PTH levels were high. In PTX rats fed the same high phosphate diet, the plasma phosphate was elevated but no change in calcium metabolism was noted. These data suggest that the effects of high dietary phosphate on parenchymal renal calcification is mediated via high PTH levels and that the protective effects of low phosphate diet might in part occur as a result of reducing endogenous PTH secretion. Future studies are needed to evaluate the role of increased PTH secretion in the development of renal parenchymal damage.

PTH IN UREMIA

PTH Immunoreactivity in Uremia

The predominance of C-terminal fragments of PTH in the plasma of uremic patients has been well established. During dialysis or hemofiltration some of these fragments leave the circulation, making the evaluation of the plasma immunoreactive PTH profile in these patients difficult. The types of PTH immunoreactivity in the filtrate of plasma from uremic patients, using an antibody both for the amino and carboxy terminal fragments, have been reevaluated recently. Tsutsumi et al. (71) examined the influence of hemodialysis and hemofiltration on the plasma PTH profile in uremic patients. Plasma from uremic patients, concentrated and fractionated by cell filtration, consisted of a large peak with C-terminal immunoreactivity and a small peak with N-terminal immunoreactivity. The immunoreactivity of the C-terminal fragment in the ultrafiltrable component of the uremic plasma consisted of at least three peaks with the same immunologic behavior but different electric charges. The elution profile in a patient undergoing chronic hemofiltration was different from the profile of two patients undergoing chronic hemodialysis. Hemofiltration was shown to be more effective than conventional hemodialysis in removing PTH fragments.

Relation Between Middle Molecules and PTH in Uremia

An important role has been attributed to middle molecules as possible uremic toxins mediating some of the uremic syndrome. Middle molecule fraction 2 (MMS FR-2) is assumed to be the most important one and has been shown to impair glucose utilization and amino acid transport in vitro. Frohling et al. (72) examined the relationship between PTH and the MMS FR-2. Ten moderately uremic and 41 severely uremic patients were studied. There was a highly significant correlation between PTH levels and the MMS FR-2, which the authors considered suggestive of a pathogenic role. It is possible that PTH is responsible for enhanced generation or diminished degradation of MMS FR-2, which in turn exerts its toxic effects. This speculation finds support in the observations made by Fürst et al. (73), who demonstrated a marked reduction of MMS FR-2 peak after parathyroidectomy. These preliminary observations serve as a link between the middle molecule hypothesis and PTH as a uremic toxin.

PRIMARY HYPERPARATHYROIDISM

Diagnosis

The diagnosis of primary hyperparathyroidism (HPT) still remains a problem in patients who do not have the classic manifestations. While some patients will present with borderline elevated serum calcium of 11.0 mg/dl and hypercalciuria, others will present with elevated serum calcium levels but normal urinary excretion of calcium. In a recent publication, Broadus et al. (74) suggested a classification of primary (HPT) using clinical and laboratory findings: (*1*) Patients with primary HPT and overt osteitis fibrosa cystica typically present with a subacute clinical history and severe hypercalcemia associated with high levels of circulating PTH. Large quantities of parathyroid gland tissue are commonly found at surgery in these patients. (*2*) Patients with primary HPT whose main compliant is renal stones demonstrate mild hypercalcemia, which is commonly intermittent, modest elevations in PTH levels, and a small mass of abnormal PTH tissue at surgery. These patients need to be differentiated from those with idiopathic hypercalcemia who do not have HPT. (*3*) Patients in the intermediate group have nonspecific clinical symptoms with only mild elevations of PTH levels; the difficult clinical decision is whether and when to submit these patients for surgery.

Subtle Primary HPT

The term *normocalcemic primary HPT* has been used for patients who have findings of nephrolithiasis, bone disease, and hypercalciuria but no evidence of persistent hypercalcemia. Since the finding of persistent normocalcemia in these patients is uncommon, the term *subtle primary HPT* has been suggested (74). Although long-term follow-up studies reveal wide fluctuations in the fasting serum calcium in these patients with only intermittent hypercalcemia, these patients manifest biochemical HPT (75). They also commonly show elevated levels of circulating 1,25 $(OH)_2D_3$, increased intestinal calcium absorption, and slow abnormal suppressibility of the PTH gland following calcium administration. Other clinical approaches helpful in the diagnosis of subtle primary HPT are a thiazide diuretic challenge and continued measurement of ionized calcium and immunoreactive PTH with a sensitive carboxy-terminal assay.

Oral Phosphate Therapy in Primary HPT

Oral phosphate therapy was shown to be effective in lowering serum calcium in patients with primary HPT but has not gained wide clinical use due to its effects on soft tissue calcification. Broadus et al. (74) have followed 10 patients with primary HPT given oral phosphate therapy (1250–1500 mg of elemental phosphorus daily) for 12 months. Intestinal calcium absorption and serum $1,25(OH)_2D_3$ levels were markedly reduced as were the bone manifestations. PTH function tended to increase during therapy. These data suggest that the $1,25(OH)_2D_3$-mediated abnormality of primary HPT and the increased bone turnover can be treated effectively with oral phosphate supplementations in some patients who are poor surgical candidates.

Dietary Calcium in Primary HPT

Increasing dietary calcium in adults with primary HPT has been associated with a marked suppression of PTH secretion. Broadus et al. (74) studied 9 patients with primary HPT 72 hours after dietary calcium intake was increased from 400 mg/day to 1000 mg/day. This increase was associated with an increase in intestinal absorption of calcium and a 20–75% suppression of parathyroid function as expressed by the 24 hour total cAMP excretion, fasting Ne cAMP, and serum PTH. These data suggest that the measured abnormalities in a given patient with primary HPT depend upon the condition of the study and at any given time a new steady state can be established by changing dietary calcium, phosphorus, and serum $1,25(OH)_2D_3$.

Variations in Plasma PTH in HPT

Many hormones are secreted episodically and the fluctuations in the plasma concentrations of the radioimmunoassayable hormone may complicate the clinical interpretation. Diurnal variations in the secretion of PTH have been described in normal individuals and in patients with primary HPT. Recent studies by Fox et al. (36) have shown episodic secretion of the hormone in the dog. Robinson et al. (76) studied the secretion of PTH in patients with primary hyperparathyroidism and in normal subjects. Frequent samplings of venous blood were examined for PTH using CH-12M antiserum, which has major immunochemical specificity for the intact hormone and does not recognize midregion or carboxy-terminal fragments. Plasma PTH varied little through the usual daylight hours, no more than could be accounted for by the intraassay variations. The authors concluded that the finding of normal PTH levels in patients with primary HPT cannot be explained on the basis of diurnal rhythms or episodic secretion. However, it is important to note that this study did not measure the levels of the biologically inert carboxy-terminal PTH. Studies with the GP-IM antiserum, which has specificity for the middle region of PTH (which includes the carboxy-terminal), also showed no diurnal periodicity of plasma PTH. These data suggest that PTH secretion in patients with primary HPT is fixed with no major variations as long as no variations in the dietary intake of calcium and phosphorus occur.

Hyperfunctioning Supernumerary Parathyroid Glands

Exploration of the neck for the treatment of primary HPT is successful in at least 95% of cases when performed by an experienced operator. In occasional cases, hypercalcemia persists despite the removal of one or more enlarged PTH glands and identification of the four glands. In these cases, the consideration of a fifth hyperfunctioning gland should be taken into account. Russell et al. (77) reported 15 patients, each of whom had HPT as a consequence of a fifth hyperfunctioning gland. Removal of the gland resulted in a reversal of the hypercalcemia. Most of the hyperfunctioning fifth glands were found in the anterior mediastinum (10 of 15 patients). Furthermore, seven of the 15 patients had enlarged supernumerary glands in the thymus gland. The authors concluded that when a diagnosis of primary HPT has been made and four normal glands are identified, a fifth gland should be suspected and exploration in the following order should be performed: (1) bilateral transcervical thymectomy; (2) the retropharyngeal and retroesophageal areas should be examined carefully; (3) the carotid sheath should be opened and explored on both sides; (4) subtotal thyroid lobectomy (sometimes bilateral) should be done. If no abnormal gland is found following the above steps, an exploration of the mediastinum is recommended.

Parathyroid Carcinoma

Carcinoma of the parathyroid gland is a rare cause of primary HPT, accounting for 3–4% of patients with hypercalcemia and elevated PTH levels. Early reports suggested that parathyroid carcinoma presents clinically somewhat differently than the much more common forms of primary HPT; there is marked and symptomatic hypercalcemia and both renal and skeletal disease are frequently present. Shane et al. (78) have examined 62 patients with parathyroid carcinoma and summarized the clinical presentation, natural history, and prognosis after surgical or medical management. In contrast to benign primary HPT, which is detected most commonly in women during the sixth decade, the patient with parathyroid carcinoma is equally likely to be a male or female and is usually one decade younger. In addition, the overwhelming majority of patients with malignant disease have moderate to severe hypercalcemia with signs and symptoms of elevated serum calcium and PTH levels. Target organ involvement is common. The simultaneous presentation of both bone and stone disease occurs commonly in parathyroid carcinoma. The patient with parathyroid carcinoma is more likely to have a palpable mass in the neck. The natural history of the carcinoma is slow and progressive. The average time from initial surgery to the first recurrence is 3 years, but intervals as long as 8 years have been reported. Only 50% of patients survive more than 5 years. Interestingly, three patients with 15-year survival were reported despite known metastatic spread. The management is based upon natural history as well as upon symptoms. Thus, although removal of local or even distant metastasis is not likely to be curative, patients, nevertheless, may improve for long periods of time. In patients with recurrent disease, aggressive management, including removal of localized lesions, is indicated. If surgery cannot be performed (e.g., in cases with metastasis) other medical approaches are indicated. Irradiation of the tumor and chemotherapy have been shown to be ineffective. Attempts to inhibit the action of PTH at the level of the target organ also have not been helpful. The key to therapy is successful surgery.

Recently, Pattillo et al. (79) cultured cells from a parathyroid carcinoma. The cells secreted PTH that had a molecular weight similar to intact highly purified bPTH and stimulated bone resorption in a manner that was equivalent and additive to synthetic bPTH 1-34.

EXTRARENAL EFFECTS OF PTH

Skeletal Activity

PTH maintains calcium homeostasis mainly by its interaction with bone. Administration of PTH causes bone resorption and calcium release and inhibits bone formation and mineralization. These metabolic effects of PTH are reflected by changes at the cellular level in the osteoclasts and osteoblasts. In addition to these mature cells, precursor cells in bone—immature osteoclasts and osteoblasts—are also affected.

Anabolic Effects

States of excess PTH are associated with enhanced bone destruction, but bone formation may be stimulated as well. Infusions of small amounts of 1-34 PTH in adult dogs for 3 weeks caused no increase in osteoclast number; hypercalcemia did not occur, but there were increments in the accretion rate of calcium. These indirect observations suggested that PTH may enhance bone formation and may possess anabolic actions.

Recently Malluche et al. (80) examined the effects of long-term infusion of physiological doses of 1-34 PTH on bone. The sustained infusion of PTH was associated with a significant increment in volume and surface density of osteoid without changes in bone mass. Mineralization of osteoid was not altered. The enhanced osteoid production was not due to augmented bone formation by individual osteoblastic or basic remodeling units but rather to increased activation frequency resulting in an increased number of remodeling units. The authors concluded that small doses of PTH do not have an anabolic effect on the bone but rather increase coupling of bone turnover. Mateska et al. (81), on the other hand, using explants of mouse radius bone, examined the effects of 1-84 PTH on osteoblastic activity. A marked increase in maturation of the cartilage and in osteoblastic activity, compatible with an in vitro anabolic effect, was demonstrated.

Slovik et al. (82) examined the effects of short-term administration of synthetic human PTH 1-34 on bone mineral metabolism in osteoporotic patients. Six patients with osteoporosis underwent detailed studies including blood and urinary measurements of calcium, phosphorus, and magnesium, ^{47}Ca kinetic studies, and calcium balance studies. ^{47}Ca kinetic studies showed increased bone accretion rate, a decrease in the transit time of calcium in the kinetic pools, and a decrease in the exchangeable pool size. The authors concluded that low doses of PTH may promote bone formation.

Parsons et al. (80) examined the effects of injecting small doses of PTH 1-34 for 6 months in patients with osteoporosis. Histologic indices of increased bone formation correlated well with those of bone resorption. Examination by polarized light showed that the new bone formed was well mineralized and of normal lamellar structure. Podbesek et al. (81) examined the effects of pulsatile versus continuous administration of 1-34 PTH on bone parameters in dogs. Pulsatile administration was much more effective than the continuous infusion of PTH.

Cellular Mechanism Mediating the Anabolic Effects of PTH

It has been established in recent years that osteoblasts and osteoclasts are derived from histogenically distinct cell lines. While the osteoblast belongs to the mononuclear system and is capable of being blood born, osteoclasts are derived from fibroblasts.

The mechanism of the functional association of these two cells is not clear. Recently, Howard et al. (85) suggested a coupling factor: Activation of the osteoclasts occurs initially and then the osteoblasts are activated. Indeed, Ashton et al. (86), using diffusion chambers in the evaluation of the effects of PTH on the differentiation of these two cells were able to comfirm that the stimulation of osteoblasts by PTH is a secondary effect of the initial osteoclast activation.

Catabolic Effects of PTH

PTH directly stimulates bone resorption and release of calcium. The mechanisms by which the release of calcium occurs are not clear. Some studies suggest that the early response to PTH is an initial uptake of calcium into the bone cell, followed by excessive calcium release.

Krieger et al. (87) used monovalent cation ionophores and neonatal mouse calvaria to evaluate the mechanisms of calcium release by bone cells. Divalent cation ionophores have previously been used to examine the role of calcium uptake in response to PTH as well as the mechanism stimulating release of calcium from bone. Low concentrations stimulated calcium release and high concentrations inhibited calcium release. Krieger et al. (87) reported that in neonatal mouse calvaria, monovalent ionophores are more potent inhibitors of stimulated bone resorption than the divalent ionophores nigericin, monensin, and X206. Each inhibited the release of calcium from calvaria stimulated with PTH in a dose-dependent response. Prolonged treatment either with ionophore alone or with PTH and ionophore caused an irreversible inhibition of the PTH-mediated calcium release. If the bones were pretreated with PTH alone for 24–48 hours, ionophore caused only a partial inhibition. Resorption stimulated by prostaglandin E_2, $1,25(OH)_2D_3$, and epidermal growth factor was also inhibited by monovalent ionophores, indicating that the inhibition is not at the PTH receptor. These results are consistent with the notion that stimulated release of calcium from bone occurs by a Na–Ca exchange mechanism. Monovalent ionophores increased intracellular Na^+, thereby decreasing the sodium gradient across bone cell membrane, leading to conditions unfavorable for calcium efflux coupled to further sodium influx.

The effect of diphosphonates on bone calcium release is well established. Since these drugs reduce calcium efflux from bone, an analog of this drug was developed to study a possible inhibiting role in the release of calcium from bone. Doppelt et al. (88) examined the effects of dichloromethane diphosphonate on 1-34 PTH-mediated hypercalcemia in the rat. Pretreatment of rats with the drug resulted in an inhibition of calcemic response to the administered PTH. These experimental data suggest a possible role for diphosphonates in the treatment of PTH-mediated hypercalcemia.

Vascular Effects of PTH

Several reports in the literature suggest effects of PTH on blood pressure. However, the conclusion from these studies is at times confusing because of different experimental designs and the length of PTH administration.

Primary HPT is commonly accompanied by elevated blood pressure, with an average of 39% prevalence. Rambausek et al. (89) have reported recently that of 77 patients with primary HPT, 42% were hypertensive. Whether the hypertension is a direct effect of the hormone or secondary to the hypercalcemia was not defined in these studies. Acute infusion of calcium resulting in hypercalcemia has been shown to cause hypertension. Marone et al. (90) have recently examined the hemodynamic changes of acute hypercalcemia-induced hypertension. High blood pressure occurred despite a decrease in blood volume and was caused primarily by an increase in total peripheral resistance with no significant changes in cardiac output. These changes could be the result of either (1) a direct effect of calcium on peripheral blood vessels or (2) secondary to reduced PTH secretion as a result of the hypercalcemia.

Recent studies have shown that PTH poses a direct vasodilatory effect. Administration of parathyroid extract or PTH were accompanied by marked hemodynamic changes. These included increase in renal blood flow and mesenteric blood flow. Administration of PTH into the renal artery was associated with a rapid increase in blood flow and a rapid increase in renin release. Administration of 1-34 PTH into the coronary blood vessels causes an immediate vasodilatory effect (91). These changes were accompanied by a marked increase in oxygen consumption and inotropic effect. McCarron et al. (92) have demonstrated a hypotensive effect of PTH in vivo. The mechanism mediating these effects of PTH remain to be defined.

Recent studies in smooth muscle cells examined the cellular effects of PTH. Rascher et al. (93) have shown a dose-dependent increase of cAMP concentration in monolayer cultures of smooth muscle cells of aortic media. This effect of PTH was not specific for vascular smooth muscle cells and was observed in other tissues. Rambausek et al. (89) examined the effects of 1-34 PTH on aortic strips preincubated with epinephrine and found a marked transient relaxation of the tonic contractions induced by epinephrine. The action of PTH was potentiated and prolonged by theophylline. Rasher et al. (93) examined the hemodynamic effect of PTH on the hind limb of the rat. Precontraction of the hind limb vasculature was induced by constant infusion of norepinephrine and PTH administration caused a dose-dependent decrease in vascular resistance. Since PTH stimulates cAMP generation in blood vessels walls, a cAMP-mediated mechanism was suggested. In addition, the authors demonstrated inhibition of the PTH-induced effect by the administration of prostaglandin synthesis inhibitors.

The cellular mechanisms mediating the PTH effect on blood vessel smooth muscle cells are not clear. Since PTH increases intracellular calcium content, and since an increase in intracellular calcium stimulates phospholipase A_2 and prostaglandin synthesis, it is possible that these actions are mediated by fluxes in cellular calcium content.

Saglikes et al. (94) examined the effects of 1-84 and 1-34 PTH on mean arterial blood pressure and vascular response to infused norepinephrine and angiotensin II. Infusion of 1-84 PTH did not alter mean arterial blood pressure; however, the infusion of 1-34 PTH led to a decrease in mean arterial blood pressure. Both 1-84 and 1-34 PTH inhibited the hypertensive response to norepinephrine and angiotensin II. Pretreatment with indomethacin abolished these effects of PTH. The authors suggested that the hypotensive effects of PTH are mediated by activation of the prostaglandin system, since calcium channel blockers did not block the hypotensive effects of PTH, whereas prostaglandin synthesis did. Mann et al. (95) evaluated the effects of PTH administration in the spontaneously hypertensive rats (SHR) and found that endogenous PTH exerted a permissive effect for development of elevated blood pressure. The relevance of these observations to the clinical observation of hypertension in patients with primary HPT is not clear. Moreoever, the well-documented disappearance of hypertension after parathyroidectomy is not in accordance with the above experimental studies. It is possible that chronic excess of the hormone has an effect opposite that of the acute elevation of PTH.

Effects of PTH on Lipid and Phospholipid Metabolism

Disturbances in lipid metabolism have been reported in patients and experimental animals with HPT. Administration of PTH to experimental rats caused a rise in blood lipids. In uremia, abnormal lipid metabolism is common. Ritz et al. (96) have demonstrated in uremic rats that parathyroidectomy prevented the increase in plasma triglycerides and cholesterol levels which was observed in uremic rats with intact parathyroid glands. Paloyan et al. (97) demonstrated that parathyroidectomy in the dog was followed by a significant decrease of serum cholesterol, while the administration of PTH led to a marked rise in both serum cholesterol and triglycerides.

Lacour et al. (98) examined the possible role of PTH in lipid metabolism. Endogenous HPT was induced by a calcium-free diet. This was associated with a marked elevation of serum cholesterol and triglyceride levels. There was a significantly reduced clearance rate of infused lipids and a significant elevation of hepatic triglyceride content. Administration of PTH to normal animals was also accompanied by elevation of serum cholesterol and triglycerides. Parathyroidectomy was associated with a significant reduction in serum cholesterol and triglyceride levels. To further evaluate the sites of these abnormalities, the authors examined the intestinal absorption of

H^3-triolein and found no change from the control group, ruling out increased intestinal absorption of lipids as a cause. The observation that both hepatic secretion and hepatic uptake of triglycerides reduced under the influence of PTH suggests a decreased peripheral removal of lipids as a possible mechanism. These data demonstrate a role for PTH in the disturbed lipid metabolism of uremia and HPT. The cellular mechanism mediating these effects remains to be elucidated.

Phospholipids are major determinants of normal membrane function and have been shown recently to be involved in transcellular transport and mediation of hormone-receptor interactions. The phosphoinositides are a group of polar phospholipids contained in the cell membrane; significant changes in their metabolism will affect the physicochemical properties of the membrane. Several hormones have been reported to stimulate turnover of phosphoinositides; the common denominator is that all of these hormones act via an increase in cellular calcium (vasopressin, serotonin, catecholamines, insulin). Mitchel et al. (99) suggested a mechanism by which all hormones that increase intracellular calcium act by increasing phosphoinositide turnover. Since PTH is known to increase intracellular calcium, it is plausible to suggest a mechanism by which PTH alters cellular phosphoinositide metabolism and affects membrane functions. Indeed, Lo et al. (100) have shown stimulation by ^{32}P incorporation into phosphatidic acid and phosphotidyl inositol following stimulation of renal cortical slices with PTH. Farese et al. (101) have shown that PTH administration to experimental animals increased the absolute contents of phosphoinositides in the renal cells. Meltzer et al. (102) have examined the effects of PTH and cyclic nucleotides on renal phosphoinositide metabolism. PTH stimulated the incorporation of ^{32}P into phosphoinositides and also caused a 50% increase in actual tissue levels of these phospholipids. These findings were independent of cAMP since incubation with cAMP did not reproduce the above observations. These data demonstrate an effect of PTH on phosphoinositide turnover. These observations may be related to the functional effects of PTH on membrane properties: (1) PTH initially increases intracellular calcium transport, which stimulates changes in phospholipid metabolism; (2) PTH directly affects changes in membrane phospholipid metabolism and in turn alters membrane fluidity and transport.

PTH and Acid-Base Balance

Several studies suggest the existence of a close relationship between PTH and acid-base changes. Wachman et al. (103) studied five normal subjects during ammonium chloride-induced acidosis and noted an increase in urinary hydroxyproline, plasma PTH levels, and phosphate clearance. These changes were reversed by administration of oral phosphate preparations. The authors suggested that the increase in PTH observed during metabolic acidosis represents a regulatory mechanism which enhances (1) the renal excretion of phosphate, which increases urinary buffer, in turn, increasing urinary hydrogen excretion, and (2) the release of phosphorus from bone, thus increasing buffer availability. The authors proposed that PTH is a hormone concerned primarily with acid-base balance homeostasis.

Hyperchloremic metabolic acidosis has been described in patients with primary and secondary HPT. The frequency of this observation is from 7% to 70%. Muldowney et al. (104) demonstrated hyperchloremic acidosis in patients with secondary hyperparathyroidism, which was reversible upon vitamin D administration or subtotal parathyroidectomy. These authors suggested that the elevated levels of PTH resulted in a depression of a proximal tubular bicarbonate reabsorption, causing the syndrome of proximal renal tubular acidosis. The effects of PTH on renal tubular bicarbonate handling and urine acidification have been extensively reviewed (105). It is well accepted from these studies that PTH increases urine bicarbonate excretion and decreases renal acid excretion. The inhibition of distal urinary acidification results from increased distal delivery of bicarbonate secondary to inhibition of proximal bicarbonate reabsorption.

The role of PTH in the extrarenal disposal of acute acid loads has been studied in nephrectomized intact and parathyroidectomized dogs and rats during acute HCl infusions (106). The intact animals developed metabolic acidosis with the administration of HCl. The same acid load given to the animals without parathyroid glands was associated with more severe metabolic acidosis and a high mortality rate. The intact animals were able to buffer 50–70% of the acid by tissue buffers, while parathyroidectomized animals buffered only 3–22%. These authors further evaluated skeletal muscle, heart, and liver pH changes and concluded that these changes could not account for the buffering of the acid loads. They suggested that PTH acts at the bone level to increase buffering capacity.

The role of PTH in extrarenal buffering during the chronic metabolic acidosis of renal failure, and the mechanism by which the hormone may mediate these changes, have been examined recently by Arruda et al. (107). The authors examined the effects of acid loads in intact or TPTX nephrectomized rats and in animals with acute and chronic renal failure. TPTX rats given PTH had significantly higher blood pH and bicarbonate values than TPTX rats not infused with PTH. Stimulation of PTH secretion by the administration of EDTA increased the buffering capacity in intact rats. Rats with chronic or acute renal failure, a state of increased PTH secretion, had a higher capacity to buffer acid load, which was abolished by the removal of the parathyroid glands. Thus, the authors demonstrated that (1) absence of PTH impairs the extrarenal buffering of acid and (2) excess PTH in the circulation is accompanied by enhanced extrarenal buffering capacity. From this study, and from the studies by Fraley et al. (106), it is possible to conclude that PTH has an important role in mediating extrarenal buffering and acid-base homeostasis and that this probably occurs at the level of bone.

The mechanism by which PTH mediates the bone buffering of an acid load was evaluated recently by Arruda et al. (107). Since carbonic anhydrase inhibitors blunt PTH-mediated bone resorption and since bone cell carbonic anhydrase was implicated in the mediation of the bone effects of PTH, the authors examined the interaction between acidosis, PTH, and carbonic anhydrase inhibitors. Administration of carbonic anhydrase inhibitors prevented the buffering capacity of administered PTH. The authors therefore concluded that carbonic anhydrase may mediate the buffering capacity of PTH at the bone cell level.

Hulter et al. (108) examined the effects of HPT on renal and systemic acid-base homeostasis in dogs. Metabolic balance studies were employed in two groups of parathyroidectomized dogs, one with endogenous acid loads and the other with chronic alkali loads. The results indicate that experimental induction of HPT caused an insignificant decrease in plasma calcium concentration and an increase in serum phosphorus concentration, but did not result in appreciable alterations in renal or systemic acid-base abnormalities. These data suggest no major role for PTH in mediating chronic acid-base disturbances but do not rule out an important role for PTH in mediating tissue buffering in acute disturbances. Madias et al. (109) evaluated the role of PTH in the acute buffering process by examining the influence of thyroparathyroidectomy on acid-base parameters in nephrectomized rats following the infusion of hydrochloric acid. The authors concluded that endogenous PTH is not necessary in the initial response to acute mineral acid loads. This conclusion contrasts with the findings of the recent studies cited above. The reason for these conflicting results may relate to the experimental design. Both Fraley et al. (106) and Arruda et al. (107) used pharmacologic doses of PTH, while Madias et al. (109) used physiologic doses. Thus, it is possible that in states of HPT where the blood levels of PTH are comparable to those of the first experiments, PTH may have a role in tissue buffering of acute acid-base changes.

Hulter et al. (108) evaluated the role of calcium movements in situations where acid-base homeostasis may be impaired. Experimental dogs were studied under three protocols: (*1*) calcium infusion, (*2*) PTH administration, (*3*) 1,25(OH)$_2$D$_3$ administration. The authors demonstrated that, depending on the direction of movement of calcium, metabolic acidosis or alkalosis will develop: (*1*) Calcium infusion causes base deposition in bone and soft tissue and brings about metabolic acidosis; (*2*) PTH administration mobilizes base from bone and causes metabolic alkalosis; (*3*) chronic 1,25(OH)$_2$D$_3$ or PTH administration increases the set point at which the plasma bicarbonate concentration is regulated by the kidney and thereby causes metabolic alkalosis to persist.

It seems from the data available to date that PTH may have extrarenal effects on acid-base homeostasis in states of excess PTH and that these effects might be in part secondary to alkali fluxes from bone to blood. The net acid-base effects in the patient, however, are dependent on several other factors which include the effect of PTH on the renal handling of bicarbonate. For further discussion of parathyroid–acid-base interactions, the reader is referred to Chapter 9 of this volume.

RENAL EFFECTS OF PTH

Is There a Role for PTH in Phosphate Homeostasis in Chronic Renal Failure?

As chronic renal failure progresses, functional adaptation takes place to increase the excretion of phosphate per nephron to maintain phosphate homeostasis. Generally, it has been thought that phosphate adaptation in uremia is the result of secondary hyperparathyroidism. However, data by Sheaser et al. have challenged that concept and showed that uremic animals can maintain phosphate homeostasis in the absence of PTH. Recent studies have shown a PTH-independent mechanism in the body's adaptation to phosphate metabolism. Caverzasio et al. (110) examined a PTH-independent mechanism in phosphate homeostasis in uremic animals. Rats were either parathyroidectomized or sham operated, and then subtotally nephrectomized. GFR and phosphate reabsorption were determined by clearance studies. The decrease in the maximal TmP/GFR in response to renal mass reduction occurred in the presence or absence of PTH; thus, the authors concluded that the phosphate adaptation in chronic renal failure is PTH independent. Wen et al. (111) examined this issue using micropuncture techniques in uremic dogs. In dogs with remnant kidney and early moderate renal failure, thyroparathyroidectomy performed 3 days before the study resulted in reduced fractional excretion of phosphate, indicating an important role for PTH in phosphate homeostasis in early renal failure. With more advanced renal failure, fractional excretion of phosphate remained high even in the absence of PTH, indicating that PTH-independent factors modulate phosphate adaptation in advanced renal failure. The nature of these factors is not clear. Indeed, recent data by Jacob et al. (112) lend further support to the notion that PTH is not a major factor in the maintenance of phosphate homeostasis in chronic renal failure. The authors showed that doses of cimetidine that restore PTH blood levels to normal in chronic renal failure result in a marked decrease in serum phosphate and tubular reabsorption of phosphate.

PTH and Glomerular Filtration Rate

Several investigators have demonstrated that glomeruli from rats and rabbits possess an adenylate cyclase enzyme system sensitive to PTH.

Ichikawa et al. (113) examined glomerular microcirculation in rats that had undergone TPTX. Using micropuncture techniques the authors evaluated the various determinants of glomerular ultrafiltration and demonstrated a marked reduction in glomerular ultrafiltering coefficient (K_f) in response to PTH administration. The authors further showed that the actions of PTH and its intermediate, cyclic AMP, on K_f are mediated by angiotensin II, via the effect of the latter on contraction of glomerular mesangeal cells. These data help to clarify prior observations of a reduced glomerular filtration rate in states of primary and secondary hyperparathyroidism.

The cellular events mediating glomerular ultrafiltration and K_f are not known. Wang et al. (114) evaluated the interaction among PTH, calcium, and cAMP on glomerular metabolism by measuring substrate oxidation in isolated glomeruli prepared from rat kidney. Increasing the calcium content of the medium inhibited CO_2 production from α-ketoglutarate and succinate, and stimulated CO_2 production from glucose and glutamate. PTH in the presence of calcium inhibited CO_2 production from α-ketoglutarate and glutamate but not from glucose. Addition of cAMP as well as hormonal agents known to act directly on the glomeruli, such as histamine, epinephrine, prostaglandin E_2, vasopressin, angiotensin II, and insulin did not alter CO_2 production from α-ketoglutarate. These data demonstrate the presence of a calcium dependent inhibitory action of PTH on the oxidation of α-ketoglutarate and glutamate, independent of cAMP.

Effects of PTH on Renal Tubular Bicarbonate Transport

Previous studies using clearance techniques have shown that PTH may inhibit overall urinary acificication. Micropuncture studies in dogs and rats identified the proximal convoluted tubule as one nephron segment in which this inhibition occurs. McKinney et al. (115) and Iino et al. (116) have shown that PTH and dibutyryl cAMP inhibit bicarbonate reabsorption in isolated perfused rabbit superficial proximal straight tubules. The mechanism of this inhibition has recently been examined by McKinney et al. (117), who found that the primary process inhibited is probably the lumen-to-bath transport.

Effects of PTH on Water Transport and Interaction with Antidiuretic Hormone

Changes in intracellular calcium content brought about by calcium ionophores and calcium channel blockers, such as verapamil, have been shown to modify ADH-stimulated sodium transport and ADH-dependent water flow across the toad urinary bladder. Since PTH increases intracellular calcium content in tubular cells, the possibility that PTH may thus interact with ADH action along the distal nephron is reasonable. Humes et al. (118) presented data to support the concept that PTH enhances the urine concentration response to ADH, and that this is inhibited by the administration of verapamil. They concluded that the potentiation of the urinary concentration response to ADH is a consequence of the ability of PTH to enhance calcium uptake by collecting duct epithelia, thereby making these cells more responsive to ADH action. The physiologic or pathophysiologic application of these observations is not clear, particularly inasmuch as hypercalcemia or nephrocalcinoses has been shown to diminish the concentration response to ADH in experimental animals and humans. These apparently conflicting results may reflect differing effects of calcium on the ascending limb of Henle and the collecting duct.

Winaver et al. (119) examined the effects of PTH on water transport in chronically TPTX dogs undergoing maximal steady-state water diuresis. The results of the study show that administration of PTH in pharmacologic doses causes a significant decrease in free water clearance and urine volume, and an increase in urine osmolality, with no changes in osmolar clearance. These effects of PTH could not be reproduced using physiologic doses of PTH. This ADH-like effect of pharmacologic doses of PTH seems to be due to both a release of endogenous ADH and a direct effect of PTH on the medullary ADH sensitive adenylate cyclase.

Cellular Mechanisms Mediating Renal Tubular Effects of PTH

The observations that administration of PTH causes a marked elevation of urinary cAMP and that renal tissue incubated with PTH showed elevated cAMP levels suggests that the cAMP–adenylate cyclase system is a major mediator of PTH action. In the last 2 years, data have accumulated to suggest that other mediators or messengers are involved in the renal tubular effects of PTH. Puschett et al. (120) have examined the effects of graded doses of PTH on the renal handling of phosphate and cAMP production and excretion. Administration of physiologic doses of 1-84 PTH produced phosphaturia and hypocalciuria but no increase in either urinary cAMP or the production of the nucleotide in cortical tissue harvested from the kidneys of these animals. When 10 times this amount of PTH was infused, phosphate excretion rose to 38% of filtered load (from 11% with physiologic dose of PTH) and urinary cAMP increased. Indeed, Nissenson et al. (121) have found that the amount of hormone needed to stimulate cAMP production in vitro is significantly lower than that necessary to produce phosphaturia. Some of the renal tubular effects of PTH may not be mediated by cAMP generation.

Preliminary studies by Gura et al. (122) have addressed the question of cellular mediation of the phosphaturic effect of PTH. The authors evaluated renal nephrogenous cAMP production and excretion in response to PTH administration in dogs and demonstrated that the phosphaturic response to PTH may not be mediated by increased renal production of cAMP and that most of the urinary cAMP is from extrarenal sources. Thus, it is possible that cellular mechanisms beyond the generation of cAMP may be critical in mediating the phosphaturic action of PTH. These data suggest that a PTH phosphaturic response independent of the cAMP system is operative.

What then is the cellular mediator of PTH tubular action? Robertson et al. (123) have recently provided evidence that calcium itself may be serving as the messenger. The possibility that changes in intracellular calcium mediate PTH transport effects in the tubule is of major interest in the light of the previously discussed observations suggesting that calcium ions produce changes in cellular membrane phospholipids, and that these in turn may cause transcellular ion transport.

CALCIUM AND METABOLIC BONE DISEASE

Clinical Application of Bone Histology

Since many of the articles and topics discussed below focus upon bone histologic features, a short introduction reviewing these features in osteoporosis, osteomalacia, and uremic bone disease is included here. The features of primary interest in evaluating a bone biopsy are bone volume and bone quality, bone formation, osteoid and osteoblasts, bone resorption and osteoclasts, bone mineralization, and marrow fibrosis.

Bone Volume and Quality
Decreased bone volume is seen in osteoporosis. Usually roentgenographic features and bone photon absorptiometry values can be used to identify osteopenia. Both primary and secondary osteoporosis have a varied histology, and only occasionally is secondary osteoporosis distinctive histologically from primary disease. Sometimes osteoporotics with several atraumatic compression fractures will have biopsies with formation, resorption, mineralization, and even bone area features within the normal range for age-matched subjects. Although biopsies are not useful for distinguishing primary from secondary osteoporosis, biopsies can still be valuable in answering three important questions: (*1*) Does the patient have osteomalacia? Bone biopsy is the only way to exclude osteomalacia. (*2*) Does the patient have a low bone turnover rate? (*3*) Does the patient have a high resorption rate? These three questions are important in determining the cause and appropriate therapy for the osteoporotic patient.

Normal trabecular bone is lamellar and displays a regular, even collagen pattern when viewed microscopically with polarized light. Woven or fibrous bone, however, shows an irregular, disorganized pattern. Woven bone occurs physiologically in fracture healing and pathologically in Paget's disease and in conjunction with certain neoplasms. Woven bone is thought to result when bone formation is abnormally rapid. It is also seen in some cases of uremic bone disease, osteogenesis imperfecta tarda, and usually in diaphyseal dysplasia, fibrous dysplasia, and melorheostosis.

Bone Formation Features

Plump, cuboidal osteoblasts are usually very active osteoblasts, and osteoid covered by such cells usually shows good tetracycline labeling. There is also usually a good correlation between osteoblast size and the rate of bone apposition (the distance between two time-spaced tetracycline administrations, divided by the number of days between administrations). Some types of uremic bone disease present with increased forming surface. A bone biopsy of a patient with a high turnover state (i.e., high forming surface and high resorbing surface) would show on Goldner's stained sections a large fraction of bone surface involved in formation, and increased osteoid area and width. An unstained section examined with ultraviolet light would show increased tetracycline-labeled surfaces with discrete double labels separated by a normal amount of matrix. This is distinct from the tetracycline-labeling features of a biopsy of advanced osteomalacia (see below). Wide osteoid with normal double labels suggests a rapid bone formation rate and not osteomalacia.

Bone Resorption

Sites of present or past bone resorption are indicated by a scalloped, crenated edge on the bone surface. Although there is at present no direct way to measure osteoclast activity, osteoclast number can be best determined by histochemical localization of acid phosphatase in osteoclasts. Osteoclasts are rich in lysosomes containing acid phosphatase. Acid phosphatase localization identifies both osteoclasts with multiple nuclei and osteoclasts with only one or no nucleus at that level of section. As mentioned previously, osteoporotics may show normal or increased osteoclast numbers. Postmenopausal osteoporotics with high osteoclast counts are good candidates for therapy with agents that decrease bone resorption, such as etidronate disodium (EHDP) and calcitonin. Crenated surface may be normal or show increased osteomalacia, depending on the cause. Crenated surface is usually normal in mild and osteomalacic forms of uremic bone disease and elevated in the fibrotic type. The mixed phase of Paget's disease also shows increased crenated surface.

Mineralization

Information on mineralization can be obtained most directly by tetracycline analysis. Most tetracycline antibiotics form stable tetracycline–calcium chelates that fluoresce intensely at wave lengths readily obtained with fluorescence microscope. These chelates only form at sites of new bone formation where the bone contains 20% or less of the maximal mineral content. These chelates remain in the bone until it is resorbed. Administration of two doses of tetracycline separated by a known time interval allows determination of the bone apposition rate (in microns of new bone matrix formed per day). The rate of osteoid maturation (in percentage per day) can then be calculated by dividing the apposition rate by the osteoid width in microns. Wide osteoid that does not abut bone containing double labels indicates a decreased rate of osteoid maturation. One type of uremic bone disease shows delayed onset of mineralization and increased osteoid area and width (malacic group).

Bone biopsy is the only conclusive way to determine if a patient has osteomalacia. As mentioned above, it is important to note that the presence of wide osteoid does not necessarily indicate osteomalacia. A biopsy with advanced osteomalacia would show increased bone surface involved in formation and increased osteoid area and width. Since mineralization is significantly delayed in osteomalacia, after double labeling only a widened single tetracycline label may be present, or no tetracycline label may be present if mineralization has halted. Tetracycline labeling should also be evaluated with attention to the discreteness of the labels, since in some conditions, such as fluoride therapy or other causes of osteomalacia, tetracycline is not properly locked into the bone and the label is diffuse and abnormally wide.

Marrow Fibrosis

The presence and extent of fibrosis in the bone marrow should also be evaluated since marrow fibrosis is usually associated with increased bone formation. In uremic bone disease, the fibrotic type of bone biopsy is characterized by increased marrow fibrosis, resorbing surface, and bone formation rate, and sometimes by woven bone. The presence of marrow fibrosis may also indicate that a hyperparathyroid state with elevated PTH has been present for several months.

Diagnostic Bone Biopsies, Osteoporosis, and Bone Aging

For clinical applications, bone biopsies have become an essential part of diagnostic and therapeutic evaluation (124), and several key histologic bone changes can be identified in a number of metabolic bone diseases (Table 2). Osteoporosis is the most common symptomatic skeletal disease and has been reviewed recently by Raisz (125). A scheme for the diagnosis of osteoporosis by the primary care physician has been outlined; it includes bone biopsy findings, typical physical examination and clinical findings, and bone mineral content data (126) (Fig. 6). In a large patient population of 150 osteoporotics, 80% were found to have primary osteoporosis; 95% of these were in the postmenopausal and senile groups. Osteoporosis, characterized by a decrease in bone volume within a normal periosteal

Table 2. Selected Trabecular Bone Features for Various Metabolic Bone Diseases

	Total Bone Area (trabecular)	Forming Surface	Osteoid Width	Resorbing Surface	Linear Rate of Matrix Formation	Rate of Osteoid Maturation	Marrow Fibrosis	Comments
Primary osteoporosis	↓ or nl[a]	nl, ↑ ↓	nl or ↓	nl	nl	nl	−	Histologic heterogeneity noteworthy
Osteomalacia	nl or ↓	↑	↑	nl or ↑ depending on cause	↓	↓	+[b] or −	Important to determine the osteoid maturation rate to distinguish osteomalacia from a high turnover state
Primary hyperparathyroidism	nl	↑	nl or ↑	↑ or nl	↓, nl or ↑	nl	±	Biopsy not usually distinctive in mild primary hyperparathyroidism
Uremic bone disease:								As a group, uremic patients have increased osteoid width, forming and resorbing surfaces and rate of bone formation compared to normals.
Mild	nl or ↓	↑	nl	nl	nl	nl	±	
Osteomalacic	nl	↑	↑	nl	↓	↓	+	
Fibrotic	nl	↑	↑	↑	↑	nl	+	

408

Paget's disease (mixed phase)	↑	↑	↑	↑	↑	+	Characteristic cement line (mosaic) pattern. Resorptive (osteolytic) & sclerotic phases.
Osteopetrosis	↑	↑ or nl	nl	nl or ↑	↑ or nl	↑ or nl	−	May be two types—one due to decreased osteoclast activity and one due to increased osteoblast activity.
Fluorosis	↑	↑	↑	↑	↑ or nl	→	−	↑ Cortical porosity and hypervascularization

SOURCE: Gruber HE et al: *Semin Hematol* 18:258–278, 1981.

[a] nl = normal.
[b] Hypophosphatemic osteomalacia.

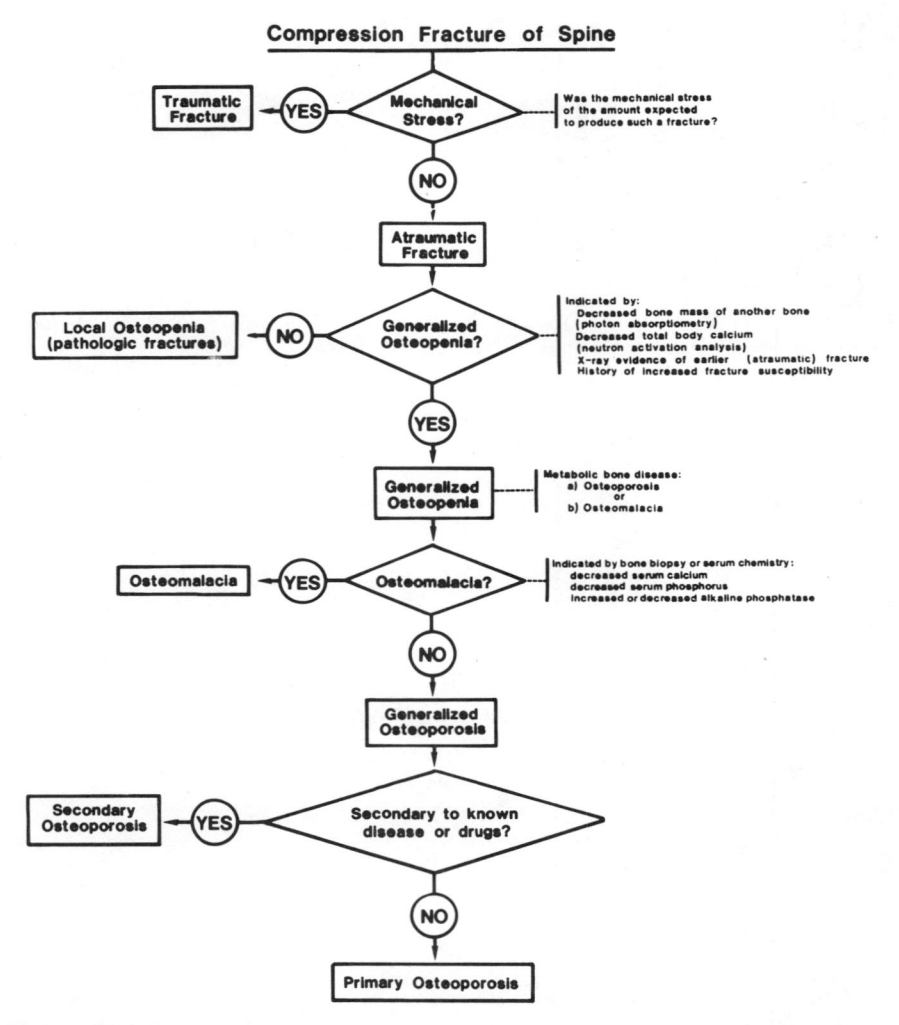

Figure 6. Schematic evaluation for the diagnostic approach to osteoporosis. (Gruber HE, Baylink DJ: *J Am Geriatr Soc* 29:490–497, 1981. Used with permission.)

perimeter, has a wide variety of causes (Table 3). The bone histologic features of osteoporosis complicate the problem of describing this metabolic bone disease because osteoporotics display great diversity with respect to cortical thickness and porosity, trabecular pattern and bone volume, and formation and resorption. The study of postmenopausal osteoporosis (PMOP) by Whyte et al. again confirmed the heterogeneity of bone features in a population of 26 postmenopausal subjects (127). As previously noted, clinical and biochemical features were not useful in predicting bone

Table 3. Osteoporosis: Classification and Tests Frequently Used for Diagnosis[a]

	Test or Comment	Results[b]
Primary osteoporosis		
Idiopathic		
Juvenile	Isolated or one or sometimes more than one child within a family may be affected	—
Young adults[b]	Urine hydroxyproline	↑
Postmenopausal	Exclude other causes of osteoporosis	—
Senile[c]	Exclude other causes of osteoporosis in patients 65 or more years old	—
Secondary osteoporosis (secondary to heritable or acquired abnormalities)		
Marfan's syndrome	Arm and leg length	↑
Morquio's syndrome	Serum hexosamine	↑
Homocystinuria	Urine homocysteine	↑
Osteogenesis imperfecta tarda	Platelet factor 3 activity	↓
Hypophosphatasia, adult form	Urine phosphoethanolamine	↑
Werner's syndrome	Obvious clincial features	—
Lactase deficiency	History; milk intolerance	—
Male hypogonadism (e.g., Klinefelter's syndrome)	Serum testosterone	↓
Gut malabsorption	Serum 25(OH)D	↓
	Serum PTH	↑
	Serum alkaline phosphatase	↑
	Urine Ca	↓
	Serum CA	↓
	Serum PO$_4$	↓
Renal Ca leak (renal hypercalciuria)	Urine cAMP	↑
Renal tubular acidosis, Type 2	Serum CO$_2$	↓
Cirrhosis: Laennec's cirrhosis or biliary	Liver function tests	↓
Immobilization	Urine hydroxyproline	↑
Multiple myeloma[d]	Serum myeloma protein	↑
Low serum PO$_4$	Serum P	
Renal PO$_4$ leak[e] associated with low serum PO$_4$, high serum 1,25(OH)$_2$D and hypercalciuria	Serum P	↓
	PTH	↓
	Urine Ca	↑
Renal PO$_4$ leak associated with low serum PO$_4$, low serum 1,25(OH)$_2$D and without hypercalciuria	Serum P	↓
	Urine Ca	↓
Treatment with PO$_4$ binders (e.g., Basojel)	Serum P	↓
	PTH	↓
	Urine Ca	↑

Table 3. (*continued*)

	Test or Comment	Results[b]
Selective deficiency of 1,25(OH)$_2$D (adult onset)	Serum Ca	↓
	Serum P	↓
	PTH	↑
	Response to 1,25(OH)$_2$D	nl
Anticonvulsant drugs	history	—
Female hypogonadism (e.g., oophorectomy or Turner's syndrome)	urine estrogen	↓
Cushing's syndrome	serum cortical	↑
Thyrotoxicosis	T$_3$, T$_4$	↑
Chronic alcoholism	history	—
Diabetes[f]	fasting blood sugar	↑
Chronic heparin treatment	history	—
Systemic mastocytosis (urticaria pigmentosa)	physical exam	—
Chronic obstructive pulmonary disease	pulmonary function tests	↓
Mild vitamin D deficiency (e.g., patients >70 years of age)	serum 25(OH)D	↓

SOURCE: Gruber HE, Baylink DJ: *J Am Geriatr Soc* 29:490–497, 1981.

[a] Use is dictated by two criteria: (*1*) if the test discloses a readily treatable disease even if not common, and (*2*) if the test is most likely to disclose an abnormality largely because the corresponding disease is relatively common.

[b] These changes indicate the changes that may occur and do not preclude the possibility of no change.

[c] Encountered in patients over 65 years of age.

[d] May present or be associated with clinical osteoporosis.

[e] In general, we find that when serum phosphorus is markedly decreased, the patient develops osteomalacia; when phosphorus is only modestly decreased, the patient develops osteoporosis.

[f] Conflicting data on whether diabetes is associated with osteopenia.

histology. Both high bone turnover (active remodeling) and low turnover (intactive remodeling) were found.

An evaluation of bone matrix and mineral abnormalities by Burnell et al. (128) has shown that osteoporotics display variable percentages of bone mineral and hydroxyproline in the bone matrix. Within the mineral, bicarbonate, calcium, and phosphorus were decreased while sodium and magnesium were increased. Four groups with different chemical composition of iliac crest bone were identified: a group with decreased matrix hydroxyproline and normal percentage of mineral (nine of 56 patients); a group with decreased matrix hydroxyproline and decreased percentage of mineral (five of 56); a group with normal matrix hydroxyproline and normal percentage of mineral (33 of 56); and a group with normal matrix hydroxyproline and decreased percentage of mineral (nine of 56).

The calcitonin response in PMOP to calcium stimulation was evaluated by Taggart et al. (129), who found that immunoreactive calcitonin levels increased significantly from baseline in normal subjects 10 and 20 minutes after calcium infusion. However, immunoreactive calcitonin levels in osteoporotics did not change significantly at any time during infusion, and the authors concluded that their data were consistent with a decreased calcitonin response to calcium infusion in PMOP, suggesting that calcitonin deficiency may be involved in the development of osteoporosis.

Aloia et al. investigated the value of a combination therapy regime of estrogen, fluoride, and calcium in nine PMOP subjects (130). A control group received fluoride and calcium but no estrogen. Significant positive slopes were found for total body calcium and bone mineral content in the combination therapy group. The change in bone mineral content was significantly different from the response of the fluoride–calcium group. In an earlier editorial, Ivey and Baylink (131) had suggested that PMOP may involve an uncoupling of the effect of estrogen deficiency superimposed upon an age-related decrease in the ability to effectively couple bone accretion and resorption.

Neutron activation analyses of the central third of the skeleton of PMOP subjects were carried out over 3 years to assess changes during a therapy regime using various combinations of NaF, calcium and vitamin D_2, and estrogens (132). Patients receiving NaF and/or estrogen showed a mean increase in calcium bone index of $5 \pm 2\%$ (SEM) compared to a negligible loss of $0.4 \pm 1.9\%$ for controls; however this difference was not significant for their small number of subjects. Eight of 16 patients treated with NaF showed adequate fluoride retention. Six of these had bone biopsies that showed histologic evidence of fluorosis. Only one of the eight subjects with fluoride retention had further fractures. This incidence was less but not statistically different from the fracture incidence in patients without NaF (five of 14). Sodium fluoride therapy for 3 years was associated with a significant increase in bone mineral.

An improved method for quantitative determination of serum alkaline phosphatase of skeletal origin has recently indicated that skeletal alkaline phosphatase activity was increased when compared with age-matched controls in seven osteoporotic patients responding to NaF therapy with increased bone formation (133). PMOP patients responding to therapy with stanozolol by increased total body calcium also showed an increase in skeletal alkaline phosphatase.

Bone mass and growth in young diabetics has been studied by Wiske et al. (134), who found that bone photon absorptiometry values were 1.24 SD below the normal mean for these subjects. Bone mass and cortical area were inversely related to disease duration. This report suggests that the reduced bone mass probably results from failure to gain normal endosteal bone mass at the appropriate age; this abnormality progresses with the diabetic condition.

Several current articles have addressed the issue of bone and aging. Mazess has reviewed noninvasive methods to evaluate aging changes in cortical and trabecular bone and concluded that the assumption of a large on-going loss of trabecular bone after the menopause may be erroneous (135). Likewise, Riggs et al. (136) have published data showing that in normal women, vertebral bone loss begins in young adulthood and does not accelerate in the immediate postmenopausal period. However, appendicular bone loss does not occur until age 50, accelerates from ages 51 to 65, and decelerates slightly after 65 years. Overall bone loss was 47% for vertebrae, 30% for the midradius, and 39% for the distal radius. Vertebral and appendicular bone loss was minimal or insignificant in normal men. By age 60, 50% of normal women (and virtually all women by age 85) had vertebral bone mineral density values below the maximum values found in osteoporotics. Thus, such subjects might be considered to have asymptomatic osteoporosis. The authors suggested that disproportionate loss of trabecular bone from the axial skeleton was a distinguishing feature of spinal osteoporosis.

Riggs et al. (137) have also used dual photon absorptiometry to assess changes in bone mineral density of the spine and proximal femur with aging. For normal women, the regression of bone mineral density and age was negative and linear. The overall decrease during life was 58% in the femoral neck, 53% in the intertrochanteric area of the femur, and 42% in the lumbar spine. For normal men, the regression was also linear, but the loss rate was two-thirds that in women for the femoral neck and intertrochanteric femur, and only one-fourth that of women for the lumbar spine. For women with nontraumatic vertebral fractures, the standard deviation from the sex specific age-adjusted normal mean was significantly lower for the lumbar spine. Thus the authors concluded that, contrary to the belief that osteoporosis is a single age-related disease, two distinct syndromes may be present: The "postmenopausal osteoporosis" group is characterized by excessive disproportionate trabecular bone loss. This type affects a small subset of women in early postmenopause with mainly vertebral fractures. The "senile osteoporosis group" is characterized by proportionate loss of both cortical and trabecular bone, involves essentially the entire population of aging women—and to a lesser degree aging men—and is associated with hip fractures and/or vertebral fractures.

Heaney has recently presented an editorial discussing the issue of calcium intake requirements and bone mass in the elderly (138). He stressed the point that evidence over the recent years has shifted to favor a role in the protection of bone mass and fracture prevention, and that the current recommended daily allowance of 800 mg calcium is too low, although it is not known what the exact optimum intake should be. Marcus (139) has also recently commented on the interrelationship of endocrinology and nutrition in the maintenance of skeletal mass and suggests an intake of 1500 mg calcium at the time of menopause.

Calcium balance in osteoporotic patients on long-term oral calcium therapy with and without sex hormones was studied by Thalassinos et al. (140). Patients on high calcium alone showed a significant increase in both total calcium balance and net calcium absorption. This effect could be sustained for periods up to 10 years (mean 3.5 years) by addition of estradiol and testosterone derivatives. Discontinuation of hormones only resulted in a significant decrease in both calcium balance and net absorption, but both were still increased as compared to initial patient values.

Two other interesting studies have looked at bone loss from less common causes. Stout (141) evaluated cortical bone features in patients with multiple sclerosis and quadriplegia resulting from poliomyelitis. Osteon densities in the femur, tibia, fibula, humerus, radius, ulna, and rib were not significantly different in the patient with multiple sclerosis. However, osteon densities were significantly lower than normal in samples from the quadriplegic in all skeletal sites except for the right arm, a skeletal region in which the patient had retained partial use. Another patient group at risk for decreased bone mineral content and increased fracture incidence is alcoholics. Johnell et al. (142) studied 38 patients with a history of abnormal alcohol intake for at least 10 years. Bone mineral content of the forearm was significantly decreased as compared with controls, with the loss rate appearing to be slightly more rapid in alcoholics who had undergone gastric surgery. Bone biopsy evaluation of osteoid surface showed an increase in this parameter above normal only in alcoholics who had undergone gastric resection. However, the number of osteoclasts was increased in alcoholics whether or not they had undergone gastric resection.

In an animal study of bone aging, Syftestad and Urist have continued their bone matrix by investigating changes in the matrix composition with aging (143). Bone matrix from senescent (28-month-old) rats was markedly deficient in the capacity to induce bone formation when compared with matrix from 13-month-old rats, suggesting that a progressive decline in matrix morphogenic activity may occur during adult life.

Renal Osteodystrophy and the Aluminum Problem

General aspects of renal bone disease have recently been reviewed by Cochran (144) and Massry (145). Torres and Moya (146) have designed a computerized tomography method to assess trabecular bone mass (TBM) in the central portion of the fourth lumbar vertebra. They have studied 29 normal subjects and 19 hemodialysis patients. Seventy-nine percent of the hemodialysis patients showed normal or high TBM. Two of the patients with increased TBM showed radiologic osteosclerosis, and four showed advanced subperiosteal resorption. The authors suggest that their vertebral tomography method may be useful in the early detection and management of renal osteodystrophy.

Bone defects in uremic osteodystrophy have been described by Weinstein and Sappington (147) who found that if accumulated osteomalacic and woven bone exceed the volume of lamellar bone removed in chronic renal insufficiency, bone density can be reduced despite an increase in trabecular bone volume. When density of iliac crest cores was measured by photon absorptiometry, patients with osteopenic uremia showed no relationship between trabecular or mineralized bone volume and core density, whereas there were significant relationships in nonuremic osteopenic subjects. Bone core density of uremic patients correlated significantly with osteoid volume and serum phosphorus.

Results from a multicenter study evaluating the effect of calcifediol in the treatment of renal failure patients have shown changes apparent on bone biopsy examination (148). The population of chronic renal failure patients on long-term dialysis consisted of two bone histologic groups: One group with active bone showed secondary hyperparathyroid bone features of increased resorption and increased formation. The second group was characterized by decreased apposition rates and decreased bone formation rates. All patients exhibited increased osteoid that decreased in volume and thickness after calcifediol treatment. The active bone group showed a reduction in hyperparathyroid features. However, the inactive group continued to show depressed formation and apposition following therapy. Osteoid that did mineralize in treated patients did so in a normal manner, increasing apposition and formation, but not to such an extent as to be normal. Both groups showed a reduction in the extent of woven bone.

Another group of dialysis patients was evaluated 24 months before and 15 months after the initiation of regular hemodialysis (149). The mean change per month in bone mineral content of the forearm was -0.43% before dialysis and $+0.08\%$ after dialysis. Patients with polycystic kidney disease had significantly lower bone mineral content values (corrected for bone width) than patients with glomerulonephritis.

Nine patients with slowly progressive renal failure have been evaluated by Brown et al. (150) for periods extending beyond 1 year. Quantitative bone histology of iliac crest bone biopsies showed that all patients had some bone abnormalities. Mild to moderate fibrosis was the most common feature, although seven patients had an increased number of osteoclasts. Eight patients showed progression of their bone disease over 1 year; the most consistent change was an increase in osteoid area. Half the patients showed evidence of HPT.

Seventeen patients with stable chronic renal failure have been recently evaluated by Christiansen et al. (151) in a study that examined serum $25(OH)D_3$, $24,25(OH)_2D_3$, $1,25(OH)_2D_3$, and bone biopsy features. Serum calcium correlated inversely with both osteoid surface and volume. No correlations were found between bone parameters and levels of the vitamin D metabolites.

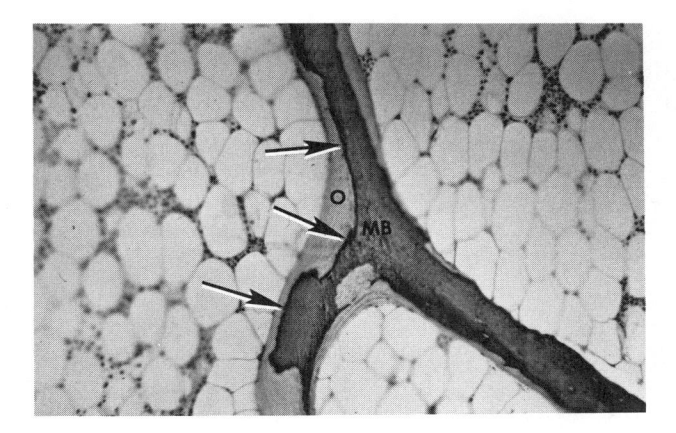

Figure 7. Bone histochemistry in a patient with aluminum overload. O, osteoid; HB, mineralized bone. Arrows are pointing to the deposition of aluminum.

The problem of bone and aluminum has received increasing attention in the last few years. In patients with aluminum intoxication, histochemical localization in bone is frequently seen along the mineralizing front between osteoid and mature mineralized bone (Fig. 7), and sometimes along cement lines. It is believed that the aluminum deposition contributes to mineralization defects. Both aluminum in water used for the dialysate preparation and aluminum contained in phosphate binders contribute to this intoxication. The dementia syndrome and the issue of aluminum intoxication have recently been reviewed by Sideman and Manor (152).

Although the aluminum problem is not completely understood, several research groups have contributed data that increase our knowledge of the problem. Ellis et al. (153) found a significant increase in the amount of aluminum (determined by neutron activation analysis) in the bone of 17 patients on hemodialysis. Eight patients on dialysis who subsequently underwent renal transplantation showed bone aluminum levels that were still significantly increased. They found no relationship between HPT and bone aluminum. In general, patients on dialysis for longer periods tended to show the highest levels of aluminum, osteomalacia, and dialysis encephalopathy.

Two groups of hemodialyzed patients, one with osteomalacia and low resorption (group 1) and one with fibrosis and no mineralization defects (group 2) were studied by Cournot-Witmer et al. (154). Group 1 showed significantly higher plasma aluminum concentrations than group 2, but no difference was found in bone aluminum content, which was elevated above normal in both groups. 25(OH) vitamin D and 1α(OH) vitamin D failed to improve the disease. In group 1 bone aluminum content showed correlation with total osteoid volume. This correlation was not found in group 2, in which iPTH, osteoclast surface, and marrow fibrosis were significantly higher than corresponding values in group 1. Aluminum could not be localized histochemically in most patients in group 2. Aluminum was seen in group 1 mainly localized along the mineralizing front; in some cases it was also found along cement lines. In group 2, only two patients showed aluminum, mainly along cement lines. The authors state that it is possible that in aluminum-intoxicated patients secondary HPT may in some way prevent the aluminum-induced mineralization defect.

Recently, aluminum histochemical staining methods using the aurine tricarboxylic acid aluminum procedure with various counterstains have been published (155–157). Maloney et al. (156) documented that the majority of the sites showing aluminum histochemically did not take up tetracycline, but in some instances, tetracycline was found at the same site as aluminum, indicating that although aluminum is usually concomitant with mineralization defects, the mineralization block may in some manner sometimes be overcome. Histochemical aluminum localization correlated well with aluminum determined by atomic absorption methods and also with osteoid width. Mineralization lag time also correlated significantly with stained aluminum. Hodsman et al. (157) found that bone aluminum was significantly higher in osteomalacic biopsies from hemodialysis patients than in biopsies from patients exhibiting osteitis fibrosa with mixed bone lesions and mild lesions. Bone aluminum correlated inversely with iPTH and crenated surface, and with the duration of dialysis for fibrosis and mixed and mild lesion patients. No correlation was found with osteomalacic subjects' aluminum levels and the duration of dialysis. In their dialysis patient population, Walker et al. (158) found that higher aluminum levels were associated with more osteomalacia. Fleming et al. (159) have concluded that oral aluminum hydroxide makes a major contribution to plasma aluminum levels in patients with renal failure. Postdialysis plasma aluminum levels were consistently higher than predialysis levels in patients both on and off aluminum therapy despite low dialysate aluminum concentration. Felsenfeld et al. (160) documented aluminum localized in bone and osteomalacia in a case report of an azotemic patient prior to initiation of dialysis, providing further evidence for the implication of binders in the etiology of aluminum bone intoxication.

The effect of aluminum on bone phosphatases in vitro was investigated by Lieberherr et al. (161) using the rat calvaria model and aluminum levels comparable to circulating aluminum concentrations in hemodialysis patients. Aluminum at concentrations from 3×10^{-11} to 1.5×10^{-6} M caused a dose-dependent increase in acid and alkaline phosphatase activities. However, concentrations of 3×10^{-6} M and greater caused a significant decrease in both enzymes' activities. The action of aluminum was modulated by medium phosphorus and calcium concentrations: phosphatase stimulated by 1.5×10^{-6} M aluminum shows higher activity in a phosphorus-free medium and lower activity in a calcium-free medium. The presence of aluminum decreased the stimulation of phosphatase by PTH and 1,25(OH)$_2$D$_3$. The action of 24,25(OH)$_2$D$_3$ on acid phosphatase was not modified by the presence of aluminum, but its stimulatory effect on alkaline phosphatase decreased at greater aluminum concentrations.

Hyperparathyroidism, Pseudohypoparathyroidism, and Hyperthyroidism

Hypercalcemic HPT following renal transplantation has recently been reviewed by Parfitt (162). Tam et al. (163) have documented increased bone apposition in primary HPT. Four of 23 patients had normal bone biopsy features of volume and surface parameters. However, bone apposition was elevated in all subjects. Following parathyroid surgery in four patients, apposition fell to normal values.

Dual photon absorptiometry assessment of midradius, distal radius, and the lumbar spine of subjects with primary HPT, hypercortisolism, and hyperthyroidism was found to show a negative deviation (suggesting bone loss) from the sex specific age regression line as compared to normal subjects (164). However, patients with secondary hypoparathyroidism due to chronic renal failure, acromegaly, and postsurgical hypoparathyroidism showed a positive deviation from normal (suggesting bone gain). For all these endocrine dysfunction patients, bone mineral density of the radius differed significantly from lumbar spine measurements, again indicating that site-specific skeletal changes occur with various endocrine abnormalities.

The effects of PTH on bone packet remodeling in patients with primary HPT were evaluated by Charhon et al. (165) in 26 patients. Mean wall thickness was significantly lower than in controls; the significant reduction appears to occur in women before the age of 50 since there is no significant difference in wall thickness in women after the age of 50 or in males at any age. Osteoblast activity is mildly depressed in HPT, and although both osteoblasts and osteoclasts are more numerous than normal, they are less active than normal.

In their study of abnormal bone and parathyroid histology in carcinoma patients with pseudohyperparathyroidism, Sharp et al. (166) found that bone histology showed increased resorption and marrow fibrosis in nine patients whose parathyroid glands were hyperplastic. Serum biochemistries suggested that bone resorption was related to a humoral substance elaborated by the tumors and distinct from PTH.

Jastrup et al. (167) investigated serum vitamin D metabolite levels and bone remodeling features in hyperthyroidism and found that 25(OH)D$_3$ was normal, 1,25(OH)$_2$D$_3$ was significantly reduced from normal, and 24,25(OH)$_2$D$_3$ levels were significantly increased. Bone histology showed enhanced turnover unrelated to vitamin D metabolites. Bone apposition and mineralization were increased and the mineralization lag time decreased apparently independently of altered vitamin D metabolite levels.

Osteopetrosis

Osteopetrosis was reviewed and 21 cases qualitatively described by Milgram and Jasty (168). In another study, two patients with increased skeletal masses were found to differ markedly with respect to acid and alkaline phosphatase, resorbing surface, bone apposition rate, and the rate of osteoid maturation. Manzke et al. (169) found that a patient with the more classic findings showed an impairment in osteoclast resorption, but normal bone formation and apposition. A second patient, however, proved to have two abnormalities: increased bone formation and apposition (resulting from increased osteoblast activity) and an impairment of a compensatory increase in bone resorption. A possible hope for therapy other than bone marrow transplantation for osteopetrotic patients has been suggested by the work of Key et al. (170), who reported promising findings in an 11-month-old child with osteopetrosis treated with calcitriol (2–16 μm/day) over 11 days. Urinary hydroxyproline and serum alkaline phosphatase increased, and the patient's monocytes, which did not liberate ^{45}Ca from labeled bone chips before therapy, were able to liberate 36% of the labeled bone (as compared to 15% for normal control monocytes).

Pregnancy, PTH, and Bone

Mineral metabolism during pregnancy has also attracted recent interest. iPTH during the third trimester has been studied by Gillette et al. (171). Creatinine clearance was increased significantly, and serum calcium and albumin decreased significantly. However, no significant differences were found for iPTH, serum phosphorus, TmP, or nephrogenous cAMP. In another study, Seino et al. (172) found that serum $1,25(OH)_2D_3$ levels were significantly elevated in maternal serum, infant serum, and cord serum at delivery. PTH was low and calcitonin higher than in maternal sera. Skeletal changes during pregnancy were thought to be mediated by a mechanism independent of vitamin D (173). Vitamin D-replete rats showed a significant loss of mineralized tissue during pregnancy and lactation. Both trabecular and cortical bone showed losses; these decreases were greatest at weaning. Similar losses were seen in vitamin D-deficient rats during pregnancy and lactation. Following weaning, there was some restoration of trabecular and cortical bone in both D-replete and D-deficient animals.

Bone GLA Protein

The vitamin K-dependent protein of bone (GLA, BGP) is one of the most abundant noncollagenous proteins in bone and is thought to first appear in calcifying bone at the time of matrix maturation to hydroxyapatite. Deftos et al. (174) have followed changes in plasma bone GLA during the treatment of various metabolic bone diseases. GLA was increased above normal in Paget's disease, primary HPT, chronic renal failure, and neoplasia involving bone. During therapy for Paget's disease with calcitonin, GLA decreased. Women with primary HPT had higher GLA levels than did men; GLA decreased following parathyroidectomy but was significantly decreased only in women. GLA did not decrease in renal failure patients during dialysis. In bone cancer patients, GLA decreased during calcitonin therapy. A general correlation was found between GLA levels and alkaline phosphatase. Further studies are necessary to more completely define the role of bone GLA levels in the management of bone disease.

Bone Tumors and the Hypercalcemia of Malignancy

Bone changes found in metastatic bone diseases have been described by Gruber et al. (124). Table 4 summarizes the histologic features in epithelial tumors, multiple myeloma, leukemia and lymphoma, and myeloproliferative syndromes. Neoplastic processes that involve bone may induce osteoblastic bone formation, osteoclastic bone resorption, marrow fibrosis, or no histologically apparent bone changes.

Quantitative bone histology from seven patients with elevated nephrogenous cAMP and the absence of bone tumors was studied by Stewart et al. (175). Compared with patients with primary HPT, the seven subjects with humoral hypercalcemia of malignancy showed a greater extent of osteoclastic surface and more frequent empty Howship's lacunae and a markedly reduced osteoblast surface and osteoid surface and volume. These results document uncoupling of osteoblasts and osteoclasts and may provide a mechanism for the marked skeletal loss seen in patients with hypercalcemia of malignancy.

A rat model for tumor-induced hypercalcemia in humans has been investigated by Berger et al. (176). This transplantable Leydig cell tumor, causing serum biochemistry features similar to those of many tumor patients, who demonstrate suppression of PTH with elevated urinary cAMP excretion, may prove a valuable model for future animal research.

Osteoblasts, Osteoclasts, and Coupling Factor

Recent findings have expanded our understanding of osteoblast and osteoclast activities and of cellular interrelationships. Gap junctions, which may have an important function in the coordination of bone cell activities, have been identified in rat studies by Doty (177). Gap junctions were found between adjacent osteoblasts and between osteoblasts and osteocytes,

Table 4. Histologic Features of Neoplastic Processes Involving Bone[a]

	Epithelial Tumors Lytic[b]	Epithelial Tumors Sclerotic[c]	Multiple Myeloma Leukemias/ Lymphomas[e]	Myeloproliferative Syndromes
Total bone	↓	↑	nl, ↓ ↑[f]	nl, ↑
Woven bone	—	↑	—	↑
Osteoblast number	nl, ↑	↑[d], occ nl	nl, ↑[f]	nl, ↑
Osteoblast size	nl, ↑	↑[d], occ nl	nl	nl, ↑
Osteoclast number	↑, occ nl	↓	nl, ↑	nl
Howship's lacunae	↑, occ nl	↓	nl, ↑	nl
Osteocyte lacunar size	nl	↑	nl	nl, ↑
Osteoid	nl	↑	nl, ↑[f]	nl, ↑ (?)
Marrow fibrosis	↑, occ nl	↑	nl, ↑[g]	↑, occ nl

SOURCE: Gruber HE et al: *Semin Hematol* 18:258–278, 1981.

[a] nl, normal.

[b] Includes squamous cell carcinomas (larynx, lung, esophagus, oral cavity, cervix), mammary carcinoma, thyroid, kidney, small cell carcinoma, lung, some gastrointestinal neoplasms.

[c] Includes prostate, urinary bladder, breast, gastric (signet ring: mucin positive), small cell carcinoma lung (occasionally), carcinoid tumors of GI tract or bronchus.

[d] Osteoblasts may be difficult to find along trabecular surfaces if entire marrow is replaced by tumor.

[e] Includes multiple myeloma, acute myelogenous leukemia, acute and chronic lymphocytic leukemia, and non-Hodgkin's lymphomas. Hodgkin's disease involving the bone marrow does not usually induce bone changes, but may have significant marrow fibrosis and occasionally may induce an osteoblastic bone reaction.

[f] Change found in plasmacytic neoplasia with osteosclerotic lesions.

[g] Marrow fibrosis is often seen in Hodgkin's disease and reticulin fibrosis is often seen in hairy cell leukemia.

providing more evidence for intercellular systems of communications between bone cells.

A number of current papers have concentrated on osteoclasts. Mills (178) has continued her ultrastructural studies of osteoclasts from patients with Paget's disease and has compared these cells with giant cells from malignant giant cell tumors. Giant cell tumors contained nuclear inclusions morphologically identical with the 12–15 nm tubules characteristic of the osteoclast nuclei in Paget's disease.

Chambers' work with osteoclasts isolated from neonatal rats (179) has shown that osteoclasts can be evaluated by following their mobility with time lapse cinematography. When calcitonin (at concentrations of 10 pg/ml and greater) is added to this in vitro system, osteoclasts show complete cessation of pseudopodial activity within minutes. This inhibition of movement can last as long as the cells are viable. However, osteoclasts regain activity when osteoblasts are added (180). This escape from the calcitonin effect is not due to calcitonin inactivation by the osteoblasts and does not occur if osteoblasts are separated from osteoclasts by a millipore filter.

Liu et al. have documented an acute reduction in osteoclast number in rats repleted with calcium following a calcium deficient diet (181). This study is the first quantitative analysis of changes in osteoclast number during calcium deprivation and the fate of osteoclasts during calcium replenishment. Twelve days of calcium deprivation resulted in a twenty-onefold increase in the number of endosteal osteoclasts. Osteoclasts disappeared completely from the endosteum after 3 days of calcium replenishment. Changes in iPTH and the production of 1,25(OH)$_2$D$_3$ could not entirely account for the decrease in osteoclast number during repletion; thus, local factors or other systemic cues contribute to the cellular decrease. Acid-positive fragments increased in the marrow space coincident with the acute osteoclast decrease early in calcium replenishment, indicating that these fragments are the products of degenerating osteoclasts. In another osteoclast study, Minkin (182) has suggested that tartrate-resistant acid phosphatase may serve as a biochemical marker of osteoclast function.

Work by Stern et al. (183) indicates that the ionophore A23187 (at a concentration of 6×10^{-7}M) and 1,25(OH)$_2$ vitamin D promote osteoclast formation in fetal rat bone cultures, suggesting that a precursor pool responds to all three agents. Using this same ionophore, Krieger et al. (184) determined that concentrations of 10^{-6}M maximally inhibits PTH-stimulated bone resorption. Other in vitro work has shown that cholera toxin (185) and amphotericin B (186) stimulate bone resorption, and that promethazine hydrochloride inhibits PTH-stimulated resorption (187).

A number of studies have investigated the effects of calcitonin. Calcitonin effects on isolated bone cells were explored by Shlossman et al (188). An isolated population of bone cells with high acid phosphatase levels and the ability to release ^{45}Ca from prelabeled bone exhibited calcitonin-induced increase in cAMP and a decrease in calcium uptake. Calcitonin had no effect on populations with a high level of alkaline phosphatase. Hormonally sensitive cells were present in 19 to 21-day-old rat fetuses and 1- and 2-day-old animals.

Kreiger et al. inhibited cell proliferation by irradiation in order to determine if the "escape" effect from calcitonin (which is apparent after the transient stimulation of bone resorption) is due to production of osteoclasts that are unresponsive to calcitonin (189). Irradiation did not affect the resorptive response caused by PTH. It did, however, induce a dose-dependent inhibition of the escape response, but this was not superimposable on the dose response inhibition of cell proliferation caused by irradiation.

Changes in calcium phosphate on bone surfaces after calcitonin administration in TPTX rat pups was studied by Norimatsu et al. (190). Their electron probe analysis data revealed that amorphous calcium phosphate clusters and globules appeared on the bone surface after a small dose of calcitonin, supporting the hypothesis that calcitonin acts directly on bone lining cells to influence calcium storage at bone surfaces.

The mechanisms of action of biphosphonates and diphosphonates, assessed in an in vitro rat model, appear to be different as studied by Reitsma et al. (191). Cl_2MDP apparently exerts its effect as a potent cytotoxin. However, APD is not cytotoxic at levels adequate to supress resorption and must, therefore, inhibit resorptive activity by another mechanism. Neither agent appeared to limit resorption by decreasing the solubility of bone matrix.

The presence of PTH receptors in four cell populations isolated from chick calvaria was evaluated by Nijewide et al. (192), who found that receptors were present on the periosteal fibroblast, osteoblast, osteoclast, and mixed cell populations, but that occupancy of the receptor induced adenylate cyclase stimulation only in osteocytes and fully differentiated osteoblasts. Biochemical and histologic characteristics of the cell populations were also reported.

The effect of 1α-hydroxy vitamin D on bone formation and PTH activity, studied by Lindholm et al (193), has been shown to result in a decreased resorption rate and increased tetracycline incorporation. Cortical and trabecular bone increased, as well as levels of bone hydroxyproline and hexosamines. Parathyroid volume was decreased and chief cells exhibited pyknosis.

In their studies on skeletal alkaline phosphatase activity, Farley et al. (194) found that neither vanadate, phenylphosphonate, nor levamisole, inhibitors of skeletal alkaline phosphatase activity, affected cellular concentrations of alkaline phosphatase during a 24-hour incubation using embryonic chick calvarial cells. Their studies indicated that alkaline phosphatase inhibition may have nonspecific effects on bone cell in vitro, and that for osteoblastlike cells an inhibition of alkaline phosphatase activity is not consistently related to a decrease in cell proliferation.

Bone formation and calcification by isolated osteoblastlike cells was reported by Nijweide et al. using chick calvaria cells (195). Their methodology showed that after 6 days of growth, 80% of the cultures transplanted onto chorioallantoic membranes of quail embryos exhibited bone-like structures. This work suggests that bone formation may need a three-dimensional structure, which may itself be necessary to stimulate bone formation or which may favor a milieu that localizes bone-forming stimulators.

Baylink et al. continue investigations of local factors influencing bone regulation. Puzas et al. have recovered an endogenous small polypeptide inhibitor of bone cell proliferation (196). Progress on an isolated human skeletal "coupling factor" continues, using in vitro bone formation and resorption assays (197–199). Further characterization will more clearly delineate this factor's role in the regulation of endosteal bone volume.

The effect of bone-derived growth factors on DNA, RNA, and proteoglycan synthesis in cultures of rabbit costal chondrocytes has been studied by Kato et al. (200). One fraction (MW 20,000–30,000) influences calvaria DNA labeling, and another (MN 6,000–13,000) influences bone collagen labeling. These studies suggest that factor(s) released by bone cells are capable of influencing cartilage metabolism and growth.

VITAMIN D AND ITS METABOLITES

For general review articles on vitamin D and its metabolites, readers are referred to a series of current publications (201–208).

Vitamin D-Binding Proteins

Haddad (209) and Bouillon and Van Baelin (210) have provided comprehensive reviews on the interesting and important subject of vitamin D-binding proteins. There is now good evidence for the existence of a high-affinity and high-capacity binding system for vitamin D and its metabolites in human plasma. This vitamin D-binding protein (DBP) is responsible for the transport of the antirachitic sterols throughout the body. The binding characteristics demonstrate high specificity for the vitamin D structure and exhibit greater preference for 25-hydroxyvitamin D [25(OH)D], 24,25-dihydroxyvitamin D [24,25(OH)$_2$D], and 25,26-dihydroxyvitamin D [25,26(OH)$_2$D], as compared to 1,25-dihydroxyvitamin D [1,25(OH)$_2$D] and the parent vitamin D. Of some interest is the observation that the greatest binding affinity demonstrated by this plasma DBP was for the recently discovered vitamin D$_3$ metabolite, 25-hydroxyvitamin D$_3$-26,23-lactone. The physiologic significance of both the new metabolite and the avid binding between the metabolite and DBP is at the moment unknown. In humans, the purified protein is an alpha-globulin of 58,000 daltons with a sedimentation coefficient of 4.0 S. It has an isoelectric point of 4.7–4.9 and is capable of binding only one molecule of vitamin D, or its metabolite, per molecule of DBP.

DBP is synthesized in liver and has minor components of sialic acid and carbohydrates. In normal individuals, the circulating concentration of this DBP is around 525 μg/ml and varies little in a wide variety of disorders of mineral homeostasis and states of vitamin D deficiency or excess. However, plasma DBP concentration does increase dramatically with pregnancy to 1254 μg/ml, while excess urinary loss in nephrotic syndrome and decreased production in liver cirrhosis may cause low DBP concentrations in plasma. It has been calculated that under normal circumstances, as much as 98% of the plasma DBP circulates with its binding sites unoccupied by any vitamin D and its metabolites. In humans the total DBP pool is estimated at around 3 g with a production rate of about 0.8

g/day, suggesting that more than half the DBP pool is replaced every 2 days and that its distribution resembles that of a typical extracellular protein. The final metabolic fate of DBP is uncertain, although it appears to bind noncovalently with high affinity and specificity to an as yet unidentified cellular protein that appears to be a major cell constituent with an estimated molecular weight of 40,000. The validity and the physiologic significance of this interaction remain to be defined.

The physiologic functions of DBP are currently under active investigation. It may play a major role in facilitating the skin production of vitamin D by removing the end product (i.e., vitamin D_3) from its equilibrium with provitamin D (i.e., 7-dehydrocholesterol and previtamin D_3). The tight binding of DBP for vitamin D and its metabolites and the remarkable excess of DBP for its sterol passengers suggest that one of the major functions of DBP is to serve as a reserve or storage mechanism providing protection against sudden onslaught of vitamin D deficiency or excess. Bouillon and Van Baelen (210) are among the proponents for the thesis that the measurement of circulating vitamin D metabolites should be separated into the free and protein-bound fractions and that it is the free hormone which crosses the cell membrane and finally activates the target cells.

Vitamin D Compounds in Milk

Human milk contains two DBPs (211): one appears to be identical to the plasma DBP and the other corresponds to a 6.0 S DBP that had previously been isolated from a number of different tissues. Characterization of this tissue DBP has revealed physical properties similar to those of plasma DBP, with the exceptions of its sedimentation coefficient and its absence from blood. The presence of two distinct DBPs has also been demonstrated in human milk whey (the soluble protein portion of milk). In contrast, bovine milk whey contains only the 6.0 S DBP, even though bovine plasma contains only the 4.0 S DBP. It is now reasonably certain that the 4.0 S DBP in milk is derived from plasma. The source of the 6.0 S tissue DBP in human and bovine milk is uncertain. However, it has been demonstrated that this DBP is formed from the association of the 4.0 S plasma DBP with a cytosolic factor derived from the homogenization of various tissues. It is thus postulated that the 6.0 S DBP in milk is formed when the 4.0 S plasma DBP comes into contact with cytosol generated from cellular disruption during lactation. Subsequent studies have demonstrated that this cytosolic factor is actin. The significance of the association between 4.0 S plasma DBP and actin remains unknown. Evidence that actin is the DBP component in human skeletal muscle has also been documented by Haddad (212).

For the past five decades, repeated analyses of human milk, using mainly the rat line bioassay technique, have revealed an estimated 20

IU/liter of vitamin D activity, which is quite low relative to the recommended daily allowance (RDA) of 400 IU/liter. This observation, coupled with the well-accepted fact that breast milk plays an important role in protecting infants against neonatal hypocalcemia, led to the postulate that there may be non-vitamin D, antirachitic factors in milk. However, other investigators, using chemical assay techniques such as the antimony trichloride method, claim that assays for vitamin D activity in the lipid fraction of milk are gross underestimates and that the water-soluble vitamin D in the form of cholecalciferol sulphate is present in both human and bovine milk whey in high concentrations. Based on the assumption that the biologic activity of vitamin D sulfate is equivalent to that of parent vitamin D, it was estimated that the antirachitic activity was 950 and 204 IU/liter in bovine and human milk, respectively. More recently, the controversy over the water-soluble vitamin D story has been put to rest by the use of more precise techniques (including high-pressure liquid chromatography and ligand-binding analysis) for the separation and measurement of vitamin D metabolites. Vitamin D sulfate was found in negligible, if any, amounts in the whey fraction of human milk. Moreover, synthetic vitamin D sulfate has demonstrated virtually no biologic activity when compared to vitamin D_3.

Reeve and associates (213) reported their recent analysis of the vitamin D components and their biologic activity in human milk. The biologic activity of each vitamin D component was measured in terms of its stimulatory action on intestinal calcium transport in the rat, rather than the traditional rat line bioassay technique. They found that human milk contained a total of 40–50 IU/liter of vitamin D activity. Vitamin D_2 and D_3 were found to be present at concentrations of 338 and 41 ng/liter, respectively, or a total equivalent of 14–16 IU/liter of vitamin D activity. The major metabolite isolated was $25(OH)D_3$, which was present at a concentration of 163 ng/l. This accounted for 33 IU/liter, or about 75% of the total vitamin D activity in human milk. $1,25(OH)_2D$ and $24,25(OH)_2D$ were present at very low levels. These authors concluded that D_2, D_3, and $25(OH)D$ are responsible for more than 90% of the total vitamin D activity in human milk. Hollis and associates (211) also analyzed human milk and confirmed that the bulk of vitamin D activity was accounted for by the parent vitamin D and $25(OH)D$. In their study the concentrations of vitamin D, $25(OH)D$, $24,25(OH)_2D$, $25,26(OH)_2D$, and $1,25(OH)_2D$ were 39 ng/liter, 311 ng/liter, 52 ng/liter, 32ng/liter, and 5.1 ng/liter, respectively. The authors also compared the concentrations of these metabolites in milk with their respective concentrations in plasma. From available information the best estimate of these metabolites in plasma 3,000 ng/liter for vitamin D, 25,000 ng/liter for $25(OH)D$, 1,500 ng/liter for $24,25(OH)_2D$, 800 ng/liter for $25,26(OH)_2D$, and 35 ng/liter for $1,25(OH)_2D$ (100 ng/liter in lactating women). Thus, with the exception of $1,25(OH)_2D$, vitamin D and its metabolites were present in milk at 1.5–3% of the levels found in plasma. This ratio was similar to that between DBP in milk and plasma. The level of 1,25(OH)$_2$D in milk was about 5–6% of that found in the plasma of lactating women. The origin of the DBP in milk is most likely the plasma, and it is reasonable to suggest that vitamin D and its metabolites cross the mammary complex attached to the DBP during the apocrine and halocrine secretion process. The reason that there is a greater milk-to-plasma ratio of 1,25(OH)$_2$D than of the other metabolites could be that mammary tissue contains a specific cytosol receptor for this metabolite. As a result, 1,25(OH)$_2$D may be secreted into milk by a dual pathway, one involving attachment to the DBP and the other to the cytosolic receptor in milk. When whole milk is allowed to stand following collection, there is a gradual transfer of vitamin D and its metabolites from the aqueous to the fat phase, reflecting the well-known ability of milk fat to "strip" the vitamin from DBP. Interestingly, [3H]-1,25(OH)$_2$D bound to its cytosol receptor in mammary tissue is much more resistant to this "stripping" action during incubation with bovine whole milk than are the metabolites attached to the DBP.

The relatively low antirachitic activity found in normal human milk has, understandably, caused some concern about its adequacy for feeding infants. This subject is further discussed in the following section. Nevertheless, the truism that, except under the most unusual circumstances, breast-fed infants do not develop hypocalcemia and rickets, requires some explanations. One possibility is that the amount of antirachitic activity required for the prevention of rickets in neonates is much lower than that needed in other age groups. Another possibility is the presence in milk of non-vitamin D factor(s) with mineral-anabolic properties. In this context it is interesting to note that several experimental studies have questioned the importance of vitamin D in the regulation of calcium absorption in neonates. Thus newborn rats have low 1,25(OH)$_2$D and high 24,25(OH)$_2$D plasma levels but are able to maintain normal plasma calcium and phosphorus concentrations, even when they are fed on milk from vitamin D-depleted mothers (214,215). Others have observed that in rat pups, orally administered 1,25(OH)$_2$D is rapidly esterified and probably inactivated (216). Also, the intestine of newborn rats lacks the capacity to produce calcium in response to intraperitoneal administration of 1,25(OH)$_2$D (217). One possible non-vitamin D metabolite in milk that may bring about a calcium anabolic response is lactose. This disaccharide is known to increase intestinal calcium absorption (218). The mechanism is uncertain, but may be related to a direct interaction between the sugar and the brush border of the enterocyte, leading to an increase in their permeability to calcium. The effect of lactose, however, cannot be attributed to a stimulation in calcium binding protein synthesis since Pansu and associates (219) have demonstrated that lactose feeding, in fact, decreased this protein in the rat duodenum. Lactose has also been shown to improve bone calcium retention and bone mass (220).

Vitamin D: Fetus, Infants, and Growth

Delvin and associates (221) measured calcium, magnesium, phosphorus, PTH, 25(OH)D, 24,25(OH)$_2$D, and 1,25(OH$_2$)D in venous cord sera from 15 preterm (after 31 weeks gestation) singletons and three twin pairs. The results were compared with those found in maternal sera. The concentrations of calcium, magnesium, and phosphorus were higher, while those of 25(OH)D and 24,25(OH)$_2$D were lower in cord sera. In each case, a correlation was observed between concentrations in fetal sera and concentrations in maternal sera. The authors suggested that the fetus depends on maternal supply of these substances, and that calcium, magnesium, and phosphorus must cross the placenta against a concentration gradient. 1,25(OH)$_2$D levels in fetal sera were also lower than those found in maternal sera, but no correlation was observed between fetal concentrations and maternal concentrations of this metabolite. Cord 1,25(OH)$_2$D was, however, significantly correlated with cord calcium concentrations. The authors therefore concluded that 1,25(OH)$_2$D was synthesized by the fetoplacental unit and was regulated by fetal needs as reflected by the fetal serum calcium concentrations. A natural extension to this informative study would be the simultaneous measurement of maternal and cord blood DBP concentrations.

Salle and associates (222) studied serum calcium, immunoreactive PTH, immunoreactive calcitonin (CT), and 25(OH)D in three groups of gestational age- and birthweight-matched premature infants supplemented, respectively, with D$_3$, 25(OH)D, and 1,25(OH)$_2$D for 5 days. All three groups of infants developed similar degrees of hypocalcemia, which reached a nadir at 48 hours followed by a progressive increase in serum calcium concentrations towards normal at 120 (sixth day) and 168 (eighth day) hours. PTH concentrations follow an opposite pattern, with peak values noted at 48 hours. CT levels peaked earlier, at 24 hours. 25(OH)D was low at birth (1.2 hours) and rose significantly after 7 days of D$_3$ or 25(OH)D administration. Not unexpectedly, the level was considerably higher in infants given the latter metabolite. The authors thus concluded that both D$_3$ and its metabolites are well absorbed when administered orally to premature infants. However, therapeutic intervention with these agents does not seem warranted, since none of them appear to favorably modify the course of neonatal hypocalcemia. This study again raises the question of the role of vitamin D and its metabolites in calcium homeostasis during the neonatal period—a problem alluded to earlier that will be discussed again at the end of this section.

Rothberg and associates (223) from South Africa, a country where commercial milk is not supplemented with vitamin D, pointed out that in winter months, breast-fed term infants may have low serum vitamin D if the nursing mothers are not given dietary vitamin D supplement. This is an interesting observation since South Africa is known for its favorable temperate climate, and the mother-infant pairs studied were from the white population and were otherwise well nourished. This study however did not provide information on whether such low serum vitamin D levels had any adverse effect on the infants.

Chan and associates (224) asked the question whether human milk is adequate for growth and bone mineralization during the first year of life. To answer the question they studied 91 term infants in three feeding groups: human milk alone, human milk with supplemental vitamin D, and Similac. No difference was observed in either the growth rate (measured by weight and length) or the bone mineral content (measured by photon absorptiometry) among the three groups of infants. However, in all feeding groups, male infants grew heavier and longer and had higher bone mineral content than corresponding female infants. Serum calcium and phosphorus concentrations were similar in all studied groups. Serum 25(OH)D was lower in the human milk alone group at 4 months and serum alkaline phosphatase was lower in the Similac group at 2 weeks. At 6 months the alkaline phosphatase concentrations in the two human milk groups were not different, although the levels in the vitamin D supplemented group were higher than those observed in the Similac group. The significance of this observation is not clear although the possibility that the supplemental vitamin D was bordering on the excess range (serum 25(OH)D levels notwithstanding) for the functional needs of the infants, deserves serious consideration. These authors also made the additional observation that maternal bone mineral content and serum 25(OH)D levels were not affected by the duration of lactation in nursing mothers who received supplemental calcium and vitamin D. Grear and associates (225) in a similar study on 18 infants found decreased bone mineral content at 12 weeks of age in infants fed breast milk alone as compared to infants fed similarly but supplemented with vitamin D. The difference, however, was no longer apparent at 6 months when the study was terminated. Likewise, no difference in body length and serum calcium, magnesium, phosphate, alkaline phosphatase, calcitonin, and PTH levels was noted between the two groups of infants. As one would expect, serum 25(OH)D levels were higher in the vitamin D supplemented infants.

Clearly there are still insufficient data to answer the question of whether human milk contains sufficient vitamin D for the functional needs of infants. The final solution would also require satisfactory answers to a number of related questions. One such question would be, is the mineral metabolism in infants as critically dependent on vitamin D as it is in adulthood? Could the free availability of minerals and other substances such as lactose in milk, during the course of evolution have reduced an infant's dependency on vitamin D? Thinking from a different angle and pursuing the concept of Bouillon and Van Baelen (210), since infants have lower levels of DBP, could they in fact have "normal" levels of free 1,25(OH)D even though the total level of the metabolite in circulation is low? Because vitamin D (and its powerful metabolites) is a two-edge sword, these reviewers feel that no widespread recommendation for its supplementation to human milk should be made until solid evidence for its need is established.

One last paper to be mentioned in this section concerns vitamin D metabolism during puberty. Aksnes and Aarskog (226) measured plasma concentrations of vitamin D metabolites in 191 adolescents representing all stages of puberty. In girls, 1,25(OH)$_2$D increased from age 11 years to a peak at 12 years. In boys, the major increase in 1,25(OH)$_2$D occurred between 13–14 years of age. When the puberty is divided into five sequential stages, the greatest increase in serum 1,25(OH)$_2$D occurred between stage 1 and stage 2 in girls and between stage 2 and stage 3 in boys, peaking in both sexes at stage 3. In both sexes the levels of 1,25(OH)D significantly decreased in subsequent stages. The ratio of 24,25(OH)$_2$D and 25(OH)D varied inversely with the concentrations of 1,25(OH)$_2$D. The lowest value for the ratio was observed at age 12 in both sexes, followed by a gradual increase to a plateau at age 15 in girls and age 17 in boys. Clearly, the role of vitamin D and its metabolites in the endocrinology of growth and puberty deserves further investigation.

Vitamin D in Other Endocrine Systems and Disorders

Thyroid

MacFarlane and associates (227) measured serum concentrations of 25(OH)D, 24,25(OH)$_2$D, and 1,25(OH)$_2$D in 21 patients with untreated hyperthyroidism. Compared to controls, 25(OH)D concentrations were not altered, 24,25(OH)$_2$D appeared elevated, but the increase did not attain statistical significance, and 1,25(OH)$_2$D concentrations were significantly lower in the hyperthyroid patients. 24,25(OH)$_2$D but not 1,25(OH)$_2$D was significantly correlated with the serum triiodothyronine (T$_3$) levels. Following oral carbimazole therapy, 25(OH)D remained unchanged, 24,25(OH)$_2$D fell significantly, and 1,25(OH)$_2$D rose significantly. The authors suggested that excess thyroid hormone may increase serum calcium and phosphate concentrations through its action on bone and mineral metabolism, leading to a state of HPT. This would in turn cause stimulation of 24-hydroxylase and suppression of 1-hydroxylase. In addition, a direct stimulatory of effect of T$_3$ on 24-hydroxylase was also suggested.

Jastrup and associates (228) in a study of 25 untreated hyperthyroid patients observed an identical pattern of changes in the three circulating vitamin D metabolites, with the exception that the 24,25(OH)$_2$D concentrations in hyperthyroid patients were significantly higher than in controls. They also attributed the changes to hypercalcemia with suppressed parathyroid secretion and hyperphosphatemia. The mean serum levels and urinary excretions of calcium and phosphorus were increased in the hyperthyroid patients as were the mean serum level of alkaline phosphatase and the mean renal excretion rate of hydroxyproline. In this study histomorphometric evaluation of iliac crest bone biopsies was also performed after in vivo tetracycline double labeling. The changes observed were characterized by an enhanced turnover in trabecular and cortical bone leading to an increased porosity of cortical bone and mobilization of bone mineral. The bone changes did not correlate to circulating levels of vitamin D metabolites. In trabecular bone the apposition rate and mineralization rate of osteoid were increased and the mineralization lag time was shortened, showing that the mineralization and formation of osteoid in the hyperthyroid state can progress with an enhanced rate in the face of reduced circulating levels of $1,25(OH)_2D$.

Emmertsen and associates (229) studied vitamin D metabolism and bone remodeling in 14 patients with medullary carcinoma of the thyroid (MCT) and hypercalcitoninemia. Serum calcium, phosphorus, immunoreactive PTH (C-terminal), and $24,25(OH)_2D$ levels were normal. $1,25(OH)_2D$ levels were increased while $25(OH)D$ levels were decreased, suggesting an enhanced activity of the renal 1-alpha-hydroxylase. A positive correlation was observed between serum $24,25(OH)_2D$ and serum $25(OH)D$ concentrations. Quantitative histomorphometric analysis of iliac crest bone biopsy after in vivo tetracycline double-labeling revealed changes similar to those seen in primary HPT. The altered vitamin D metabolism was thought to be either a result of a direct action of hypercalcitoninemia on renal 1-alpha-hydroxylase or an adaptive change in calcium–phosphorus homeostasis. The bone changes were attributed to an enhanced sensitivity to circulating PTH induced by the increased $1,25(OH)_2D$ concentrations.

Diabetes and Insulin
Frazer and associates (230) studied vitamin D metabolism and metacarpal cortical thickness in 45 white, insulin-dependent diabetic subjects, 7–18 years of age. Serum calcium and phosphorus concentrations were normal, serum immunoreactive PTH was in the low normal range, and serum alkaline phosphatase was elevated compared to age- and sex-matched controls. Metacarpal cortical thickness was low in 87% of the patients studied. $24,25(OH)_2D$ levels were elevated while $1,25(OH)_2D$ levels were reduced. The increase in $24,25(OH)_2D$ was greater in patients with the greatest reduction in metacarpal cortical thickness and was maximally increased in the first 5 years of clinical diabetes. No correlation was observed between diabetes control, as measured by hemoglobin A1C and urine and plasma glucose concentrations, and the circulating levels of vitamin D metabolites. Thus, despite insulin therapy, alterations in vitamin D metabolism and reduction in metacarpal cortical thickness develop in young, insulin-dependent diabetic patients.

Glucocorticoids

Findling and associates (231) measured vitamin D metabolites and PTH levels in seven patients with spontaneous ACTH-dependent Cushing's syndrome. Remission of hypercortisolism was associated with an increase in serum phosphorus concentration paralleled by an increase in tubular reabsorption of phosphate. Serum calcium concentration was unchanged, while daily urine calcium excretion was reduced. Although iPTH and 1,25(OH)$_2$D levels before treatment were not different from normal, the levels of both hormones fell significantly following remission. The authors interpreted these data as suggesting a state of relative excess of these hormones in their patients. 25(OH)D levels were normal before treatment and remained unchanged after remission of the disorder. No correlation was observed between changes in iPTH and changes in either serum phosphorus or serum 1,25(OH)$_2$D concentrations. However, change in 1,25(OH)$_2$D was inversely correlated with change in serum phosphorus concentration. The authors suggested that bone loss in endogenous hypercortisolism may be a result of multiple hormonal excess: PTH, 1,25(OH)$_2$D, and adrenocorticosteroids. They also concluded that the known impairment of intestinal calcium absorption in Cushing's syndrome cannot be attributed to a decrease in the circulating levels of 1,25(OH)$_2$D.

Chronic Renal Failure

Christiansen and associates (232) studied the effect of administering either vitamin D$_3$ or 1,25(OH)$_2$D on serum immunoreactive PTH in 17 undialysed adult patients with chronic renal failure. Both forms of treatment led to significant reduction in iPTH, although the magnitude was clearly greater in the 1,25(OH)$_2$D group. Vitamin D$_3$ administration was associated with clear increases in serum 25(OH)D and 24,25(OH)$_2$D levels, while that of 1,25(OH)$_2$D was unchanged. In patients given 1,25(OH)$_2$D, the reverse pattern of changes was observed (i.e., increase in serum 1,25(OH)$_2$D with no change in serum 25(OH)D or 24,25(OH)$_2$D. Furthermore, in 1,25(OH)$_2$D-treated patients, the change in iPTH was related to the increment in serum calcium concentrations, whereas in vitamin D$_3$-treated patients, no such relationship was observed since the mean serum calcium levels did not appear to change with treatment. The authors suggested that 24,25(OH)$_2$D may be used as an alternative metabolite to 1,25(OH)$_2$D in suppressing uremic HPT. It has the potential advantage of suppressing parathyroid secretion without inducing significant hypercalcemia. However, it needs to be pointed out that this study did not exclude the possibility that 25(OH)D or, less likely, vitamin D$_3$ may have participated in the observed parathyroid suppression.

Delmez and associates (233) reported the effect of continuous ambulatory peritoneal dialysis (CAPD) on iPTH removal, serum 25(OH)D, and DBP, and net fluxes of calcium, phosphorus, and magnesium into or out of the body in 10 patients. Both the intact hormone and the carboxy-terminal fragment of PTH were measured and an estimated 13.6 ± 3.2% of total extracellular PTH was removed per day through the dialysate fluid. The proportion of the intact hormone and the carboxy-terminal fragment in the dialysate was similar to that found in the plasma. Serum 25(OH)D and DBP levels were normal before and 6 months after the initiation of treatment with CAPD. Daily calcium gain from the dialysate was 9.9 ± 9.7 mg, while the phosphorus and magnesium removal by the dialysate were 308.4 ± 15.5 mg and 31.2 ± 15.5 mg, respectively. The authors considered the removal of phosphorus and magnesium inadequate and suggested the additional use of intestinal phosphate binders and the possibility of lowering the dialysate magnesium concentrations. They also suggested an increase in dialysate calcium levels for better mineral homeostasis.

Chesney and associates (234) measured serum vitamin D metabolites in children with renal disease who had not been treated with glucocorticoids. In patients with endogenous creatinine clearance of 75–150 ml/min/1.73 m^2, 1,25(OH)$_2$D, 25(OH)D, and 24,25(OH)$_2$D levels were not different from those of normal controls. Eighteen children were studied in this group, and all except one (who had Alport syndrome) had glomerular disease. In a second group of children with definitely impaired renal function (creatinine clearance 0–48 ml/min/1.73 m^2) there was a significant reduction in 1,25(OH)$_2$D but the levels of 25(OH)D remained normal. A total of 24 children were included in this group, and all except three had tubulointerstitial disease. Within this group of patients, a direct correlation was observed between glomerular filtration rate and serum 1,25(OH)$_2$D levels. 24,25(OH)$_2$D levels were low only in patients with markedly reduced creatinine clearance (i.e., less than 13 ml/min/1.73 m^2). Thus, 1,25(OH)$_2$D is not reduced until greater than 50% of functional renal mass is lost. Decrease in 24,25(OH)$_2$D only becomes apparent when 90% of glomerular filtration is lost, and 25(OH)D remains normal even in children with severe renal failure.

Vitamin D and Metabolic Bone Disease

Osteomalacia

Cunningham and associates (235) reported the effect of alkali on bone morphology and vitamin D metabolism in two patients with chronic metabolic acidosis and osteomalacia secondary to urinary diversion. Alkali treatment alone led to good clinical, biochemical, and bone histologic response in both patients, one of whom had markedly impaired glomerular filtration. Plasma 25(OH)D and 1,25(OH)$_2$D concentrations were normal before and during treatment in one patient, while in the other patient, these metabolites were low before and normal during treatment. These observations suggest that osteomalacia in these patients is not always attributable to low circulating levels of vitamin D metabolites and that the bone abnormalities can be adequately treated with alkali alone, even in patients with impaired glomerular filtration. Furthermore, the healing of bone with alkali treatment is not necessarily accompanied by changes in the plasma levels of vitamin D metabolites.

Mason and colleagues (236) measured vitamin D metabolites in 21 patients with hypophosphatemic osteomalacia of juvenile onset. In eight patients who had not received any antirachitic treatment, serum $1,25(OH)_2D$ and $25(OH)D$ concentrations were normal while that of $24,25(OH)_2D$ was low. In 13 patients who were receiving vitamin D_2 and oral phosphate, serum $25(OH)D$ and $24,25(OH)_2D$ levels were high, while $1,25(OH)_2D$ levels were low. The authors pointed out available evidence that suggests that hypophosphatemia causes repression of 24-hydroxylase and enhancement of 1-hydroxylase activities. They therefore argued that an abnormality in vitamin D metabolism exists in their patients, since their $1,25(OH)_2D$ levels were within the normal range, rather than high as one might expect. They further reasoned that since D_2 and oral phosphate treatment resulted in a reduction in serum $1,25(OH)_2D$, the need for the use of $1,25(OH)_2D$ itself in the treatment of these patients should be seriously considered. Of relevance to such considerations was the observation that the bone histologic improvement in their patients was not as complete as that reported by others who employed $1,25(OH)_2D$ in the treatment of similar patients. Clearly, the lively debate on this fascinating disorder will continue. It should be pointed out that the assay used for $1,25(OH)_2D$ in this study may not be as sensitive for detecting $1,25(OH)_2D_2$ as it is for $1,25(OH)_2D_3$. Thus the possibility exists that the total 1,25D measured may be an underestimate because of the incomplete detection of 1,25D2.

Loeffler and Sherman (237) reported their experience in treating hypophosphatemic vitamin D-resistant rickets with low doses of vitamin D (50,000 u/day) and oral phosphate (1.6 g/day). The progress of 13 patients was reviewed over an average period of 10 years; all patients were on the treatment protocol for an average of 5 years. The authors pointed out that although previous studies using traditional high-dose vitamin D and phosphate have reported initial accelerated growth, the final heights of these patients were not different from those reported for untreated patients. Some patients from the present study also had initial acceleration in growth, but the final overall growth rate remained suboptimal and not different from that reported for untreated patients. Since the "low-dose" vitamin D patients have less vitamin D toxic episodes, the authors recommended this treatment regimen over the more conventional "high-dose" vitamin D regimen. For reasons not immediately apparent from the paper, the authors also concluded that the addition of oral phosphate imparted no further benefit over low-dose vitamin D and, therefore, is not recommended. They also noted that osteotomies for correction of lower extremity deformities performed before maturity all required revision, whereas osteotomies performed after maturity did not require revision.

Lund and associates (238) examined a group of patients who presented with fractures of the proximal femur and found a surprisingly high (25%) incidence of histologic osteomalacia. 25(OH)D levels were normal in these patients, and although 1,25(OH)$_2$D was low in the group as a whole, the levels of this metabolite in patients with histologic osteomalacia were normal. The authors postulated a state of reduced sensitivity to 1,25(OH)$_2$D as a possible cause for the osteomalacia observed.

Compston and associates (239) studied vitamin D metabolism and quantitative bone histology in 10 patients with privational osteomalacia (reduced exposure to ultraviolet irradiation with or without low dietary vitamin D intake) and 10 patients with malabsorption (following gastrointestinal surgery and bypass operations) bone disease. The authors pointed out that anticonvulsant medications and hospitalization are factors that may alter the basic pattern of circulating vitamin D metabolites in these disorders. Thus they cited the less well known observations that anticonvulsants may increase serum 1,25(OH)$_2$D through increased hydroxylation of 25(OH)D. Hospitalization may lead to rapid vitamin D repletion, expecially in patients with privational osteomalacia, both through the availability of this vitamin D in hospital diets and possibly also through a reduction in cereal fiber intake. Patients with privational osteomalacia often consume a diet with high fiber content, and it has been postulated that such a diet may interrupt the enterohepatic circulation of vitamin D metabolites. In any case, the data from this study demonstrated an inverse correlation between 1,25(OH)$_2$D levels and the osteoid volume, surface, and seam thickness index (tetracyline labeling was not done in this study) in all patients not receiving anticonvulsants. In addition, the circulating 1,25(OH)$_2$D levels were low in all patients with privational osteomalacia who were not hospitalized or receiving anticonvulsants. The authors therefore suggested that deficiency of 1,25(OH)$_2$D may play an important role in the development of the osteomalaciclike bone disease in their patients. However, exceptions to this general observation were found in the several malabsorption patients who were neither hospitalized nor on anticonvulsant medications, but in whom the presence of bone disease was associated with normal levels of plasma 1,25(OH)$_2$D. In these patients the authors postulated the existence of target-organ resistance to active vitamin D metabolites in the abnormal or diseased intestine.

Osteoporosis

Rickers and associates (240) studied the effect of 24 weeks of treatment with pharmacologic doses of prednisone on bone mineral content and vitamin D metabolism in 31 patients. The patients were divided into two similar groups with regard to age, sex, and prednisone dose. Group A received prednisone plus "triple-treatment" (i.e., vitamin D_2 45,000 IU twice weekly, sodium fluoride 50 mg/day and calcium phosphate 4.5 g/day) while group B received prednisone only. Serum $25(OH)D_2$, $25(OH)D_3$, and $1,25(OH)_2D$ were unchanged in group B. In group A $25(OH)D_2$ increased enormously, $25(OH)D_3$ was suppressed, and $1,25(OH)_2D$ was reduced by half. The suppression of $25(OH)D_3$ was attributed to possible substrate competition for hydroxylation in the liver, and the reduction in $1,25(OH)_2D$ was thought to be a result of a marked increase in circulating levels of $25(OH)D_2$, either alone or in combination with corticosteroid excess. Bone mineral content fell rapidly and similarly in both groups, suggesting that the triple-treatment has no preventive effect on corticosteroid-induced osteopenia.

Sorensen and associates (241) studied $1,25(OH)_2D$ levels and their increment following an acute intravenous injection of parathyroid extract in elderly osteopenic patients. $1,25(OH)_2D$ concentrations were lower in the osteopenic subjects as compared to age-matched nonosteopenic controls. The increment following parathyroid extract injection, however, was not different between the two groups. The authors concluded that the reduction in $1,25(OH)_2D$ levels in these patients is not due to a primary defect in $1,25(OH)_2D$ formation but is attributable to alteration in factors that normally stimulate the formation of this metabolite.

Van Kesteran and associates (242) demonstrated that the addition of fluoride to the therapeutic regimen of calcium and dihydrotachysterol led to clear improvement in bone histology in patients with primary osteoporosis. Volumetric density and surface percentage covered with osteoid and with osteoblasts increased in patients whose serum fluoride concentration was maintained between 0.20 and 0.25 $\mu m/ml$ and whose bone fluoride content was greater than or equal to 0.20%.

Epstein and associates (243) studied the effect of vitamin D, hydroxyapatite, and calcium gluconate treatment on cortical bone thinning in postmenopausal women with primary biliary cirrhosis. This disorder is known to be associated with malabsorption of calcium, phosphate, and vitamin D and the development of accelerated cortical bone thinning. Patients were divided into three groups: one group received no mineral supplement, a second group received hydroxyapatite, and a third group received calcium gluconate. All patients were given vitamin D_2 100,000 units monthly. Patients were followed for 14 months and before and after treatment hand radiographs were used to assess changes in metacarpal cortical thickness using the technique of caliper radiogrammetry. Cortical bone loss occurred in the control group. The hydroxyapatite group demonstrated significant increase in cortical bone thickness. No significant change in cortical bone thickness was observed in the calcium gluconate group. The authors concluded that vitamin D_2 did not prevent the metacarpal cortical bone thinning of primary biliary cirrhosis. The addition of calcium gluconate prevents bone thinning, and the addition of hydroxyapatite promotes positive cortical bone balance.

Hypophosphatasia

Opshaug and colleagues (244) reported on a 4-month-old boy with infantile hypophosphatasia followed for 9 months. During the initial hypercalcemic stage, the patient had hypophosphatasia, low $1,25(OH)_2D$, normal $25(OH)D$, and elevated $24,25(OH)_2D$ and $25,26(OH)_2D$. Urinary cAMP excretion was also low. The patient developed vitamin D-deficiency rickets at 9 months of age attributed to a combination of restricted vitamin D intake and lack of sun exposure. Alkaline phosphatase rose makedly as did the urinary cAMP, but serum $25(OH)D$ concentration became very low. Following the institution of vitamin D therapy, serum $1,25(OH)_2D$ showed a brisk rise to a considerably elevated value. With the healing of rickets, alkaline phosphatase returned to its characteristic low levels.

Miscellaneous Findings

Measurements in Serum and Food Items

Clemens and associates (245) reported details of their assay for circulating vitamin D, while Thompson and associates (246) documented the technique of measuring vitamin D in fortified milk, margarine, and infant formulas. Clemens and associates (245) noted that the normal range for circulating vitamin D in 30 Boston subjects ranged from less than 0.5 ng/ml to 25 ng/ml. Subjects sampled during summer months had higher concentrations of vitamin D than those sampled during winter months. Single exposure to a given quantity of ultraviolet radiation led to increases in circulating vitamin D_3 by 30–50 times in the first several days with a return to basal levels by 1 week.

Antituberculosis Treatment

Brodie and associates (247) reported the effect of a combination of rifampicin 600 mg/day and isoniazid 300 mg/day on serum PTH, $25(OH)D$, and $1,25(OH)_2D$ in eight normal subjects and nine tuberculous patients. In normal subjects, serum PTH, $25(OH)D$, and $1,25(OH)_2D$ decreased significantly by 57%, 34%, and 23% after a 14-day course of treatment. Serum calcium and phosphorus concentrations did not change. In tuberculous patients, both $25(OH)D$ and $1,25(OH)_2D$ were reduced while PTH increased after 1 month of treatment. At the end of 6 months of treatment, $25(OH)D$ decreased further while $1,25(OH)_2D$ and PTH levels demonstrated no further change. The authors suggested that patients under antituberculosis treatment should be closely monitored.

Sodium Loading and Hypercalciuria

Breslau and associates (248) examined the basis for previous observations that oral sodium loading could lead to hypercalciuria in previously normocalciuric subjects and an increase in intestinal calcium absorption. In eleven normal subjects, oral sodium loading was associated with significant increases in the following parameters: urinary sodium and calcium excretion, serum PTH and 1,25(OH)$_2$D, and fractional intestinal calcium absorption. Serum calcium levels corrected for total protein did not change. In two postsurgical HPT patients maintained on vitamin D, similar sodium loading also led to increased urinary excretion of sodium and calcium. However, there was no increase in PTH, 1,25(OH)$_2$D, and fractional intestinal calcium absorption. Corrected serum calcium concentration decreased. The authors concluded that sodium-induced renal hypercalciuria is accompanied by increased 1,25(OH)$_2$D synthesis and enhanced intestinal calcium absorption. Since this adaptive mechanism did not occur in two patients with hypoparathyroidism, mediation by PTH is suggested.

Treatment of Hypoparathyroidism
Okano and associates (249) studied the relative efficacy of different vitamin D metabolites in the treatment of patients with pseudohypoparathyroidism, idiopathic hypoparathyroidism, and postsurgical hypoparathyroidism. The average pretreatment serum calcium levels and clinical manifestations were indistinguishable among the three groups of patients. The minimum dose of 1,25(OH)$_2$D$_3$ which controlled all the clinical symptoms and maintained serum calcium at approximately 8.5 mg/dl was not different among the three groups of patients. On the other hand, patients with pseudohypoparathyroidism required less 1-α-D$_3$ than patients with idiopathic hypoparathyroidism, who in turn require less of the metabolite than patients with postsurgical hypoparathryoidism. No significant difference was found in the optimal maintenance dose of dihydrotachysterol or vitamin D$_2$ in the three patient groups. The authors postulated that the lower 1-α-D$_3$ requirement in pseudohypoparathyroid patients may be attributed to the known increased PTH levels in these patients, thus facilitating the conversion of 1-α-D$_3$ to 1α=25(OH)D$_3$. The PTH concentrations in the other two types of hypoparathyroid patients are either low or absent.

Perforating Granuloma Annulare
Aliaga and colleagues (250) reported the occurrence of perforating granuloma annulare (PGA) in a 10-year-old boy who was being given 600,000 IU of vitamin D every week for prophylaxis against rickets. The lesions developed a few weeks after the initiation of vitamin D therapy, showed no evidence of resolution through the two years of treatment, and disappeared shortly after the withdrawal of vitamin D. Individual lesions usually started as small red papules that, after a few days, began to enlarge, developing a central umbilication, a reddish halo, and a small crust which detached itself from time to time. Histologic studies revealed

a perforating epidermic column consisting of necrobiotic tissue and mucinous material arising in the papillary dermis and communicating with the epidermic surface. At the upper border of the column there were atrophy of the epidermis and zones of interruption by extruding bundles of collagenous tissue with abundant fibroblasts. The lower border of the plug was surrounded by palisading histiocytes and a dense lymphocytic infiltrate. Multinucleated giant cells were also present. It was not mentioned whether calcium deposits were noted in the lesion. This report should serve to alert physicians to some of the less well known complications of vitamin D therapy.

The Fifth International Workshop on Vitamin D

The fifth international workshop on vitamin D was held at Williamsburg, Virginia, February 14–19, 1982. The complete proceedings have already been published (251). Papers and discussions were grouped under the following headings: Vitamin D Metabolism and Catabolism; Receptors for $1,25(OH)_2D_3$; Biological Actions of $24,25(OH)_2D_3$; Calcium Binding Proteins (CaBP)—Chemistry and Molecular Biology; Intestinal Calcium Transport—Physiology and Molecular Actions; Skeletal Actions of Vitamin D Metabolites; Renal Actions of Vitamin D Metabolites: Regulation of Hepatic and Renal Vitamin D-Hydroxylases; Parathyroid Hormone-Vitamin D Interactions; Vitamin D Nutrition (Human and Animal); Vitamin D Metabolism in Humans; Pregnancy/Neonatology; Assay Methodology: Vitamin D and Metabolites; Renal Osteodystrophy; Clinical Observations and New Disease States; Chemistry of Vitamin D Steroids; Photobiology: Vitamin D Binding Proteins (DBP).

DISORDERS OF PHOSPHATE METABOLISM

Phosphorus and the Cell

Most intracellular phosphorus is in organic form. A major understanding of the clinical and physiologic effects of abnormalities of phosphate metabolism depends on our ability to measure accurately the changes in cellular inorganic phosphorus and high energy phosphate.

The last 2 years have witnessed major advances in the ability to measure accurately the concentration of these changes in vivo and in vitro as a result of the advancement of two methods, namely phosphorus-31 nuclear magnetic resonance (^{31}P NMR) and high pressure liquid chromatography and ashing for phosphate analysis.

Clinical Applications of ^{31}P NMR

Application of NMR to biology and medicine is new. It is based on the magnetic properties of nuclei, whereas ultraviolet and visible spectroscopies are based on properties of electronic states in the molecule. Nuclei that have odd atomic number behave as spinning electrical charges and therefore have a magnetic moment. The ^{31}P nucleus has an odd atomic number so that when it is placed in a magnetic field its magnetic moment aligns either parallel or antiparallel to the external magnetic field. If energy is provided at the proper frequency in the radio frequency range, energy will be absorbed, and a transition from the lower to higher energy states will take place. As nuclei return to the low energy state, a signal at the same frequency as the one absorbed is omitted. Thus, using a high resolution magnetic field will allow the use of NMR in the measuring of in vivo intracellular inorganic phosphorus, ATP, ADP, and creatine phosphate.

Chance et al. (252) have demonstrated recently that NMR is useful in following the changes in skeletal muscle energy metabolism and inorganic phosphate during exercise in humans. Gadian et al. (253) utilized NMR to study skeletal forearm muscles of a 16-year-old boy with myopathy, ophthalmoplegia, and raised basal metabolic rate by examining the skeletal muscles of the forearm. The muscles of the forearm showed an abnormal spectrum with a high inorganic phosphorus content in relation to phosphocreatine. This resting high inorganic phosphorus level is a direct consequence of impaired mitochondrial oxidative phosphorylation. These workers demonstrated that NMR is useful as a noninvasive tool in the clinical diagnosis and study of muscle metabolism in relation to cellular energetics and inorganic phosphorus.

Newman et al. (254) studied six patients with muscular dystrophy and examined cellular energetic and inorganic phosphorus metabolism using NMR. The phosphorus spectrum was abnormal in that the ratios of phosphocreatine to adenosine triphosphate and to inorganic phosphate were reduced. Absolute quantification suggested a reduced phosphocreatine peak.

NMR has been used to evaluate the change in ATP, creatine phosphate, and inorganic phosphate as well as intracellular pH during ischemia. Using the surface coil, Grove et al. (255) examined the time course changes in myocardial ATP, creatine phosphate, and inorganic phosphate during ischemia and found an initial (10 minutes) marked reduction of creatine phosphate, followed by a fall in ATP (17 minutes), and an accumulation of inorganic phosphorus.

Using this direct method, values for ATP and creatine phosphate content of both heart and skeletal muscle are higher when compared to established enzymatic methods. The reason for this difference rests in the methodology of obtaining biopsies. The duration of the freezing process must be minimized to obtain the highest values of ATP and creatine phosphate. Thus, it seems that the NMR method provides an improved noninvasive in vivo clinical tool in the research of cellular phosphate metabolism.

Several problems are still unresolved with this methodology. Due to the high baseline noise, this method has value only for the determination of phosphorylated components available in the cell in high concentrations (i.e., ATP, CP, ADP, Pi). Sugar phosphates, for instance, cannot be determined by this method. The values for inorganic phosphorus calculated using this method are 10 times lower than those found by using the enzymatic methods. The reason for this discrepancy is not clear but may be the result of the NMR being unable to detect intramitochondrial phosphate stores. Finally, the operational expense and high cost of the equipment are a major deterrent to using this methodology. One has to calculate carefully the cost effectiveness of this method against the more widely available enzyme methods.

High Pressure Chromatography
Biopsy samples obtained by liquid nitrogen freezing and perchloric acid extraction are applied to a resin column, and all phosphorylated intermediates are separated and analyzed qualitatively and quantitatively. Up to 32 phosphate intermediates can be separated by this method (256). The ability to separate and quantify inorganic phosphorus, creatine phosphate, ATP, ADP, as well as sugar phosphates, NAD, and phospholipid precursors allows the investigators to draw conclusions about the energy state of the sample as well as its relation to phosphate and intermediary metabolism. Brautbar et al. (257) have recently used this method in the evaluation of various aspects of cellular inorganic phosphate and intermediary metabolism in phosphate depletion. In a recent monograph (258) these workers demonstrated the major inportance and applicability of this method to the clinical evaluation of phosphate metabolism derangements.

Clinical Conditions Associated with Hypophosphatemia

Several clinical conditions are associated with hypophosphatemia and have been recently reviewed (53).

Hypophosphatemia in the Surgical Patient
Hypophosphatemia in the surgical patient has been examined by Swaminathan et al. (259), who reported that 29% of surgical patients have serum phosphorus levels of less than 2.4 mg/dl. Most of these patients were receiving glucose infusions and no dietary phosphate. The hypophosphatemia commonly occurs 24–28 hours postoperatively and is frequently the result of administration of hypertonic glucose or amino acid solution. The authors suggest that the fall in plasma phosphate is related to the changes in phosphate metabolism after the trauma of surgery, anesthesia, and starvation. These changes are commonly transient and without any major side effects. Chronic profound hypophosphatemia is more likely to occur

during intravenous feedings in patients who were previously nutritionally depleted. Following elective surgery the majority of patients who receive constant intravenous therapy recover quickly and do not need routine intravenous phosphate supplements.

The evaluation of postsurgical hypophosphatemia and its prevention has been recently studied (260). Nineteen patients undergoing surgery were studied on the day of surgery and the first 3 postoperative days. Patients were infused with 100 g glucose at a rate of 0.3 g/kg/hr. A significant decrease in fasting blood phosphorus was found in the first 3 postoperative days and was most pronounced on the second day: 2.3 ± 0.21 mg/dl as compared to 3.6 ± 0.15 mg/dl ($p < 0.01$). There was also a significant correlation between the changes in serum phosphorus and urinary phosphorus: as urinary phosphorus excretion increased, plasma phosphorus levels fell. Administration of intravenous phosphorus (10 mmol/100 g glucuose/5 hr) did not prevent the fall in serum phosphorus levels. The authors conclude that two major mechanisms mediate the hypophosphatemia of the immediate postoperative period: (*1*) increased tissue metabolism and secondary shifts of phosphate from blood to soft-tissue compartments and (*2*) excessive renal losses of phosphate secondary to osmotic diuresis.

Thus, it appears from these two studies that postsurgical hypophosphatemia is transient and may not be of major concern. Therefore, if hypophosphatemia occurs in the late postsurgical period, another mechanism should be looked for.

Burn Injury

Hypophosphatemia is commonly associated with severe burn injury with the lowest levels reported on the fifth day. The fatal outcome of some of these patients has been attributed to hypophosphatemia. The mechanism by which the hypophosphatemia develops in severe burn injury is not clear. Several investigators suggested respiratory alkalosis secondary to gram-negative septicemia and rapid tissue build-up as a cause. This issue was examined recently by Lennquist et al. (261). Thirty-three severely burned patients were evaluated, and urinary and serum phosphorus levels, blood calcitonin and PTH, and urinary epinephrine and norepinephrine were measured. In all patients, serum phosphorus levels decreased significantly to 0.74 mM on the fourth day after the burn injury and gradually returned to normal levels thereafter. The duration of the hypophosphatemia varied from 2 to 10 days with a mean of 3 days. Serum PTH levels were normal, whereas serum calcitonin levels were markedly elevated. Urinary phosphate decreased and reached a nadir on the seventh day after injury; thereafter, it returned to normal levels. Urinary epinephrine was usually above the normal levels, and urinary norepinephrine was significantly and markedly elevated. The observation that in the face of marked hypophosphatemia, urine was not free of phosphate, as expected in hypophosphatemia of extrarenal origin, suggests a renal loss of phosphate in these patients. The authors attributed this inappropriate urinary loss of phosphate to the increased calcitonin levels found in these patients. This study suggests an increased urinary phosphate loss as a contributing mechanism to the hypophosphatemia of the severely burned patients. The roles of respiratory alkalosis, hyperalimentation, and increased cortisol secretion in the hypophosphatemia of these patients have not been examined.

Posttransplantation Hypophosphatemia

Renal transplant patients often present with moderate hypophosphatemia. Recently, Garabedian et al. (262) reported that 60% of children with a transplanted kidney develop hypophosphatemia. Usually, the hypophosphatemia develops during the immediate posttransplant period, but persistent hypophosphatemia for a period of up to 1½ years has been reported. This hypophosphatemia has been attributed to several mechanisms: (*1*) persistent HPT; (*2*) glucocorticoid-induced phosphaturia; (*3*) renal phosphate leak; and (*4*) excessive use of antacids. Garabedian et al. (262) concluded from their recent study that the hypophosphatemia is usually moderate and is well tolerated. This hypophosphatemia was correlated with a tubular phosphate leak.

Interestingly, serum levels of $1,25(OH)_2D_3$ were lower in the transplanted patient despite the fact that hypophosphatemia is a powerful stimulus of renal hydroxylase. The authors, and Farrington et al. (263) and Walker et al. (264), suggested an additional mechanism for the posttransplant hypophosphatemia: reduced intestinal absorption of phosphate. After transplantation, most patients have a dramatic improvement in calcium absorption, but phosphorus absorption may remain impaired. The authors suggested that the steroids used in these patients constitute the major mechanism mediating posttransplantation hypophosphatemia, and they advocate large doses of vitamin D to correct the steroid-induced phosphate intestinal malabsorption. Kovarik et al. (265) evaluated phosphate handling by the transplanted kidney in 42 patients with long-term and stable transplant function. Only 19% of these patients showed a normal renal handling of phosphate as determined by normal TmP/GFR and a normal PTH and plasma phosphate. Eighty-one percent of the patients studied demonstrated a reduced TmP/GFR, suggesting a renal phosphate leak. In 15 patients, this phosphate leak was caused by persistent high levels of PTH, whereas in the remaining 19 patients, the renal phosphate leak was PTH independent, as demonstrated by low levels of PTH. In the latter, the possibility of chronic subclinical rejection of the transplanted kidney, which may bring about proximal tubular as well as distal tubular lesions, was suggested. As prolonged hypophosphatemia is a most serious risk factor for the development of osteomalacia, it is recommended that the mechanisms be evaluated in each posttransplant patient and that correct therapy be planned accordingly.

Rosenbaum et al. (266) studied 73 patients with transplants 6 months after transplantation. All patients had stable renal function. Twenty-three patients had fasting serum phosphorus levels of less than 2.5 mg/dl. While the average serum phosphorus of the total transplant recipient group was 3.1 mg/dl, the hypophosphatemic transplant patient had a serum phosphorus of 2.1 mg/dl. The hypophosphatemic patients had similar fractional reabsorption of phosphate as compared with the total transplant recipient population, and their renal phosphate threshold (TmP/GFR) was reduced from 3.1 ± 0.1 mg/100 ml in the total population to 1.4 ± 0.2 mg/100 ml. Although PTH levels correlated inversely with the TmP/GFR in the total transplant group, the hypophosphatemic patients appeared to have lower renal TmP/GFR than did the normophosphatemic transplant patients with similar PTH levels. Calcium infusion tests and phosphate titration studies were performed in 11 hypophosphatemic transplant patients. Five of the 11 had only mildly elevated PTH levels and failed to decrease the rate of phosphate excretion during calcium infusions. These data indicate a renal tubular defect in phosphate transport independent of PTH. Another possible explanation for the presence of hypophosphatemia and decreased phosphate reabsorption in the presence of relatively normal PTH levels is a hyperresponsiveness to the phosphaturic action of PTH.

Hypophosphatemia of Respiratory Alkalosis

A marked reduction of serum phosphorus and associated hypophosphaturia occurs during acute hyperventilation respiratory alkalosis. The fall of serum phosphorus has been attributed to increased trapping of phosphate by soft tissues. Recent studies by Brautbar et al. (267) have examined the effects of acute hyperventilation on serum phosphorus and skeletal muscle phosphorylated intermediates. The authors examined muscle biopsies from dogs during a control period and during 2 and 3 hours of acute hyperventilation. A marked increase in cellular inorganic phosphorus and phosphorylated nucleotides as well as glucose-6-phosphate accompanied the fall in serum phosphorus, and demonstrated that the hypophosphatemia seen during acute hyperventilation is the result of shifts of phosphate from blood to skeletal muscle (Figs. 8–10). A marked fall in serum phosphorus occurred only when the hyperventilation was accompanied with low-dose glucose administration. It is common to find that patients with some degree of hyperventilation secondary to alcoholic liver disease, gram-negative sepsis, or central nervous system abnormalities display marked hypophosphatemia with no evidence of urinary losses of phosphate. Whether the hypophosphatemia in these patients is the result of prolonged hyperventilation and increased muscle glycolytic activity or

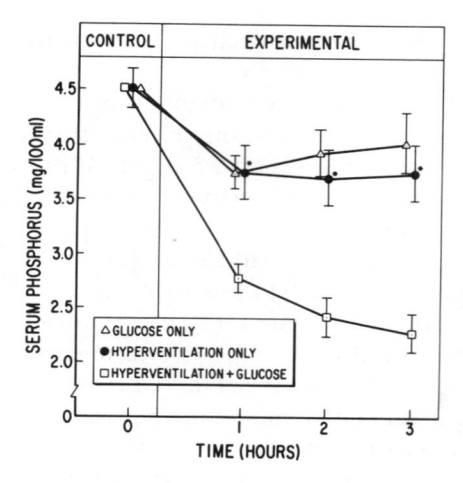

Figure 8. Changes in serum phosphorus during experimental acute hyperventilation in dogs. Hyperventilation in conjunction with glucose administration causes a marked fall in serum phosphorus. (Brautbar N et al: *Min Elect Metab* 9:45–50, 1983. Used with permission.)

whether other factors such as poor dietary intake of phosphate or administration of antacids contribute has not been evaluated.

Hypophosphatemia in Alcoholic Patients

The most common clinical entity accompanied by marked hypophosphatemia is chronic alcoholism and alcoholic withdrawal. Serum phosphorus levels may be normal when patients are first admitted to the hospital but subsequently decline.

The mechanism for the hypophosphatemia in the chronic alcoholic has been reviewed by Knochel (268). Structural, electrochemical, and biochemical abnormalities of skeletal muscle are common in the alcoholic patient.

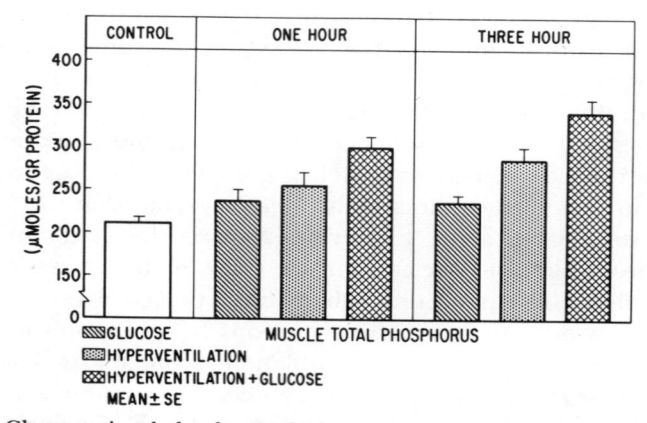

Figure 9. Changes in skeletal muscle biopsy total phosphorus during acute hyperventilation in dogs. (Brautbar N et al: *Min Elect Metab* 9:45–50, 1983. Used with permission.)

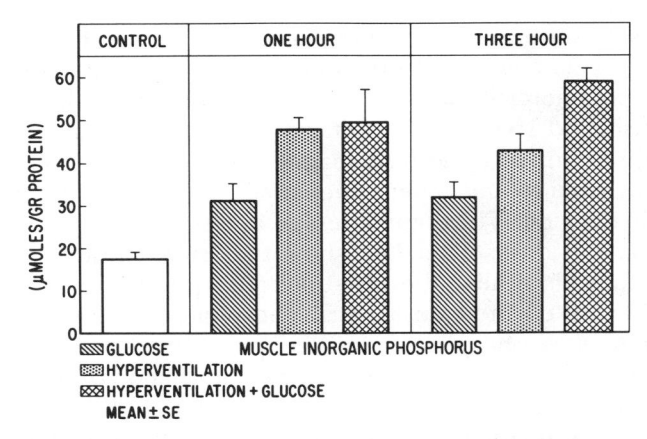

Figure 10. Changes in skeletal muscle biopsy inorganic phosphate contents during acute hyperventilation in dogs. (Brautbar N et al: *Min Elect Metab* 9:45–50, 1983. Used with permission.)

The mechanism for the myopathy in the chronic alcoholic patient is believed to be mediated in part by hypophosphatemia, since isolated dietary phosphate depletion is associated with skeletal myopathy. Ferguson et al. (269) examined the effects of chronic alcoholism in an experimental model in the dog to avoid the problem of malnutrition, which commonly complicates the understanding of alcoholic myopathy. The authors examined the effect of chronic alcoholism on chemical composition and active sodium transport of skeletal muscle. After 1 month of ethanol intake, skeletal muscle phosphorus content declined markedly. This was associated with a marked decline in skeletal muscle magnesium content. Sodium content rose significantly while chloride content increased. Measurements of transmembrane potential difference (Em) and Na-K-ATPase activity increased significantly after 1 month of ethanol administration. Total tissue oxygen consumption increased after 1 month of alcoholism and remained elevated. Reduction in tissue content of magnesium and phosphorus occurred in the face of normal serum levels of these ions. These data suggest a direct effect of alcohol on skeletal muscle membrane and ionic contents, unrelated to the measured serum phosphate. Whether these abnormalities are mediated via primary changes in intracellular phosphorus cannot be concluded from this study since inorganic phosphorus was not measured and since total phosphorus measurements do not represent inorganic phosphorus.

Hypophosphatemia Associated with Antacid Ingestion
The effects of prolonged ingestion of antacids on phosphate homeostasis and the development of severe hypophosphatemia have been described in the past. A recent study by Spencer et al. (270) examined the effects

of low doses of aluminum-containing antacids on phosphate and calcium balance. Metabolic balance studies were performed in 17 human volunteers. Four commercially available antacids were studied: Maalox, Amphojel, Gelusil, and Mylanta. The antacids Maalox, Mylanta I, and Mylanta II contain aluminum hdroxide and magnesium hydroxide; Gelusil contains aluminum hydroxide and magnesium trisilicate; and Amphojel contains aluminum hydroxide. Thirty milliliters of antacids were given three times daily over 18–30 days. The data show that small doses of aluminum-containing antacids inhibit the intestinal absorption of phosphorus, evidenced by a marked increase in fecal phosphate contents and a distinct reduction in urinary phosphorus. Urinary phosphorus returned to normal upon cessation of antacids, suggesting that no major depletion in body phosphorus stores occurred with the above regimen of treatment. Interestingly, there was no difference in phosphate balance between the control group and the patients on low-dose antacids. Thus, low-dose antacids are recommended in order to prevent the development of phosphate depletion.

Hypophosphatemia in the Diabetic Patient
It has been known for many decades that diabetics formed the second most common group of hypophosphatemic patients and that uncontrolled diabetes mellitus and diabetic ketoacidosis caused a marked loss of body phosphorus by excessive urinary phosphate excretion. Prior to therapy, the serum phosphorus is usually normal but will fall to extremely low levels during fluid, insulin, and nonphosphate electrolyte replacement therapy. Indeed, Atchley et al. (271) reported hypophosphatemia in diabetic patients on withdrawal of insulin. Franks et al. (272) reported an improvement in the mental state and a decrease in fatality rate with administration of phosphate. The benefits of oral or parenteral phosphate therapy during treatment of severely uncontrolled diabetes mellitus still have not been resolved. Although Sterling (273) recommended phosphate supplementation, Gibby et al. (274) did not find phosphate supplements to be beneficial. Since the red blood cell concentration of 2,3-DPG in diabetic ketoacidosis has been shown to be reduced (275), and since reduced 2,3-DPG will impair tissue oxygenation, it was suggested that administration of phosphate to these phatients would improve red blood cell 2,3-DPG and thus improve tissue oxygenation.

Keller and Berger (276) have examined the effect of phosphate replacement therapy on the course of diabetic coma in 24 patients with diabetic ketoacidosis and 16 patients with nonketotic hyperosmolar coma, and found no evidence to advocate phosphate administration during the treatment of these patients. Measurements of multiple parameters of brain, myocardial, and skeletal muscle oxygenation prior to the administration of supplemental phosphorus in a large series of patients are not available, and this issue remains controversial.

It is commonly believed that the administration of insulin lowers the concentration of phosphate in the blood by promoting cellular influx of phosphorus from the circulation to the soft-tissue compartments. This effect might have an important role during the treatment of diabetic ketoacidosis. Since insulin also augments directly the renal tubular reabsorption of phosphorus, the former action of insulin might be opposed by the latter. Since severe glycosuria in these patients is associated with hypercalciuria and possibly with secondary HPT, it appears that the opposing forces may influence serum phosphate levels in patients with uncontrolled diabetic ketoacidosis. Raskin et al. (277) examined the effects of chronic insulin therapy on phosphate metabolism in 21 patients with diabetes mellitus. The institution of optimal diabetic control over 4–10 days increased the concentration of serum phosphorus and decreased the urinary excretion of phosphate. The authors attributed the decrease in urinary phosphorus excretion to several factors: (1) elimination of glucose from the urine by optimal insulin therapy; (2) elimination of hyperglucagonemia, which has a direct effect on renal tubular phosphate transport and causes hyperphosphaturia; (3) suppression of secondary HPT, which may occur secondary to "renal leak" of calcium during the glycosuria. Indeed, the authors showed a marked reduction in iPTH levels during optimal treatment. The finding of increased circulating concentrations of phosphorus during optimal insulin therapy is paradoxical since insulin itself has a hypophosphatemic effect. The suggestion that several other mechanisms are operative during the above therapeutic regimen may help to explain this paradox. Gertner et al. (278) examined changes in phosphate homeostasis accompanying the treatment of diabetes mellitus and reached the same conclusions.

Hypophosphatemia after Parathyroidectomy in Chronic Renal Failure

Serum phosphate levels often fall after parathyroidectomy in patients with chronic renal failure but frank hypophosphatemia is uncommon. Farrington et al. (279) reported 13 patients with chronic renal failure who developed severe hypophosphatemia 3–52 weeks after parathyroidectomy. Prior to surgery, these patients had a high level of alkaline phosphatase activity and significantly higher values of bone resorption activity as measured by iliac crest bone biopsies than those patients who underwent parathyroidectomy but remained normophosphatemic.

There are several possible causes for the decrease in plasma phosphate in these patients: a reduction in the mobilization of phosphate from bone under the influence of reduced immunoreactive PTH concentrations and increased accretion of phosphate into healing bone. In patients developing hypophosphatemia while receiving dialysis, other factors may be important, including phosphate-binding antacids, low dietary intake of phosphate, repeated dialysis with phosphate-free dialysate, and reduced absorption of phosphate due to oral calcium supplements.

The authors demonstrated here that patients developing hypophosphatemia after parathyroidectomy had significantly greater preoperative plasma alkaline phosphatase activities, and their plasma phosphate and hydroxyproline concentrations were also substantially higher. Hypophosphatemic patients also had greater histologic indices of bone turnover, having significantly higher values for active resorption surfaces and active formation surfaces than the normophosphatemic group. A higher proportion of hypophosphatemic patients also had radiologic erosions and osteosclerosis. These data indicate that hypophosphatemia tends to occur in patients with more severe hyperparathyroid bone disease and therefore the major cause of hypophosphatemia is likely to be either reduced mobilization of phosphate from bone or its increased accretion into bone.

Phosphate is considered to be an important modulator of bone mineralization, and a significant inverse correlation exists between plasma phosphate values and histologic indices of osteomalacia in patients with chronic renal failure. Severe osteomalacia has also been described in patients with hypophosphatemia receiving hemodialysis. Hypophosphatemia after parathyroidectomy may lead to delayed healing of bone lesions. Careful postoperative monitoring of plasma phosphate as well as plasma calcium concentrations is necessary in these patients so that appropriate treatment may be instituted. In many of these patients adding phosphate to the dialysis fluid did not prevent persistent hypophosphatemia; oral phosphate supplements may be necessary in such patients.

Clinical and Metabolic Consequences of Hypophosphatemia and Phosphate Depletion

Several laboratories have recently examined the effects of phosphate depletion on various organ systems. Although most of the models are experimental, the underlying mechanisms provide an explanation for the organ system dysfunction in phosphate depletion in patients.

Myocardium
The effects of pure phosphate depletion on cardiac function in patients have been described (280). Three patients who were ingesting excessive amounts of phosphate-binding antacids presented with congestive heart failure and profound hypophosphatemia. Physical findings, x-ray, and echocardiographic evaluation suggested severe myocardial dysfunction. These abnormalities reversed with restoration of serum phosphate to normal, suggesting an important role for phosphate in myocardial metabolism.

O'Connor et al. (281) evaluated the effect of phosphate depletion on cardiac function in seven patients. They found that stroke work was reduced but returned to normal after phosphate administration The authors showed that with correction of the hypophosphatemia, left ven-

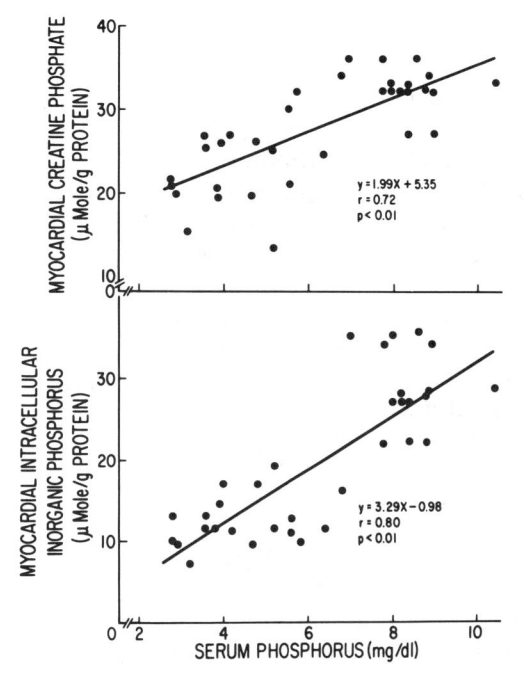

Figure 11. Changes in myocardial cellular inorganic phosphates and creatine phosphate concentration in phosphate depletion. These changes are correlated with the fall in serum phosphate levels. (Brautbar N et al: *Am J Physiol* 242:F699-F704, 1982. Used with permission.)

tricular stroke volume improved and pulmonary artery wedge pressure decreased. Fuller et al. (282) studied cardiac function in dogs before and during phosphate depletion. During phosphate depletion, stroke volume, maximum ascending aortic blood flow, and maximum left ventricular time rate of change of pressure decreased significantly; all these changes disappeared upon phosphate repletion.

In all the above studies, the biochemical mechanism has not been elucidated. The effects of phosphate depletion on myocardial energy production transport and utilization have been examined by Brautbar et al. (257). Both cellular inorganic phosphorus and creatine phosphate concentrations were markedly reduced in phosphate-depleted animals, while ATP fell only late in the course. The fall in creatine phosphate and inorganic phosphate correlated strongly with the fall in inorganic phosphorus, suggesting that the latter has a major role in the development of metabolic derangements (Fig. 11). Phosphate depletion is associated with an impaired mitochondrial oxygen consumption, reduced energy transport via the creatine phosphate shuttle, and reduced myofibrillar energy utilization. These summarized data demonstrated an effect of phosphate depletion on all steps of myocardial energetics regulated by the creatine phosphokinase isoenzymes (257,282).

Kreusser et al. (283) examined the effects of experimental phosphate depletion on myocardial hemodynamics and metabolism. These studies demonstrated impaired myocardial contractile force and impaired inotropic response of the heart to catecholamines as well as impaired vasoconstrictor response to angiotensin II. These hemodynamic changes were associated with reduced cardiac muscle content of ATP, creatine phosphate, and total phosphorus. Thus, in addition to reduction in myocardial performance during phosphate depletion, evidence was presented to suggest vascular resistance to pressor agents. Indeed, Saglikes et al. (284) reported a lower resting mean arterial blood pressure in phosphate-depleted rats and resistance to the pressor effects of angiotensin II and catecholamines. These arterial changes were associated with a marked reduction in arterial wall ATP, creatine phosphate, and inorganic phosphate. These data may explain the anecdotal reports of hypotension in patients with severe hypophosphatemia and may further support the rationale for treatment, since these abnormalities are reversible upon repletion with phosphate.

Skeletal Muscle
Phosphorus depletion in experimental studies has been shown to cause severe muscle weakness and creatinuria. Fuller and associates (285) examined the effect of phosphate depletion and repletion on skeletal muscle in the dog. Resting muscle membrane potential and muscle content of potassium and total phosphorus fell, while muscle sodium, chloride, and water content rose with phosphate depletion. Serum CPK activity, however, remained normal in these animals. All these abnormalities returned to, or towards, normal with phosphate repletion. Further studies by the same group of investigators demonstrated that overt rhabdomyolysis may be precipitated by the superimposition of severe hypophosphatemia on preexisting subclinical myopathy induced in the dog by feeding a low-phosphorus and low-calorie diet. The production of severe and acute hypophosphatemia in these subclinically phosphorus-depleted dogs by total parenteral nutrition with a solution deficient in phosphate content brought about clinical, biochemical, and histologic evidence of rhabdomyolysis. Unfortunately, the study did not include the effect of administering hyperalimentation at the same dosage to the non-phosphorus-depleted control animals. Thus, the exact role of subclinical phosphorus depletion, per se, cannot be rigorously defined. However, the resemblance between this experimental model and clinical rhabdomyolysis seen in the malnourished chronic alcoholic is striking. These malnourished patients are usually given large amounts of carbohydrate and other nutrients following hospitalization. Within a few days they develop muscle pain and profound weakness associated with severe hypophosphatemia and gross elevation in CPK and aldolase. We have recently examined the cellular molecular mechanism mediating the skeletal myopathy of phosphate depletion (286). Abnormalities in the creatine phosphate energy shuttle for energy transport, mitochondrial oxidative phosphorylation, and myofibrillar energy

use were found. All these events were preceded by a marked reduction in cellular inorganic phosphorus stores.

From these experimental studies, we suggested a mechanism by which the primary event leading to the cellular impairment in energy metabolism is the reduction in intracellular inorganic phosphorus stores as a consequence of prolonged hypophosphatemia.

Respiratory Muscle
Several studies in adult patients have shown that pulmonary muscle weakness may occur as a consequence of hypophosphatemia (287). Recently, a patient who developed severe hypophosphatemia during parenteral hyperalimentation was found to have severe respiratory failure secondary to respiratory muscle weakness. Planas et al. (288) examined pulmonary function and respiratory muscle performance during experimental phosphate depletion. The authors demonstrated no change in basal pulmonary muscle function in phosphate-depleted dogs but found a marked reduction in performance following fatiguing stimulations of the diaphragm. These observations may have important clinical applications, since many of our hypophosphatemic patients are either alcoholics with poor nutrition and recurrent pulmonary infections, or uncontrolled diabetics who are immune compromised and have a higher tendency for pulmonary infections.

Effects of Phosphate Depletion on Intermediary Metabolism

Carbohydrate Metabolism
Since phosphate is essential for glucose uptake by the cell, and since glycolysis is stimulated by high intracellular inorganic phosphorus and is inhibited when cellular inorganic phosphorus concentration is low, it was reasonable to suggest an abnormality in carbohydrate metabolism in phosphate depletion. Indeed, the early studies of Gold et al. (289) and Harter et al. (290) demonstrated hyperglycemia in the face of hyperinsulinemia in phosphate-depleted dogs. The authors suggested insulin resistance secondary to hypophosphatemia.

Davis et al. (291) evaluated the effects of acute and chronic hypophosphatemia on glucose uptake by skeletal muscle in the rat. Acute hypophosphatemia had no effect, but chronic hypophosphatemia caused a direct and linear correlation between glucose uptake and plasma phosphorus. These data were confirmed recently in hypophosphatemic patients (292).

Brautbar et al. (293) recently examined glucose and glycogen pathways in liver, skeletal muscle, and heart from normal and phosphate-depleted rats. The hypophosphatemia was associated with a marked and significant reduction in intracellular inorganic phosphorus, glucose-6-phosphate, fructose-6-phosphate, and glycogen concentration. The changes in gly-

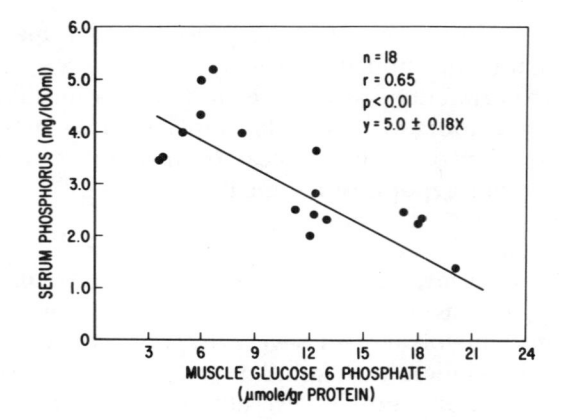

Figure 12. Changes in skeletal muscle glucose-6-phosphate and serum phosphorus during phosphate depletion. (Brautbar N et al: *Clin Res* 30:52A, 1981. Used with permission.)

cogen and glucose-6-phosphate were correlated with the changes in intracellular inorganic phosphorus (Fig. 12). These data demonstrate reduced glycolytic activity secondary to the reduction in intracellular inorganic phosphorus concentration. This is not surprising, since phosphofructokinase, an allosteric enzyme that is a major regulator of glycolysis, is inhibited by low intracellular inorganic phosphorus concentration. The reduced glycogen concentration is probably the result of reduced glycogen synthesis, but increased glycogen breakdown could not be ruled out by these studies.

Recent studies by Horl et al. (294) evaluated glycogen concentration and glycogen synthetase and phosphorylase activity in the hearts of phosphate-depleted rats. Glycogen concentration and glycogen synthetase activity were significantly reduced and glycogen phosphorylase activity was increased, compatible with reduced glycogen synthesis as well as increased glycogen breakdown.

Horl et al. (295) also examined the effects of phosphate depletion on gluconeogenesis in isolated hepatocytes, and the effects of various gluconeogenic stimuli. Glucose production from pyruvate by isolated hepatocytes from phosphate-depleted rats was markedly diminished. Glucagon caused an increased glucose production in control rats with no change in the phosphate-depleted group.

The above findings may have important clinical implications. Impaired gluconeogenesis and hypoglycemia have been reported in the past in patients with phosphate depletion who also developed liver dysfunction. It is possible that the resistance to insulin and impairment in carbohydrate metabolism seen in phosphate depletion may play a role in the uncontrolled diabetic patient with severe hypophosphatemia, and again points out the question of phosphate supplements in the management of these patients.

Membrane Integrity, Phospholipid Metabolism, and Fatty Acid Oxidation

The possibility of a functional and/or structural abnormality of the cellular membrane was suggested by Fuller et al. (282). They demonstrated a reduced membrane resting potential in skeletal muscle of phosphate-depleted dogs. Since cellular membrane integrity is dependent on a normal synthesis of phospholipids, and since inorganic phosphate and glycerol phosphate are major precursors in the biosynthetic pathway of phospholipids, it is plausible to suggest an impairment in phospholipid synthesis during phosphate depletion. Indeed, Ramsay and Douglas (296) recently found a decrease in total lipids, sterol esters, and triacyl glycerol, as well as in phosphatidyl serine, in cell walls of bacteria grown on a phosphate-free medium. Brautbar et al. (297) reported recently a significant and marked reduction in the content of acid-extractable water-soluble phospholipids in kidney, liver, and cardiac muscle but not skeletal muscle in the phosphorus-depleted state.

Analysis of major cellular phospholipid composition has shown a marked reduction in the contents of phosphatidylcholine and phosphatidylethanolamine as a consequence of impairment at various steps of phospholipid biosynthesis.

Since fatty acids are a major source for myocardial energy production, it was plausible to suggest an impairment in fatty acid metabolism. Indeed, Brautbar et al. (298) reported recently a marked impairment in the oxidation of long-chain and short-chain fatty acids by heart mitochondria from phosphate-depleted rats.

Treatment of Hypophosphatemia

Should Hypophosphatemia be Treated?

Treatment of hypophosphatemia remains controversial since carefully controlled studies have not been performed. A current approach to this issue has been reviewed by Kleeman (299). Phosphate treatment is necessary when hypophosphatemia is part of a true phosphate depletion syndrome (PDS). However, hypophosphatemia, even as low as 1.0–2.0 mg/dl in adults or 2.0–3.0 mg/dl in preadolescent children, does not necessarily mean or cause PDS. There are many examples in adult and pediatric medicine of chronic hypophosphatemia caused by a high renal clearance of phosphorus (low TmP/GFR) (i.e., liberal amounts of phosphorus in the urine with low serum phosphorus. These do not develop in PDS unless there is superimposed a true lack of available phosphorus for the metabolic and growth needs of the patients. In the latter setting, phosphorus excretion decreases markedly or disappears completely from the urine. This intense tubular reabsorption of phosphorus is an invariable feature of true phosphate depletion.

The biochemical consequences (depletion of intracellular high energy phosphates) and the clinical manifestations of severe phosphorus depletion probably do not occur in children unless the concentration of phosphorus in the plasma falls below 1.5 mg/dl Knochel (300) has emphasized that these changes in phosphorus metabolism are more apt to produce overt PDS when they occur in an individual who is already sick from some form of acute or chronic debilitating illness; that is, they start off with "sick cells" upon which phosphorus depletion is superimposed. This is consistent with our own personal experience and observations.

When, under these circumstances, the patient develops one or more of the varied clinical syndromes ascribed to phosphorus depletion, oral or parenteral administration is necessary. This categorical statement is based on the innumerable clinical studies in the literature in which one or more of these abnormalities is reversed or totally corrected only by phosphorus replacement and correction of the profound hypophosphatemia. It is true that many of these patients have associated electrolyte, acid-base, and nutritional abnormalities that are often simultaneously corrected, and that very few controlled studies with and without phosphorus administration are available. However, in most of the reported experimental and clinical studies the probability is so strong that the phosphorus administration is primarily responsible for correction of the specific disorder that we believe we can accept the basic correctness of this conclusion.

In most of the reported cases, the dysfunction caused by the phosphate depletion is of such seriousness that it would not be justified to withhold phosphorus replacement. However, randomized studies with and without phosphorus therapy are still necessary. Recently, a study along these lines was carried out during the treatment of patients with diabetic ketoacidosis and nonketotic hyperosmolar coma. Keller and Berger (276) randomly assigned a total of 40 cases to either standardized conventional treatment alone or combined with phosphate infusions from the beginning of therapy. The patients were appropriately matched for age, sex, and clinical characteristics. The initial concentration of inorganic phosphate in the serum was normal or elevated in almost every patient. In those receiving phosphorus, the serum level fell to a low of 2.8–3 mg/dl by 8 hours, while in the control group a low of 1.8 mg/dl was seen. These values persisted over the next 24–48 hours, and the patients were followed very closely for at least 96 hours. Food was permitted ad libitum in both groups after the second day of treatment. The authors concluded that a favorable effect of phosphate therapy on the clinical course of diabetic ketoacidosis or hyperosmolar coma could not be demonstrated. We are all aware of the fact that profound hypophosphatemia almost always develops during recovery from these conditions, and the vast majority of clinical centers have not given (during the past 4–5 decades) parenteral phosphorus replacement. The most likely explanation for the failure to see a PDS in this setting is the fact that the oral intake of phosphorus-containing nutrients is begun early in the course of treatment, usually by the end of the first 24 hours.

Administration of Parenteral Phosphate

Parenteral phosphate administration to the patient with phosphate depletion should be done cautiously. These individuals have a state of physiologic HPT and, independent of that their renal tubules continue to reabsorb almost all the filtered phosphorus despite the development of hyperphosphatemia. The longer the duration of the phosphorus depletion, the more persistent is this physiologic dysfunction. Therefore, the absence of a normal increase in phosphorus excretion signifies that the kidney cannot play its essential role of preventing an abnormal rise of serum phosphate concentration. When the latter occurs, it immediately causes a decrease in calcium ion concentration, at times to profoundly hypocalcemic levels. Thus, in a matter of hours we may transform a phosphate depletion state into a phosphate "excess" one, with its hazardous consequences. We recommend that elemental phosphorus not be parenterally administered at a rate greater than 1 g/24 hr and that serum phosphorus and the rate of rise in urinary phosphorus be followed closely.

Vannetta et al. (301) examined the efficacy and safety of intravenous phosphate administration to patients with severe hyphophosphatemia. Ten adult patients with severe hypophosphatemia (serum phosphorus below 1 mg/dl) and normal renal function were studied prospectively. They were treated with a solution containing 9 mmol of phosphorus as monobasic phosphate potassium (KH_2PO_4), infused over a period of 12 hours. Serum phosphate, calcium, and potassium values and urinary excretion of phosphate were measured every 12 hours. The serum phosphorus levels were significantly improved at 12 hours, by more than 1 mg/dl in all patients after 36 hours, and to normal in six patients in 48 hours. Serum potassium levels were never above normal and serum calcium levels declined in only one patient. These data demonstrate that intravenous administration of phosphate at a rate of 9 mmol over a period of 12 hours is both safe and efficient in adult patients with normal renal function.

DISORDERS OF MAGNESIUM

Measurements of Cellular Magnesium

Studies of the concentration of magnesium inside the cell have been carried out for a number of years. Estimates of the concentration of the free unbound magnesium were made based on the amount required for various enzymatic reactions and the known binding constants, such as for ATP or creatine phosphate. Total magnesium measurements have been done utilizing atomic absorption spectroscopy. The concentration of magnesium in the kidney was found to be 10.4 mmol/kg wet weight. The above methods are crude and do not yield the crucial information affecting cellular magnesium transport—the free ionized magnesium. A method using calculation of the equilibrium constant of aconitate hydratase has been described.

Since most of the intracellular magnesium is bound to protein and since only a small fraction is soluble and determines many of the reactions in the cell, it has been of major importance to try to determine the concentration of free intracellular magnesium in various conditions (e.g., ischemia), its depletion, and its interactions with various hormones.

Recently, high resolution NMR has been used to allow measure free intracellular magnesium. This method measures the changes in phosphocreatine and calculates the concentration of free cellular magnesium, which was found to be 3.0–4.4 mmol/kg wet weight. Wu et al. (302) examined the changes in intracellular free magnesium in the perfused heart in response to ischemia by ^{31}P NMR. The concentration of intracellular free magnesium in the beating heart cell was found to be 2.5 ± 0.7 mM with no significant changes during ischemia. This study demonstrates the importance of ^{31}P NMR in the determination of in vivo free magnesium concentration. This major development in methodology hopefully will increase our knowledge and understanding of intracellular magnesium changes in various pathologic conditions.

Magnesium and the Cardiovascular System

The relationship between the magnesium ion and myocardial function has been reviewed by Brautbar et al. (53). Cardiac rhythm abnormalities have frequently been documented in hypomagnesemic patients, and magnesium therapy has even been suggested to improve mechanical recovery after myocardial infarction. The availability of isolated perfused heart muscle preparations, and the ability to measure transcellular ^{28}Mg fluxes, have added to our understanding of magnesium effects on the heart. Indeed, early studies have advocated the use of a high Mg concentration in coronary infusate prior to ischemia. Although the mechanisms by which magnesium protects against ischemia are not clear, several have been suggested: (1) a "membrane stabilizing" effect of increased divalent cation concentration; (2) a negative inotropic effect of increased magnesium causing ATP sparing; and (3) intracellular effects of elevated magnesium concentration protecting ATP levels. Bersohn et al. (303) studied isolated perfused hearts and measured coronary flow and oxygen consumption. The authors examined the effects of magnesium on recovery from ischemia and demonstrated that elevated magnesium protects ischemic myocardium only under circumstances in which it has a negative inotropic effect before the onset of ischemia. Magnesium may mediate sparing of ATP and thus protect the heart from ischemia.

Recently, Iseri and Bures (304) reported on two patients who displayed life-threatening cardiac arrhythmias with severe hypomagnesemia secondary to chronic alcoholism. The arrhythmias were corrected by magnesium therapy. The authors concluded that magnesium deficiency may be the hidden factor in intractable ventricular arrhythmias, especially in patients with a strong history of alcoholism. Although more studies are required to further substantiate these conclusions, it is our feeling that patients who have a condition that predisposes to magnesium depletion (e.g., diabetic ketoacidosis, cirrhosis, malabsorption syndrome, protracted postoperative course, and recurrent pancreatitis) and who display ventricular arrhythmias should be evaluated carefully for severe hypomagnesemia and treated accordingly.

Several investigators have shown a relationship between decreased magnesium content of cardiac muscle and coronary arteries and the incidence of mortality from nonocclusive coronary artery disease. The incidence of nonocclusive coronary artery disease has been found to be highest in geographic areas with soft drinking water or soil poor in magnesium (305). The observation that heart tissue and coronary vessels have a significantly reduced magnesium level in patients with sudden death caused by nonocclusive coronary heart disease suggests a role for chronic hypomagnesemia in the genesis of this entity.

Manthry et al. (306) measured serum levels of magnesium in 106 patients undergoing coronary angiography. The patients were classified into three groups according to the severity of the coronary heart disease: no lesions on angiography (31), moderate lesions (34), and severe lesions (41). Patients with severe coronary heart disease had lower mean serum magnesium and higher serum copper and manganese than those without the disease. In contrast, patients with moderate disease did not show any alterations in the concentration of the above trace metals. The authors concluded that a deficiency of magnesium, but not of other trace metals studied, may be present in patients with severe coronary heart disease. These findings support the theory that magnesium deficiency may contribute to the development of serious cardiac rhythm disturbances in these patients.

Several investigators have evaluated the concentration of magnesium in the cardiovascular tissue of patients with cardiac pathology. When the magnesium content of myocardium, aorta, and myocardial necrotic zones in patients with myocardial infarction was measured, the infarcted zone showed markedly less magnesium. Also, magnesium is strikingly reduced in the noninfarcted portions of the heart in patients with myocardial infarction as compared to controls.

Saetersdal et al. (307) examined heart mitochondrial contents of magnesium in normal patients and in patients with evidence of right ventricular overload. No differences were found in the content of magnesium. However, the authors did not examine the total myocardial content of magnesium in these patients, and therefore the interpretation of these findings is not clear.

It is a well-documented observation that immediately after the onset of myocardial infarction, there is a marked rise in the blood levels of long-chain free fatty acids. A reduction in magnesium levels with a rise to normal after recovery has also been reported. Flink et al. (308) examined plasma magnesium and long-chain free fatty acid levels in 16 patients with acute myocardial infarction. In each patient, there was a sharp fall in magnesium levels and a sharp rise in free fatty acid levels shortly after the onset of pain. Both magnesium and free fatty acids returned to normal. This regularly occurring lowering of the magnesium levels early in myocardial infarction could be very important in the production of myocardial irritability, especially if the baseline magnesium levels are already low. Since urinary losses of magnesium were minimal and since the timing of the lower magnesium values was identical to that of the rise in free fatty acid levels, the authors suggested that lipolysis secondary to ischemia causes release of free fatty acid to the circulation and this in turn causes lowering of magnesium levels in the blood. These findings may be of major clinical importance, especially in patients who have been treated with diuretics or who have been consuming alcohol. Indeed, the use of antilipolytic measures in patients with myocardial infarction has been advocated by Sodipallares et al. (309), who administered intravenous solutions of glucose, insulin, and potassium salts as a "polarizing" solution. The addition of magnesium to this mixture has been advocated by Lim et al. (310). Future studies are needed to further examine these findings and to develop a therapeutic regimen. It is our feeling from the data available to date that magnesium supplementation might be indicated in patients with acute myocardial infarction and who have previously been on diuretics. Even if they may not show clear evidence of hypomagnesemia, they may still be total body magnesium deficient.

Furukawa et al. (311) examined recently the effects of magnesium chloride on sinoatrial nodal pacemaker activity and atrial contractility, utilizing the isolated blood perfused canine atrial preparation. Magnesium chloride injected directly into the sinus node artery produced dose-related negative chronotrophic and inotropic effects. Moreover, magnesium chloride produced a uniform depression of contraction amplitude at all frequencies examined. These observations may help explain the protective effects of magnesium on the heart. Magnesium directly reduces heart rate and contractility and in turn will reduce energy utilization and have relative sparing effects on ATP levels.

Magnesium and Blood Vessels

Acute hypomagnesemia in animals and humans is often associated with rises in blood pressure and elevation in peripheral vascular resistance in a variety of regions in the circulation. Several disease entities associated with hypomagnesemia, and at times magnesium depletion, are commonly associated with elevated blood pressure (diabetes mellitus, alcoholism, essential hypertension). Hypermagnesemia has been associated with reduction in blood pressure levels, and early studies by Hazard et al. (312) have shown that acute elevations of serum magnesium are associated with hypotension. The mechanism mediating this effect of magnesium on blood pressure has been recently evaluated. Altura et al. (313) examined in vitro the influence of various mangesium levels on blood vessel contractility and reactivity. Hypermagnesemia induced rapid vasodilation and depressed the reactivity to contractile agonists, while lowering magnesium levels was associated with increased reactivity to pressor agonists. The authors show that, in addition to modulating drug and hormone induced contractions in smooth muscle cells, magnesium can alter the baseline tension or tone. In addition, the authors showed that magnesium can directly influence the uptake, content, binding, and distribution of calcium in smooth muscle cells.

Diabetes mellitus is commonly associated with marked hypomagnesemia and also a high incidence of hypertension. Recent in vitro experiments in alloxan diabetic rats (313–316) suggest that the altered vascular tone noted in these experimental animals may in part be due to modification in the Mg–Ca exchange sites at the vascular smooth muscle cell membranes. Although a sudden withdrawal of magnesium is accompanied by potent contractions in the aorta of normal rats, aorta from alloxan diabetic rats showed little or no response. Relaxation is commonly seen in response to magnesium administration but is missing in the aorta from alloxan diabetic rats. These data indicate that in alloxan diabetic rats membrane permeability to calcium might be decreased, cellular or membrane calcium is present in a more tightly bound form, and the functional Mg–Ca exchange sites are fewer in number or are altered. These data are consistent with the notion that magnesium and, in particular, membrane-bound magnesium may exert a regulatory role in vascular tone, vascular reactivity, and peripheral vascular resistance, and may have a functional role in calcium fluxes and compartmentalization. Certain disease entities associated with hypomagnesemia, such as diabetes mellitus, are also associated with vascular tone changes; these alterations may be partly mediated via changes in magnesium homeostasis.

A role for hypomagnesemia in essential hypertension has been suggested. Recent in vitro experiments in rats with spontaneous hypertension have shown impaired response in vascular smooth muscle responsiveness to agonists and to removal or administration of magnesium (313,315,316). Both clinical and experimental evidence suggest that verapamil can produce peripheral vasodilatation, decrease in arterial blood pressure, and lower systemic vascular resistance. The basic mechanism mediating these effects of verapamil are thought to be via its inhibition of calcium influx into the vascular smooth muscle. Turlapaty et al. (317) examined the possible interactions of verapamil and magnesium on tone and contraction of vascular smooth muscle. Thoracic aorta and portal vein were examined in vitro. The authors demonstrated that magnesium and verapamil have synergistic effects on the amplitude of contraction via the effects on inhibition of calcium fluxes, and probably by decreasing cytosolic calcium contents. These data may suggest an important role for magnesium as a calcium channel blocker, and possibly in potentiating the hypotensive effect of verapamil on the peripheral vasculature.

These observations may have important clinical implications in hypertensive and cardiac patients who are treated with diuretics (which have a tendency to cause hypomagnesemia) and verapamil at the same time. Further evidence that magnesium directly affects vascular smooth muscle cells has been submitted by Moreland et al. (318). The authors have examined the influence of varying free magnesium levels on Ca-stimulated ATPase activity and phosphorylation of Ca-sensitive actomyosin. Both the calcium-stimulated ATPase and actomyosin phosphorylation exhibited an optimal magnesium level. These experimental data demonstrate a major role for magnesium in the regulation of vascular smooth muscle tone and contraction.

Magnesium and Skeletal Muscle

The myopathy of chronic alcoholism, in which magnesium depletion is a hallmark, resembles the morphologic changes described in experimental magnesium deficiency in the rat. Stendig-Lindberg et al. (319) examined 10 patients with hypomagnesemia and myopathic symptoms, seven of whom were chronic alcoholics and three of whom had hypomagnesemia secondary to malabsorption syndrome. In the hypomagnesemic patients, muscle strength was significantly reduced, as was creatine phosphate content. Anderson et al. (320) evaluated skeletal muscle total phosphorus and magnesium content in 13 patients with acute alcoholic myopathy. Total muscle phosphorus and magnesium content were significantly and markedly reduced. These findings suggest that the myopathy of alcoholism is in part a result of chronic magnesium depletion.

The effects of magnesium depletion on skeletal muscle function and structure is difficult to study since severe isolated magnesium deficiency is commonly associated with hypokalemia, hypophosphatemia, and hypocalcemia. Cronin et al. (321) examined the effects of magnesium depletion on transmembrane electrical potential difference of skeletal muscle and muscle cell morphology in magnesium deficient dogs. Magnesium content of skeletal muscle fell only modestly despite prolonged magnesium deficiency (10 weeks). The most pronounced muscle compositional change was a marked loss of muscle total phosphorus and gain of calcium, sodium, and chloride with no changes in cellular potassium levels and only a slight change in magnesium levels. Muscle histology showed abnormal findings of focal necrosis in four of nine dogs with muscle cell hyperpolarization developing after 10 weeks of magnesium depletion. The authors concluded that intracellular depletion of phosphorus secondary to magnesium depletion is the major derangement leading to the skeletal muscle abnormalities of magnesium depletion. Interestingly, serum phosphorus levels were normal in these dogs while muscle total phosphorus content was reduced. Several major problems exist, however, with the interpretation of these studies: (*1*) The results of skeletal muscle content of the various electrolytes were expressed per dry weight but not per milligram of protein or DNA. Since it is not possible to rule out an effect of magnesium depletion on protein synthesis, which would further change the distribution of magnesium and phosphorus in the cell, it is possible that, if expressed per milligram protein, there might be no fall in magnesium or phosphorus. (*2*) Analysis of total phosphorus does not relate to either inorganic phosphorus or nucleotide phosphorus. A reduction in total phosphorus may be limited to changes in total nucleotide phosphorus or protein phosphorus with no change in cellular inorganic phosphorus. (*3*) The observation that muscle magnesium fell only slightly may not be relevant since most of the active magnesium in the cell is unbound and cannot be detected by tissue ashing methods.

Potter et al. (322) have reviewed the role that the magnesium ion may play in the regulation of muscle contraction via its effects on the cellular calcium-binding proteins troponin, parvalbumin, myosin, and calmodulin. The major effect of magnesium is to greatly reduce the rate of calcium binding to sites that bind magnesium and calcium competitively. Thus, during a transient increase in magnesium (similar to that seen during muscle activation), these sites would bind very little calcium and consequently play a regulatory role. These data indicate a role for intracellular magnesium in the regulation of the high affinity calcium-binding proteins and suggest a mechanism by which magnesium depletion may affect muscle function.

Stephenson et al. (323) examined the effects of magnesium on the activation of skinned fibers from skeletal muscle. In skinned muscle fibers the internal composition can be manipulated directly and calcium movements estimated from isometric force transients, net changes in sarcoplasmic reticulum (SR) calcium, and ^{45}Ca flux between fiber and bath. The authors show that magnesium can stimulate the SR active calcium transport system, inhibit a calcium-dependent calcium efflux pathway for SR, and shift the isometric force–Ca relation by reducing calcium-binding to myofilament-regulating sites. These observations suggest a mechanism by which magnesium depletion may alter skeletal muscle excitation–contraction coupling. Indeed, Hasselbach et al. (324) demonstrated the dependence of SR calcium transport on magnesium. Thus, it is possible that the initial event in magnesium depletion is an impairment in the SR uptake of calcium and in turn inhibition of the excitation-contraction coupling. Studies of SR function in magnesium depletion are needed to further extend observations to our patients.

Magnesium Metabolism in Diabetes Mellitus

Decreased serum magnesium concentration has been demonstrated in patients with diabetes mellitus. Mather et al. (325) found hypomagnesemia to occur in 25% of a group of out-patients with diabetes mellitus. The pathogenesis of hypomagnesemia in diabetic patients is not clear. Several factors have been suggested, including the effects of osmotic diuresis and renal losses, poor nutritional intake, and increased deposition in soft tissue in response to insulin administration and biosynthesis of new protein. McNair et al. (326) evaluated the interrelation between glucose metabolism and magnesium in 215 insulin-treated diabetic out-patients. All patients had normal creatinine clearance and no other diseases. A definite hypomagnesemia and hypermagnesuria occurred in 38.6% and 55% of all patients, respectively. In the presence of hypermagnesuria, the serum magnesium concentration was inversely correlated with urinary magnesium excretion rate. Urinary magnesium excretion correlated with urinary glucose excretion. The authors conclude that (1) hypomagnesemia is common in uncontrolled diabetes mellitus; (2) the mechanism is probably reduced tubular transport of magnesium in the presence of elevated tubular glucose content secondary to hyperglycemia. It is necessary to note that insulin administration initially corrected the hyperglycemia and glycosuria but not the hypermagnesuria. No explanation for this observation is evident. The long-term effect of this hypomagnesemia in diabetic patients is not clear since both skeletal muscle and red and white blood cell magnesium were found to be normal in diabetic patients with hypomagnesemia. However, it is important to note here that although total magnesium content was not reduced, the concentration of free cellular magnesium was not measured and might have been lower in hypomagnesemic diabetic patients.

Recently, Hoskins et al. (327) examined renal magnesium transport in experimental diabetes mellitus. The uptake of ^{28}Mg was measured in slices of kidney cortex from rats with alloxan diabetes. ^{28}Mg uptake was significantly increased over uptake measured in kidney cortex slices from control rats. Immediate institution of insulin therapy to the diabetic rats prevented the diabetes-induced increased uptake of ^{28}Mg. Moreover, the in vitro studies showed a direct effect of insulin on ^{28}Mg uptake by the kidney, suggesting that the in vivo effect of insulin might be partially a direct effect on renal tubular site(s) and that insulin deficiency (diabetes mellitus) may alter tubular magnesium transport regardless of the serum or tubular glucose levels.

Clinical Assessment of Intestinal Absorption of Magnesium

The evaluation of intestinal absorption of magnesium has clinical importance in renal lithiasis and states of impaired vitamin D metabolism (e.g., uremia). One of the difficulties that has hindered research on magnesium metabolism is the lack of a satisfactory tracer isotope. The radioisotope ^{28}Mg has a short half-life of 21.3 hours, and thus, has been regarded as a relatively safe radioisotope for use in human subjects. Upon injection, ^{28}Mg rapidly disappears from the circulation and is initially concentrated in the soft tissues. However, over 80% of magnesium in the human body appears to be contained in slowly exchanging compartments that are not accessible to measurement by the use of ^{28}Mg. The potential role of ^{26}Mg has been explored recently by Schwartz (328), using neutron activation and mass spectrometry for detection. The authors have shown that net magnesium absorption can be measured by evaluation of fecal excretion. Although this method appears to be safe and accurate, its practical use for clinical research is not feasible. Nicar et al. (329) developed an oral magnesium load test for the assessment of intestinal magnesium absorption. An oral dose of 25 mmol of magnesium was given to patients. Fasting blood and urinary magnesium were obtained at 2-hour collection periods from control patients and patients with primary HPT, absorptive hypercalciuria, and hypoparathyroidism. Following the oral magnesium load, urinary magnesium increased significantly from the fasting levels, with every individual showing a rise. Mg absorption was measured in this study indirectly from the increment in urinary magnesium following an oral magnesium load. Its reliability was shown by good physiological correlation with findings from other methods used for magnesium absorption. Although easy to perform, this method has some major difficulties: (*1*) the patients must be in magnesium balance; (*2*) the patients must not have magnesium depletion; (*3*) large variability of individual data renders interpretation difficult.

The Effects of Diet, Hyperalimentation, and Fasting on Magnesium Metabolism

The nutritional importance of magnesium and the consequences of magnesium depletion have been reviewed recently by Flink (330). The 1980 recommended daily dietary allowances of magnesium by the National Academy of Sciences and National Research Council are shown in Table 5. These recommendations mean that a 70 kg man needs 350 mg/day, while infants, lactating women, or patients recovering from a serious disease need almost three times the amount recommended. The guidelines, preparations, and doses for magnesium supplementation are shown in Table 6.

Acute and chronic fasting produce a negative magnesium balance through carbohydrate deprivation and increased urinary ketones. Indeed,

Table 5. Daily Nutritional Requirements for Magnesium

Period of Life	Age (years)	Daily Amount of Magnesium (mg/day)
Infants	0–0.5	50
	0.5–1.0	70
Children	1–3	150
	4–6	200
	7–10	250
Males	11–14	350
	15–18	400
	19 and older	350
Females	11–14	300
	15 and older	300
	During pregnancy	300 + 150
	During lactation	300 + 150

SOURCE: Adapted from Flink EB: *Western J Med* 133:304–312, 1980.

refeeding with carbohydrates increases the reabsorption of magnesium by 80%. The effects of a liquid protein diet on magnesium metabolism was examined recently (331). Six obese subjects treated with liquid protein diet supplemented with vitamins and potassium chloride were studied for 40 days. While serum magnesium levels did not change, a negative magnesium balance developed as a result of marked urinary magnesium losses. These studies indicate that a liquid protein fast results in depletion of intracellular and skeletal stores of magnesium. Since abnormalities in cardiac rhythm have been demonstrated with this diet, and since magnesium depletion can precipitate or trigger cardiac arrhythmias, a relationship between this negative magnesium balance and the fatalities reported recently with the liquid protein diet has been suggested.

The importance of magnesium supplementation in patients receiving peripheral hyperalimentation has been reexamined. Freeman et al. (332) evaluated the effects of magnesium infusions on urinary and fecal magnesium excretion, serum magnesium, and nitrogen balance in seven well-nourished and three nutritionally depleted adult surgical patients on hyperalimentation. They were maintained on constant nitrogen and calorie intake for 14 ± 2 days. Magnesium doses ranged from 0 to 664 mg/day and were given in varying crossover patterns. In both groups, urinary magnesium excretion increased as the amount of magnesium infused increased but, at comparable magnesium infusion, depleted patients excreted significantly less magnesium. Renal conservation was most pronounced in well-nourished patients on magnesium-free intake and in depleted patients given 70 mg magnesium daily. Endogenous fecal mag-

Table 6. Guidelines for Treatment of Magnesium Deficiency

1. It is important to determine that the kidneys are producing urine and that blood urea nitrogen and creatinine values are normal. Magnesium may be needed and may be administered even in the presence of severe renal insufficiency, but the treatment must be monitored by measuring serum or plasma levels frequently. Note that $MgSO_4$ (magnesium sulfate) is the heptahydrate $MgSO_4$. Ampules containing 1.0 gram of $MgSO_4$ or 8.1 mEq of magnesium are convenient to use. Parenterally given Mg doses recommended below refer to $MgSO_4$.

    General requirements: On the first day of therapy at least 1 mEq of Mg per kg of body weight (lean body mass) should be given parenterally. Subsequently, at least 0.5 mEq of Mg per kg of body weight per day should be given for three to five days. If parenteral fluid therapy continues after this, at least 0.1 mEq per kg per day should be given. Infants and young children need twice as much.

2. The following schedule for an average adult is safe and effective.
    Intramuscular route:
        Day 1—2 grams (16.3 mEq) every four hours for five doses.
        Days 2–5—1.0 gram (8.1 mEq) every six hours.
    Intravenous route (this is the preferred route if intravenous infusion is being used already):
        Day 1—5 grams (41 mEq) per liter of fluid and at least two liters or 82 mEq.
        Days 2–5—A total of 6 grams (49 mEq) distributed equally in total fluids of the day.

3. For a sudden emergency such as convulsions or tachyarrhythmia.[a]
    Intravenous dose: 2 grams of $MgSO_4$ as 20 percent solution (10 ml of 20 percent $MgSO_4$) given in one minute. This should be followed by 5 grams of $MgSO_4$ in 500 ml solution over five to six hours and, finally, followed with the intramuscular schedule for days 2–5 as listed above.

4. Oral therapy. Most Mg salts can cause diarrhea, which can be a limiting factor (other preparations than the ones listed below can also used).
    Liquid milk of magnesia: one teaspoonful four times a day as tolerated, or
    Magnesium hydroxide tablets: 300 mg tablets four times a day as tolerated; increase to two tablets four times a day as tolerated, or
    Magnesium acetate (9.35 mEq per gram) as 10 percent solution: 10 ml in water four times a day as tolerated.

5. Monitor therapy. Magnesium repletion of tissues is slow. Magnesium levels need to be checked from time to time. As satisfactory blood levels are obtained, the dose can be adjusted to the lowest dose needed to maintain normal levels. Obviously, therapy should be stopped if the acute episode that caused the disturbance in the first place has been corrected. Under certain circumstances, such as renal or gastrointestinal wasting of magnesium, the oral dose should be continued indefinitely.

[a] Adapted from Iseri LT et al: *Am J Med* 58:837–846, 1975.

nesium excretion was minimal and ranged from 2 to 38 mg/day. At each level of magnesium intake, serum levels of well-nourished patients were normal. With infusions of less than 200 mg/day, serum magnesium concentrations in depleted subjects averaged 1.6 mg/dl. Reduced urinary magnesium excretion as well as borderline serum levels measured in depleted adults suggest that the magnesium dosage should be higher than that usually recommended during total parenteral nutrition. In both groups a positive correlation between magnesium and nitrogen balance was noted.

Diuretics and Magnesium Metabolism

A common cause for magnesium losses and negative magnesium balance is prolonged use of diuretics, mainly the loop diuretics. Diuretic-induced renal magnesium losses have been implicated in the frequent finding of magnesium depletion and hypomagnesemia in patients with congestive heart failure, where ventricular ectopic beats and digitalis toxicity may be potentiated.

Recent studies by Leary et al. (333) support the view that biologically important magnesium losses may result from chronic administration of diuretics, with loop diuretics causing more profound depletion than thiazides. Administration of piretanide (a thiazide) at a dose of 12 mg/day to nine patients over a period of 12 weeks resulted in a marked fall in serum magnesium. When hydrochlorothiazide at a dose of 100 mg/day was administered with amiloride, 10 mg/day, to 15 hypertensive patients, the amiloride blunted the fall in serum magnesium. This observation underscores the importance of adding potassium- and magnesium-sparing diuretics (such as amiloride and triamterene) to chronic diuretic therapy.

Widman et al. (334) examined the effects of diuretic induced hypomagnesemia on skeletal muscle content of magnesium. By using long-term therapy with potassium and magnesium-sparing diuretics (aldactone and triamterene), the authors were able to prevent the fall in skeletal muscle content of magnesium.

Magnesium is an important cofactor and a critical determinant of Na-K-ATPase activity in several tissues, including the heart, skeletal muscle, and kidney. This enzyme is necessary to release energy for the Na-K pump that actively incorporates potassium into the cells, and thus, maintains intracellular potassium. Decrease in tissue magnesium may affect the pump and reduce intracellular potassium content. Such changes may be associated with serious cardiac arrhythmias, which are usually ascribed to hypokalemia, but are in fact provoked by a decrease in intracellular potassium due to magnesium depletion. The effects of magnesium supplementation on intracellular potassium levels during diuretic therapy have not been critically and carefully studied, although such an approach may be theoretically indicated. A schematic representation of the mecha-

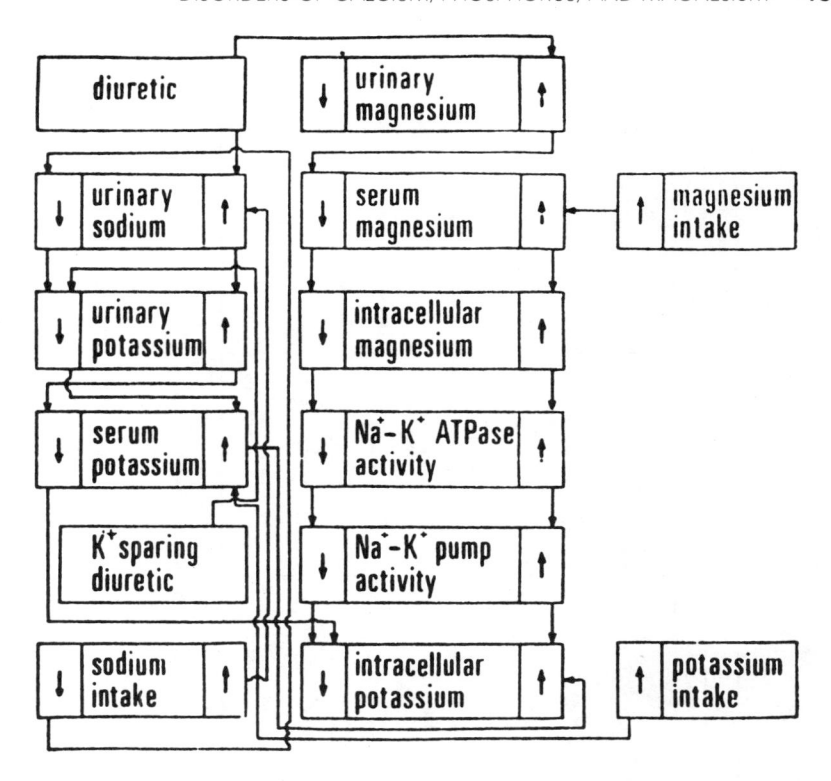

Figure 13. A schematic representation of a possible role for changes in intracellular magnesium on cellular function, and the importance of magnesium supplementation, and the superiority of magnesium and potassium sparing diuretics. (Leary WP, Reyes AJ: *South African Med J* 61:279–280, 1982. Used with permission.)

nism whereby magnesium supplementation might be effective is shown in Figure 13.

It is our impression that magnesium depletion should be looked for in any patient who is on prolonged diuretic therapy (mainly with loop diuretics) and who may have other conditions that may precipitate cardiac arrhythmias.

Guidelines for Diagnosis and Therapy of Magnesium Depletion

Unfortunately, there is no one single laboratory test that unequivocally reveals a magnesium deficiency. It is well accepted that normal serum magnesium levels do not rule out magnesium depletion. Thus, white blood cell, red blood cell, and skeletal muscle magnesium content have been used in clinical research centers. Serum magnesium levels are not without value in day-to-day clinical medicine. They should be determined

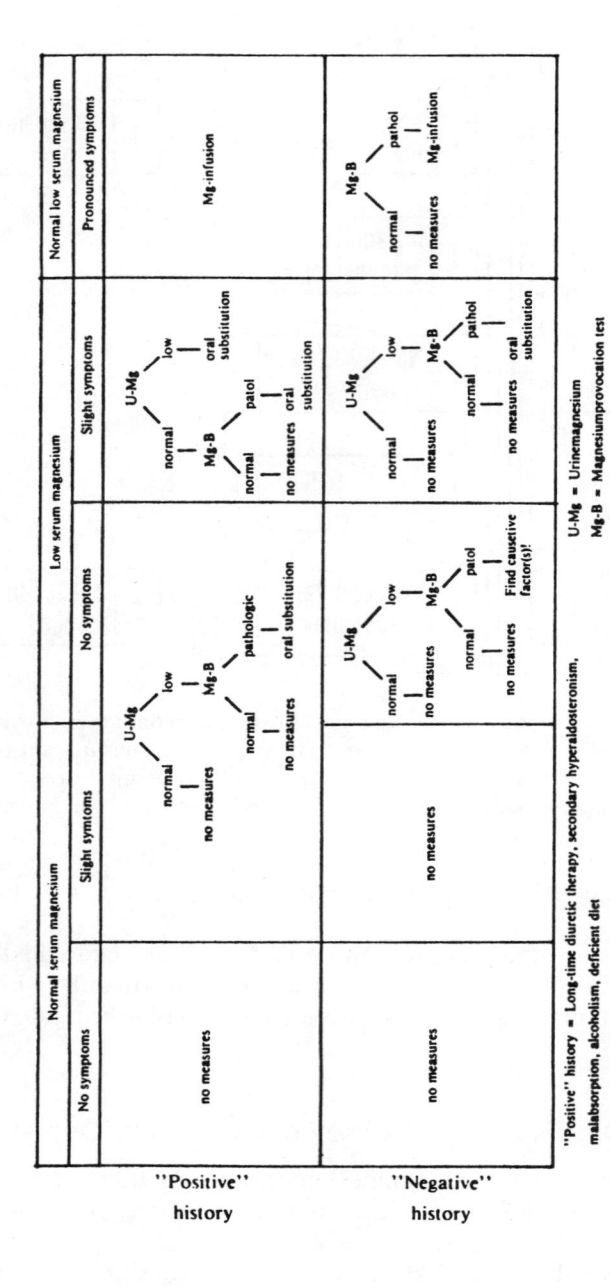

Figure 14. A schematic representation of the diagnostic evaluation of magnesium depletion. (Dyckner T, Wester PO: *Acta Med Scand* (Suppl)661:37–39, 1981. Used with permission.)

in any patient who is on long-term diuretic therapy, who has cardiac arrhythmias, or who has prolonged Q-T intervals on ECG. If serum magnesium levels are normal in these conditions, magnesium depletion still cannot be ruled out and each patient should be evaluated according to clinical presentation and symptoms. Recently, Dyckner et al. (335) formulated a protocol to help in the diagnosis of magnesium deficiency and suggest some guidelines for therapy (Fig. 14). The authors use the magnesium provocative test, which consists of administering 30 mmol of $MgSO_4$ in 500 ml of 5% dextrose over 12 hours, with measurement of the urinary excretion of magnesium over the 24 hours before and after the test. A retention of less than 20% indicates that magnesium depletion is unlikely. The test should not be used in any patient with renal insufficiency, hypotension, or respiratory disease. The judicial clinical evaluation of the patient within the guidelines shown in Figure 14 will increase our detection of patients with magnesium depletion but with normal serum magnesium.

REFERENCES

1. Habener JF, Potts JT Jr: Biosynthesis of parathyroid hormone (first of two parts). *N Engl J Med* 229:580–585, 1978.
2. Habener JF, Potts JT Jr: Subcellular distributions of parathyroid hormone, hormonal precursors, and parathyroid secretory protein. *Endocrinology* 104:265–275, 1979.
3. Habener JF, Kronenberg HM, Potts JH: Biosynthesis of preproparathyroid hormone in Hand AR, Oliver C (eds): *Methods in Cell Biology*. New York, Academic Press, 1981, vol 23, pp 51–70.
4. Morrissey JJ, Cohn DV: The effects of calcium and magnesium on the secretion of parathormone and parathyroid secretory protein by isolated procine parathyroid cells. *Endocrinology* 103:2081–2090, 1978.
5. Majzoub JA, Dee PC, Habener JF: Cellular and cell-free processing of parathyroid secretory proteins. *J Biol Chem* 257:3581–3588, 1982.
6. Raisz LG: Effects of calcium on uptake and incorporation of amino acids in the parathyroid glands. BBA, 148:460–465, 1967.
7. Hamilton JW, Cohn DV: Studies on the biosynthesis in vitro of parathyroid hormone. *J Biol Chem* 244:5421, 1969.
8. Hamilton JW, MacGregor RR, Chu LH, et al: The isolation and partial purification of a non-parathyroid hormone calcemic fraction from bovine parathyroid glands. *Endocrinology* 89:1440, 1969.
9. Chu LLH, MacGregor RR, Anast CS, et al: Studies on the biosynthesis of rat parathyroid hormone and proparathyroid hormone: Adaptation of the parathyroid gland to dietary restriction of calcium. *Endocrinology* 93:915, 1973.
10. Moran JR, Born W, Tuchschmid CR, et al: Calcium regulated biosynthesis of the parathyroid secretory protein, parathyroid hormone, and parathyroid hormone in dispersed bovine parathyroid cells. *Endocrinology* 108:2264–2268, 1981.
11. Martin KJ, Hruska KA, Freitag JJ, et al: The peripheral metabolism of parathyroid hormone. *N Engl J Med* 301:1097–1098.

12. D'Amour P, Segre GV, Roth SI, et al: Analysis of parathyroid hormone and its fragments in rat tissues. *J Clin Invest* 63:89–98, 1979.
13. Hruska KA, Korkor A, Martin K, et al: Peripheral metabolism of intact parathyroid hormone. Role of liver and kidney and the effect of chronic renal failure. *J Clin Invest* 67:885–892, 1981.
14. Segre GV, D'Amour P, Hultman A, et al: Effects of hepatectomy, nephrectomy, and nephrectomy/uremia on the metabolism of parathyroid hormone in the rat. *J Clin Invest* 64:439–448, 1981.
15. Segre GV, Perkins AS, Witters LA, et al: Metabolism of parathyroid hormone by isolated rat kupffer cells and hepatocytes. *J Clin Invest* 67:449–457, 1981.
16. Olgaard K, Arbelaez M. Schwartz J, et al: Abnormal skeletal response to parathyroid hormone in dogs with chronic uremia. *Calcified Tissue Int* 34:403–407, 1982.
17. Rothstein M, Morrissey J, Slatopolsky E, et al: The role of Na-Ca exchange in parathyroid hormone secretion. *Endocrinology* 111:225–230, 1982.
18. Bruce BR, Anderson NC Jr: Hyperpolarization in mouse parathyroid cells by low calcium. *Am J Physiol* 236:C15, 1979.
19. Dempster DW, Tobler PH, Olles P, et al: Potassium stimulated parathyroid hormone release from perfused parathyroid cells *Endocrinology* 111:191–195, 1982.
20. Hove K, Sand O: Evidence for a function of calcium influx in the stimulation of hormone release from the parathyroid gland in the goat. *Acta Physiol Scand* 113:37–43, 1981.
21. Wild P, Bitterli D, Becker M: Quantitative changes of membranes in rat parathyroid cells related to variations of serum calcium. *Lab Invest* 47:370–374, 1982.
22. Morrissey JJ, Hruska K: Effects of cations on parathyroid secretion and phospholipid metabolism. Proc. 63rd Ann. Meet. Endocrine Society, Cincinnati, 1981, Abstract No. 579.
23. Bellorin-Font E, Martin KJ, Fretag JJ, et al: Altered adenylate cyclase kinetics in hyperfunctioning human parathyroid glands. *J Clin Endocrinol Metabol* 52:409–507, 1981.
24. Onties DA, Mahafee DD, Wells SA: Adenylate cyclase activity in human parathyroid tissues: Reduced sensitivity to suppression by calcium in parathyroid adenomas as compared with normal glands from hyperparathyroid patients. *Metabolism* 30:406–411, 1981.
25. Brown EM: Relationship of 3'5'-adenosine monophosphate accumulation to parathyroid hormone release in dispersed cells from pathological human parathyroid tissue. *J Clin Endocrinol Metabol* 52:961–968, 1981.
26. Willgoss D, Jacobi JM, de Jersey J, et al: Effect of calcium on cyclic nucleotide phosphodiesterase in parathyroid tissue. *Biochem Biophys Res Commun* 94:763–768, 1980.
27. Oldham SB, Lipson LG, Tietjen GE: Presence of calmodulin in parathyroid adenomas. *Min Elect Metabol* 7:273–280, 1982.
28. Mahaffee DD, Copper CW, Ramp WK, et al: Magnesium promotes both parathyroid hormone secretion and adenosine 3'5' monophosphate production in rat parathyroid tissues and reverses the inhibitory effect of calcium on adenylate cyclase. *Endocrinology* 110:487–495, 1982.
29. Brown EM: Lithium induces abnormal calcium-regulated PTH release in dispersed bovine parathyroid cells. *J Clin Endocrinol Metabol* 52:1046–1048, 1981.
30. Wallace J, Scarpa A: Regulation of parathyroid hormone secretion in vitro by divalent cations and cellular metabolism. *J Biol Chem* 257:10613–10616, 1982.
31. Brown EM: PTH secretion in vivo and in vitro. *Min Elect Metabol* 8:130–150, 1982.

32. Habener JF, Potts JT Jr: Relative effectiveness of magnesium and calcium on the secretion and biosynthesis of parathyroid hormone in vitro. *Endocrinology* 98:197–202, 1976.
33. Mayer GP, Hurst JG: Sigmoidal relationship between parathyroid hormone secretion rate and plasma calcium concentration in calves. *Endocrinology* 102:1036–1042, 1978.
34. Segre GV, Harris ST, Neer R, et al: Plasma parathyroid hormone and calcium concentration in man. 3rd Annual Scientific Meeting, American Society of Bone Mineral Research, Cincinnati, 1981, p. 30A.
35. Fox J, Heath H: The "calcium clamp": Effect of constant hypocalcemia on parathyroid hormone secretion. *Am J Physiol* 240:E649–E655, 1981.
36. Fox J, Offord KP, Heath H: Episodic secretion of parathyroid hormone in the dog. *Am J Physiol* 241:E171–177, 1981.
37. Gittes RF, Radde IC: Experimental model for hyperparathyroidism: Effects of excessive numbers of transplanted isologous parathyroid glands. *J Urology* 95:595–603, 1966.
38. Mayer GP, Habener JF, Potts JT Jr: Parathyroid hormone secretion in vivo: Demonstration of a calcium independent, nonsuppressible component of secretion. *J Clin Invest* 57:678–683, 1976.
39. Brown EM, Wilson RE, Thatcher JG, et al: Abnormal calcium-regulated PTH release in normal parathyroid tissue from patients with adenoma. *Am J Med* 71:565–570, 1981.
40. Brown EM, Brennan MF, Hurwitz S: Dispersed cells prepared from human parathyroid glands: Distinct calcium sensitivity of adenomas vs. primary hyperplasia. *J Clin Endocrinol Metabol* 46:267–276, 1978.
41. Brown EM, Wilson RE, Eastman RC, et al: Abnormal regulation of parathyroid hormone release by calcium in secondary hyperparathyroidism due to chronic renal failure. *J Clin Endocrinol Metabol* 54:172–179, 1982.
42. McMahon MJ, Woodhead JS, Hayward RD: The nature of hypocalcemia in acute pancreatitis. *Br J Surg* 65:216–218, 1978.
43. McMahon MJ, Heyburn PJ, Playforth MS, et al: Parathyroid function during acute pancreatitis. *Br J Surg* 69:95–98, 1982.
44. Llach F, Felsenfeld AJ, Haussler MR: The pathophysiology of altered calcium metabolism in rhabdomyolysis. *N Engl J Med* 305:117–123, 1981.
45. Saxe AW, Chen SL, Marx SJ, et al: In vitro studies of parathyroid hormone release: Effect of cimetidine. *Surgery* 92:793–798, 1982.
46. Mallett RB, Sainsbury R, Benton K: Failure of cimetidine to suppress immunoreactive parathyroid hormone and hypercalcemia in primary hyperparathyroidism. *Postgrad Med J* 57:242–243, 1981.
47. Findling JW, Adams ND, LeMann J Jr, et al: Vitamin D metabolites and parathyroid hormone in Cushing's syndrome: Relationship to calcium and phosphorus homeostasis. *J Clin Endocrinol Metabol* 54:1039–1044, 1982.
48. Martin KJ, Hruska K, Freitag J, et al: Clinical utility of radioimmunoassay for parathyroid hormone. *Min Elect Metab* 8:263, 1980.
49. Nissenson RA, Abbott SR, Teitelbaum AP, et al: Endogenous biologically active human parathyroid hormone: Measurement by a guanyl nucleotide—amplified renal adenylate cyclase assay. *J Clin Endocrinol Metabol* 52:840, 1981.
50. Diamond B, Yelton DE, Scharff MD: Monoclonal antibodies. *N Engl J Med* 304:1344, 1981.
51. Reiss E, Canterbury JM: A radioimmunoassay for parathyroid hormone in man. *Proc Soc Exp Biol Med* 128:501–504, 1968.
52. Kao PCK: Parathyroid hormone assay. *Mayo Clin Proc* 57:596–598, 1982.

53. Brautbar N, Lee DBN, Kleeman CR: The divalent ions: Calcium phosphorus, magnesium and vitamin D, in Freinkel N (ed): *Contemporary Metabolism*. New York, Plenum Press, 1982, pp 441–509.
54. Goldstein DA, Chui LA, Massry SG: Peripheral nerve calcium and motor nerve conduction velocity in acute renal failure. *J Clin Invest* 62:88, 1978.
55. Goldstein DA, Massry SG: Effect of parathyroid hormone administration and withdrawal on brain calcium and electroencephalogram. *Min Elect Metabol* 1:84, 1978.
56. Akmal M, Goldstein DA, Multani S, et al: Role of uremia, increased serum calcium (Ca) and parathyroid hormone (PTH) on changes in encephalogram (EEG) in chronic renal failure. American Society Nephrology 15th Annual Meeting, Chicago, 1982, p 17A.
57. Meytes D, Bogin E, Ma A, et al: Effects of parathyroid hormone on erythrocytes. *J Clin Invest* 67:1263–1269, 1981.
58. Zevin D, Levi J, Bessler H, et al: Effect of parathyroid hormone and 1,25 dihydroxyvitamin D_3 on RNA and heme synthesis by erythroid precursors. *Min Elect Metabol* 6:125–129, 1981.
59. Shasha SM, Better OS, Winaver J, et al: Improvement in the anemia of hemodialyzed patients following subtotal parathyroidectomy. *Isr J Med Sci* 14:328–337, 1978.
60. Bogin E, Massry SG, Levi J, et al: Effect of parathyroid hormone on osmotic fragility of human erythrocytes. *J Clin Invest* 69:1017–1025, 1982.
61. Bogin E, Massry SG, Harary I: Effect of parathyroid hormone on rat heart cells. *J Clin Invest* 67:1215–1227, 1981.
62. Drueke T, Fleury I, Toure Y: Effects of parathyroidectomy on left ventricular function in hemodialysis patients. *Lancet* 1:112, 1980.
63. Baczynski R, Brautbar N, Carpenter C, et al: Effect of parathyroid hormone on energy metabolism of heart. 14th Annual Meeting of the American Society of Nephrology, 1981, Washington, DC, p 1A.
64. Bogin E, Levi J, Harary I, et al: Effects of parathyroid hormone on oxidative phosphorylation of heart mitochondria. *Min Elect Metabol* 7:151–156, 1982.
65. Brautbar N, Baczynski R, El-Belbessi S, et al: Effect of PTH on skeletal muscle: Role of PTH in uremic myopathy. 15th Annual Meeting, American Society of Nephrology, 1982, Chicago, p 119A.
66. Remuzzi G, Dodesini P, Livio M, et al: Parathyroid hormone inhibits human platelet function. *Lancet* 2:1321–1323, 1981.
67. Massry SG, Doherty CC, Kimball P, et al: Effect of intact parathyroid hormone (PTH) and its fragments on human polymorphonuclear leucocytes: Implications in uremia. 15th Annual Meeting, American Society of Nephrology, 1982, Chicago, p 12A.
68. Palmieri MAG, Nutting DE, Bhattcharya SK, et al: Parathyroid ablation in dystrophic hamsters. *J Clin Invest* 68:646–654, 1981.
69. Tomford RG, Karlinsky ML, Buddington B, et al: Effect of thyroparathyroidectomy and parathyroidectomy on renal function and the nephrotic syndrome in rat nephrotoxic serum nephritis. *J Clin Invest* 68:655–664, 1981.
70. Borle AB, Clark I: Effects of phosphate included hyperparathyroidism and parathyroidectomy on rat kidney calcium in vivo. *Am J Physiol* 241:E136–E141, 1981.
71. Tsutsumi M, Fukase M, Fujita T, et al: Parathyroid hormone in the plasma filtrate of uremic patients. *Min Elect Metabol* 7:146–150, 1982.
72. Frohling PT, Kokot F, Cernacek P, et al: Relation between middle molecules and parathyroid hormone in patients with chronic renal failure. *Min Elect Metabol* 7:48–53, 1982.
73. Furst P: Personal communications.

74. Broadus AE: Primary hyperparathyroidism viewed as a bihormonal disease process. *Min Elect Metabol* 8:199–214, 1982.
75. Broadus AE, Horst RL, Littledike ET, et al: Primary hyperparathyroidism with intermittent hypercalcemia: Serial observations and simple diagnosis by means of an oral calcium tolerance test. *Clin Endocrinol* 12:225, 1980.
76. Robinson MF, Body JJ, Offord KP, et al: Variation of plasma immunoreactive parathyroid hormone and calcitonin in normal and hyperparathyroid man during daylight hours. *J Clin Endocrinol Metabol* 55:538–544, 1982.
77. Russell CF, Grant CS, Van Heerden J: Hyperfunctioning supernumerary parathyroid glands. *Mayo Clin Proc* 57:121–124, 1982.
78. Shane E, Bilezikian JP: Parathyroid carcinoma: A review of 62 patients. *Endocrine Rev* 3:218–228, 1982.
79. Pattillo RA, Ruckett ACF, Wilson SD, et al: A human parathyroid carcinoma that produces parathyroid hormone: Long term maintenance in tissue culture. *J Clin Endocrinol Metabol* 53:641–644, 1981.
80. Malluche HH, Sherman D, Meyer W, et al: Effect of long term infusion of physiologic doses of 1-34 PTH on bone. *Am J Physiol* 242:F197–F201, 1982.
81. Podbesek R, Stevenson RW, Zanelli GD, et al: Treatment with human parathyroid hormone fragments (hPTH 1-34) stimulates bone formation and intestinal calcium absorption in the greyhound, in Cohn DN, Talmadge RV, Matthews JL (eds): *Hormonal Control of Calcium Metabolism*. Amsterdam, Excerpta Medica, 1981.
82. Slovik DM, Neer RM, Potts JT Jr: Short term effects of synthetic human parathyroid hormone (1-34) administration on bone mineral metabolism in osteoporotic patients. *J Clin Invest* 68:1261–1271, 1981.
83. Parsons JA, Meunier P, Podebesek R, et al: Pathological and therapeutic implications of the cellular and humoral responses to parathypin *Biochem Soc Trans* 9:383–386, 1981.
84. Podbesek R, Stevenson RW, Zanelli GD, et al: in Cohn DV, Talmage RG, Matthews JL(eds): *Hormonal Control of Calcium Metabolism*. Amsterdam, Excerpta Medica, 1981.
85. Howard GA, Drivadahl RH, Baylink DJ: Evidence for production and partial characterization of a coupling factor in bone metabolism. *Calcif Tiss Int* 131:53, 1980.
86. Ashton BA, Owen MR, Eagleson CC, et al: Inhibitory action of PTH on the differentiation of osteogenic precursor cells, in Cohn DV, Talmage RV, Matthews JL (eds): *Hormonal Control of Calcium Metabolism*. Amsterdam, Excerpta Medica, 1981.
87. Krieger NS, Tashjian AH Jr: Inhibition of parathyroid stimulated bone resorption by monovalent cation ionophores. *Calcif Tissue Int* 34:239–244, 1982.
88. Doppelt SH, Neer RM, Potts JT Jr: Human parathyroid hormone 1-34 mediated hypercalcemia in a rat model and its inhibition by dichloromethane diphosphate. *Calcif Tissue Int* 33:649–654, 1981.
89. Rambausek M, Ritz E, Rascher W, et al: Vascular effects of parathyroid hormone (PTH), in Massry SG, Letteri J, Ritz E (eds): Advances in Experimental Biology and Medicine. New York, Plenum Press, 1982, vol 131, pp 619–632.
90. Marone C, Beretta-Piccoli C, Weidmann P: Acute hypercalcemic hypertension in man: Role of hemodynamics, catecholamines and renin. *Kidney Int* 20:92– , 1981.
91. Hashimoto K, Nakagana Y, Shibaya T, et al: Effects of parathyroid hormone and related polypeptides on the heart and coronary circulation of dogs. *J Cardiovas Pharmacol* 3:668–676,1981.
92. Ellison DH, McCarron DA: Renal and cardiovascular response to Ca^{2+} infusion at varying Na^+ intakes in hypertensive humans. 15th Annual Meeting American Society Nephrology, 1982, Chicago, p 76A.

93. Rascher W, Rambauser M, Kreusser W, et al: Are prostaglandins and the sodium potassium pump involved in the vasodilatations induced by parathyroid hormone? 9th Scientific Meeting of the International Society for Hypertension, Mexico, 1982.
94. Saglikes Y, Campese VM, Massry SG: Mechanism of the hypotensive action of the intact and aminoterminal fragment of parathyroid hormone (PTH). 15th Annual Meeting, American Society Nephrology, 1982, Chicago, p 83A.
95. Mann JFE, Becker M, Ritz E: Effects of parathyroidectomy (PTX) on blood pressure (BP), body fluid and electrolyte homeostasis in normotensive and spontaneously hypertensive rats (SHR). 15th Annual Meeting, American Society of Nephrology, 1982. Chicago, p 79A.
96. Ritz E, Heuck CC, Boland R: Phosphate, calcium and lipid metabolism, in Massry SG, Ritz E, Jahn H, (eds): Advances in Experimental Biology and Medicine. New York, Plenum Press, vol 128, pp 405–416, 1980.
97. Paloyan E, Kolar J, Castles J, et al: The role of the parathyroids in lipid metabolism. *Fed Proc* 22:676, 1963.
98. LaCour B, Basile C, Drueke T, et al: Parathyroid functional lipid metabolism in the rat. *Min Elect Metabol* 7:157–165, 1982.
99. Michell RH: *Biochim Biophys Acta* 415:81–147, 1975.
100. Lo H, Lehotay DC, Katz D, et al: *Endocrine Res Commun* 3:377–385, 1976.
101. Farese RV, Bidot-Lopez P, Sabir A, et al: Parathyroid hormone acutely increases polyphosphoinostitides of the rabbit kidney cortex by a cyclohexamide-sensitive process. *J Clin Invest* 65:1523–1526, 1980.
102. Meltzer V, Weinreb S, Bellorin-Font E: Parathyroid hormone stimulation of renal phosphoinositide metabolism is a cyclic nucleotide-independent effect. *Biochim Biophys Acta* 712:258–267, 1982.
103. Wachman A, Bernstein DS: Parathyroid hormone in metabolic acidosis. Its role in PH homeostasis. *Clin Orthop Relat Res* 69:252–263, 1970.
104. Muldowney FP, Freaney R, McGeeny D: Renal tubular acidosis and aminoaciduria in osteomalacia of dietary or intestinal origin. *Q J Med* 37:517–539, 1968.
105. Arruda JAL, Nascimento L, Westenfelder C, et al: Effect of parathyroid hormone on urinary acidification. *Am J Physiol* 232:F429–F433, 1977.
106. Fraley DS, Adler S: An extrarenal role for parathyroid hormone in the disposal of acute acid loads in rats and dogs. *J Clin Invest* 63:985–997, 1979.
107. Arruda JAL, Alla V, Rubinstein M, et al: Parathyroid hormone and extrarenal acid buffering. *Am J Physiol* 239:F533, 1980.
108. Hulter HN, Sebastian A, Toto RB, et al: Renal and systemic acid base effects of the chronic administration of hypercalcemia-producing agents: Calcitriol, PTH and intravenous calcium. *Kidney Int* 21:445–458, 1982.
109. Madias EN, Johns CA, Homer SA: Independence of the acute acid buffering response from endogenous parathyroid hormone. *Am J Physiol* 243:F141–F149, 1982.
110. Caverzasio J, Hans-Jakob G, Fleisch H, et al: Parathyroid hormone-independent adaptation of the renal handling of phosphate in response to renal mass reduction. *Kidney Int* 21:471–476, 1982.
111. Wen SF, Stoll RW: Renal phosphate adaptation in uremia dogs with a remnant kidney. *Clin Sci* 60:273–282, 1981.
112. Jacob AI, Lanier D, Canterbury J, et al: Reduction by Cimetidine of serum parathyroid hormone levels in uremic patients. *N Engl J Med* 302:671–674, 1980.
113. Ichikawa I, Humes DH, Dousa TP, et al: Influence of parathyroid hormone on glomerular ultrafiltration in the rat. *Am J Physiol* 234:F393–F401, 1978.

114. Wang MS, Kurokawa K: Effects of parathyroid hormone and calcium ions on substrate oxidation by isolated glomeruli of the rat. *Biochim Biophys Acta* 677:397–402, 1981.
115. McKinney TD, Meyers P: Bicarbonate transport by proximal tubules: Effects of parathyroid hormone and dibutyryl cyclic AMP. *Am J Physiol* 138:F166–F174, 1980.
116. Lino Y, Burg MB: Effects of parathyroid hormone on bicarbonate reabsorption by proximal tubules in vitro. *Am J Physiol* 236:F387–F351, 1979.
117. McKinney DT, Myers P: PTH inhibition of bicarbonate transport by proximal convoluted tubules. *Am J Physiol* 239:F127–F134, 1980.
118. Humes HD, Simmons CF, Brenner BM: Interaction between antidiuretic hormone and parathyroid hormone on urine concentration. *Am J Physiol* 239:F244–F249, 1980.
119. Winaver J, Chen TC, Fragola J, et al: Alterations in renal tubular water transport induced by parathyroid hormone. *J Lab Clin Med* 99:457–473, 1982.
120. Puschett JB: Are all of the renal tubular actions of parathyroid hormone mediated by the adenylate cyclase system. *Min Elect Metabol* 7:281–285, 1982.
121. Nissenson RA, Kugal N, Arnaud CD: The parathyroid hormone receptor-adenylate cyclase in chicken renal plasma membrane. *J Biol Chem* 254:1469–1475, 1979.
122. Gura V, Friedler RM, Leibovici H, et al: On the role of nephrogenous cyclic AMP in the renal handling of sodium during PTH and diuretic administration. *Min Elect Metabol* 5:39, 1981.
123. Robertson JS, Winaver J, Syck DB, et al: Restoration of parathyroid hormone action on proximal tubular function by calcium repletion. 12th Annual Meeting, American Society Nephrology, 1979, Boston, p 64A.
124. Gruber HE, Stauffer ME, Thompson ER, et al: Diagnosis of bone disease by core biopsies. *Semin Hematol* 18:258–278, 1981.
125. Raisz L: Osteoporosis. *J Am Geriatr Soc* 30:127–138, 1982.
126. Gruber HE, Baylink DJ: The diagnosis of osteoporosis. *J Am Geriatr Soc* 29:490–497, 1981.
127. Whyte MP, Bergfeld MA, Murphy WA, et al: Postmenopausal osteoporosis. A heterogeneous disorder as assessed by histomorphometric analysis of iliac crest bone from untreated patients. *Am J Med* 72:193–202, 1982.
128. Burnell JM, Baylink DJ, Chesnut CH III, et al: Bone matrix and mineral abnormalities in postmenopausal osteoporosis. *Metabolism* 31:1113–1120, 1982.
129. Taggart H, Chesnut CH III, Ivey JL, et al: Deficient calcitonin response to calcium stimulation in postmenopausal osteoporosis? *Lancet* 1:475–478, 1982.
130. Aloia JF, Zanzi I, Vaswani A, et al: Combination therapy for osteoporosis with estrogen, fluoride and calcium. *J Am Geriatr Soc* 30:13–17, 1982.
131. Ivey JL, Baylink DJ: Postmenopausal osteoporosis: Proposed roles of defective coupling and estrogen deficiency. *Metabol Bone Dis Rel Res* 3:3–7, 1981.
132. Harrison JE, McNeill K, Sturtridge W, et al: Three-year changes in bone mineral mass of postmenopausal osteoporotic patients based on neutron activation analysis of the central third of the skeleton. *J Clin Endocrinol Metabol* 52:751–758, 1981.
133. Farley JR, Chesnut CH III, Baylink DJ: Improved method for quantitative determination in serum of alkaline phosphatase of skeletal origin. *Clin Chem* 27:2002–2007, 1981.
134 Wiske PW, Wentworth SM, Norton JA Jr, et al: Evaluation of bone mass and growth in young diabetics. *Metabolism* 31:848–854, 1982.
135. Mazes RB: On aging bone loss. *Clin Orthoped Rel Res* 165:239–252, 1982.
136. Riggs B, Wahner H, Dunn W, et al: Differential changes in bone mineral density of the appendicular and axial skeleton with aging: Relationship to spinal osteoporosis. *J Clin Invest* 67:328–335, 1981.

137. Riggs B, Wahner H, Seeman E, et al: Changes in bone mineral density of the proximal femur and spine with aging. Differences between the postmenopausal and senile osteoporosis syndromes. *J Clin Invest* 70:716–723, 1982.
138. Heaney RP: Calcium intake requirement and bone mass in the elderly. *J Lab Clin Med* 100:309–312, 1982.
139. Marcus R: The relationship of dietary calcium to the maintenance of skeletal integrity in man-an interface of endocrinology and nutrition. *Metabolism* 31:93–101, 1982.
140. Thalassinos N, Gutteridge D, Joplin G, et al: Calcium balance in osteoporotic patients on long-term oral calcium therapy with and without sex hormones. *Clin Sci* 62:221–226, 1982.
141. Stout DS: The effects of long-term immobilization on the histomorphology of human cortical bone. *Calc Tiss Int* 34:337–342, 1982.
142. Johnell O, Nilsson BE, Wiklund PE: Bone morphometry in alcoholics. *Clin Orthop Rel Res* 165:253–258, 1982.
143. Syftestadt GT, Urist MR: Bone aging. *Clin Orthoped Rel Res* 162:228–297, 1982.
144. Cochran M: Aspects of renal bone disease. *Aust N Z J Med* 11 (Suppl 1):33–37, 1981.
145. Massry SG: Mechanism of secondary hyperparathyroidism in renal failure: Role of phosphate retention, skeletal resistence to the calcimic action of parathyroid hormone and altered vitamin D metabolism, in Silberman M, Slavkin H (eds): *Current Advances in Skeletogenesis—Development, Bio-mineralization, Mediators and Metabolic Bone Disease*. Proceedings of the 5th International Workshop on Calcified Tissues. Excerpta Medica, Amsterdam, 1982, pp 467–474.
146. Torres A, Moya M: A new method for the assessment of bone mass in renal osteodystrophy. Usefulness of computerized tomography in hemodialysis patients. *Nephron* 30:231–236, 1982.
147. Weinstein RS, Sappington LJ: Qualitative bone defect in uremic osteosclerosis. *Metabolism* 31:805–811, 1982.
148. Frost HM, Griffith DL, Jee WS, et al: Histomorphometric changes in trabecular bone of renal failure patients treated with calcifediol. *Metabol Bone Dis Rel Res* 2:285–295, 1981.
149. Lindergard B: Changes in bone mineral content evaluated by photon absorptiometry before the start of active uremia treatment. *Clin Nephrol* 16:126–130, 1981.
150. Brown DJ, Dawborn JK, Thomas DP, et al: Assessment of osteodystrophy in patients with chronic renal failure. *Aust N Z J Med* 12:250–254, 1982.
151. Christiansen C, Christensen MS, Melsen F, et al: Mineral metabolism in chronic renal failure with special reference to serum concentrations of 1,25(OH)$_2$D. *Clin Nephrol* 15:18–22, 1981.
152. Sideman S, Manor D: The dialysis dementia syndrome and aluminum intoxication. *Nephron* 31:1–10, 1982.
153. Ellis HA, McCarthy JH, Herrington J: Bone aluminum in haemodialysed patients and in rats injected with aluminum chloride: Relationship to impaired bone mineralisation. *J Clin Pathol* 32:832–844, 1979.
154. Cournot-Witmer G, Zingraff J, Plachot J, et al: Aluminum localization in bone from hemodialyzed patients: Relationship to matrix mineralization. *Kidney Int* 20:375–385, 1981.
155. Buchanan M, Ihle B, Dunn C: Haemodialysis related osteomalacia: A staining method to demonstrate aluminum. *J Clin Pathol* 34:1352–1354, 1981.
156. Maloney N, Ott S, Alfrey A, et al: Histological quantitation of aluminum in iliac bone from patients with renal failure. *J Lab Clin Med* 99:206–216, 1982.
157. Hodsman A, Sherrard D, Alfrey A, et al: Bone aluminum and histomorphometric features of renal osteodystrophy. *J Clin Endocrinol Metabol* 54:539–546, 1982.

158. Walker GS, Aaron JE, Peacock M, et al: Dialysate aluminum concentration and renal bone disease. Kidney Int 21:411–415, 1982.
159. Fleming L, Stewart W, Fell G, et al: The effect of oral aluminum therapy on plasma aluminum levels in patients with chronic renal failure in an area with low water aluminum. Clin Nephrol 17:222–227, 1982.
160. Felsenfeld AJ, Gutman R, Llach F, et al: Osteomalacia in chronic renal failure: A syndrome previously reported only with maintenance dialysis. Am J Nephrol 2:147–154, 1982.
161. Lieberherr M, Grosse B, Cournot-Witmer G, et al: In vitro effects of aluminum on bone phosphatases: A possible interaction with bPTH and vitamin D_3 metabolites. Calc Tiss Int 34:280–284, 1982.
162. Parfitt AM: Hypercalcemic Hyperparathyroidism following renal transplantation: Differential diagnosis, management, and implications for cell population control in the parathyroid gland. Min Elect Metabol 8:92–112, 1982.
163. Tam CS, Bayley A, Cross EG, et al: Increased bone apposition in primary hyperparathyroidism: Measurements based on short interval tetracycline labelling of bone. Metabolism 31:759–765, 1982.
164. Seeman E, Wahner W, Offord K, et al: Differential effects of endocrine dysfunction on the axial and the appendicular skeleton. J Clin Invest 69:1302–1309, 1982.
165. Charhon S, Edouard C, Arlot ME, et al: Effects of parathyroid hormone on remodelling of iliac trabecular bone packets in patients with primary hyperparathyroidism. Clin Orthop Rel Res 162:255–263, 1982.
166. Sharp C, Rude R, Terry R, et al: Abnormal bone and parathyroid histology in carcinoma patients with pseudohyperparathyroidism. Cancer 49:1449–1455, 1982.
167. Jastrup B, Mosekilde L, Melsen F, et al: Serum levels of vitamin D metabolites and bone remodelling in hyperthyroidism. Metabolism 31:126–131, 1982.
168. Melgram JW, Jasty M: Osteopetrosis. J Bone Joint Surg 64A:912–929, 1982.
169. Manzke E, Gruber HE, Hiness RW, et al: Skeletal remodelling and bone related hormones in two adults with increased bone mass. Metabolism 31:25–32, 1982.
170. Key F, Cole F, Teitelbaum SL, et al: Osteopetrosis: Response to high-dose calcitriol. Calc Tiss Int 34(Suppl 1):S32, 1982 (abstract).
171. Gillette ME, Insogna KL, Lewis AM, et al: Influence of pregnancy on immunoreactive parathyroid hormone levels. Calc Tiss 34:9–12, 1982.
172. Seino Y, Ishida M, Yamaoka K, et al: Serum calcium regulating hormones in the perinatal period. Calc Tiss Int 34:131–135, 1982.
173. Miller SC, Holloran BP, DeLuca HF, et al: Role of vitamin D in maternal skeletal changes during pregnancy and lactation: A histomorphometric study. Calc Tiss Int 34:245–252, 1982.
174. Deftos LJ, Parthemore JG, Price PA: Changes in plasma bone GLA protein during treatment of bone disease. Calc Tiss Int 34:121–124, 1982.
175. Stewart AF, Vignery A, Silverglate A, et al: Quantitative bone histomorphometry in humoral hypercalcemia of malignancy: Uncoupling of bone cell activity. J Clin Endocrinol Metabol 55:219–227, 1982.
176. Berger ME, Golub MS, Sowers JR, et al: Hypercalcemia in association with a Leydig cell tumor in the rat: A model for tumor-induced hypercalcimia in man. Life Sci 30:1509–1515, 1982.
177. Doty SB: Morphological evidence of gap junctions between bone cells. Calc Tiss Int 33:509–512, 1981.
178. Mills BG: Comparison of the ultrastructure of a malignant tumor of the mandible containing giant cells with Paget's disease of bone. J Oral Pathol 10:203–215, 1981.

179. Chambers TJ, Dunn CJ: Osteoclast activity is determined by intracellular cAMP levels, in Silberman M, Slavkin H (eds): *Current Advances in Skeletogenesis—development, Biomineralization, Mediators and Metabolic bone disease.* Proceedings of the 5th International Workshop on Calcifice Tissues. Amsterdam, Excerpta Medica, 1982, pp 154–159.

180. Chambers TJ: Osteoblasts release osteoclasts from calcitonin-induced quiescence. *J Cell Sci* 57:247–260, 1982.

181. Liu CC, Rader JI, Gruber HE, et al: Acute reduction in osteoclast number during bone repletion. *Metabol Bone Dis Rel Res* 4:201–209, 1982.

182. Minkin C: Bone acid phosphatase: Tartrate-resistant acid phosphatase as a marker of osteoclast function. *Calc Tiss Int* 34:285–290, 1982.

183. Stern PH, Orr M, Brull E: Ionophore A23187 promotes osteoclast function in bone organ culture. *Calc Tiss Int* 34:31–36, 1982.

184. Krieger NS, Tashjian AH Jr: Inhibition of parathyroid hormone-stimulated bone resorption by monovalent cation ionophores. *Calc Tiss Int* 34:239–244, 1982.

185. Tashjian AH Jr, Ivey JL: Stimulation of bone resorption in organ culture by cholera toxin. *Biochem Biophys Res Comm* 102:1055–1064, 1981.

186. Rabadjija L, Goldhaber P: Amphotericin B: Stimulation of bone resorption in organ culture. *Proc Soc Exp Bio Med* 169:326–333, 1982.

187. Goldhaber P, Rabadjija L: Effect of promethazine hydrochloride on bone resorption in tissue culture. *Proc Soc Exp Bio Med* 169:105–109, 1982.

188. Shlossman M, Brown M, Shapiro E, et al: Calcitonin effects on isolated bone cells. *Calc Tiss Int* 34:190–196, 1982.

189. Krieger NS, Feldman RS, Tashjian AH Jr: Parathyroid hormone and calcitonin interactions in bone: Irradiation-induced inhibition of escape in vitro. *Calc Tiss Int* 34:197–203, 1982.

190. Norimatsu H, Yamamoto T, Ozawa H, et al: Changes in calcium phosphate on bone surfaces and in lining cells after the administration of parathyroid hormone or calcitonin. *Clin Orthop Rel Res* 164:271–277, 1982.

191. Reitsma PH, Tietelbaum SL, Bijvoet OLM, et al: Differential action of the biphosphonates (3-amino-1-hydroxypropylidine)-1,1-biphosphonate (APD) on rat macrophage-mediated bone resorption in vitro. *J Clin Invest* 70:927–933, 1982.

192. Nijweide PJ, van der Plas A, Scherft JP: Biochemical and histological studies on various bone cell preparations. *Calc Tiss Int* 33:529–540, 1981.

193. Lindholm TS, Nilsson OS, Lindholm TC: New bone formation and parathyroid activity effected by 1αhydroxyvitamin D₃. *Clin Orthoped Rel Res* 162:264–269, 1982.

194. Farley JR, Puzas JE, Baylink DJ: Effect of skeletal alkaline phosphatase inhibitors on bone cell proliferation in vitro. *Min Elect Metabol* 7:316–323, 1982.

195. Nijweide P, van Iperen-van Gent A, Kawailarang-de Haas E, et al: Bone formation and calcification by isolated osteoblastlike cell. *J Cell Biol* 93:318–323, 1982.

196. Puzas JE, Drivdahl RH, Howard GA, et al: Endogenous inhibitor of bone cell proliferation. *Proc Soc Exp Bio Med* 166:113–122, 1981.

197. Baylink DJ, Farley J, Howard GA, et al: Coupling factor, in Massry S, Letteri J, Ritz E (eds): *Regulation of Phosphate and Mineral Metabolism.* New York, Plenum Press, 1982, pp 409–421.

198. Howard GA, Bottemiller B, Turner R, et al: Parathyroid hormone stimulated bone formation and resorption in organ culture: Evidence for a coupling mechanism. *Proc Natl Acad Sci* 78:3204–3208, 1981.

199. Howard GA, Bottemiller BL, Baylink DJ: Evidence for the coupling of bone formation to bone resorption in vitro. *Metabol Bone Dis Rel Res* 2:131–135, 1980.

200. Kato Y, Watanabe R, Nomura Y, et al: Effect of bone derived growth factor on DNA, RNA and proteoglycan synthesis in cultures of rabbit costal chondrocytes. *Metabolism* 31:812–815, 1982.
201. Deluca HF: The vitamin D system: A view from basic science to the clinic. *Clin Biochem* 14:213–222, 1981.
202. DeLuca HF: The transformation of a vitamin into a hormone: The vitamin D story. *Harvey Lect* 75:333–379, 1979.
203. DeLuca HF: Subcellular mechanisms involving vitamin D. *Subcell Biochem* 8:251–272, 1981.
204. Koshy KT: Vitamin D: An uptake. *J Pharm Sci* 71:137–153, 1982.
205. Haussler HR, Cordy PE: Metabolites and analogues of vitamin D. Which for what? *JAMA* 247:841–844, 1982.
206. Vitamin D preparations up-to-date. *Drug Ther Bull* 19(26):103–104, 1981.
207. Chesney RW: Current clinical applications of vitamin D metabolite research. *Clin Orthop* 161:285–314, 1981.
208. Lee DBN, Brautbar N, Massry SG: Renal production and biologic actions of vitamin D metabolites. *Sem Nephrol* 1:335–355, 1981.
209. Haddad, JG: Vitamin D binding proteins. *Adv Nutr Res* 4:35–58, 1982.
210. Bouillon R, Van Baelen H: The transport of vitamin D: Significance of free and total concentrations of vitamin D metabolites, in Norman AW, Schaefer K, Herrath DV (eds): *Vitamin D. Chemical, Biochemical and Clinical Endocrinology of Calcium Metabolism.* Berlin, Walter de Gruyter, 1982, pp 1181-1186.
211. Hollis EW, Roos BA, Lambert PW: Vitamin D compounds in human and bovine milk. *Adv Nutr Res* 4:59–75, 1982.
212. Hadd JG: Human serum binding protein for vitamin D and its metabolites (DEP): Evidence that actin is the DBP binding component in human skeletal muscle. *Arch Biochem Biophys* 213:538–544, 1982.
213. Reeve LE, Chesney RW, DeLuca HF: Vitamin D of human milk: Identification of biologically active forms. *Am J Clin Nutr* 36:122–126, 1982.
214. Halloran BP, DeLuca HF: Vitamin D deficiency and reproduction in rats. *Science* 204:73, 1979.
215. Halloran BP, Barthell EN, DeLuca HF: Vitamin D metabolism during pregnancy and lactation in the rat. *Proc Natl Acad Sci USA* 76:5549, 1979.
216. Noff D, Edelstein S: Vitamin D and its hydroxylated metabolites in the rat. Placental and lacteal transport, subsequent metabolic pathways and tissue distribution. *Horm Res* 9:292, 1978.
217. Ueng TH, Golub EE, Bronner F: The effect of age and 1,25-dihydroxyvitamin D_3 treatment on the intestinal calcium-binding protein of suckling rats. *Arch Biochem Biophys* 196:624, 1979.
218. Ambrecht HJ, Wasserman RH: Enhancement of Ca^{++} uptake by lactose in the rat small intestine. *J Nutr* 106:1265, 1976.
219. Pansu D, Bellaton C, Bronner F: Effect of lactose on duodenal calcium-binding protein and calcium absorption. *J Nutr* 109:508, 1979.
220. Schaafsma G, Visser R: Nutritional interrelationships between calcium, phosphorus and lactose in rats. *J Nutr* 110:1101, 1980.
221. Delvin EE, Glorieux FH, Salle BL, et al: Control of vitamin D metabolism in preterm infants: Feto-maternal relationships. *Arch Dis Child* 57:754–757, 1982.
222. Salle BL, David L, Glorieux FH, et al: Early oral administration of vitamin D and its metabolites in premature neonates. Effect on mineral homeostasis. *Pediatr Res* 16:75–78, 1982.

223. Rothberg AD, Pettifor JM, Cohen DF, et al: Maternal-infant vitamin D relationships during breast-feeding. *J Pediatr* 101:500–503, 1982.
224. Chan GM, Roberts CC, Folland D, et al: Growth and bone mineralization of normal breast-fed infants and the effects of lactation on maternal bone mineral status. *Am J Clin Nutri* 36:438–443, 1982.
225. Greer FR, Searcy JE, Levin RS, et al: Bone mineral content and serum 25-hydroxyvitamin D concentrations in breast-fed infants with and without supplemental vitamin D: One year follow-up. *J Pediatr* 100:919–922, 1982.
226. Aksnes L, Aarskog D: Plasma concentrations of vitamin D metabolites in puberty: Effect of sexual maturation and implications for growth. *J Clin Endocrinol Metab* 55:94–101, 1982.
227. MacFarlane IA, Mawer EB, Berry J, et al: Vitamin D metabolism in hyperthyroidism. *Clin Endocrinol* 17:51–59, 1982.
228. Jastrup B, Nosekiloe L, Melsen F, et al: Serum levels of vitamin D metabolites and bone remodelling in hyperthyroidism. *Metabolism* 31:126–132, 1982.
229. Emmertsen K, Melsen F, Mosekilde L, et al: Altered vitamin D metabolites and bone remodelling in patients with medullary thyroid carcinoma and hypercalcitoninemia. *Metabol Bone Dis Rel Res* 4:17–23, 1982.
230. Frazer TE, White NH, Hough S, et al: Alterations in circulating vitamin D metabolites in the young insulin-dependent diabetic. *J Clin Endocrinol Metab* 53:1154–1159, 1981.
231. Findling JW, Adams ND, Lemann J Jr, et al: Vitamin D metabolites and parathyroid hormone in Cushing's syndrome: Relationships to calcium and phosphorus homeostasis. *J Clin Endocrinol Metab* 54:1039–1044, 1982.
232. Christiansen C, Rodbro P, Nestoft J, et al: A possible direct effect of 24,25-dihydroxycholecalciferol on the parathyroid gland in patients with chronic renal failure. *Clin Endocrinol* 15:237–242, 1981.
233. Delmez JA, Slatopolsky E, Martin KJ, et al: Minerals, vitamin D, and parathyroid hormone in continuous ambulatory peritoneal dialysis. *Kidney Int* 21:862–867, 1982.
234. Chesney RW, Hamstra AJ, Mazess RB, et al: Circulating vitamin D metabolites concentrations in childhood renal diseases. *Kidney Int* 21:65–69, 1982.
235. Cunningham J, Fraher LJ, Clemens TL, et al: Chronic acidosis with metabolic bone disease. Effect of alkali on bone morphology and vitamin D metabolism. *Am J Med* 73:199–204, 1982.
236. Mason RS, Rohl PG, Lissner D, et al: Vitamin D metabolism in hypophosphatemic rickets. *Am J Dis Child* 136:909–913, 1982.
237. Loeffler RD, Sheman FC: The effect of treatment on growth and deformity in hypophosphatemic vitamin D-resistant rickets. *Clin Orthop* 162:4–10, 1982.
238. Lund B, Sorensen OH, Lund B, et al: Vitamin D metabolism and osteomalacia in patients with fracture of the proximal femur. *Acta Orthop Scand* 53:251–254, 1982.
239. Compston JE, Vedi S, Merrett AL, et al: Privational and malabsorption metabolic bone disease: Plasma vitamin D metabolite concentrations and their relationship to quantitative bone histology. *Metabol Bone Dis Rel Res* 3:165–170, 1981.
240. Rickers H, Dedling A, Christiansen C, et al: Corticosteroid-induced osteopenia and vitamin D metabolism. Effect of vitamin D_2, calcium phosphate and sodium fluoride administration. *Clin Endocrinol* 16:409–415, 1982.
241. Sorensen OH, Lumholtz B, Lund B, et al: Acute effects of parathyroid hormone on vitamin D metabolism in patients with bone loss of aging. *J Clin Endocrinol Metab* 54:1258–1261, 1982.
242. van Kesteren RG, Duursma SA, Visser WJ, et al: Fluoride in serum and bone during treatment of osteoporosis with sodium fluoride, calcium and vitamin D. *Metabol Bone Dis Rel Res* 4:31–37, 1982.

243. Epstein D, Kato Y, Dick R, et al: Vitamin D, hydroxyapatite, and calcium gluconate in treatment of cortical bone thinning in postmenopausal women with primary biliary cirrhosis. *Am J Clin Nutr* 36:426–430, 1982.
244. Opshaug O, Maurseth K, Howlid H, et al: Vitamin D metabolism in hypophosphatasia. *Acta Paediatr Scand* 71:517–521, 1982.
245. Clemens TL, Adams JS, Nolan JM, et al: Measurement of circulating vitamin D in man. *Clin Chim Acta* 121:301–308, 1982.
246. Thompson JN, Hatina G, Maxwell WB, et al: High performance liquid chromatographic determination of vitamin D in fortified milks, margarine and infant formulas. *J Assoc Off Anal Chem* 65:624–631, 1982.
247. Brodie MJ, Boobis AR, Hillyard CJ, et al: Effect of rifampicin and isoniazid on vitamin D metabolism. *Clin Pharmacol Ther* 32:525–530, 1982.
248. Breslau NA, McGuire JL, Zerwekh JE, et al: The role of dietary sodium on renal excretion and intestinal absorption of calcium and on vitamin D metabolism. *J Clin Endocrinol Metab* 55:369–373, 1982.
249. Okano K, Furukawa Y, Morii H, et al: Comparative efficacy of various vitamin D metabolites in the treatment of various types of hypoparathyroidism. *J Clin Endocrinol Metab* 55:238–243, 1982.
250. Aliaga A, Serrano G, de la Cuadra J, et al: Perforating granuloma annulare and vitamin D. *Dermatologica* 164:62–66, 1982.
251. Norman AW, Schaefer K, Herrath D-V, et al (eds): *Vitamin D—Chemical, Biochemical and Clinical Endocrinology of Calcium Metabolism*. Berlin, Walter de Gruyter, 1982.
252. Chance B, Eleff S, Leigh JS, et al: Mitochondrial regulation of phosphocreatine/inorganic phosphorus ratios in exercising human muscle: A gated ^{31}P NMR study. *Proc Nat Acad Sci USA* 78:6714–6718, 1981.
253. Gadian D, Ross B, Bore P, et al: Examination of a myopathy by phosphorus nuclear magnetic resonnance. *Lancet* 2:774–777, 1981.
254. Newman RJ, Bore PJ, Chan L, et al: Nuclear magnetic resonnance studies of forearm muscle in Duchene dystrophy. *Br Med J* 284:1072–1074.
255. Grove TH, Ackerman JH, Radda GK, et al: Analysis of rat heart in vivo by phosphorus nuclear magnetic resonnance. *Proc Nat Acad Sci USA* 77:299–302, 1980.
256. Bessman SP, Grieger PJ, Sung-Cho-Lu T, et al: Separation and automated analysis of phosphorylated metabolic intermediates. *Ann Biochem* 53:533–546, 1974.
257. Brautbar N, Baczynski R, Carpenter C, et al: Impaired energy metabolism in rat myocardium during phosphate depletion. *Am J Physiol* 242:F699–F704, 1982.
258. Brautbar N, Geiger PJ: Rapid method for separation of phosphorylated intermediates. Application to biopsy specimens. *Biochem Med* (in press).
259. Swaminathan R, Bradley P, Morgan DB, et al: Hypophosphatemia in the surgical patient. *Surg Gynecol Obstet* 148:448–454, 1979.
260. Hessov I, Jensen NG, Rasmussen A: Prevention of hypophosphatemia during postoperative routine glucose administration. *Acta Chir Scand* 146:109–114, 1980.
261. Lenquist S, Lindell B, Nordstrom N, et al: Hypophosphatemia in severe burns. *Acta Chir Scand* 145:1–6, 1979.
262. Garabedian M, Silve C, Levy D, et al: Chronic hypophosphatemia in kidney transplanted children and young adults in health and disease, in Massry SG, Ritz E, Jahn H (eds): *Phosphate and Minerals in Health and Disease*. New York, Plenum Press, 1980, pp 249–254.
263. Farrington K, Varghese Z, Newman SP, et al: Dissociation of absorption of calcium phosphate after successful cadaveric transplantation. *Br Med J* 1:712–714, 1979.
264. Walker GS, Peacock M, Marshall DH, et al: Factors influencing the intestinal absorption of calcium and phosphorus following renal transplantation. *Nephron* 26:225–229, 1980.

265. Kovarik J, Grad H, Stummvoll HK, et al: Tubular phosphate handling after successful kidney transplantation. *Klin Wochensch* 58:763–869, 1980.
266. Rosenbaum RW, Hruska KA, Korkor A, et al: Decreased phosphate reabsorption after renal transplantation: Evidence for a mechanism independent of calcium and parathyroid hormone. *Kidney Int* 19:568–578, 1981.
267. Brautbar N, Leibovici H, Massry SG: On the mechanism of hypophosphatemia during acute hyperventilation: Evidence for increased muscle glycolysis. *Min Elect Metabol* 9:45–50, 1983.
268. Knochel JP: Hypophosphatemia. *West J Med* 134:15–26, 1981.
269. Ferguson ER, Blanchley JD, Knochel JP: Experimental alcoholism induces phosphorus and magnesium deficiency in skeletal muscle, in Massry SG, Letteri J, Ritz E (eds): *Advances in Experimental Biology and Medicine*. New York, Plenum Press, 1982, pp 291–302.
270. Spencer H, Kramer L, Norris C, et al: Effect of small doses of aluminum-containing antacids on calcium and phosphorus metabolism. *Am J Clin Nutr* 36:32–40, 1982.
271. Atchley DW, Loeb RF, Richards DW, et al: On diabetic acidosis. A detailed study of electrolyte balances following the withdrawal and reestablishment of insulin therapy. *J Clin Invest* 12:297, 1933.
272. Franks M, Berris RF, Kaplan NO, et al: Metabolic studies in diabetic acidosis. II. The effect of administration of sodium phosphate. *Arch Intern Med* 81:42, 1948.
273. Sterling MA: Diabetic keto acidosis in childhood. *Pediatr Clin North Am* 26:152, 1979.
274. Gibby OM, Veale KEA, Hayes TM, et al: Oxygen availability from the blood and the effect of phosphate replacement on erythrocyte 2,3-diphosphoglycerate and hemoglobin-oxygen affinity in diabetic ketoacidosis. *Diabetologia* 15:381–385, 1978.
275. Kanter Y, Gerson JR, Bessman AN: 2,3-Diphosphoglycerate, nucleotide phosphate, and organic and inorganic phosphate levels during the early phases of diabetic ketoacidosis. *Diabetes* 26:429–433, 1977.
276. Keller U, Berger W: Prevention of hypophosphatemia by phosphate infusion during treatment of diabetic ketoacidosis and hyperosmolar coma. *Diabetic* 29:87–95, 1980.
277. Raskin P, Pak CYC: The effect of chronic insulin therapy on phosphate metabolism in diabetes mellitus. *Diabetologia* 21:50–53, 1981.
278. Gertner JM, Tamborlane WV, Horst RL, et al: Mineral metabolism in diabetes mellitus: Changes in accompanying treatment with a probable subcutaneous insulin infusion system. *J Clin Endocrinol Metabol* 50:862–866, 1980.
279. Farrington K, Varghese Z, Baillod RA, et al: Hypophosphatemia after parathyroidectomy in chronic renal failure. *Br Med J* 284:856–885, 1982.
280. Darsee JR, Nutter DO: Reversible severe congestive cardiomyopathy in three cases of hypophosphatemia. *Ann Intern Med* 89:867, 1978.
281. O'Connor LR, Wheeler WS, Bethune JE: Effect of hypophosphatemia on myocardial performance in man. *N Engl J Med* 297:901–903, 1977.
282. Fuller TJ, Nichols WW, Brenner BJ, et al: Reversible depression in myocardial performance in dogs with experimental phosphorus deficiency. *J Clin Invest* 62:1194–1200, 1978.
283. Kreusser W, Vetter HO, Mittman U, et al: Haemodynamics and myocardial metabolism of phosphorus depleted dogs: Effect of catecholamines and angiotensin II. *Eur J Clin Invest* 12:219–228, 1982.
284. Campese VM, Saglikes Y, Brautbar N, et al: Effect of phosphate depletion in blood pressure. 15th Annual Meeting, American Soc. of Nephrology, Chicago, 1982, p 4A.
285. Fuller TJ, Carter NW, Barcenas C, et al: Reversible changes of the muscle cell in experimental phosphorus deficiency. *J Clin Invest* 57:1019, 1976.

286. Brautbar N, Carpenter C, Baczynski R, et al: Impaired skeletal muscle energetics in phosphate depleted rats. *Kidney Int* (in press).
287. Newman JH, Neff TA, Ziporin P: Acute respiratory failure associated with hypophosphatemia. *N Engl J Med* 296:1101–1103, 1933.
288. Planas RF, McBrayer RH, Koen PA: Effects of hypophosphatemia on pulmonary muscle performance, in Massry SG, Letteri J, Ritz E (eds): *Advances in Experimental Biology Medicine*. New York, Plenum Press, 1981, pp 283–290.
289. Gold LN, Massry SG, Friedler RM: Effect of phosphate depletion in renal tubular reabsorption of glucose. *J Lab Clin Med* 89:554, 1977.
290. Harter HR, Santiago JU, Rutherford WE, et al: The relative role of calcium, phosphorus and parathyroid hormone in glucose and tolbutamide mediated insulin release. *J Clin Invest* 58:359–367, 1976.
291. Davis JL, Lewis SB, Schultz TA, et al: Acute and chronic phosphate depletion as a modulator of glucose uptake in rat skeletal muscle. *Life Sci* 24:629–632, 1979.
292. Defronzo RA, Lang R: Hypophosphatemia and glucose intolerance: Evidence for tissue insensitivity to insulin. *N Engl J Med* 303:1259, 1980.
293. Brautbar N, Moser S, Finander P, et al: Effect of phosphate depletion on cell membrane phospholipids and glucose pathway in kidney, liver and skeletal muscle. *Clin Res* 30:52A, 1981c.
294. Horl WH, Kreusser W, Heidland A, et al: Abnormalities of glucose metabolism in cardiomyopathy of phosphorus depletion, in: Massry SG, Ritz E, Jahn H (eds): *Advances in Experimental Biology Medicine*. New York, Plenum Press, 1980, pp 343–350.
295. Horl WH, Kreusser W, Heidland A, et al: Defective hormonal stimulation of isolated hepatocytes in phosphorus depleted rats, in Massry SG, Letteri J, Ritz E (eds): *Advances in Experimental Biology Medicine*. New York, Plenum Press, 1982, pp 303–308.
296. Ramsay AM, Douglas LJ: Effects of phosphate limitation of growth on the cell-wall and lipid composition of Saccharomyces cerevisiae. *J Gen Microbiol* 110:185–191, 1979.
297. Brautbar N, Moser S, Massry SG: Effect of phosphate depletion on cell membrane phospholipids and glucose pathway in kidney and skeletal muscle. 14th Annual Meeting, American Society of Nephrology, Washington, DC, 1981, p 125A.
298. Brautbar N, Tabernero-Romo J, Coato J, et al: Myocardial fatty acid oxidation and phospholipid metabolism during phosphate depletion. *Clin Res* 31:52A, 1983.
299. Kleeman, CR: Should hypophosphatemia be treated? in Massry SG, Letteri J, Ritz E (eds): *Advances in Experimental Biology Medicine*. New York, Plenum Press, 1982, pp 309–318.
300. Knochel JP: Hypophosphatemia in the alcoholic. *Arch Intern Med* 140:613–614, 1980.
301. Vannatta JB, Whang R, Papper S: Efficacy of intravenous phosphorus therapy in the severely hypophosphatemic patient. *Arch Intern Med* 141:885–887, 1981.
302. Wu TS, Pieper GM, Salhany JM, et al: Measurement of free magnesium in perfused and ischemic arrested heart muscle. *Biochemistry* 20:7399–7403, 1981.
303. Bershon MM, Shine KI, Sterman WD: Effect of increased magnesium on recovery from ischemia in rat and rabbit hearts. *Am J Physiol* 242:H89–H93, 1983.
304. Iseri LT, Bures AR: Serious ventricular arrhythmias due to magnesium deficiency, in Cantin M, Seelig MS (eds): *Magnesium in Health and Disease*. New York, Spectrum Publications, 1980, pp 559–563.
305. Seelig MS, Heggtreit HA: Magnesium interrelationship in ischemic heart disease. *Am J Clin Nutr* 27:59, 1974.
306. Manthey J, Stoeppler M, Morgenstern W, et al: Magnesium and trace methods: Risk factors for coronary heart disease? *Circulation* 64:722–729, 1981.

307. Saetersdal T, Engedal H, Roli J, et al: Calcium and magnesium levels in isolated mitochondria from human cardiac biopsies. *Histochemistry* 68:1–8, 1980.
308. Flink EB, Brick JE, Shane SR: Alterations of long chain free fatty acid and magnesium concentration in acute myocardial infarction. *Arch Intern Med* 141:441–443, 1981.
309. Sodi-Pallares D, Testelli MR, Fishleder BL: Effects of an intravenous infusion of a potassium-glucose-insulin solution on the electrocardiographic signs of myocardial infarction. *Am J Cardiol* 9:166–181, 1962.
310. Lim P, Jacob E: Magnesium deficiency in patients on long-term diuretic therapy for heart failure. *Br Med J* 3:620, 1972.
311. Furukawa Y, Chiba S: Effects of magnesium on the isolated blood perfused atrial and ventricular preparations of dog heart. *Jap Heart J* 22:239–246, 1981.
312. Hazard R, Wurmser L: Action de selts de magnesium sur les vasoconstricteurs ranaux. *CR Soc Biol* 110:525–528, 1932.
313. Altura BM, Altura BT: Magnesium ion and contraction of vascular smooth muscles: Relationship to some vascular diseases. *Fed Proc* 40:2672–2679, 1981.
314. Turlapaty, PDMV, Altura BM: Magnesium deficiency produces spasms of coronary arteries: Relationship to etiology of sudden death ischemic heart disease. *Science* 208:198–200, 1980.
315. Turlapaty PDMV, Altura BM: Magnesium ions and contractions of alloxan diabetic vascular muscle artery. *Artery* 6:375–384, 1980.
316. Turlapaty PDMV, Altura BT, Altura BM: Ca uptake and distribution in alloxan diabetic rat arterial and venous smooth muscle. *Experientia* 36:1298–1299, 1980.
317. Turlapaty PDMV, Weiner R, Altura BM: Interactions of magnesium and verapamil on tone and contractibility of vascular smooth muscle. *Eur J Pharm* 76:268–272, 1981.
318. Moreland RS, Ford GD: The influence of magnesium on calcium-activated, vascular smooth muscle actomyosin ATPase activity. *Arch Biochem Biophys* 208:325–333, 1981.
319. Stendig-Lindberg G, Bergström J, Hultman E: Hypomagnesemia, muscle electrolytes and metabolites. *Acta Med Scand* 201:273–280, 1977.
320. Anderson R, Haller R, Elms J, et al: Skeletal muscle phosphorus and magnesium deficiency in alcoholic myopathy. *Min Elect Metabol* 4:106–112, 1980.
321. Cronin RE, Ferguson ER, Shannon WA, et al: Skeletal muscle injury after magnesium depletion in the dog. *Am J Physiol* 243:F113–F120, 1982.
322. Potter JD, Robertson SP, Johnson JD: Magnesium and the regulation of muscle contraction. *Fed Proc* 40:2653–2656, 1981.
323. Stephenson E: Magnesium effect on activation of skinned fibers from striated muscle. *Fed Proc* 40:2662–2666, 1981.
324. Hasselbach W, Fassold E, Migala A, et al: Magnesium dependence of sarcoplasmic reticulum calcium transport. *Fed Proc* 40:2657–2661, 1981.
325. Mather HM, Nibet JA, Burton GH, et al: Hypomagnesemia in diabetes. *Clin Chim Acta* 95:235–242, 1979.
326. McNair P, Christensen SM, Transbol IB: Renal hypomagnesium in human diabetes mellitus: Its relation to glucose homeostasis. *Eur J Clin Invest* 12:81–85, 1982.
327. Hoskins B: Altered magnesium transport in slices of kidney cortex from chemically-induced diabetic rats. *Res Commun Chem Pathol Pharmacol* 34:29–45, 1981.
328. Schwartz R: ^{26}Mg as a probe in research on the role of magnesium in nutrition and metabolism. *Fed Proc* 41:2709–2713, 1982.
329. Nicar MJ, Pak CY: Oral magnesium load test for the assessment of intestinal magnesium absorption. *Min Elect Metabol* 8:44–51, 1982.
330. Flink EB: Nutritional aspects of magnesium metabolism. *West J Med* 133:304–312, 1980.

331. Licata AA, Lantigga R, Amatruda J, et al: Adverse effects of liquid protein fast on the handling of magnesium, calcium, and phosphorus. *Am J Med* 71:767–772, 1981.
332. Freeman JB, Wittine MT, Stegnik CD, et al: Effects of magnesium infusions on magnesium and nitrogen balance during parenteral nutrition. *Can J Surg* 25:570–572, 1982.
333. Leary WP, Reyes AJ: Diuretics, magnesium, potassium and sodium. *S Afr Med J* 61:279–280, 1982.
334. Widman L, Dyckner T, Wester PO: Effects of moduretic and aldactone on electrolytes in skeletal muscle in patients on long-term diuretic therapy. *Acta Med Scand* 661 (Suppl):33–36, 1981.
335. Dyckner T, Wester PO: Magnesium deficiency—Guidelines for diagnosis and substitution therapy. *Acta Med Scand* 661 (Suppl):37–39, 1981.
336. Iseri CT, Freed J, Bures AL: magnesium deficiency of cardiac disorder. *Am J Med* 58:837–846, 1975.

CHAPTER 11
Physiology and Disorders of Water Metabolism

Ronald Skowsky
Marshal P. Fichman

This chapter discusses and summarizes the published literature on the physiology and disorders of vasopressin (ADH) and water metabolism for the review years. Since minimal space will be allotted for background review of earlier data, the reader is encouraged to consult the previous volumes of this series for additional information.

THIRST

Regulation of total water balance in the intact organism requires the integration of several dipsogenic factors to enable the perceived thirst sensation to initiate water-seeking behavior, as well as to stimulate release of hormonal factors to conserve existing body fluids. Three major pathways—osmotic, hypovolemic, and renin-angiotensin II (AII)—have been proposed for initiation of thirst; the stimuli for each appears to be separate and additive (1) (Fig. 1).

Dehydration-induced drinking is believed to be based upon the concept that relative extracellular hyper- and hypo-osmolality produces intracellular hyper- and hypo-osmolality, respectively, since stimuli effecting extracellular fluid (ECF) volume or osmolality (hemorrhage, dehydration, hypertonic saline administration) can initiate drinking behavior via cerebral osmoreceptors and cerebral sodium receptors. Unlike most other mammals (except the rat and monkey), humans have a slower fluid intake during

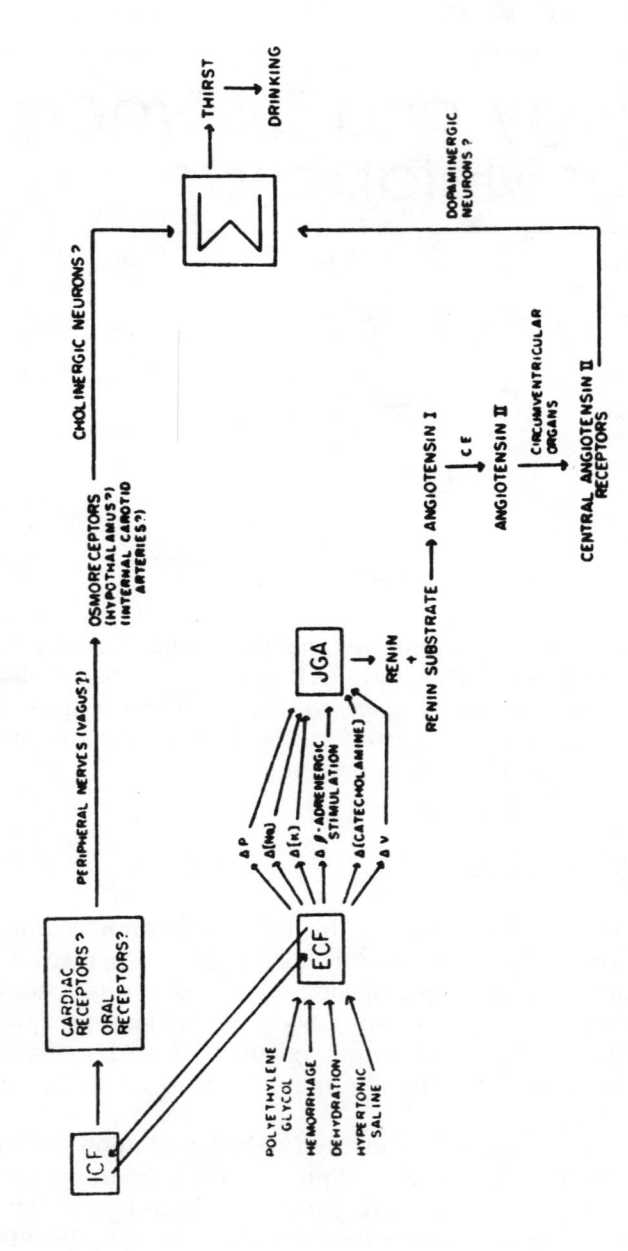

Figure 1. The major pathways (osmoreceptors and angiotensin) and associated factors for induction of fluid intake. (Greenleaf JE, Fregly MJ: *Fed Proc* 41:2507–2508, 1982. Reprinted with permission.)

and after fluid loss (involuntary dehydration). The two factors most likely responsible for this phenomenon are (1) the upright posture, producing postural hypovolemia and an increase in the renin-angiotensin system, and (2) extracellular fluid and electrolyte loss by sweating from exercise and heat exposure which increases drinking via mechanisms unrelated to changes in plasma volume, osmolality, or AII (2). Water deprivation leads to both intracellular and extracellular fluid depletion and stimulates thirst and arginine vasopressin (AVP) secretion. Wood et al. (3) have suggested that in the nonhuman primate, cellular dehydration is a much more potent stimulus for thirst than vascular hypovolemia. Following 24-hour fluid deprivation and a 5.8% increase in plasma osmolality, intravenous administration of water to restore plasma osmolality to normal reduced drinking by 85% while intravenous isotonic saline infusion (to correct only the hypovolemia) reduced drinking by only 3.2%. In addition, studies by Thrasher (4) are more compatible with osmoreceptor mediation of thirst rather than regulation via sodium receptors adjacent to the third cerebral ventricle lying within the blood-brain barrier (BBB) and responding to cerebrospinal fluid (CSF) sodium concentrations. Systemic intravenous infusions of urea, glucose, glycerol, or galactose elevate CSF sodium concentrations significantly yet fail to stimulate drinking behavior or plasma AVP concentrations.

The AII pathway also plays a role in mediating thirst sensation. Drinking behavior can be induced by decreasing blood pressure and/or plasma volume, decreasing plasma sodium concentration, increasing plasma potassium concentration, or pharmacologic administration of β-adrenergic agonists, all of which will augment renin release and generation of AII, an extremely potent CNS dipsogen.

The role of AII in mediating dehydration-induced thirst has been challenged on the basis of inadequate plasma levels achieved during fluid deprivation. Epstein's earlier studies showed minimal water consumption in animals following an infusion of 8 ng AII/min (5). Recently, Phillips et al. (6) have calculated this amount to yield about 500 pg AII/ml, which can be considered a threshold stimulatory concentration and correlates well with the amount of endogenous AII produced after 48-hour dehydration (399 pg AII/ml plasma) which induces considerable fluid intake. Infusion studies with the AII antagonist, saralasin (Sar^1Ala^8-angiotensin II), have yielded contradictory results, producing a decrease in thirst only in some studies. These conflicting results may be explained by the recent observations that certain CNS neurons respond to AII alone, acetylcholine alone, or a combination of both neurotransmitters, which suggests that parallel neural circuits exist for stimulation of thirst (7). It requires a combination of both the cholinergic antagonist, atropine, plus saralasin to produce a decrease in water consumption in fluid-deprived animals.

Schelling et al. (8) recently demonstrated that AII does not cross the BBB from plasma in rats and dogs, and any central effect of systemic AII

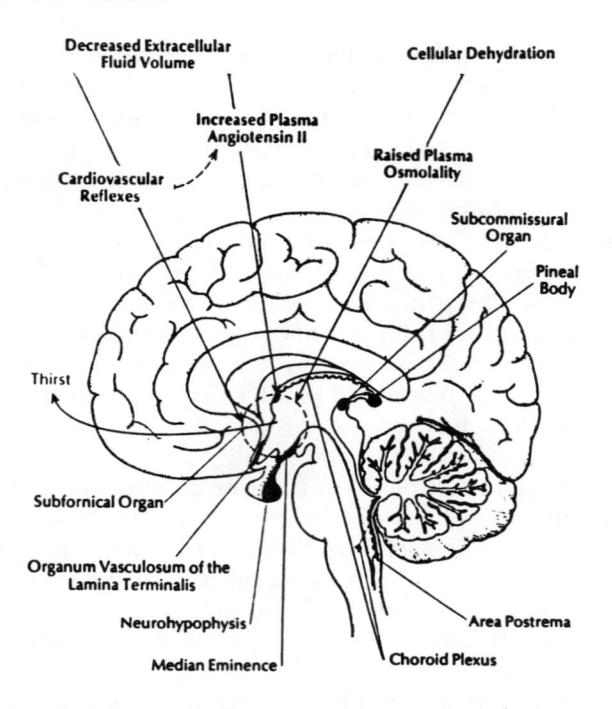

Figure 2. Interactions within the central nervous system modulating osmotic and hemodynamic mechanisms of AVP secretion. (Ramsay PJ, Ganong WF, in Krieger DT, Hughes JC (eds): *Neuroendocrinology*. New York, HP Publishing Co, 1980, pp 123–129. Reprinted with permission.)

must be limited to the circumventricular organs, which have fenestrated capillaries (without tight junctions) and lie functionally outside of the BBB (Fig. 2). Brain receptors for AII have been identified on the surface of the organum vasculosum laminae terminalis (OVLT) and subfornical organ (SFO) (9). Autoradiographic studies following systemic AII infusion document binding sites in both the SFO and the OVLT (10), while fluorescent-labeled AII given intracerebroventricularly reaches only receptors on the OVLT surface (11). Lesion experiments following a discrete knife cut to separate the SFO and OVLT in vivo showed no significant decrease in AII-induced drinking, but the pressor effect of central AII was reduced, suggesting separate central nervous system (CNS) pathways for thirst and blood pressor responses (6). In addition, following destruction of the OVLT in the dog, osmotically induced drinking is decreased and osmotic control of AVP secretion is disrupted, suggesting the presence of osmoreceptors as well as AII receptors on the OVLT (12). In sheep (13), ablation of the OVLT markedly diminishes osmoreceptor-stimulated fluid intake without reducing AII-induced drinking or daily food and water intake. Weanling infant animals with hypothalamic lesions in the dorsomedial nuclei become hypodipsic and hypophagic. However, despite the decrease in fluid intake, they respond to osmotic stimuli better than control animals, suggesting that the hypothalamic lesion has "reset" regulation of drinking and eating behavior (14).

Vasopressin itself may possess a central dipsogenic action. Injection of 0.10–0.15 mU of AVP into the third ventricle of conscious dogs caused a significant increase in water intake, although no effect was observed following ingestion into either the lateral cerebral ventricle or carotid artery (15).

Termination of drinking and satiety of thirst depends on several factors that appear to vary among species. Alimentary satiety can be partially mimicked via gastric distention, but it is distinct from that relieved by passage of water through the pharynx. Two other types include volume receptors and tissue receptors (recovering from dehydration) within the lateral or medial hypothalamus, both producing cessation of drinking behavior and fluid intake (16).

SYNTHESIS OF AVP

Similar to other polypeptide hormones, AVP—and oxytocin (OT)—and their associated neurophysins (NP) appear to be synthesized first as part of a larger prohormone molecule. Using a pulse-chase paradigm to examine hypothalamic AVP biosynthesis, Gainer et al. (17) suggested that a 20,000 dalton protein was first produced; this was synthesized as either an OT precursor or as an AVP precursor. A pI 5.4 fraction synthesized in the homozygous Brattleboro rat (with hereditary diabetes insipidus) has been identified as NP-oxytocin (NO-OT) and a pI 6.1 fraction in normal rats has been identified as NP-vasopressin (NP-VP). Using immunoprecipitation and electrophoretic separation of purified bovine posterior pituitary glands, Beguin et al. (18) isolated a single polypeptide chain of 80,000 daltons that showed immunologic reactivity with NP antibodies and which, upon further peptide bond cleavage, separated into a 68,000 dalton and a 10,000 dalton fragment. The latter smaller peptide was identical to NP. Although the investigators could not determine if the 80,000 dalton molecule was related to NP-VP or to NP-OT, it appeared that only one NP fragment existed per 80,000 dalton molecule, since the 68,000 fragment had no immunoreactivity. Subsequent work by the same group of investigators with further fractionation of the 80,000 dalton molecule resulted in the remarkable demonstration that immunoreactive adrenocortiocotropic hormone (ACTH) and β-endorphin are associated with this large peptide NP precursor and are included within the 68,000 dalton fragment (19). This fragment is much larger than the well-described 35,000 dalton protein, pro-opiomelanocortin (containing α-melanotropin, ACTH, and β-lipotropin—the latter including the endorphin peptide sequence) and may represent a hypothalamic precursor common to both NP-VP and ACTH/β-endorphin. In addition, these investigators identified two distinct 80,000 dalton fragments representing propeptides for both NP-VP and NP-OT, and proposed the name *neurohypophyseal coenophorin* (from the Greek word for *common*) for this class of large molecular eight peptides.

Rosenior et al. (20) have further examined the posttranslational cleavages of these NP-VP precursors in rat hypothalamic extracts and have isolated several large molecular weight peptide precursors of NP-VP (35,000 and 20,000 daltons) and NP-OT (28,000 and 17–18,000 daltons). They have suggested that the common NP-VP precursor of 35,000 daltons is split into an AVP precursor peptide (13–15,000) and an NP-VP precursor peptide (20–24,000) which subsequently proceed along separate biosynthetic pathways. Although the presence of two biosynthetic pathways for AVP is still debatable, the existence of the 20,000 dalton NP-VP precursor has been confirmed by several laboratories. Land et al. (21) have shown that this 166-amino acid precursor molecule has a signal peptide of 19 amino acids followed by AVP connected to NP by a Gly-Lys-Arg sequence. The carboxy terminal of this precursor contains 39 amino acids and has been immunocytochemically identified within the AVP-synthesizing cells in the magnocellular nuclei of normal rats but absent in tissues from the homozygous Brattleboro rat (22). Russell et al. (23) have clearly established that the 20,000 dalton NP-VP and NP-OT precursors do indeed release immunologically active AVP and OT upon limited trypsin proteolysis. They have proposed the names *propressophysin* and *prooxyphysin* for these peptide precursors.

SECRETION OF AVP

Neurophysiology

The synthesis and release of AVP in mammals is mediated by a multitude of mechanisms acting upon the hypothalmic-supraoptic-paraventricular-neurohypophyseal system (Fig. 3, Table 1). The neurosecretory magnocellular neurons have the morphological, electrical, and chemical characteristics shared by other neurons and show some degree of correlation between frequency of action potentials and neurotransmitter release at nerve terminals. Norepinephrine nerve terminals ending on the supraoptic nucleus (SON) neurons can be anatomically demonstrated and adrenergic mechanisms have been implicated in AVP biosynthesis, generally as inhibitory effects. Although very few dopaminergic and serotoninergic neurons are immunocytochemically demonstrable within the paraventricular nucleus (PVN), some ventral hypothalamic dopaminergic cell bodies extend dorsally into the PVN. Acetylcholine and its appropriate enzymes, acetylcholinesterase and choline acetyltransferase, are present in high

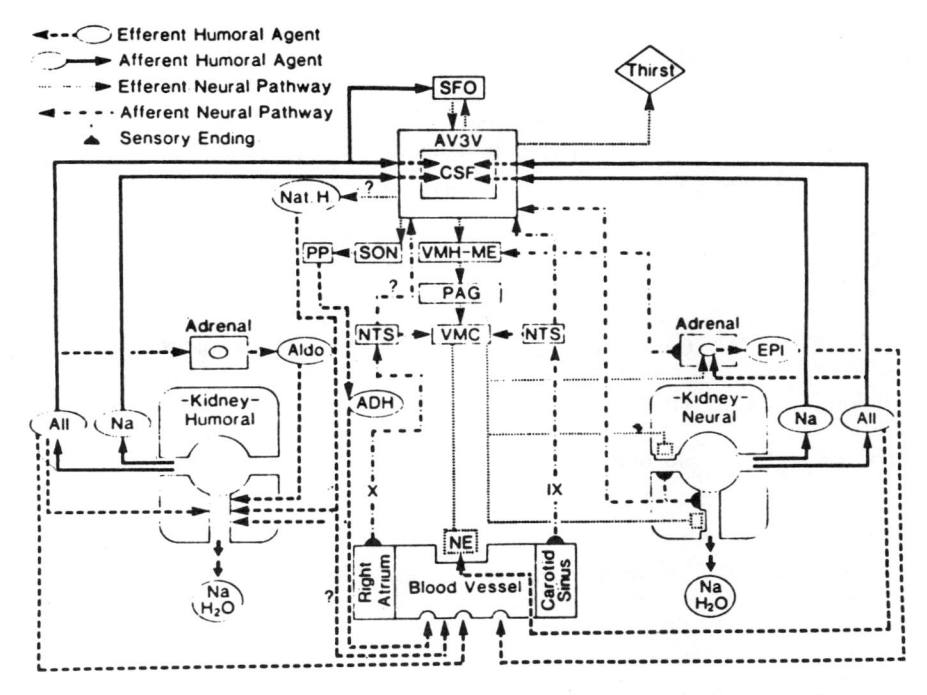

Figure 3. Humoral and neural mechanisms regulating osmotic and hemodynamic stimulation of AVP secretion. *Humoral agents*: AII, angiotensin II; Na, sodium; Aldo, aldosterone; ADH, antidiuretic hormone; Nat H, natriuretic hormone; EPI, epinephrine. *Neural structures*: SFO, subformical organ; CSF, cerebrospinal fluid of the third ventricle; AV3V, anteroventral third ventricle; VMH-ME, ventromedial hypothalamus-median eminence region; SON, supraoptic nucleus; PP, posterior pituitary; PAG, periaqueductal gray; VMC, vasomotor center; NTS, nucleus of the tractus solitarius; NE, norepinephrine stored in sympathetic nerve terminal. (Brody MJ, Johnson AK, in Martini L, Ganong WF, (eds): *Frontiers in Neuroendocrinology, Vol 6*. New York, Raven Press, 1980, pp 249–292. Reprinted with permission.)

concentrations in the SON, and studies suggest two populations of cholinergic receptors: muscarinic receptors that produce depression of neuronal unit activity and nicotinic receptors that produce excitation.

Gouzek et al. (24) recently demonstrated that administration of the alpha-adrenergic agonist, methoxamine, to dehydrated rats augmented the tissue depletion of AVP in the SON and PVN hypothalamic areas as well as in the neurohypophysis. This is in contrast to their findings in normally hydrated animals of increased tissue content (presumably secondary to decreased secretion) and suggests a modification of CNS monoamine effect dependent upon the state of hydration. In addition, CNS monoamine depletion studies by Lenard and Hahn (25) emphasize

Table 1. Factors Influencing Secretion of Arginine Vasopressin and Thirst

Stimulus	Site of Action	Effect on AVP
Osmolality	Osmosensitive neurons of the anterior hypothalamus	Increased tonicity stimulates AVP and thirst; decreased tonicity suppresses AVP and thirst
Volume	Left atrial stretch receptors	Volume depletion stimulates AVP and thirst; volume expansion suppresses AVP and thirst
	Carotid baroreceptors, Aortic arch baroreceptors	Hypotension stimulates AVP and possibly stimulates thirst
Angiotensin II	Hypothalamus (SFO and OVLT)	All stimulate AVP and thirst
Hypoxia	Carotid chemoreceptors	Extreme hypoxia stimulates AVP secretion; milder degrees of hypoxia have no consistent effect
Pain and noxious stimuli	Emetic center, vagus baroreceptors	Stimulates AVP only or produces vasovagal reaction, hypotension, or emesis
Psychosis		Psychosis stimulates AVP and is occasionally associated with exaggerated thirst
Hormonal and metabolic influences	Hypothalamus	B-endorphin, TRH, prostaglandins, adrenal insufficiency, sex steroids, hypothyroidism, hypoglycemia, and porphyria stimulate AVP
Nausea and emesis	Emetic center	These factors stimulate AVP
Temperature	Hypothalamic thermoreceptors, and possibly peripheral thermoreceptors.	High ambient temperature stimulates AVP release
Drugs	Hypothalamus and possibly other sites	Clofibrate, chlorpropamide, carbamazepine, opiate alkaloids, vincristine, cyclophosphamide, furosemide, thiazides (?), nicotine, and isoproterenol stimulate AVP
		Oxilorphan, butorphenol, alcohol, dilantin, and norepinephrine inhibit AVP

the importance of CNS monoamines in AVP biosynthesis. Hypothalamic damage to the amygdalar mesolimbic pathways with 6-hydroxydopamine (a norepinephrine neurotoxin) produces hyperphagia and hyperdipsia while treatment with 6-hydroxydopamine and desmethylimipramine (producing selective destruction of dopamine nerve terminals) induces hypophagia and hypodipsia, emphasizing the importance of overall balance of hypothalamic monoamines.

Opioid Mediated Secretion of AVP

The opioid peptides are derived from the precursor peptide, β-lipotropin, and are present in high concentration in the hypothalamus and the pituitary gland; endorphins are mostly localized within the adenohypophysis and pars intermedia, and enkepholins are localized primarily within the neurophypophysis. Martin and Voight (26) recently reported finding in the neurohypophysis of the rat, immunoreactive methionine-enkephalin in OT-containing fibers and immunoreactive leucine-enkephalin in AVP-containing fibers; the leucine enkephalin antisera used was not specific. Using an affinity purified antisera, Watson et al. (27) have subsequently demonstrated that at least one component of the "leucine-enkephalinlike immunoreactivity" in AVP neurons is the opioid peptide, dynorphin (700 times more potent by bioassay than leucine-enkephalin). These investigators showed that dynorphin and AVP occur in the same magnocellular neurons, while dynorphin and OT occur in separate cells.

Data from earlier work have suggested that morphine and other opioid peptide analogs produce an antidiuresis by stimulation of AVP, but conflicting data exists favoring an inhibitory role of opioids upon AVP secretion. Some of this contradictory data may be explained by the observation that the opioid can affect AVP release at several neural sites. In rats, both morphine and β-endorphin inhibit the calcium-dependent AVP secretion following in vitro electrical stimulation of the pituitary stalk (28,29) or medial basal hypothalamus (30). Likewise, most studies support an in vivo inhibitory effect of opioids upon AVP release. This is seen as a decrease in electrical activity of magnocellular neurons in rats receiving intracerebroventricular morphine, and is abolished by naloxone (31). It is also demonstrated in vivo following electrical foot shock-induced stress in rats (32). This procedure evokes increases in plasma concentration of β-endorphin, but plasma AVP is increased only in animals receiving naloxone. Likewise, dexamethasone pretreatment abolishes the stress-induced β-endorphin rise and will produce elevations in plasma AVP, consistent with an inhibitory role of opioids in the final pathways for AVP secretion in the rat.

Other data do not appear to support an inhibitory role of opioids in the rat. Christensen et al. (33) were unable to demonstrate an effect of either β-endorphin or met-enkephalin, leu-enkephalin, or morphine on in vitro electrically evoked release of AVP from the isolated rat neurohypophysis. Indeed, earlier studies suggested an antidiuretic effect of opioids in rats. This discrepancy may be reconciled by the observation of Aziz et al. (34) that intracerebroventricular (ICV) administration of high doses of morphine produces a biphasic effect on AVP release, as initial stimulatory effect followed by a later inhibitory effect, while low dose injection produces only inhibition; both stimulatory and inhibitory effects of morphine were naloxone-reversible and stereospecific and possibly may be explained by different opiate receptor affinities.

In humans the effect of opioids upon AVP secretion clearly appears to be dependent upon the conditions of stimulation involved—osmotic or nonosmotic. Lightman et al. (35) demonstrated that when AVP is stimulated by a phyperosmolar stimulus (hypertonic saline infusion), neither naloxone nor the long lasting synthetic agonist analog of methionine enkephalin, DAMME [D-Ala^2, MePhe^4, Met (O)-ol) enkephalin] had any effect on plasma AVP. However, when AVP is stimulated by the nonosmotic hemodynamic volume stimulus of a passive 65° head-up tilt, infusion of DAMME inhibits the expected elevation of plasma AVP (36). This tilt stimulus to AVP arises in volume receptors in the left atrium and pulmonary great vessels outside the BBB and suggests that alternate pathways exist to the magnocellular neurons which may or may not be blocked by opioid peptides. Other human studies also support an inhibitory role of opiate peptides upon AVP release. Metkephamid acetate, another synthetic agonist analog of methionine enkephalin, suppresses plasma AVP values in normal human volunteers (37), and the rise in plasma AVP after intravenous nicotine in human subjects is potentiated following the opiate antagonist naloxone (38).

In vivo studies in the conscious rat model, however, fail to demonstrate a clear-cut distinction of opioid peptide action upon osmotic and nonosmotic release of AVP. Ishikawa and Schrier (39) showed that treatment with either naloxone (relatively pure narcotic antagonist) or oxilorphan (possessing both narcotic agonist and antagonist properties) produced lower plasma AVP values than in control studies following both hypertonic saline infusion (osmotic stimulus) as well as induced plasma hypovolemia (nonosmotic stimulus). This occurred in the absence of changes in mean arterial blood pressure, glomerular filtration rate, or solute excretion and suggests a stimulatory effect of opioids upon AVP secretion. The studies by Knepel et al. (40) in the conscious rat model, however, are closer to the human model. Naloxone administration augmented the plasma AVP response to both AII infusion and induced nonhypotensive, isomolar hypovolemia, yet was without effect upon plasma AVP following hypertonic saline infusion or induction of hypotension following ganglionic blockade. This suggests that an inhibitory effect by opiates is involved in some, but not all, of the AVP stimulatory neural pathways. The discrepancies between the rat and human model remain unexplained.

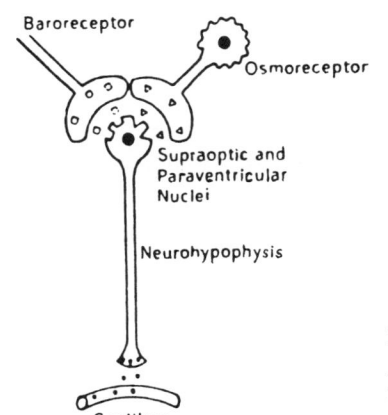

Figure 4. Osmotic and nonosmotic control of AVP secretion. (Schrier RW et al: *Am J Physiol* 236:321–332, 1979. Reprinted with permission.)

Osmotic and Volume (Nonosmotic) Mediated Secretion of AVP

It is well known that changes in plasma osmolality as well as alterations in baroreceptor tone are the predominant regulators of AVP secretion, albeit via separate anatomical pathways. Specific monophasic cells lying in the perinuclear zone of the magnocellular neurons respond to osmotic changes across the capillaries of the BBB (Fig. 4). In addition, another set of "primitive osmoreceptors" exists within the limbic, amygdaloid, and olfactory areas which is responsive to various nonspecific noxious stimuli as well as to changes in plasma osmolality. Many variables are believed to affect the sensitivity of the osmoreceptors, including the type of solute producing the osmotic change, individual variations in osmoreceptor threshold, rate of change of the osmotic stimulus, age, and nonosmotic stimuli.

The second major control mechanism for AVP release is the hemodynamic response to nonosmotic stimuli, which involves the autonomic nervous system by way of baroreceptors within the vascular bed responding to volume-induced changes in arterial pressure and communicating to the hypothalamus via parasympathetic pathways. High pressure (carotid, aortic arch) arterial baroreceptors as well as low pressure (left atrium) baroreceptors are important in modifying systemic volume change. Alterations in the balance between sympathetic and parasympathetic tone in the absence of blood pressure changes, may also participate in the release of AVP; this includes the acute stress of pain, hypoxia, and severe psychological abnormalities. However, it appears that pain and other noxious stimuli must produce a vasovagal reaction, hypotension, or emesis in order to evoke AVP release. The reader is referred to the following recent reviews of osmotic and nonosmotic control mechanisms of AVP secretion (41–44).

The relationship between plasma osmolality and plasma AVP is believed to be either linear or log-linear in humans and other mammals. Reaves et al. (45) studied this relationship in the cat and demonstrated a higher osmotic threshold (314 mOsm/kg in cats versus 280 mOsm/kg in man) and an increased sensitivity (increased slope) of the osmoreceptors. These findings may be related to neural and vascular hypothalamic anatomic changes unique to the cat, including a new lateral hypothalamic nucleus-containing AVP and the presence of a carotid rete arterial plexus (in lieu of an internal carotid artery) with changes in CNS thermoregulation. An altered osmotic threshold for AVP has also been reported in humans with Kallman's syndrome (hypogonadotropic hypogonadism with anosmia secondary to agenesis of the olfactory bulb). In a series of seven patients (46), five had abnormal Uosm/Posm relationships, with the calculated osmotic threshold decreased in one (270.6 mOsm/kg) and elevated in two others ($\geq$ 294 mOsm/kg), suggesting extensive hypothalamic involvement.

Recent data strongly implicate the participation of AII (probably of CNS origin) in the osmoregulation of AVP from the magnocellular neurons. Using the laboratory model of the organ-cultured rat hypothalamo-neurohypophyseal explant, Sladek et al. (47) demonstrated that AVP release was significantly greater when a 5 mOsm/kg increment in perfusate osmolality was combined with AII than with either stimulus alone. Addition of saralasin, an AII antagonist, prevented the release of AVP in response to increased tissue culture medium osmolality. Antiserum against AII also blocked osmotically induced AVP release in this in vitro system (48). Additional studies (49) demonstrated that AI augmented the osmotic release of AVP, but the response was blocked by simultaneous addition of saralasin, suggesting that AI must be converted to AII in order to potentiate AVP release. Thus, one role of AII appears to be to increase the sensitivity of the osmoreceptor and augment AVP release to osmotic stimuli.

Endogenous CNS prostaglandins also appear to modulate the sensitivity of the osmoreceptor for AVP secretion. Hoffman et al. (50) demonstrated that ICV administration of the prostaglandin synthetase inhibitor, indomethacin, markedly blunted the rise in plasma AVP following systemic hypertonic saline infusion; ICV perfusion with PGE_2 produced elevations in plasma AVP. Ethanol also appears to affect osmoreceptor sensitivity. In a study by Eisenhofer and Johnson (51), oral ingestion of 75 ml of ethanol produced a biphasic response of plasma AVP, which included a fall in the first hour followed by a subsequent rise in AVP, despite increasing ethanol blood levels and a slight rise in plasma osmolality (corrected for the effect of ethanol). Ethanol also blunted the plasma AVP response to intravenous infusion of hypertonic saline, suggesting an effect upon osmoreceptor sensitivity.

Pregnancy in the rat appears to be another physiologic state associated with a reset osmotic threshold (52). Pregnant rats tended to have lower basal plasma osmolalities and sodium levels but normal basal plasma AVP and urinary osmolalities. The AVP/Osm regression curve was shifted to the left with an osmotic threshold about 11 mOsm/liter lower in pregnant animals compared to normal animals; the osmotic threshold for thirst also appeared to be lowered. The reason for this regulatory change is not apparent since it cannot be reproduced in virgin rats receiving progesterone and/or estrone. However, it may be related to the increases in plasma renin and angiotensin known to occur during gestation.

Changes in systemic hemodynamics can modulate AVP secretion via either baroreceptors or left atrial stretch receptors, the latter exerting a negative feedback with increased intraatrial volume and distention. Menninger (53) has demonstrated the presence of *right* atrial stretch receptors in the cat that will diminish electrical activity of SON neurons and lower plasma AVP values (acting alone and/or synergistically with left atrial stretch receptors).

Earlier studies on volume-mediated changes in AVP release emphasized the hypovolemic effects following hemorrhage and suggested that high pressure rather than low pressure receptors have the primary role in regulating AVP; decreases in plasma volume of less than 6–10% are generally not sufficient to augment AVP secretion. Fewer studies have examined the effects of hypervolemia, although earlier results have suggested that expansion of extracellular volume lowers plasma AVP, which is related more to increases in left atrial pressure rather than to changes in arterial blood pressure. Epstein et al. (54) have utilized the water immersion model which induces a central volume expansion of approximately 700 ml of extracellular fluid without significant alterations of heart rate, blood pressure, or plasma composition, and which produces a natriuresis, kaliuresis, and diuresis. In dehydrated normal human volunteers, 4 hours of immersion suppresses plasma AVP and plasma renin activity without concomitant changes in plasma osmolality. PRA returned to basal levels in the hour following immersion but AVP tended to remain suppressed in some subjects, an unusual example of PRA-AVP dissociation. Greenleaf et al. (55) also used the water immersion model and they were able to document mild hemodilution and decreases in osmolality of 4 mOsm/kg by the second hour of immersion, which were associated with suppression of plasma AVP and PRA and were believed to be due to transfer of hypotonic fluid into the vascular compartment. It appears that monkeys are less sensitive to changes in atrial pressure as reflected in modulation of AVP secretion. Gilmore et al. (57) infused isotonic, isosmotic high molecular weight dextran to monkeys sufficient to increase left ventricular end-diastolic pressure but could not alter mean plasma AVP levels nor mean arterial blood pressure, suggesting a primacy of high pressure arterial baroreceptors over volume receptors in this species.

Just as physiologic aging may affect the sensitivity of the osmoreceptor regulation of AVP, it may also affect the AVP response to hemodynamic stimuli. Rowe et al. (56) compared the plasma AVP response to orthostasis after overnight recumbency in young subjects (19–31 years of age) with that in old subjects (62–80 years of age). Despite no significant difference in mean arterial blood pressure, pulse rate, or basal recumbent AVP levels, the elevation in plasma AVP following upright posture was significantly lower in half of the elderly subjects, despite a normal orthostatic rise in plasma norepinephrine.

Stress is another known nonosmotic stimulus for AVP secretion. Insulin-induced hypoglycemia, whether acting as a nonspecific stress or via unknown pathways, appears to be another nonosmotic stimulator of AVP release which, in humans, produces a sevenfold rise in AVP and a 2 mEq/liter elevation of plasma sodium without affecting mean arterial blood pressure or blood volume (estimated from hematocrit) (58). Beta-adrenergic blockade with propranolol before insulin-induced hypoglycemia suppresses PRA but does not alter the plasma AVP response. In the rat, insulin-induced hypoglycemia similarly produces a fivefold rise in plasma AVP, but with a 2% fall in plasma osmolality, a 10% fall in blood volume, and no significant change in mean arterial blood pressure (59). In addition, water loading decreases and hypertonic saline infusion increases the hypoglycemic augmentation of plasma AVP, suggesting that this stimulus of AVP acts synergistically with the CNS osmoreceptors. Additional studies in rats (60) and humans (61) demonstrated augmented AVP release following administration of 2-deoxy-D-glucose, a hexokinase inhibitor, causing CNS intracellular glycopenia and increased epinephrine secretion, but causing extracellular hyperglycemia. This elevation in AVP was not mediated by osmotic or hypovolemic stimuli and was inhibited by prior treatment with propranolol, which suggests a different mechanism of action. However, hyperglycemia in the streptozotocin diabetic rat is associated with higher plasma AVP basal concentration and an augmented release after hypertonic saline (62).

The stress of surgery stimulates release of AVP and this has been documented during cardiac valve or coronary bypass surgery (63). It appears that pulsatile perfusion during cardiopulmonary bypass is more physiologic and attenuates the AVP stress response, producing less vasoconstriction, a higher extracorporeal flow rate, and a decreased natriuresis (64). In addition, surgery performed under extradural anesthesia almost completely suppresses the release of AVP as compared to general anesthesia, apparently by blocking specific neural conduction pathways (65).

CNS EFFECTS OF AVP

In addition to the well-known effects of AVP on the kidney and the cardiovascular system, several other roles have been proposed for vasopressin, including that of a significant neurotransmitter. Acting as a central neuromodulator, studies have suggested that AVP influences memory, behavior, ACTH release, and tissue growth via its effect on tissue catecholamine concentrations and turnover in various areas of the brain.

AVP within the brain is not confined to the magnocellular neurohypophyseal neurons but has been identified in the postmortem adult human brain in several extrahypothalamic sites, including the locus coeruleus, periaqueductal grey, substantia nigra, and globus pallidus (66). In addition, AVP has been identified in several hypothalamic sites in human fetuses between 15–34 weeks of gestation (67).

One possible role for AVP that has been postulated is that of an antipyretic neuromodulator, since AVP is released into the blood and brain during fever (68). Kasting et al. (69) examined the effects of hemorrhage (20% of blood volume) on the endotoxin-induced febrile response. This procedure elevated plasma AVP and was associated with significantly lower body temperature. Sheep hemorrhaged in the cold had temperature changes similar to control sheep. In addition, homozygous Brattleboro rats as well as Long-Evans rats treated with ICU anti-AVP antisera, when subjected to hyperthermia, either convulsed at higher temperature or did not convulse at all (70). This suggests that deficiency of AVP increases the seizure threshold and that AVP may act as a releasing factor to maintain homostasis in febrile states. In addition, intravenous vasopressin, but not oxytocin, produces moderate analgesia in mice which is not abolished by opiate antagonists but is diminished by vasopressin antagonists. ICV administration of AVP does not produce analgesia which suggests a peripheral site of action (71).

AVPs action as a neurotransmitter may result from its effect on monoamine metabolism. AVP has been demonstrated to increase serotonin synthesis in vitro from hippocampal brain slices (72), although in vivo lysine vasopressin administration appears to decrease hippocampal serotonin, dopamine, and norepinephrine (73); the reasons for this discrepancy are not apparent. In addition, intravenous administration of vasopressin (but not oxytocin) has been reported to elevate plasma prolactin both in normal non-estrogen-primed male rats as well as in hypophysectomized rats with the adenohypophysis implanted under the renal capsule (74).

AVPs role as putative neurotransmitter is strengthened by its presence within the cerebrospinal fluid (CSF), resulting from either diffusion from sites within the central nervous system (CNS) or by direct secretion into the ventricles. Potential CNS sites of direct secretion into the CSF include the magnocellular neurons of the SON and PVN, the parvocellular perikarya of the PVN, and the parvocellular neurons of the suprachiasmatic nuclei. AVP (as well as oxytocin and estrogen-stimulated neurophysins) exhibits a rhythmic circadian pattern in CSF, but not in plasma, with highest concentrations occurring during the daylight period (75,76). However, there appears to be an effective blood-brain barrier against plasma-CSF or CSF-plasma transport of these neurohypophyseal peptides. Intravenous infusion of hypertonic saline increases plasma and CSF osmolality and plasma AVP but not CSF AVP concentration, and ICV infusion of a hypertonic solution increased CSF osmolality and AVP but caused no change in plasma values (77–80). However, one study has reported that the hypovolemia of hemorrhage increases the AVP concentration in both plasma and CSF (81). In the human, CSF levels of AVP are significantly higher in patients with benign intracranial hypertension and other miscellaneous neurological diseases than in control subjects despite normal plasma AVP levels (82). This suggests a different origin of CSF vasopressin from that released into the blood.

AVP, acting within the median eminence and/or within the adenohypophysis, has been regarded as one of the possible stimulators for ACTH release, although it appears unlikely that it is the only corticotropin releasing factor (CRF). Chromatographic separation of hypothalamic median eminence extracts have revealed the presence of one (83) or two (84) high molecular weight CRFs and one low molecular weight CRF, the latter being similar in size to AVP. Since nerve terminal endings in the median eminence appear to originate from the PVN rather than the SON, Dornquist et al. (85) quantitated changes in plasma ACTH and AVP following separate electrical stimulation of each magnocellular nucleus. Stimulation of the caudal pole of the SON increased AVP but decreased ACTH, while PVN stimulation increased both AVP and ACTH. This anatomic distribution has been confirmed by other immunocytochemical studies of hypothalamic tissue (86,87). In addition, following ICV administration of antivasopressin antiserum, PVN stimulation no longer releases ACTH, although electrical stimulation of areas ventral to the PVN still induce plasma ACTH elevations, suggesting existence of CRFs other than AVP (88). Studies using median eminence-neural lobe extracts from the homozygous Brattleboro rat suggest the presence of a non-AVP substance with CRF activity in concentrations that have been reported to be equal (89) or less (90) than that of the normal rat. Thus, it appears reasonable that several peptides exist that possess CRF activity, only one of which is AVP. However, Beny et al. (91) quantitated the in vitro release of both AVP and CRF from incubated microdissected rat median eminences and estimated that AVP accounted for at least 85% of released CRF activity.

An increasing body of evidence suggests that the neurohypophyseal peptides are involved in acquisition, consolidation, and retention of learned behavior. Following surgical removal of the neurohypophysis, extinction of two-way active avoidance behavior is markedly facilitated, which is restored to normal by AVP administration. AVP treatment of intact rats increases the resistance to extinction of both active and passive conditioned behavior and improves consolidation as well as retrieval of learned material. Oxytocin appears to have opposite effects of AVP and tends to facilitate active avoidance behavior as well as increasing retention of passive avoidance behavior. Recent reviews have summarized the earlier data (92,93).

Vasopressin administration has been shown to improve facilitation of learned tasks in food-deprived animals (94) as well as reversing drug-induced amnesia and facilitating memory retrieval (95). Cooper et al. (96) reported that vasopressin therapy improved the conditioned flavor aversion behavior in old rats versus young control rats, significantly reducing the age difference in extinction of this learned behavior. Kovacs et al. (97) injected AVP antiserum intracerebrally into the hippocampus and lessened passive avoidance behavior, suggesting that endogenous AVP in the septohippocampal system is involved in cognitive memory. In addition, systemic or ICV injection of a synthetic antagonistic analog of AVP induces a behavioral effect opposite that of AVP, that is, a facilitation of extinction of active avoidance response (98).

Finally, it should be appreciated that all CNS mechanisms regulating AVP secretion have not been fully elucidated. Kilcoyne et al. (99) demonstrated immunoreactive AII in the hypothalamic SON and PVN, the median eminence, and the neurohypophysis; and the results suggested the presence of both AVP and AII within the same neuron in certain sites. In addition, immunoreactive cholecystokinin, gastrin (100), and glucagon (101) have been detected within the neurohypophysis of the rat. And in vitro incubation of neurohypophyseal tissue with potassium induces release of both cyclic AMP and cyclic GMP prior to peak secretion of AVP (102). The significance of these other peptides and cyclic nucleotides in controlling AVP release remains to be determined.

AVP AND THE CARDIOVASCULAR SYSTEM

It appears that there are at least two distinct types of vasopressin receptors. The classic renal receptors in the collecting ducts modulating free water reabsorption have been termed V_2 receptors, which are cyclic AMP-dependent, antidiuretic selective. The other vasopressin receptors are cyclic AMP-independent, pressor-sensitive V_1 receptors, which mediate the AVP effects of contraction of vascular smooth muscle, glycogenolysis in hepatocytes, and prostaglandin synthesis in renal tissue. In addition, V_1 receptors attenuate ACTH release and may be involved in prolongation of extinction of active avoidance behavior (although this neurotransmitterlike action may be mediated through V_2 receptors). AVP is believed to have two separate effects upon blood vessels: a direct pressor action, which is prostaglandin-independent, and an indirect action of augmenting the effects of other pressor agents, which is prostaglandin-dependent. In large doses, AVP infusion will increase mean systemic blood pressure, left atrial pressure, left ventricular systolic and diastolic pressures, and total pulmonary and coronary peripheral resistance; it will decrease heart rate, pulmonary arterial pressure, cardiac output, portal venous pressure, and coronary blood flow. AVP also decreases myocardial oxygen uptake, myocardial contractility, and left ventricular efficiency.

In addition to a direct pressor effect upon peripheral vessels, AVP is believed to have a direct CNS action on central regulation of systemic blood pressure, possibly mediating the pressor effect to ICV administration of AII, and to be regulated by CNS monoamines. Hypophysectomized animals have an impaired ability to maintain their blood pressure following hemorrhage or pharmacologic blockage of AVP. Pittman et al. (103) demonstrated that ICV injection of picomole amounts of AVP produced short latency, dose-related increases in systemic blood pressure. Since these changes also occurred in the homozygous Brattleboro rat, the hypertension does not occur through release of pituitary AVP. Although systemic AVP infusion induces elevation in the blood pressure, Liard et al. (104) showed that intravertebral arterial administration of AVP induces a greater reflex bradycardia than the same dose injected into the vena cava, suggesting CNS modulation of the baroreceptor reflex. In addition, local destruction of the AI noradrenergic neurons in the ventrolateral medulla of the rabbit induces elevation of plasma AVP and hypotension (105).

Further support for a central catecholamine role in augmenting CNS AVP release and blood pressure control is provided in a study by Kimura et al. using dogs (106). Following ICV administration of norepinephrine with predominant α-adrenergic action, or clonidine, an α-adrenergic agonist, they observed a marked reduction of plasma AVP as well as a drop in systemic blood pressure and heart rate; pretreatment with the alpha-adrenergic blocking agent, phenoxybenzamine, abolished the cardiovascular effect of norepinephrine and significantly inhibited the fall of AVP by 80%, supporting the importance of central α-adrenergic receptors in the regulation of AVP.

In addition to the role of CNS catecholamines in regulating AVP and blood pressure, the central cardiovascular effects of AII appear to be mediated through stimulation of AVP. Unger et al. (107) demonstrated that the dose-dependent elevations of blood pressure following ICV injection of AII in the rat could be partially inhibited by pretreatment of the animal with either prazosin (α-adrenoreceptor blocker) or a synthetic AVP antagonist. Combined pretreatment with both pharmacologic blockers completely inhibited the pressor response of AII, suggesting that both endogenous release of AVP as well as stimulation of the sympathetic nervous system contribute to the cardiovascular effects of centrally administrated AII. This concept is further supported by the observation that angiotensin-converting enzyme is higher in the pars intermedia and neurohypophysis of the homozygous Brattleboro rat than in normal control animals, and the high concentration is reversed by vasopressin therapy (108). This suggests a close inverse relationship between AVP and AII in the intermediate and posterior lobes of the pituitary gland.

Studies emphasizing systemic changes in plasma levels of AVP, catecholamines, and plasma renin activity tend to reflect the peripheral vasopressor effects of these agents more so than the central effects, although both may be operative. Zerbe et al. (109) tried to determine whether the subnormal blood pressure recovery following hemorrhage in Brattleboro rats was due to a disturbance in the renin-angiotensin or sympathetic systems or whether it was secondary to the AVP deficiency per se. Despite prolonged recovery from the induced hypotension, both plasma epinephrine and PRA in the Brattleboro rat were significantly higher before bleeding and increased more after hemorrhage than in control animals, suggesting intact sympathetic and renin-angiotensin systems. Vasopressin deficiency appears to be the cause of the impaired hemodynamic response to hemorrhage, although passive contribution from the angiotensin system cannot be ruled out. Use of potent specific antagonists of the vasoconstrictor effects of vasopressin have been extremely helpful in this type of investigation, since they will lower the blood pressure in fluid-deprived animals (with elevated plasma AVP) but not in the Brattleboro rat or water-replete animal (110,111). They do not inhibit the pressor effect of noreprinephrine or AII.

Gavras et al. (112) examined this problem by subjecting rats sequentially to catecholamine depletion followed by AVP blockade. Initial catecholamine depletion significantly decreased systemic blood pressure and elevated plasma AVP in all animals. Infusion of either a vasopressin antagonist or an angiotensin converting enzyme inhibitor produced only transient falls in blood pressure, suggesting that the sympathetic nervous system is more involved in maintenance of blood pressure in the resting state, while AVP and renin are backup systems.

Other investigators have examined the role of AVP in the renin-angiotensin contribution to blood pressure regulation. Vasopressin is known to have an inhibitory effect on renin secretion in normal rats and animals with elevated PRA, although its physiologic significance is not clear. Malayan et al. (113) examined the effects of continuously increasing infusion rates of AVP in normal conscious dogs to determine the range of plasma concentration needed to affect PRA, blood pressure, and heart rate; plasma AVP values varied from a basal level of 2.7 pg/ml to 33.5 pg/ml. Only the highest infusion rate of AVP produced a rise in blood pressure or a fall in heart rate, while an increase in plasma AVP of 4.2 pg/ml maximally suppressed PRA by 34%. Comparable plasma AVP levels achieved following 24 hours of dehydration or nonhypotensive hemorrhage were 7.4 pg/ml and 47.4 pg/ml, respectively. The results suggest that fluid deprivation can elevate plasma AVP sufficiently to affect PRA, while higher concentrations are required for cardiovascular blood pressure changes.

Schwartz et al. (114) also examined the effect of AVP on PRA in dogs subjected to mild hemorrhage in the face of vasopressin blockade by a selective AVP pressor antagonist. In the absence of AVP blockade, blood pressure and heart rate did not change, although PRA increased from 3.8 to 10.8 ng/ml 3 hr. Following AVP blockade, the same blood loss significantly lowered blood pressure, increased heart rate, and increased PRA from 7.1 to 30.3 ng/ml/3 hr. The increase in PRA following the AVP antagonist was greater, reflecting either the inhibition of renin by AVP or decreased renal perfusion. In any event, the results support a physiologic role for AVP in maintenance of blood pressure during hemorrhage. However, it appears that elevated plasma concentrations of AVP are a prerequisite for cardiovascular effects, since a 4-day continuous infusion of vasopressin at a rate of 0.067 mU/kg/min (to keep plasma levels within the physiologic range) failed to change blood pressure, PRA, or plasma aldosterone concentration (115).

Studies of human subjects also suggest that the pressor effects of catecholamines and AVP are modulated by endogenous AII. Normal human volunteers received pharmacologic infusions of norepinephrine, angiotensin II, and vasopressin in amounts sufficient to produce elevations in blood pressure (116,117). Pretreatment with an angiotensin converting enzyme inhibitor significantly blunted the pressor response to norepinephrine and to vasopressin but not to AII. However, the angiotensin converting enzyme inhibitor did not attenuate the pressor response to norepinephrine if the subject received a simultaneous infusion of AII in a subpressor dose. The results suggest that endogenous AII modulates the peripheral pressor effects of catecholamines and AVP, which is blunted by angiotensin converting enzyme inhibition.

Vasopressin has been incriminated in the pathogenesis of hypertension, although most animal studies have used the model of spontaneous hypertension in rats, deoxycorticosterone (DOC) salt-treated rats, and two-kidney Goldblatt hypertension. Berecek et al. (118) evaluated the role of vasopressin in the development of DOC salt-induced hypertension. Homozygous Brattleboro rats did not develop elevated arterial pressures with DOC salt treatment unless they were treated with AVP. Likewise, normotensive Brattleboro rats without AVP treatment did demonstrate decreased in vitro renal vascular pressor responsiveness to norepinephrine or AII during DOC salt-induced hypertension, while normal rats or AVP-replete Brattleboro rats showed increased renal pressor responsiveness, suggesting a role for AVP in the pathogenesis of DOC hypertension, possibly increasing vascular reactivity. Similar findings have been demonstrated in rats with lesions in the anteroventral region of the third cerebral ventricle, an area that controls AVP release and produces central diabetes insipidus. The animals required AVP replacement to develop DOC-induced hypertension (119). The Brattleboro rat with one-clip kidney-induced hypertension has less blood pressure elevation than the Long-Evans rat, which is restored by administration of DDAVP (120).

Matsuguchi et al. (121,122) evaluated the relative roles of AVP and catecholamines in the maintenance of elevated vascular resistance in the DOC hypertensive rat. Vascular resistance was lowered by 40% following infusion of an AVP pressor antagonist and was lowered by 43% following sympathetic denervation. Hatzinikolaou et al. (123) also demonstrated that the hypertensive response induced by DOC and saline was partially abolished by pretreatment with an AVP pressor antagonist and completely reversed by a combined pretreatment of an AVP antagonist plus alpha- and beta-adrenergic blockers. Other investigators (124), however, have failed to document enhanced pressor responsiveness to infused AVP in DOC hypertensive rats, suggesting that elevated blood pressure results from continued sustained exposure to elevated plasma levels of AVP. In any event, it appears that both AVP and an intact sympathetic nervous system are important.

Disturbances in CNS content of AVP and plasma AVP have been documented in the stroke-prone spontaneously hypertensive rat (SHRSP). Rascher et al. (125) demonstrated elevated plasma concentrations of AVP only in adult animals over 24 weeks of age, while significantly lower plasma levels of AVP than controls were found in young animals. In the adult SHRSP, tissue AVP content was reduced up to 70% in the hypothalamus amygdala, the septum, and the brain stem, versus control animals, while neurohypophyseal AVP content was increased by 26% (126–128). When subjected to 24–48 hours of fluid deprivation, the adult SHRSP responded with a greater increase in plasma AVP although there appeared to be an end organ tissue sensitivity to vasopressin (possibly secondary to down regulation of receptors) because the hypertensive rats are unable to increase urinary concentration and had a greater loss of water and sodium (129). Thus it appears that reduced CNS content of AVP may contribute to the experimental hypertension that is associated with further disturbance in plasma fluid and electrolytes.

The role of AVP in human hypertension is clearly an unsettled issue despite observed abnormalities in AVP homeostasis. The majority of studies have reported normal basal plasma levels in patients with benign essential hypertension, although this may be inappropriately elevated in the presence of increased baroreceptor stimulation from the raised arterial pressures, which should act to inhibit AVP secretion. DeLima et al. (130) quantitated plasma AVP in patients with low renin essential hypertension during furosemide-induced acute volume reduction (averaging a 10% plasma volume decrease over 2 hours). Basal plasma AVP was not significantly different between hypertensive and normotensive groups. In normotensive subjects, plasma AVP rose progressively during the study while it remained unchanged in the hypertensive subjects. Since low renin hypertension is believed to be characterized by extracellular and plasma volume expansion and appropriate AVP suppression, normal basal AVP concentrations could represent increased secretion rates. However, this does not explain the blunted response to volume depletion. In addition, Trimarco et al. (131) reported that hypertensive patients also show an abnormal AVP response to hemodynamic postural changes. Following overnight bed rest, head-up tilt normally induces a decrease in effective plasma volume and an increase in plasma AVP; hypertensive subjects showed a paradoxical drop in plasma AVP (despite an appropriate decrease in plasma volume).

Cowley et al. (132) reported plasma AVP concentrations about twice as high in hypertensive patients than in normotensive subjects, which strongly correlated with the degree of urinary sodium excretion, suggesting a direct renal pressor effect of the elevated AVP levels. In addition, in older hypertensive subjects excreting sodium in excess of 250 mEq/day, plasma AVP levels were twice those of age-matched hypertensives excreting less than 150 mEq/day, suggesting a direct effect of AVP upon intravascular volume or a failure of AVP suppression in the face of volume expansion.

AVP SECRETION IN THE FETUS AND NEONATE

Vasopressin and oxytocin are present in the mammalian fetal neurohypophysis during the latter half of gestation and appear to be readily released upon appropriate stimuli, although their roles in fetal homeostasis have not been defined. Earlier studies have reviewed and summarized previous data (44).

The late gestational-age sheep fetus increases fetal plasma AVP up to 300 times during acute asphyxial stress which is associated with a massive expulsion of meconium into the amniotic fluid, although maternal plasma AVP remains unchanged (133–135). Fetal hypoxic stress is important but does not appear to be the sole factor in augmenting fetal AVP secretion. Daniel et al. (136) also studied the late gestational-age sheep fetus and found a strongly significant nonlinear correlation between fetal plasma AVP concentrations and osmolality, as well as between fetal plasma AVP and urine osmolality. Although there was no transplacental passage of AVP, there was a significant linear correlation between maternal and fetal plasma osmolality and sodium concentrations, suggesting that the fetal neurohypophysis and kidney may be active in regulating fetal osmolar and volume homeostasis.

Rose et al. (137) compared the hemodynamic stress of hemorrhage in newborn lambs and weanling lambs (3–4 weeks of age). In newborns, 15% hemorrhage does not change blood pressure but causes a delayed rise in ACTH and AVP, while in weanling lambs, hemorrhage of the same degree induces a fall in blood pressure, a prompt rise in ACTH, but a delayed rise in AVP, suggesting age-related maturational differences in the response to hemorrhagic stress.

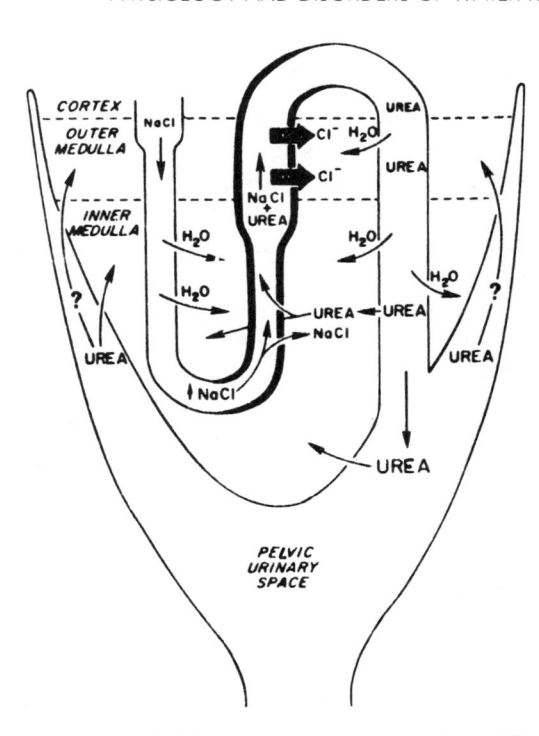

Figure 5. Kokko-Rector model for urinary concentration. (Hogg RJ, Kokko JP: *Rev Physiol Biochem Pharmacol* 86:95–135, 1979. Reprinted with permission.)

In the human newborn, whether delivered vaginally or by cesarean section, the concentration of AVP in arterial cord plasma is higher than in venous cord plasma, suggesting fetal hypersecretion (138). AVP levels are also elevated in infants subjected to stress during pregnancy, labor, and/or delivery and were associated with the presence of meconium in amniotic fluid, which suggests a causal effect by the stressed fetus.

RENAL CONCENTRATING AND DILUTING MECHANISMS

The presence of a countercurrent multiplier system and a hyperosmolar milieu in the renal medulla is the basis for urinary concentration and dilution (Fig. 5). This classic model has been altered by Kokko and Rector and by Stephenson to conform to more recent microperfusion and micropuncture data, and the reader is referred to earlier volumes of this series as well as to recent reviews (139–141) for a comprehensive and detailed explanation. According to the Kokko-Rector model, active transport of sodium and chloride from the thick ascending limb produces a hypotonic tubular fluid. In the presence of AVP, water (but not urea) moves passively from the cortical and outer medullary collecting ducts increasing the concentration of urea in the inner medullary collecting ducts. Urea, perhaps facilitated by AVP, diffuses along the gradient from the inner medullary collecting ducts into the interstitium by the descending limb of Henle's loop. The recycled urea increases the gradient for water reabsorption from the descending limb, which leads to an increase in the sodium chloride concentration of the tubular fluid entering the papillary tip and ascending limb.

Since the thin ascending limb is impermeable to water but permeable to salt and urea, and since the salt concentration within the thin segment is greater than in the surrounding medullary interstitium, salt will diffuse out faster than urea can diffuse in, and a hypotonic tubular fluid will be formed with an increase in medullary tonicity. In the thick ascending limb, salt is removed, leaving a more hypotonic fluid containing primarily urea. The greatest dilution occurs in the cortical diluting segment. Finally, within the distal tubule and collecting ducts, luminal fluid will be progressively concentrated in the presence of AVP, with urea diffusion proceeding from the inner medullary and papillary ducts. Kokko and Rector's model stresses the recycling of urea to produce a hyperosmolar medullary interstitium, while Stephenson emphasizes the passive or active transport of salt out of the thin ascending limb, in addition to "trapped" medullary urea, to yield a hyperosmolar gradient.

The strengths and weaknesses of the active and passive models have been recently reviewed (141). An integrative hypothesis assumes that the tubular fluid at the junction of the outer and inner medulla of the descending limb is slightly hyperosmolar to the fluid leaving the inner medulla in the interstitial vasa recta compartment (142). Even assuming there is no active transport out of the ascending limb, a difference of 33 mOsm/kg of tubular over interstitial fluid could account for an increase in urine osmolality from 530 to 2,200 mOsm/kg.

It was demonstrated in the rat that ureteral perfusion of high concentrations of urea increases urine osmolality (143). Interruption of the ureter from the renal pelvis in the rat markedly lowers maximal urine concentration at the papillary tip, probably due to loss of ureteral reflux of urea (144).

In partially nephrectomized rats, urine osmolality is much lower than normal in the remnant kidney (145). A greater percentage of filtered water is delivered to and reabsorbed by the papillary collecting duct of the remnant kidney. Dilution of urea in the collecting duct and increased vasa recta flow may account in part for the concentration defect in uremia. In addition, urea may be secreted into the medullary collecting tubule during water or mannitol diuresis in the rat (146). Exposure of the renal papilla of the rat decreases urine osmolality by greater than 50% due to failure of urea recycling (147).

Thus, the ability to concentrate the urine depends upon the reabsorption of solute delivered to the loop of Henle, the relative solute excretion or solute loss, and the renal response to AVP. The ability to dilute the urine depends upon the delivery of salt and water to the cortical diluting segment of the ascending limb, salt reabsorption by the ascending limb, and the lack of AVP response, mediating back diffusion of water out of the collecting duct.

RENAL EFFECTS OF AVP

The antidiuretic response to vasopressin by the kidney involves several mechanisms:

1. The activation of collecting tubular cell adenylate cyclase and formation of cyclic adenosine monophosphate (AMP), which ultimately facilitates the transport of H_2O from the tubular lumen to the hypertonic medullary interstitium;
2. the activation of adenylate cyclase in the ascending limb of the tubular cell, which facilitates the transport of Cl^- and accordingly Na^+ into the interstitium and increases medullary hyperosmolality;
3. the facilitation of reabsorption of urea from the inner medullary collecting tubule to the interstitium, which further enhances the medullary osmolar gradient for back diffusion of water;
4. the vasoconstrictive effect of AVP on vasa recta renal medullary blood flow, which lessens the washout of medullary solute.

There has been considerable data accumulated showing that AVP sensitive adenylate cyclase is present in the thick ascending limb as well as in the collecting tubule in the rat (148), the mouse, and the rabbit, but is present only in the collecting tubule in man (149) (Fig. 6). In turn, AVP and cyclic AMP have been shown to increase chloride transport from the lumen to the interstitium in the medullary thick ascending limb (150–152), but not in the cortical ascending limb (150) or the thin ascending limb (153) of the mouse. The transport of sodium appears to be secondary to AVP-induced chloride transport, increasing medullary interstitial tonicity (151, 152). Hypertonicity of the peritubular fluid induced by urea, mannitol, or hypertonic saline inhibits AVP-induced adenylate cyclase generation and chloride transport, providing a modulating effect on medullary hypertonicity (154). AVP and cyclic AMP stimulated water transport have been demonstrated not only in isolated collecting tubules of rats (155) but also in cortical collecting tubules of man (156).

The action of antidiuretic hormone (ADH) on the renal collecting tubule cell involves occupancy and activation of an adenylate cyclase receptor on

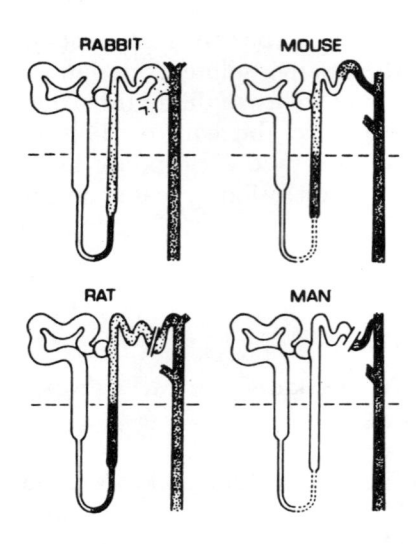

Figure 6. Distribution of AVP action sites in renal tubules from four different species. (Morel F: *Am J Physiol* 9:159–164, 1981. Reprinted with permission.)

the serosal side of the cell. This binding is facilitated by a cyclic guanosine monophosphate (GMP) regulatory subunit, and the cellular uptake of calcium is facilitated by means of a calmodulin protein complex. ADH-stimulated cyclic AMP is degraded by a phosphodiesterase to an inactive nucleotide 5'AMP. ADH-stimulated cyclic AMP in turn induces the production of a protein kinase, leading to the phosphorylation of a protein that ultimately interacts with the cell membrane at the mucosal surface. The transport of this protein is probably aided by the aggregation of microtubules and the action of microfilaments which compose the cellular cytoskeleton. The interaction of the protein with the mucosal cell surface leads to increased transport of water and small solutes, such as urea, by independent and separate mechanisms. Hydroxine, a stimulator of cyclic GMP, enhances vasopressin-induced water flow, adenylate cyclase, cyclic AMP-dependent protein kinase, and luminal membrane aggregrate frequency in the toad bladder but has no effect on Na^+ or urea permeability. Methohexital inhibits ADH-induced water flow, adenylate cyclase, and cyclic AMP-dependent protein kinase activation (Fig. 7) (157).

The antidiuretic action of AVP is associated with dose-related increases in particle aggregate clusters on the mucosal surface of the toad bladder and isolated collecting ducts of the Brattleboro rat (158). The water permeability response to AVP in the granular cells involves the shuttling and translocation to the luminal membrane of cytoplasmic tubular vacuoles containing particle aggregates. This translocation is probably mediated by microtubules and microfilaments. The aggregates are the site of transmembranous water channels, and fusion of tubular vacuoles with the luminal membrane inserts the aggregates and increases water premeability (159). The action of AVP produces morphologic evidence of marked swelling of the granular cells, elongation of microvilli, formation of

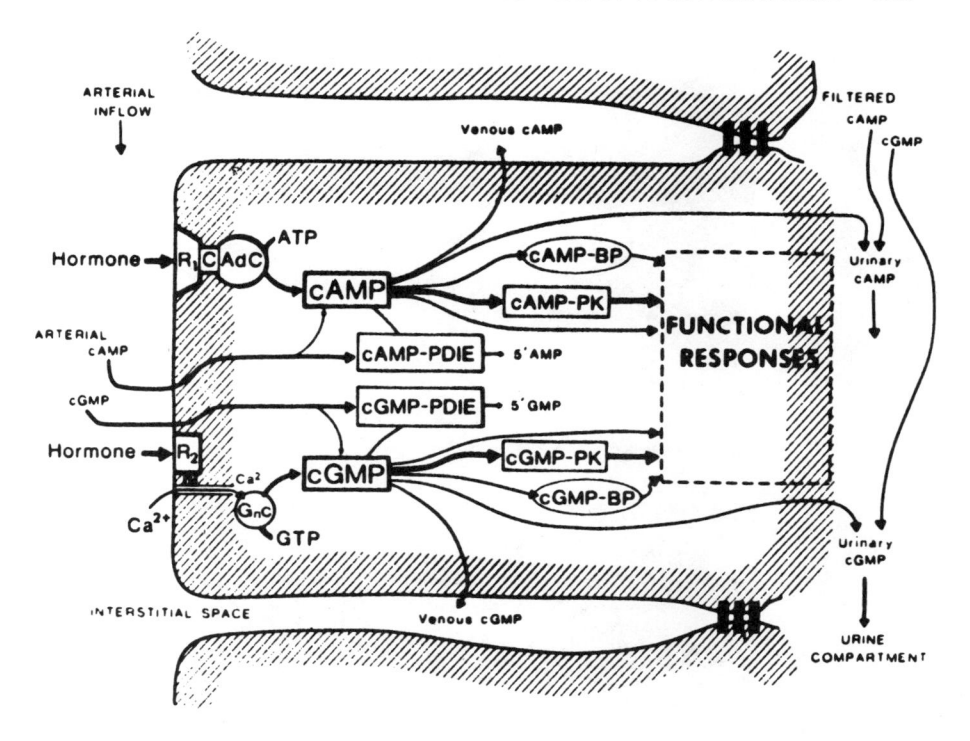

Figure 7. Cellular actions of AVP in renal tubular cells. (Dousa TP, in Brenner BM, Stein JH (eds): *Contemporary Issues in Nephrology, Vol 4, Hormonal Function and the Kidney*. New York, Churchill Livingstone, 1979, pp 251–285. Reprinted with permission.)

intracellular lakes, increased pinocytotic vesicles on the basal surface of the cell, and numerous extracellular multivesicular bodies in the dilated intracellular space (Fig. 8a,b) (160). Lowering the temperature decreases the fluidity. Vasopressin effects on water transport and particle aggregation are not inhibited by cold-induced decreases in fluidity, while AVP-induced urea transport is inhibited (161).

Trifluoperazine, an inhibitor of calmodulin, inhibits AVP and cyclic AMP-induced water flow but not urea or short circuit current response in the toad bladder, which suggests that calmodulin facilitates AVP-induced water transport distal to cyclic AMP generation (162).

Phosphodiesterase may regulate AVP responsiveness since isolated collecting tubules and thick ascending limbs in the rat have significant quantities of both cyclic AMP and cyclic GMP phosphodiesterase (163), and increasing interstitial osmolality of isolated papillary collecting ducts from 200 to 800 mOsm/kg increases AVP-stimulated adenylate cyclase and inhibits phosphodiesterase (164) (Fig. 8).

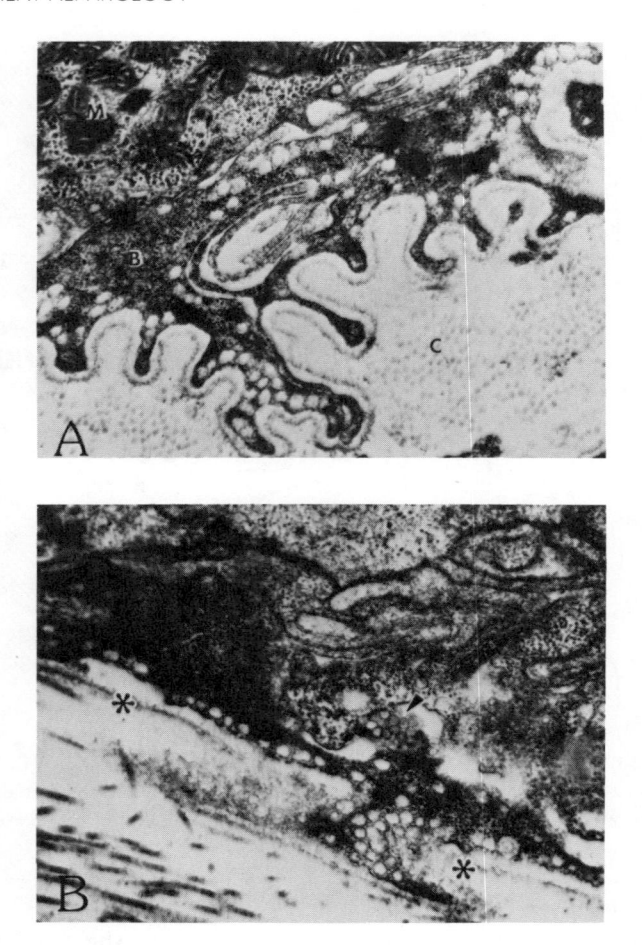

Figure 8. Transmission electron micrographs of the effects of AVP on toad urinary bladder cell. (*a*) TEM showing increased basal pinocytosis post-AVP. (*b*) An extracellular multivesicular body is seen (arrow). Asterisks show basal lamina. Note the presence of numerous basal vesicle. (Davis WL et al: *Ann N Y Acad Sci* 372:121, 1981. Reprinted with permission.)

Physiologic studies on the action of AVP on water and solute transport have generally utilized the toad bladder or in vitro micropuncture models. Changes in ionic intracellular composition of the serosal cell appear to dramatically affect osmotic water. Mendoza et al. (166) demonstrated that intracellular sodium regulates the magnitude of the hydrostatic response to both vasopressin and cyclic AMP. Likewise, Hardy et al. (167) showed that reduction of serosal calcium concentration inhibits by more than 60% vasopressin-stimulated osmotic water flow which affects diffusional permeability to water. Slight increases in the serosal hydrostatic pressure gradient of only 1 cm H_2O also significantly inhibits vasopressin-induced osmotic water flow, presumably by back flux of water through a paracellular pathway (168). A rise in temperature in the perfusate of isolated collecting tubules will inhibit the effect of AVP on water permeability (169).

The endogenous kallikrein-kinin system also appears to play some role in AVP-induced water flow since inhibition of this system by aprotinin increases both vasopressin- and cyclic AMP-stimulated water transport. Potentiation of endogenous kinin (by kininase II inhibitor, captopril) decreases vasopressin- and cyclic AMP-induced water flow. However, vasopressin-stimulated urea and sodium transport is decreased by aprotinin (170,171) and increased by captopril, while AVP may increase urinary kallikrein excretion (172), suggesting separate and divergent effects on these cellular actions of AVP.

Potassium depletion induces a reversible vasopressin-resistant polyuria. Kim et al. (173) examined the renal effects of potassium depletion using microdissected medullary collecting tubular (MCT) and thick medullary ascending limbs (MAL). AVP-sensitive adenylate cyclase activity was decreased in the MAL but increased in the MCT, and the latter actually had a higher accumulation of tissue cyclic AMP following vasopressin exposure than did normokalemic control subjects. Thus, the intracellular AVP resistance to urinary concentration in hypokalemic states appears to exist distal to the generation of cyclic AMP.

Further studies on the polyuria of hypokalemia were reported in vitro using potassium deplete dogs (174). The polyuria and decrease in concentrating ability was associated with a blunting of AVP secretion and an increase in urinary prostaglandin PGE_2 excretion. Indomethacin treatment partially normalized the osmotic responsiveness of AVP but did not alter the decrease in urine concentration, suggesting an inhibitory role of PGE on AVP osmoreceptors during potassium depletion but not on mammal urine concentrating ability. In addition potassium depleted rat kidney shows a decrease in PGE_2 and an increase in thromboxane B_2 which would tend to enhance renal concentrating ability (175). Thus, the defect in hypokalemia appears to reside both at the neurohypophysis as well as at the renal collecting duct, albeit by separate pathophysiologic mechanisms. In addition, Nadvornikova et al. (176) has resported that administration of synthetic AVP analogs to human volunteers is associated with an increased fractional excretion of potassium (possibly by increased tubular secretion) that is more pronounced in younger than in older subjects, and may become clinically significant with continued therapy.

Defects in urine concentration are frequently observed following therapeutic administration of the antineoplastic drug *cis*-dichlorodiamine platinum (cisplatin). Gordon et al. (177) evaluated this effect in rats and observed an initial decrease in effective AVP release immediately after starting the drug (1 day), while at 8 days the concentrating defect appeared to be due to diminished interstitial solute in renal medullary tissue secondary to "washout" from the initial polyuria. High concentrations of intracellular copper also appear to inhibit the renal response to AVP at a site proximal to cyclic AMP production, possibly by altering the sulfhydryl content of the cell membrane since reducing agents reverse the inhibition (178,179).

Exposure of cell receptors to high concentrations of vasopressin induces refractoriness of the renal response, undoubtedly by a down regulation of the membrane receptor. Handler et al. (180) investigated this phenomenon in the toad bladder and suggested that under different conditions, this refractoriness results from a reduced vasopressin-sensitive adenylate cyclase activity, a reduced tissue accumulation of cyclic AMP, and a refractoriness of water transport in response to exogenous cyclic AMP.

Aging is also associated with an impaired urine concentrating ability with a failure to increase papillary cyclic AMP following exogenous AVP (181,182).

AVP is removed from the plasma by both hepatic and renal clearance. Much of the AVP cleared by the kidney is biologically and immunologically intact. Kimura et al. (183) have utilized the stop-flow techniques to characterize the renal handling of AVP in the dog. Their data suggests that AVP is reabsorbed from or degraded in the proximal nephron and secreted into the distal nephron so that urinary clearance closely matches the glomerular filtration rate, although they could not estimate the amount of AVP taken up and degraded in the peritubular capillaries.

Finally, AVP physiology appears to be abnormal in patients with chronic renal disease. In end-stage renal disease patients undergoing hemodialysis, predialysis plasma AVP concentrations are inappropriately elevated in the face of expanded plasma volumes and moderately elevated blood pressure, despite normal plasma volumes and osmolality (184). In addition to an abnormality in osmoreceptor function, the hemodynamic AVP stimulation to plasma volume reduction also appears dysfunctional. Patients with chronic renal failure on hemodialysis were subjected to isosmolar volume reduction via intensified hemofiltration (185). Despite a decrease in mean arterial blood pressure, plasma AVP showed a paradoxical drop at 1 hour in eight out of eight subjects and at 2 hours in five out of eight subjects. This decrease in plasma AVP is not secondary to removal by the dialysis procedure since no change in plasma AVP concentration could be documented after routine hemofiltration nor could any detectable immunoassayable AVP be measured in the hemofiltrate samples (186).

PROSTAGLANDIN REGULATION OF AVP

Prostaglandins appear to have a diversified role in modulating several aspects of renal function including water transport, sodium transport, regulation of renal blood flow, renin release, glomerular filtration, and

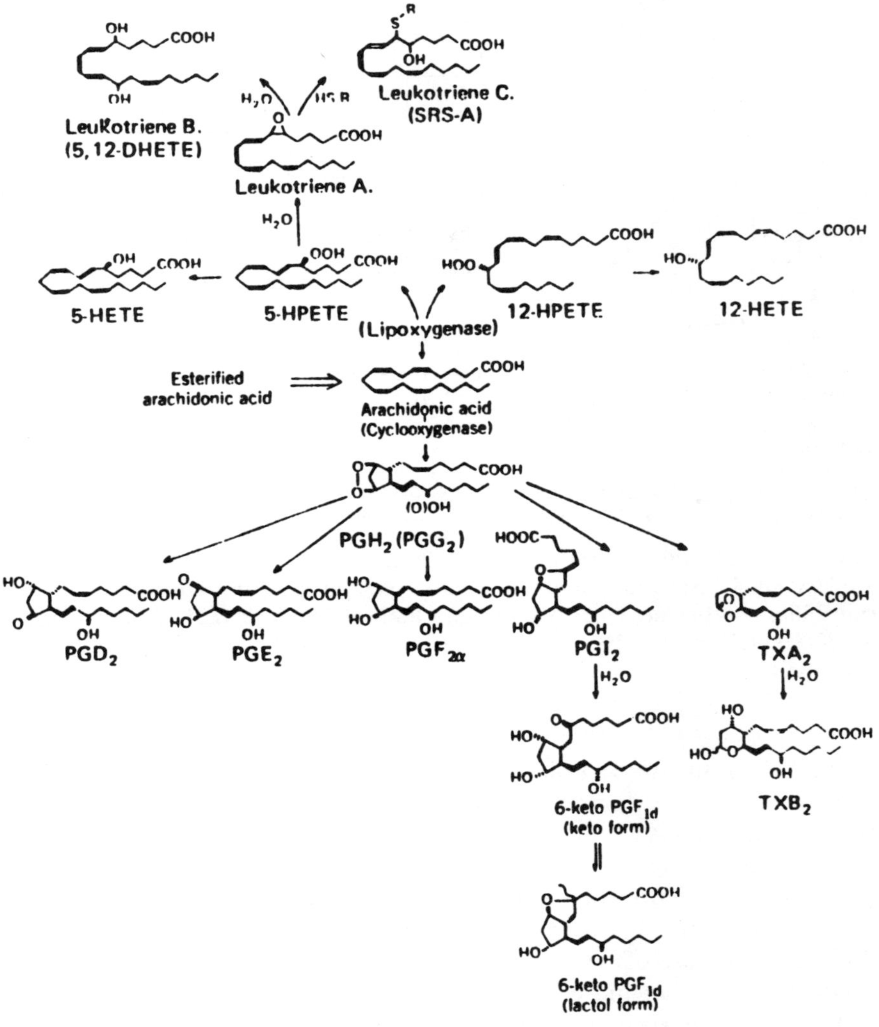

Figure 9. Scheme of biologically active compounds derived from arachidonic acid. (Anggard E, Oliw E: *Kidney Int* 19:773, 1981. Reprinted with permission.)

erythropoietin production. The major active prostaglandin compounds are prostaglandin E_2 (PGE_2), prostacyclin, and thromboxane A_2, although medullary synthesis of PGE_2 appears most significant in regulating renal effects (Fig. 9). The role of prostaglandin A_2 and D_2 in renal function is not clear. The action of PGE_2 on water excretion is still controversial and evidence exists that prostaglandins act as a negative feedback modulator of AVP action, that is, AVP stimulates PGE_2 synthesis which subsequently

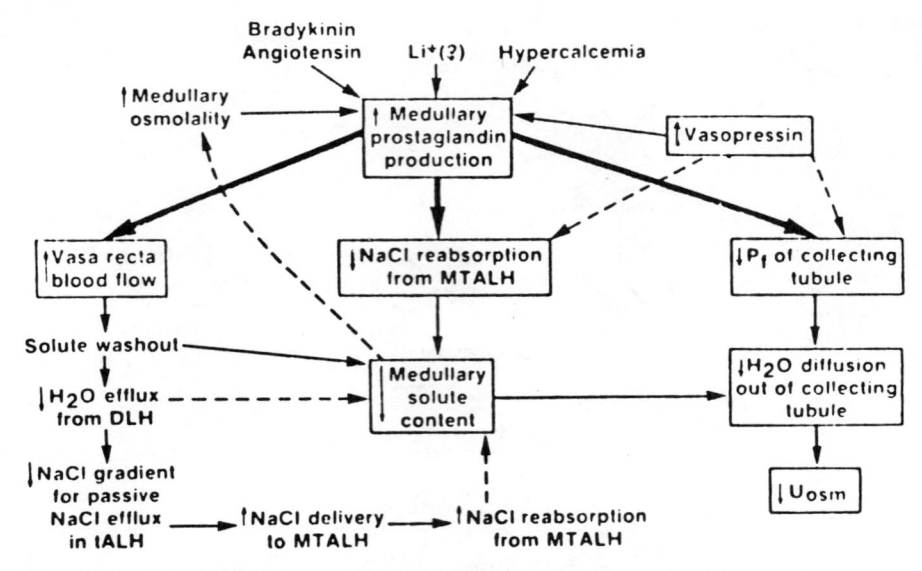

Figure 10. Regulation of water metabolism by medullary prostaglandins. MTALH, medullary thick ascending limb of Henle; P_f; vasopressin-dependent osmotic permeability coefficient; DLH, descending limb of Henle; tALH, thin ascending limb of Henle. (Stokes JB: *Am J Physiol* 240:471–480, 1981. Reprinted with permission.)

inhibits AVP-stimulated cyclic AMP and water transport. However, conflicting studies have demonstrated both increased and decreased PGE_2 excretion following AVP, and human experiments have reported increased urinary PGE_2 during both increased and decreased urinary flow rates. It appears that the action of renal medullary prostaglandins in controlling water excretion reflects their antagonism of AVP effect at four levels, including a decrease of AVP-dependent osmotic water permeability of the collecting tubules, an increase of renal medullary blood flow, inhibition of salt absorption from the thick ascending limb of Henle's loop, and inhibition of urea reabsorption from the collecting tubule (Fig. 10) (187,188). The reader is referred to recent reviews of the role of prostaglandins in regulation of water excretion (187,189–191).

Forrest et al. (192) studied the mechanisms underlying the acidosis inhibition of the hydroosmotic response to AVP and suggested this was secondary to increased production of local PGE_2 synthesis. In addition, prostaglandin synthesis inhibitors block the pH-dependent inhibition of AVP action. This effect may contribute to the polyuria and hyposthenuria noted in hemorrhagic shock. Selkurt (193) suggests that the large amounts of PGE produced by the renal medulla and other tissues during the hypotensive period are incompletely metabolized by the pulmonary circulation. They appear in the systemic circulation and contribute toward potentiation of the hypotension by their vasodilatory effects.

Jones et al. (194) compared the renal effects of prostaglandin E_2 and I_2. Both compounds increase renal blood flow, urine flow, and PRA, and decrease systemic blood pressure. PGE_2 was, however, more effective in augmenting sodium excretion. Their results suggest that both PGE_2 and PGI_2 exert their effects by promoting vasodilation, while PGE_2 also has a direct action on renal tubular function. The synthesis of thromboxane A_2 (TXA_2) is stimulated by vasopressin in the toad bladder as measured by its stable product TXB_2. Imidazole, a TXA_2 synthesis inhibitor, suppressed vasopressin-stimulated water flow while analogs of TXA_2 enhance vasopressin-stimulated water flow (195).

Recent human studies have continued to produce conflicting results regarding the relationship between AVP, urine flow rates, and PGE_2. Walker et al. (196) reported that urinary PGE_2 excretion varied directly with the urine flow rate in normal subjects as well as in central and nephrogenic diabetes insipidus, increasing during water loading and decreasing following administration of the synthetic AVP analog DDAVP (desamino, D-arginine vasopressin). They suggest that PGE_2 excretion is not directly dependent on AVP or state of hydration since inhibition of prostaglandin synthesis with indomethacin blunted free water clearance while it suppressed the rise in PGE_2 urinary excretion. The increase in urinary PGE_2 with polyuria may facilitate water excretion by AVP antagonism.

Dusing et al. (197) reported contradictory results. They found that patients with central diabetes insipidus have low urinary excretion of PGE_2 in their basal, untreated, polyuric state. Urinary PGE_2 is markedly stimulated following administration of DDAVP with a resultant decrease in urine flow rates. Therapy with indomethacin, in addition to DDAVP, suppresses urinary PGE_2 and increases urinary concentrating ability as compared to DDAVP alone, suggesting urine flow rate itself is not a significant determinant of PGE_2 excretion. Belch et al. (198) also report an increased release of prostacyclin (PGI_2) following administration of DDAVP. Finally, Padfield et al. (199) have reported that indomethacin treatment for 3 days (sufficient to reduce endogenous prostaglandin production) does not alter the renal response to infused AVP, suggesting that prostaglandin may have little activity in the day-to-day renal effects of AVP.

Some of the confusing and contradictory results on the relationship between AVP and renal PGE_2 may be clarified by the recent study of Zipser et al. (200). In normal volunteers, pharmacologic doses of vasopressin injection (Pitressin) stimulates urinary PGE_2 excretion, while administration of the nonpressor AVP analog, DDAVP, or 8-hour dehydration failed to decrease PGE_2 excretion despite a similar antidiuretic response. Infusion of AII, however, did increase urinary PGE_2. These results suggest that it is not the antidiuretic effect of AVP that increases PGE_2 synthesis, but rather that AVP has two opposite effects on PGE_2 urinary excretion: a stimulation by the pharmacologic pressor properties, and an inhibition by the antidiuretic effects. Other studies, however, fail to show a stimulation of PGE_2 by AVP or DDAVP (201).

The inhibitory effect of urea on AVP stimulation of PGE_2 in renal medullary slices could account for the effect of increased urine volume on increasing urine PGE. Inner medullary urea would fall during water diuresis due to medullary washout, which could thereby increase urine PGE while dehydration would do the opposite (202).

Schlondorff et al. (203) have shown that prostaglandin inhibition by naproxin stimulates and therefore endogenous PGE inhibits AVP-stimulated cyclic AMP, protein kinase, and water flow in the toad bladder. On the other hand, exogenous PGE_2 and PGE_1 actually stimulate cyclic AMP and protein kinase and may inhibit the effects of cyclic AMP and cyclic AMP-dependent protein kinase on water flow. The stimulatory effect of PGE on cyclic AMP may account for its inhibitory effect on NaCl reabsorption in the toad bladder or collecting tubule. AVP initially increases and then more steadily decreases NaCl flow across the isolated cortical collecting duct of the rabbit (204). This latter effect is blocked by prostaglandin inhibition by meclofenamate and reintroduced by PGE_2. AVP also inhibits reabsorption of and stimulates secretion of calcium and phenylate, and this action is also blocked by prostaglandin inhibition and restored by PGE_2 (205). Thus, the inhibitory effects of AVP on ion transport may be mediated by AVP stimulation of PGE_2 production.

There have been several studies attempting to relate the polyuric effects of hypercalcemia and AVP antagonism by prostaglandins. Calcium ionophore stimulates while calmodulin inhibition inhibits PGE response to hyperosmolality (202). Calcium channel blockade by verapamil inhibits the enhancing effort of prostaglandin inhibition on ADH-induced water transport in the toad bladder (206), suggesting that ADH stimulation of PGE_2 is dependent on cellular uptake of calcium.

Calcium infusion in the renal artery of the dog increases urine PGE_2 markedly; indomethacin inhibits this effect (207). Hypercalcemic rats develop vasopressin-resistant polyuria and high urine PGE, both reversed by indomethacin (208). Berl et al. (209) have shown that indomethacin increases the antidiuretic response to vasopressin in hypercalcemic dogs. On the other hand, hypercalcemia blunted the antidiuretic response to vasopressin in indomethacin-treated dogs. Thus, the polyuric effect of hypercalcemia is not dependent on PGE_2. Increased cytosolic calcium enhances vasopressin action, while increased extracellular calcium inhibits vasopressin action. PGE_2 appears to inhibit calcium entry into cells, which may account for its opposing effect on the antidiuretic action of vasopressin (210).

The antidiuretic effects of cyclooxygenase inhibitors may be in part independent of AVP action. Since both indomethacin and meclofenamate increase urine osmolality in the diabetes insipidus rat devoid of vasopressin (211), these drugs increased papillary Na^+, urea, and osmolality, probably by interfering with PGE_2 inhibition of ascending limb reabsorption of NaCl, collecting tubule reabsorption of urea, and renal medullary washout.

Thromboxane A_2 has a faciliatory effect on AVP-induced water transport in contrast to PGE_2. Synthetic prostaglandin endoperoxide analogs, EPA I and EPA II, inhibit AVP-induced water transport in the toad bladder, while another analog EPA III reversed EPA I but not PGE_2 inhibitory activity (212). Potassium depletion in the rat stimulates thromboxane B_2 and inhibits PGE_2 (175).

In obstructive uropathy, there is increased production of PGE_2 and thromboxane A_2, which could mediate the vasoconstrictive effects of unilateral ureteral obstruction (213). Imidazole blockade of TXA_2 generation in the unilaterally obstructed rat kidney produced no increase in renal blood flow on the obstructed side, however (214). Glomerular synthesis of PGF_2, the major metabolite of PGI, 6 keto-PGF_1 and TXB_2 were increased following ureteral ligation in the ligated kidney, while PGE_2 production increased in the contralateral kidney (215).

Osmotic diuresis by mannitol in the rat kidney is associated with increased renal blood flow. Thus, response is blocked by indomethacin and restored by prostacyclin but not by PGE_2 (216). In isolated rat kidney collecting tubules, volume expansion, inhibition of NaCl, and water reabsorption are blunted by indomethacin (217). Thus, prostaglandins could mediate volume expansion-induced diuresis by increasing medullary blood flow, inhibiting collecting tubule Na^+ or Cl^- reabsorption, and antagonizing AVP generation of cyclic AMP.

HORMONAL REGULATION OF WATER BALANCE

Sex Steroid Hormones

The chronic administration of estrogen produces sodium retention in laboratory animals and in humans. Recent studies of rats have suggested that estrogens have a stimulatory effect on AVP and elevate plasma levels on the morning of proestrus administration and following estradiol administration to ovariectomized animals (218). Forsling et al. (219) reported changes in AVP in normal adult women followed throughout the menstrual cycle with nadir values at the onset of menses and peak values at midcycle around the day of ovulation, shortly after the preovulatory rise in estradiol. This parallels the findings in rats. In addition, Stromberg et al. (220) reported a fourfold increase of plasma AVP in women with primary dysmenorrhea at the time of menses. Although treatment with a prostaglandin synthesis inhibitor decreased the abdominal pain, it did not alter plasma AVP concentration, suggesting that the elevated AVP was not related to the nonosmotic stress stimulus. Finally, Cavicchia et al. (221) demonstrated a rise in plasma AVP in male rats following copulation that persisted for at least 60 minutes. It is uncertain whether this reflects the stress stimulus or CNS modulation by other neurotransmitters.

PARATHYROID HORMONE

Hypercalcemia is a well-known metabolic disturbance associated with a vasopressin-resistant polyuric state. Hammer et al. (222) examined the effects of calcium infusion upon pituitary secretion of AVP in normal subjects and in uremic patients on hemodialysis (nephrectomized and nonnephrectomized). While no effects were observed in normal individuals, plasma AVP was elevated during the infusion in uremic patients and was directly related to the rise in ionized calcium. The authors suggest this augmented AVP response results from the secondary hyperparathyroidism in the dialysis patients and the biological effect of PTH enhancing entry of calcium into the neurohypophysis. A similar finding was reported by Baylis et al. (223). They examined the osmoregulation of AVP in hypercalcemic hyperparathyroid nonuremic patients. All patients in this study had a reversible decreased renal concentrating ability. Following hypertonic saline administration, the patients demonstrated an exaggerated AVP response. Although the subjects had normal renal function, this augmented rise in AVP may reflect a stimulatory effect of PTH. Finally, Berl et al. (209) have examined the renal effects of hypercalcemia by quantitating the antidiuretic effect of exogenous AVP in dogs with and without prostaglandin inhibition. Acute hypercalcemia diminished the AVP-induced renal concentration in the prostaglandin-inhibited animals, suggesting that the renal defect is not dependent upon the synthesis of medullary prostaglandins.

Insulin

Szczepanska-Sadowska et al. (224) examined the integrated effects of insulin and vasopressin on renal water and electrolyte excretion in fluid-loaded ethanol treated rats. Insulin by itself increased urinary volume, decreased urinary osmolality, and in low doses increased urinary sodium excretion. Vasopressin by itself was antidiuretic and slightly natriuretic. Simultaneous administration of insulin and vasopressin produced no change in urinary volume or osmolality but induced a prolonged and significant natriuresis, suggesting a synergistic effect between these two peptide hormones.

Somatostatin

Somatostatin may also be a regulator of vasopressin-stimulated water flow, since it inhibits vasopressin and theophylline, but not cyclic AMP-mediated water flow. Immunoreactive somatotropin releasing inhibitory factor is present in the toad bladder and renal distal and collecting tubule and probably acts as an inhibitor of vasopressin at the adenylate cyclase catalytic subunit (225).

Glucocorticoids

The presence of glucocorticoids is required for the normal capacity of the kidney in the formation of dilute urine and the excretion of free water. Numerous studies in the past have attempted to elucidate the role of vasopressin in the impaired water excretion of glucocorticoid insufficiency. Linas et al. (226) demonstrated that mineralocorticoid-replaced, adrenalectomized rats had elevated levels of plasma AVP 1 day after withdrawal of cortisol and excreted only 70% of a 30 ml/kg water load in 3 hours, and only 40% of the water load 14 days after cortisol withdrawal. In the heterozygous Brattleboro diabetes insipidus rat, water excretion was impaired 14 days after but not 1 day after cortisol withdrawal. Cardiac index and renal blood were decreased at 14 days. Thus, the impaired water diuresis in glucocorticoid insufficiency was due to elevated vasopressin at day 1, but independent of vasopressin at day 14. The elevation of vasopressin is probably due to nonosmotic stimulation via the baroreceptor in response to a decrease in cardiac stroke volume.

Thyroid Hormone

Thyroid hormone deficiency is also associated with an impairment in urinary dilution. Again, there appears to be an AVP-dependent mechanism due to enhanced AVP release secondary to decrease in cardiac output in hypothyroidism, as well as an AVP-independent mechanism involving enhanced proximal tubule reabsorption of $NaCl^-$ and limited delivery of urine to the cortical diluting segment (227).

HYPONATREMIC DISORDERS

Hyponatremic disorders can be physiologically categorized by quantitating plasma tonicity, as well as by clinically assessing extracellular fluid volume or total body sodium. The hyponatremias are thus divided into hypertonic, isotonic, and hypotonic categories, and the large number of hypotonic hyponatremias are subclassified into hypovolemic, normovolemic, and hypervolemic groups. The differential diagnosis or etiology of these

Table 2. Conditions and Causes of Hyponatremic Disorders

Conditions	Possible Causes
Hypertonic hyponatremia	Hyperglycemia
	Hypertonic infusions (glucose, mannitol, glycine)
Isotonic hyponatremia	Pseudohyponatremia
	hypertriglyceridemia
	paraproteinemia (myeloma, etc.)
	Isotonic infusions—acutely (glucose, mannitol, glycine)
Hypotonic hyponatremia	
Hypovolemic hypotonic hyponatremia	Urine Na$^+$ > 20 mEq/liter because of
	adrenal insufficiency
	hypoaldosteronism
	Bartter's syndrome
	diuretics
	diabetes mellitus out of control
	chronic renal salt wasting
	renal tubular acidosis
	Urine Na$^+$ < 10 mEq/liter because of
	gastrointestinal losses
	excessive sweating
	third spacing (e.g., burns, pancreatitis)
	bronchorrhea

various types of hyponatremia are summarized in Table 2 and have been discussed in detail in the previous volumes of this series.

Syndrome of Inappropriate ADH Secretion (SIADH)

SIADH is undoubtedly the most common form of hypotonic normovolemic hyponatremia observed and diagnosed in clinical practice (Table 3). Although the patient appears clinically euvolemic without manifestation of edema, these syndromes are usually associated with excessive body water of 4–5 liters; hyponatremia will never develop unless the patient is ingesting or receiving some source of free water. This syndrome is best defined by the criteria listed in Table 3 and generally refers to primary defects in AVP function causing continued secretion and/or action of the hormone that cannot be ascribed to known osmotic or nonosmotic stimuli. Semantic problems may arise in defining particular cases of hypotonic normovolemic hyponatremia as "inappropriate" or "appropriate" elevations of AVP since AVP is known to have some causative role in increasingly more hyponatremic disorders. Some investigators prefer the classification of "excessive" vasopressin secretion for these reasons. Readers are referred to recent comprehensive reviews of this topic (41–44,228,229).

Table 2. (continued)

Conditions	Possible Causes

Normovolemic hypotonic hyponatremia	Syndrome of inappropriate antidiuretic hormone secretion (SIADH)
	Osmoregulatory reset variant
	Pregnancy
	"Beer drinker's" hyponatremia
	Exacerbated psychosis
	Hypopituitarism
	Hypothyroidism
	Glucorticoid deficiency (early)
	Psychogenic polydipsia
	Polydipsic vomiting
	Diuretic-induced
	Antidiuretic drugs
	  vincristine
	  cyclophosphamide
	  general anesthetics
	  morphine
	  barbiturates
	  carbamazepine
	  clofibrate
	  amitriptyline
	  thioridazine
	  desipramine
	  tranylcypromine
	  chlorpropamide
	  tolbutamide
	  phenformin
	  acetaminophen
	  indomethacin
	  oxytocin
	  vasopressin (DDAVP, etc.)
	  haloperidol
	  chlorthalidone
	  centozolone
	  adenine arabinoside

Hypervolemic hypotonic hyponatremia	Urine $Na^+ > 20$ mEq/liter because of
	  acute tubular necrosis
	  chronic renal failure, endstage
	Urine $Na^+ < 10$ mEq/liter because of
	  congestive heart failure
	  cirrhosis with ascites
	  nephrotic syndrome

Table 3. Syndrome of Inappropriate Antidiuretic Hormone Secretion

Diagnostic Criteria for SIADH
  Exclusion of the other causes of hyponatremia such as cardiac, renal, hepatic, thyroid, pituitary, or adrenal disease in which there is appropriate although nonosmotic stimulation of AVP release. Drug-induced AVP release should also be excluded.
  Hyponatremia and serum hypoosmolality.
  High urine Na^+.
  Urine that is more concentrated than is appropriate for the degree of serum hypoosmolality.
  Normovolemia, that is, no signs of either edema or extracellular fluid volume contraction.
  Normal renal function.
  Normal thyroid function.
  Normal adrenal function (glucocorticoid and mineralocorticoid).
  Impaired excretion of water load.
  Correction of the hyponatremia by fluid restriction (with the exception of the Osmoregulatory Reset variant).
Mechanisms (based on radioimmunoassay)
  Vasopressin levels elevated and unrelated to plasma osmolality.
  Vasopressin levels and plasma osmolality elevated in parallel, with the osmotic threshold for vasopressin release *reset* below normal.
  Vasopressin levels elevated at low plasma osmolality, but, above the threshold for vasopressin release, plasma vasopressin increases normally (i.e., vasopressin "leak").
  Vasopressin levels are normal and increase normally with increased plasma osmolality (i.e., increased renal sensitivity to vasopressin).
Etiology
  Tumors producing vasopressin as determined by radioimmunoassay or bioassay of tissues, blood, urine:
  Bronchogenic carcinoma, (oat cell is most common)
  Pancreatic carcinoma
  Duodenal carcinoma
  Colonic carcinoma
  Hodgkin's disease and lymphoma
  Leukemia
  Prostatic carcinoma
  Nasopharyngeal carcinoma
  Thymoma
  Carcinoid
  Neuroblastoma
  Tuberculoma
  Ureteral carcinoma
  Ewing's sarcoma
  Other chest lesions
    Tuberculosis
    Pneumonia
    Pulmonary abscess

Table 3. (*continued*)

Other chest lesions (*continued*)
    Cystic fibrosis
    Cavitary lesions (*Aspergillosis*)
    Acute respiratory failure
    Chronic obstructive pulmonary disease
    Acute pneumothorax
    Acute bronchitis
    Acute bronchiolitis
    Status asthmaticus
    IPPB
  Idiopathic
  Central nervous system disorders
    Trauma
    Meningitis
    Subdural hematoma
    Cerebral abscess
    Encephalitis
    Subarachnoid hemorrhage
    Cerebral thrombosis
    Acute psychoses
    Acute intermittent porphyria
    CNS lupus
    Guillain-Barré syndrome
    Cerebral atrophy
    Primary and metastatic tumors
    Hypoplastic corpus callosum
    Rocky Mountain spotted fever
    Multiple sclerosis
    Cavernous sinus thrombosis
    Malignant histiocytosis
    Wernicke's encephalopathy
    Polyarteritis nodosa
    Epilepsy
  Drugs

Reductions in serum uric acid concentrations have been recommended as a screening procedure in patients with hyponatremia secondary to SIADH. The mechanism of hypouricemia appears to be an increase in uric acid excretion secondary to a decrease in distal tubular reabsorption. This effect seems to be induced by volume expansion, since the direct effect of AVP is a reduction in the fractional renal clearance of urate. Ducobu et al. (230) examined 22 hyponatremic patients and claimed hypouricemia was a reliable method of detecting SIADH. However,

Osterlind et al. (231) studied 69 patients with bronchogenic small cell carcinoma and coexistent SIADH in 25 patients, and concluded that use of the serum uric acid lacks both sensitivity and specificity for making the diagnosis; hypouricemia appears to be present in any volume expanded state.

Yamaji et al. (232) examined the immunoreactive neurophysins isolated from five subjects with oat cell bronchogenic carcinoma and SIADH. Vasopressin and nicotine stimulated neurophysin could be isolated in all samples, primarily as a 10,000 dalton peptide, although 6.5–8.7% of the total immunoreactivity was contained in a 20,000 dalton high molecular weight peptide, felt to represent an AVP neurophysin precursor similar to that isolated from the hypothalamus. The entity SIADH has also been reported in patients with malignant histiocytosis (233) and nasal neuroblastoma (234). In addition, Ginsberg et al. (235) have reported that the combination of three potent antineoplastic drugs—vinblastine, cisplatin, and bleomycin—used as chemotherapy for metastatic germ cell tumors appear to act synergistically to produce hyponatremia secondary to impaired water handling.

An unusual case of intermittent, episodic SIADH was reported by Sato et al. (236) in an 8-year-old girl with documented periodic and simultaneous hypersecretion of both ACTH and AVP. These episodes occurred at approximately monthly intervals and were associated with elevated excretion of epinephrine and norepinephrine but lowered cerebrospinal fluid concentration of homovanillic acid, suggesting a periodic CNS dysfunction of catecholamine metabolism. Clinical SIADH has also been reported in patients with Wernicke's encephalopathy (237), Guillain-Barré syndrome (238), and in psychiatric subjects receiving haloperidol (239).

AVP Secretion in Pulmonary Disease

Low pressure volume receptors modulating AVP secretion reside within the pulmonary great vessels, and intrathoracic pathology has been associated with nonosmotic hypersecretion of vasopressin. Farber et al. (240) studied a group of hypercapnic, hypoxic, edematous subjects with chronic obstructive pulmonary disease and observed a high incidence of elevated plasma AVP concentration, as well as high PRA and aldosterone levels. They suggested that the hypercapnia increased renal sodium absorption and postulated stimulation of the renin-angiotensin system and neurohypophysis to induce clinical edema and hyponatremia. They did not elaborate on the mechanisms involved. Szatalowicz et al. (241) also documented excessive water retention and hypoosmolality secondary to elevated plasma AVP concentrations in 13 patients with acute respiratory failure. Excessive AVP secretion and fluid retention has been reported in numerous other types of pulmonary disease, including acute pneumothorax in the neonate (242), acute bronchitis (243), acute bronchiolitis (244), and legionnaires disease (245). It appears that this problem may be unrecognized during acute respiratory infections in the pediatric age group (246). One explanation may be a decreased erythrocyte Na^+, K^+, ATPase activity which leads to increased intracellular sodium accumulation, reducing the extracellular sodium concentration (247). PEEP ventilation may facilitate the development of hyponatremia in respiratory disorders since it increases plasma AVP levels in the dog (248).

MISCELLANEOUS HYPONATREMIC DISORDERS

Tarnow-Mordi et al. (249) described newborn hyponatremia in a series of 136 deliveries. Of the 41 mothers who received only oral fluids during labor, 24 delivered infants with normal cord plasma sodium concentrations. Of the 95 mothers who received intravenous fluids (usually 5% or 10% glucose in water), only 14 delivered infants with normal cord plasma sodium and 31 had cord plasma sodium concentrations below 130 mEq/liter. There was a positive correlation between the degree of hyponatremia and the rate of fluid administration, which suggests that the hypoosmolar fluid in combination with augmented fetal AVP secretion contributed to these findings.

Emesis has been suggested as another nonosmotic stimulus for AVP secretion. Fisher et al. (250) described acute elevation of plasma AVP concentration following chemotherapy-induced emesis in patients with metastatic malignancies.

Drug-Induced Hyponatremia

Diuretic-induced hyponatremia is usually mild and has been ascribed to hypokalemia, which facilitates the intracellular movement of sodium, mild volume contraction, excessive AVP release, and primary polydipsia, or increased natriuresis, in association with fluid overload. Ashraf et al. (251) have described the rapid (less than 3 weeks) onset of thiazide-induced severe hyponatremia in seven previously healthy patients, leading to death or residual permanent paralysis. Metabolic studies suggested that an underlying defect in urinary dilution, as well as hypokalemia, induces a state of susceptibility to thiazide-related hyponatremia.

Drug-induced hyponatremia is probably the factor producing hypoosmolality in mentally disturbed patients receiving psychotropic agents. Gleadhill et al. (252) reports a 5–8% incidence of hyponatremia in patients with schizophrenia related to excessive polydipsia and antipsychotic and anticholinergic medication. In addition, Brent et al. (253) reported SIADH in a patient with depressive psychosis whose hyponatremia was refractory

Table 4. Agents Modifying the Release or Peripheral Action of AVP

Augmentation of AVP Release

Isoproterenol	Vincristine	Haloperidol
Prostaglandin E	Cyclophosphamide	Glycine
Halothane	Amitriptyline	Chlorthalidone
Ether	Thioridazine	Centozolone
Cyclopropane	Desipramine	Thiothixene
Thiopental	Tranylcypramine	Amitryptyline
Nitrous oxide	Chlorpropamide	Fluphenazine
Barbiturates	Histamine	Clomipramine
Nicotine	GABA	Adenine arabinoside
Acetylcholine	Carbachol	
Carbamazepine	Substance P	
Clofibrate	Neurotensin	

Facilitation of Peripheral Action of AVP

Chlorpropamide	Oxytocin (large doses)
Tolbutamide	Triiodothyronine
Phenformin	Aldosterone
Acetaminophen	Theophylline
Thiazides	Griseofulvin
Indomethacin	

Inhibition of AVP Release

Ethanol	Dopamine
Diphenylhydantoin	Glucocorticoids
Norepinephrine	Clonidine
Phenothiazines	Opioid Peptides
Atropine	

Inhibition of Peripheral Action of AVP

Diatrizoate	Ethacrynic acid	Thioglycolate
Hypercalcemia	Furosemide	Glutathione
Hypermagnesiumia	Ovalain	Glyceride
Hypokalemia	Colchicine	Acetohexamide
Lithium	Amphotericin B	Tolazamide
Prostaglandin E	Dinitrophenol	Dopamine
Phenocetin	Indocetic acid	Isophosphamide
Propoxyphene	Fluroacetic acid	Vasopressinoid acid
Demethylchlortetracycline	N-ethylmaleimide	Gentamycin
Methoxyfluorane	Cysteine	Vinblastine
	Trifluoperazine	Somatostatin

to fluid restriction yet corrected during the course of electroshock therapy (ECT). Demeclocycline, a competitive inhibitor of AVP at the renal tubules, has been used to correct the hyponatremia associated with psychogenic polydipsia (254), although the side effects are not mentioned. Other drugs are summarized in Table 4.

Arginine Vasopressin

```
 1   2   3   4   5   6   7   8   9
Cys-Tyr-Phe-Gln-Asn-Cys-Pro-Arg-Gly-NH2
 |_____|
```

Vasopressor Antagonist: d(CH$_2$)$_5$Tyr(Me)AVP

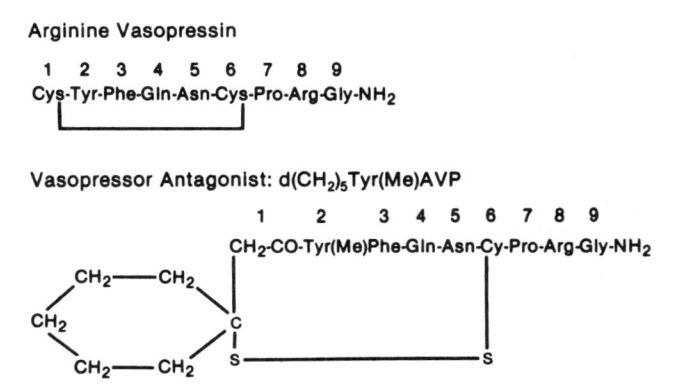

Figure 11. Structure of AVP and a vasopressor antagonist. (Manning M, Sawyer WH: *Ann Int Med* 96:520–522, 1982. Reprinted with permission.)

THERAPY OF HYPONATREMIC STATES

After initial, logical attempts to treat any underlying disease or to eliminate any offending drug that may have precipitated the excessive secretion of AVP and the ensuing hypoosmolar state, the physician is left with the therapeutic modalities of fluid restriction, hypertonic saline, mannitol, furosemide, and possibly end organ AVP antagonism with demeclocycline or lithium. Decaux et al. (255) have recommended urea administration (60–90 g orally over 24 hours or 80 g intravenously over 6 hours) in addition to fluid restriction and salt supplementation as therapy for severe hyponatremia that requires rapid correction of the serum sodium concentration. The urea promotes an osmotic diuresis, restores the medullary toxicity, and induces sodium retention. Weizman et al. (256) have proposed another therapeutic approach for the rapid correction of hyponatremia in SIADH by adding deoxycorticosterone acetate (DOCA) (4 mg/m^2/24 hours) to the established use of 3% hypertonic saline and furosemide (257).

Recently, however, investigators have reported that correction of hyponatremia that is done too rapidly causes central pontine myelinolysis (CPM), a demyelinative disorder with lesions in the gray matter of the brain (258,259) in humans and in experimental animals. Although the pathophysiology is unknown, possible explanations include rapid osmotically induced damage to oligodendrocytes (the myelin forming cells of the CNS) or vasogenic edema which produces demyelination in the vascular gray matter of the brain.

Possible future therapeutic agents for treatment of AVP-induced hyponatremia are synthetic vasopressin analogs with intrinsic antidiuretic antagonism (Figs. 11 and 12). Manning and Sawyer have pioneered this

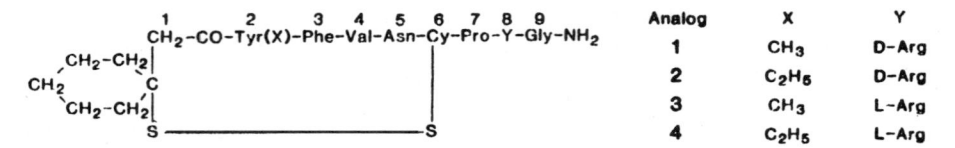

```
         1       2    3   4   5   6 7 8  9
      CH₂-CO-Tyr(X)-Phe-Val-Asn-Cy-Pro-Y-Gly-NH₂
    CH₂-CH₂|                     |
CH₂      C                       |
    CH₂-CH₂|                     |
         S ──────────────────────S
```

Analog	X	Y
1	CH₃	D-Arg
2	C₂H₅	D-Arg
3	CH₃	L-Arg
4	C₂H₅	L-Arg

Figure 12. Structure of four antidiuretic antagonists of AVP. (Sawyer WH et al: *Science* 212:49–51, 1981. Reprinted with permission.)

research area and have described three types of antagonists of vasopressor and antidiuretic responses: (*1*) pure vasopressor antagonists with varying degrees of antidiuretic agonism, (*2*) both pressor and antidiuretic antagonists with weak antidiuretic agonism, and (*3*) pure antidiuretic antagonists with some degree of pressor antagonism (260–262). Position 1 and 2 modification of the AVP molecule produces pure antagonists to the vasopressor response, while position 2 and 4 alterations yield analogs with antidiuretic antagonism (263–265). If these antidiuretic antagonists prove successful against endogenous and exogenous AVP in humans with minimal side effects, they will certainly open a new therapeutic door.

AVP SECRETION IN CONGESTIVE HEART FAILURE AND CIRRHOSIS

Hypervolemic, hypotonic hyponatremia is classically associated with the clinical state of decompensated congestive heart failure and hepatic cirrhosis. These endematous states are secondary to accumulation of both sodium and water, but hyponatremia develops due to inadequate excretion of ingested free water. Hemodynamic alterations and disturbances in the renin-angiotensin system characterize these conditions, but since the liver accounts for about half of vasopressin metabolic clearance, it seems logical to postulate an AVP contribution to the observed hyponatremia.

Linas et al. (266) produced cirrhosis in rats with carbon tetrachloride, resulting in elevated AVP levels, decreased renal blood flow, and impaired water excretion. In contrast, cirrhotic Brattleboro rats had no dysfunction in water excretion, suggesting a role for AVP in this hyponatremic disorder.

Bichet et al. (267) studied 12 stable cirrhotic patients with ascites. Seven patients demonstrated abnormal fluid retention following an oral water load, excreting only 27% of the administered challenge, and exhibited elevated plasma AVP concentration which did not completely suppress during the water challenge. The patients also had higher PRA and plasma aldosterone, suggestive of a decreased effective blood volume acting as a nonosmotic vasopressin stimulus and contributing to the dilutional hyponatremia.

Riegger et al. (268) studied 20 subjects with severe congestive heart failure, using prazocin to lower left atrial pressure (and lessen AVP inhibition) by increased stimulation of stretch receptors. Two subgroups of patients could be identified. One group had elevated basal plasma AVP despite decreased osmolality, and the other group had relatively normal values. Only the patients with normal osmoreceptor control demonstrated a rise in AVP following prazocin, which suggests that the elevated AVP was controlled by nonosmotic stimuli. The same group of investigators also induced congestive heart failure in dogs by rapid pacemaker stimulation for 2 weeks (269), reducing cardiac output by 54% and doubling pulmonary artery pressure. These changes were accompanied by increasing concentrations of PRA, AII, aldosterone, catecholamines, and AVP, suggesting a hormonal role in the fluid retention of heart failure.

POLYURIC DISORDERS

The various diseases, disorders, and renal abnormalities associated with the polyuric state are listed in Table 5 and have been discussed in detail in earlier volumes of this series.

Central Diabetes Insipidus

The animal model for central or neurogenic diabetes insipidus is the homozygous Brattleboro rat, which is incapable of synthesizing physiologic amounts of AVP. Boer et al. (270) have described impaired brain development in this animal in addition to the previously described impaired body growth. In the neonatal homozygous Brattleboro rat, there is marked maldevelopment of the cerebellum and medulla oblongata as well as slight changes in the cerebral cortex. The role of absent CNS stores of vasopressin in this developmental malformation is still speculative. Durr et al. (271) examined vasopressin integrity in the experimental obese rat model, with hyperphagia and weight gain induced by stereotaxically lesioning the ventromedial hypothalamus. These animals developed polyuria and were unable to increase urinary AVP concentrations following fluid deprivation, suggesting the presence of partial diabetes insipidus.

Histiocytosis X is a well-recognized cause of central diabetes insipidus with onset in childhood. Grimaldi et al. (272) have described the onset of diabetes insipidus secondary to granulomatous histiocytosis in a 70-year-old woman. Other unusual causes of central diabetes insipidus recently reported include postpartum pituitary necrosis (273), multiple staphylococcal brain abscesses (274), hypoxia following cardiopulmonary arrest (275), and systemic blastomycosis (276).

The DIDMOAD syndrome describes the combination of central diabetes insipidus, diabetes mellitus, optic atrophy, and high-tone deafness and is transmitted by an autosomal recessive mode. Bartelheimer et al. (277) have described two siblings with this syndrome and emphasize the simul-

Table 5. Conditions and Causes of Polyuric Hypernatremic Disorders

Conditions	Possible Causes
Central diabetes insipidus	Head trauma, skull fractures, orbital trauma
	Pituitary surgery
	Craniopharyngioma, cerebral tumors
	Metastatic tumors (e.g., breast)
	Granulomas
	Sarcoid
	Tuberculosis
	Lues
	Wegener's granulomatosis
	Histiocytosis X
	Sickle cell disease
	Encephalitis
	Meningitis
	Vascular, aneurysms, thrombosis
	Idiopathic (50%)
	Hypoxic "brain death"
	Optic atrophy, nerve deafness, diabetes, mellitus, and diabetes insipidus
	Leukemia
	Septooptic dysplasia
	Familial
	Hypothalamic obesity
	Brain abscesses
	Postpartum pituitary necrosis (Sheehan syndrome)
	Hydrocephalus
	Cerebroventricular cysts
	Internal carotid ligation
	Blastomycosis

taneous occurrence of atonia and dilatation of the urinary tract which is present in 46% of the cases, often with fatal complications, yet is not included in the acronym *DIDMOAD*. Kehl et al. (278) reported the diagnosis of this syndrome in a 32-year-old female who had, in addition to the classic features and urinary tract dilatation, regional atrophy of the cerebellum and pons, and hydrocephalus internus. This was associated with disturbances in personality and mental function and may represent a more generalized CNS malformation.

Kaplowitz et al. (279) quantitated plasma AVP and osmoreceptor sensitivity in two brothers with familial central diabetes insipidus. Following elevation of the plasma osmolality from hypertonic saline, one subject had undetectable plasma AVP concentration while his sibling had a measurable but subnormal AVP response, suggesting intrafamilial variability in the genetic expression of inherited diabetes insipidus. Block et al. (280)

Table 5. (*continued*)

Conditions	Possible Causes
Nephrogenic diabetes insipidus	Congenital nephrogenic diabetes insipidus
	Hypercalcemia
	Hypokalemia
	Colchicine toxicity
	Lithium intoxication
	Phenacetin nephropathy
	Dimethylchlortetracycline
	Propoxyphene intoxication
	Methoxyflurane
	Oxalosis
	Uric acid nephropathy
	Medullary cystic disease
	Relief of urinary tract obstruction
	Successful renal transplant
	Diuretic phase of acute tubular necrosis
	Hypergammaglobulinemic disorders
	Multiple myeloma
	Sarcoid
	Sjögren's syndrome
	Amyloidosis
	Sickle cell anemia
	Interstitial nephritis
	Lupus nephritis
	Acute renal artery stenosis
	Malnutrition (protein depletion)
Osmotic diuresis	Mannitol
	Urea
	Chronic renal failure
	Diuretic phase of acute tubular necrosis
	Relief of urinary tract obstruction
	Successful renal transplant
	High protein tube feeding
	Intravenous hyperalimentation
	Glucose
	Diabetes mellitus out of control
	Nonketotic hyperglycemic hyperosmolar coma
	Sodium
	Diuretics
	Excessive administration of Na-containing intravenous fluids
	Chloride and other anions
	Hypertonic enemas
	Cholestyramine
Mineralocorticoid excess states	Primary hyperaldosteronism
	Cushing's syndrome

measured the binding affinity kinetics of AVP to mononuclear phagocytes from the blood of three patients with familial diabetes insipidus, before and following initiation of DDAVP therapy. Receptor binding was elevated (compared to normal control subjects) prior to treatment but significantly decreased following DDAVP, suggesting down regulation of the receptor affinity and number.

Differential Diagnosis of the Polyuric State

Diagnostic studies usually attempt to reproduce osmotic and/or hemodynamic stimuli for AVP secretion which are quantitated by changes in renal concentration or direct measurement of plasma AVP. The results of the classic dehydration tests have to be interpreted in light of the observations that persistent polyuria will wash out the renal medullary concentration gradient and lower maximal urinary concentration ability. Patients with partial central diabetes insipidus possess an augmented sensitivity to low levels of AVP which may obscure results obtained during prolonged dehydration. Zerbe et al. (281) compared the results obtained following dehydration and urinary response to exogenous vasopressin with the results obtained by including plasma AVP measurements. In severely polyuric patients who are unable to concentrate their urine following dehydration, the single study with the renal response to exogenous vasopressin will establish the diagnosis of *severe* central or severe nephrogenic diabetes insipidus. However, patients who are able to increase urine osmolality greater than 9% following fluid deprivation will need further studies to reliably exclude primary polydipsia (or possibly partial nephrogenic diabetes insipidus) even though the majority (75%) of this group will represent partial central diabetes insipidus.

Vasopressin Therapy

The introduction of the synthetic AVP analog DDAVP has markedly improved the therapy of central diabetes insipidus with its prolonged half-life and absent pressor activity. Although side effects are remarkably low, Itabashi et al. (282) have reported hypersensitivity to chlorobutanol in the DDAVP solution. Laszlo et al. (283) have compared DDAVP with another long-acting vasopressin analog, dVDAVP (1-desamino, 4-valine, 8-D-arginine vasopressin) in treatment of 14 patients with central diabetes insipidus and concluded that both were effective forms of therapy. Finally, Moses et al. (284) have reported that DDAVP, originally introduced as a nasal spray, is also effective in patients with diabetes insipidus when administered subcutaneously in doses of 1–2 µg every 12–16 hours. Subcutaneous administration appears to be approximately 10 times more effective than intranasal administration.

Therapeutic use of lithium in psychiatric patients may be associated with the dose-dependent side effect of a vasopressin-resistant polyuria secondary to inhibition of AVP effect on the collecting duct. Christensen (285) investigated this phenomenon in rats with lithium-induced polyuria treated with constant infusion of either AVP or DDAVP for 7 days. Although AVP had little effect on reversing the polyuria, DDAVP restored urine volume and osmolality almost to normal, suggesting that the high renal affinity of DDAVP may reverse the lithium-induced renal concentrating defect.

DDAVP has been used to treat nocturnal enuresis in double-blind studies (286, 287). There was a significant decrease in the incidence of enuresis during therapy which increased upon discontinuation of the DDAVP. Therapeutic response appeared better in children over the age of 10. No increase in morning urine osmolalities and no side effects were reported. The authors suggest that the functional cognitive effects of DDAVP may be as active as the antidiuretic action in this problem. Recently DDAVP has been shown to shorten the prolonged bleeding time in uremic patients associated with an increase in Factor VIII coagulant activity and larger von Willebrand factors (288). DDAVP has been used in conjunction with high fluid intake and diuretics to treat sickle cell crisis by inducing hyponatremia and water transports intracellularly reducing the concentration of hemoglobin 5 (289). This therapy was successful in reducing the incidence and severity of crises if the serum sodium was maintained between 120–125 mEq/liter.

Nephrogenic Diabetes Insipidus

The causes of congenital and acquired vasopressin-resistant diabetes insipidus are listed in Table 5. Postulated mechanisms of hypercalcemic- and hypokalemic-induced polyuric states are covered in previous sections, but in both instances, stimulation of thirst as well as production of a vasopressin-resistant nephrogenic diabetes insipidus may contribute to the polyuric state.

Lithium-induced polyuria occurs commonly in the psychiatric population and is primarily the result of inhibition of cyclic AMP generated by vasopressin (290) and is accompanied by elevated plasma vasopressin levels despite low urine osmolalities. The concentrating defect is most common in long-term users whenever a distal acidification defect occurs (291). Usage for several years is associated with the development of a tubulointerstitial nephropathy, including cortical fibrosis (292), dilated tubules, and microcysts. On electron microscopy, abnormal epitheleal cells with elongated and dense spherical mitochondria are seen (293).

Cisplatin produces a polyuric state in many patients subjected to its therapeutic use. Its use in the rat is accompanied by polyuria and decreased papillary Na^+ and urea content due to failure of urea recycling (177).

Table 6. Conditions and Causes of Nonpolyuric Hypernatremia

Conditions	Possible Causes
Water deprivation in postoperative or comatose patient	—
Gastrointestinal water loss in excess of sodium (osmotic diarrhea)	Infantile diarrhea Lactose intolerance Lactulose
Cutaneous water loss	Betadine treatment of burns Heat stroke Seborrheic dermatitis
Primary adipsia (complete or partial)	Osmoreceptor damage
Essential hypernatremia	Osmoreceptor damage but intact baroreceptors
Osmoregulatory reset at a high level	—
Hypernatremia with increased total body sodium	Congestive heart failure with pneumonia or tracheotomy Cirrhosis with ascites and water restriction, lactulose Hypertonic sodium chloride intravenously in renal failure Hypertonic sodium chloride enemas to infants Breastfeeding malnutrition Inadvertent hypertonic sodium chloride dialysate Hypertonic sodium chloride abortions Hypertonic sodium bicarbonate postcardiac arrest or in treatment of metabolic acidosis Hypertonic sodium phosphate administration Saltwater drowning Saline emetic Exchange transfusions

After 1 day of cisplatin therapy, post water-deprivation levels of vasopressin are diminished, and the concentrating defect responds to vasopressin. However, after 8 days, vasopressin levels were normal and there was no reduction in polyuria following exogenous vasopressin. Interstitial solute was markedly reduced (294), probably accounting for the concentrating defect.

HYPERNATREMIC STATES

The causes of hypernatremia include all of the polyuric disorders in Table 4 as well as the nonpolyuric hypernatremic conditions listed in Table 5.

Since patients with hypernatremia are always hyperosmolar, the subgrouping of this category is only on the basis of their extracellular fluid status—hypovolemic, normovolemic, and hypervolemic (229). These disorders have been thoroughly discussed in earlier volumes of this series. Recent attention has been focused on the increased incidence of unrecognized breast feeding malnutrition leading to infantile hypernatremic dehydration (295–297). Increased breast milk sodium content as well as inadequate hydration is believed to be responsible for this life-threatening situation.

At the other end of the age spectrum, asymptomatic hypernatremia was reported in six elderly patients with adipsia following a cerebrovascular accident (298), with serum sodium concentrations ranging from 152–172 mEq/liter. These cases emphasize that hypernatremia develops only if there is a dysfunctional thirst mechanism or if the patient is physically unable to obtain a source of free water, (for example, infants and bedridden geriatric patients). Thus, it is appropriate to conclude this review with the same emphasis with which it was initiated—the primacy of thirst in maintaining homeostasis of the body fluids.

REFERENCES

1. Greenleaf JE, Fregly MJ: Dehydration-induced drinking: Peripheral and central aspects. Fed Proc 41:2507–2508, 1982.
2. Greenleaf JE: Dehydration-induced drinking in humans. Fed Proc 41:2509–2514, 1982.
3. Wood RJ, Rolls ET, Rolls BJ: Physiological mechanisms for thirst in the nonhuman primate. Am J Physiol 242:423–428, 1982.
4. Thrasher TN: Osmoreceptor mediation of thirst and vasopressive secretion in the dog. Fed Proc 41:2528–2532, 1982.
5. Epstein AN: Consensus, controversies, and curiosities. Fed Proc 37:2711–2716, 1978.
6. Phillips MI, Hoffman WE, Bealer SL: Dehydration and fluid balance: Central effects of angiotensin. Fed Proc 41:2520–2527, 1982.
7. Knowles WD, Phillips MI: Angiotensin II responsive cells in the organism vasculosum lamina terminalis (OLVT) recorded in hypothalamus brain slices. Brain Res 195:256–259, 1980.
8. Schelling P, Ganten P, Sponer G, et al: Component of the renin angiotensin system in the cerebrospinal fluid of rats and dogs with special consideration of the origin and the fate of angiotensin II. Neuroendocrinology. 31:297–308, 1980.
9. Phillips MI: Biological effects of angiotensin in the brain, in Gross F, Vogel G, (eds): Enzymatic Release of Vasoactive Peptides. New York, Raven Press, 1980, pp 337–364.
10. Van Houten M, Schiffrin E, Mann JFE, et al: Radiographic localization of specific binding sites for blood-borne angiotensin II in the rat brain. Brain Res 186:480–485, 1980.
11. Landas S, Phillips MI, Stamler JF, et al: Visualization of angiotensin II receptor sites in the brain by fluorescent microscopy. Science 210:791–793, 1980.
12. Thrasher TN, Keil LC, Ramsey DJ: Lesions of the organism vasculosum of the lamina terminalis (OVLT) attenuate osmotically-induced drinking and vasopressin secretion in the dog. Endocrinology 110:1837–1839, 1982.

13. McKinley MJ, Denton DA, Leksell LG, et al: Osmoregulatory thirst in sheep is disrupted by ablation of the anterior wall of the optic recess. *Brain Res* 236:210–215, 1982.
14. Bellinger LE, Bernardis LL: Water regulation in weaning hypodipsic dorsomedial hypothalamic-lesioned rats. *Am J Physiol* 242:285–295, 1982.
15. Szczepanska-Sapowska E, Sobocinska J, Sadowski B: Central dipsogenic effect of vasopressin. *Am J Physiol* 242:372–379, 1982.
16. Adolph EF: Termination of drinking: Satiation. *Fed Proc* 2533–2535, 1982.
17. Gainer H, Sarne Y, Brownstein MJ: Neurophysin biosynthesis: Conversion of a putative precursor during axonal transport. *Science* 195:1354–1356, 1977.
18. Beguin P, Pierre N, Boussetta H, et al: Characteristic of the 80,000 molecular weight form of neurophysin isolated from bovine neurohypophysis. *J Biol Chem* 256:9289–9294, 1981.
19. Lauber M, Pierre N, Bousetta H, et al: The M_r 80,000 common forms of neurohypophysis have corticotropin- and B-endorphinlike sequences and liberate by proteolysis biologically active corticotropin. *Proc Natl Acad Sci USA* 78:6086–6090, 1981.
20. Rosenior JC, North WG, Moore GJ: Putative precursors of vasopressin, oxytocin, and neurophysins in the rat hypothalamus. *Endocrinology* 109:1067–1072, 1981.
21. Land H, Schutz G, Schmale M, et al: Nucleotide sequence of cloned $_c$DNA encoding bovine arginine vasopressin-neurophysin II precursor. *Nature* 295:299–303, 1982.
22. Watson SJ, Siedah NG, Chretien M: The carboxyterminus of the precursor to vasopressin and neurophysin: Immunocytochemistry in rat brain. *Science* 217:853–855, 1982.
23. Russell JT, Brownstein MJ, Gainer H: Biosynthesis of vasopressin, oxytocin, and neurophysin: Isolation and characterization of two common precursors, (propressophysin and prooxyphysin). *Endocrinology* 107:1880–1891, 1980.
24. Gozek JW, Ciosek J, Janus J: The release of neurohypophysial hormones as influenced by stimulation of alpha-adrenergic transmission in long-term dehydrated male white rats. Information 1: Hypothalamus and neurohypophysial vasopressor activity. *Acta Physiol Pol* 32:127–136, 1981.
25. Lenard L, Hahn Z: Amygdalar noradrenergic and dopaminergic mechanisms in the regulation of hunger and thirst-motivated behavior. *Brain Res* 233:115–132, 1982.
26. Martin R, Voight KH: Enkephalin co-exists with oxytocin and vasopressin in nerve terminals of rat neurohypophysis. *Nature* 289:502–504, 1981.
27. Watson SJ, Akil H, Fischli W, et al: Dynorphine and vasopressin: Common localization in magnocellular neurons. *Science* 216:85–87, 1982.
28. Iversen LL, Iverson JD, Bloom FE: Opiate receptors influence vasopressin release from nerve terminals in rat neurohypophysis. *Nature* 284:350, 1980.
29. Lightman SL, Iversen LL, Forsling J: Dopamine and (D-Ala², D-Leu⁵) enkephalin inhibit the electrically stimulated neurohypophysial release of vasopressin in vitro: Evidence for calcium-dependent opiate action. *J Neurosci* 2:78–81, 1982.
30. Knepel W, Reimann W: Inhibition by morphine and beta-endorphin of vasopressin release evoked by electrical stimulation of the rat medial basal hypothalamus in vitro. *Brain Res* 238:484–488, 1982.
31. Clarke G, Lincoln PW, Wolp P: Inhibition of vasopressin neurons by intraventricular morphine. *J Physiol* 303:59, 1980.
32. Knepel W, Nutto P, Hertting G: Evidence for inhibition by beta-endorphin of vasopressin release during foot shock-induced stress in the rat. *Neuroendocrinology* 34:353–356, 1982.
33. Christensen JD, Fjalland B: Lack of effect of opiates on release of vasopressin from isolated rat neurohypophysis. *Acta Pharmacol Toxicol* 50:113–116, 1982.

34. Aziz LA, Forsling ML, Woolf CJ: The effect of intracerebroventricular injections of morphine on vasopressin release in the rat. *J Physiol* 311:401–409, 1981.
35. Lightman SL, Langdon N, Forsling ML: Effects of the opiate antagonist naloxone and the enkephalin analogue DAMME on the vasopressin response to a hypertonic stimulus in man. *J Clin Endocrinol Metab* 51:1447–1449, 1980.
36. Lightman SL, Forsling ML: The effect of the methianine enkaphalin analogue DAMME on the vasopressin response to tilt in man. *Clin Sci* 59:501–503, 1980.
37. Zerbe RL, Henry DP, Robertson GL: A new Met-enkaphalin analogue supresses plasma vasopressin in man. *Peptides* 3:199–291, 1982.
38. Lightman S, Langdon N, Todd K, et al: Naloxone increases the nicotine stimulated rise of vasopressin secretion in man. *Clin Endocrinol* 16:353–358, 1982.
39. Ishikawa S, Schrier RW: Evidence for a role of opioid peptides in the release of arginine vasopressin in the conscious rat. *J Clin Invest* 69:666–672, 1982.
40. Knepel W, Nutto P, Anhut H, et al: Vasopressin and beta-endorphin release after osmotic and nonosmotic stimuli: Effect of naloxone and dexamethasone. *Eur J Pharmacol* 77:299–306, 1982.
41. Robertson GL, Aycinena P, Zerbe RL: Neurogenic disorders of osmoregulation. *Am J Med* 72:339–353, 1982.
42. Skorecki KL, Brenner BM: Body fluid homeostasis in congestive heart failure and cirrhosis with ascites. *Am J Med* 72:323–388, 1982.
43. Schrier RW, Bichet DG: Osmotic and nonosmotic control of vasopressin release and the pathogenesis of impaired water excretion in adrenal, thyroid and edematous disorders. *J Lab Clin Med* 98:1–15, 1981.
44. Forsling M: *Antidiuretic Hormone*, Vol 5. London, Eden Press, Inc, 1982, pp 39–55.
45. Reaves TA, Liu H, Qasim MM, et al: Osmotic regulation of vasopressin in the cat. *Am J Physiol* 240:108–111, 1981.
46. Hochberg Z, Moses AM, Miller M, et al: Altered osmotic threshold for vasopressin release and impaired thirst sensation: Additional abnormalities in Kalman's syndrome. *J Clin Endocrinol Metab* 55:779–782, 1982.
47. Sladek CD, Joynt RJ: Role of angiotensin in the osmotic control of vasopressin release by the organ-cultured rat hypothalamo-neurohypophyseal system. *Endocrinology* 106:173–178, 1980.
48. Slader CD: Osmotic control of vasopressin release: Role of acetylcholine and angiotensin, in Yoshida S, Shore L, Yogi K (eds): *Antidiuretic Hormone*. Baltimore, University Park Press, 1980, p 117.
49. Slader CD, Blair M, Ramsay DJ: Further studies on the role of angiotensin in the osmotic control of vasopressin release by the organ-cultured rat hypothalamo-neurohypophysial system. *Endocrinology* 111:599–607, 1982.
50. Hoffman PK, Share L, Crafton JT, et al: The effect of intracerebroventricular indomethacin on osmotically stimulated vasopressin release. *Neuroendocrinology* 34:132–139, 1982.
51. Eisenhoffer G, Johnson RH: Effect of ethanol ingestion on plasma vasopressin and water balance in humans. *Am J Physiol* 242:522–527, 1982.
52. Purr JA, Stamoutsos B, Lindheimer MD: Osmoregulation during pregnancy in the rat: Evidence for resulting of the threshold for vasopressin secretion during gestation. *J Clin Invest* 68:337–346, 1981.
53. Menninger RP: Right atrial stretch decrease supraoptic neurosecretory activity and plasma vasopressin. *Am J Physiol* 241:44–49, 1981.
54. Epstein M, Preston S, Weitzman RE: Isosmotic central blood volume expansion supresses plasma arginine vasopressin in normal man. *J Clin Endocrinol Metab* 52:256–262, 1981.

55. Greenleaf JE, Shevartz E, Keil LC: Hemodilution, vasopressin suppressive and diuresis during water immersion in man. *Aviat Space Environ Med* 52:329–336, 1981.
56. Rowe JW, Minaker KL, Sparrow D, et al: Age-related failure of volume-pressure-mediated vasopressin release. *J Clin Endocrinol Metab* 54:661–664, 1982.
57. Gilmore JP, Zucker IH, Ellington MJ, et al: Failure of acute intravascular volume expansion to alter plasma vasopressin in the nonhuman primate, Macaca fascicularis. *Endocrinology* 106:979–982, 1980.
58. Bayus PH, Zerbe RL, Robertson GL: Arginine vasopressin response to insulin-induced hypoglycemia in man. *J Clin Endocrinol Metab* 53:935–940, 1981.
59. Bayus PH, Robertson GL: Rat vasopressin response to insulin-induced hypoglycemia. *Endocrinology* 107:1975–1979, 1980.
60. Bayus PH, Robertson GL: Vasopressin response to 2-deoxy-D-glucose in the rat. *Endocrinology* 107:1970–1974, 1980.
61. Thompson BA, Campbell RG, Lulivivat U, et al: Increased thirst and plasma arginine vasopressin levels during 2-deoxy-D-glucose induced glucoprivation in humans. *J Clin Invest* 67:1083–1093, 1981.
62. Van Itallie CM, Fernstrom JD: Osmolal effects on vasopressin secretion in the streptozotocin diabetic rat. *Am J Physiol* 5:411–417, 1982.
63. Oka Y, Wakayama S, Oyama T, et al: Cortisol and antidiuretic hormone responses to stress in cardiac surgical patients. *Can Anaesth Soc J* 28:334–338, 1981.
64. Levine FH, Philbin DM, Kone K, et al: Plasma vasopressin levels and urinary sodium excretion during cardiopulmonary bypass with and without pulsatile flow. *Ann Thoracic Surg* 32:63–67, 1981.
65. Bonnet F, Harari A, Thibonnier M, et al: Suppression of antidiuretic hormone hypersecretion during surgery by extrodural anesthesia. *Br J Anesth* 54:29–36, 1982.
66. Rossor MN, Iverson LL, Hawthorn J, et al: Extrahypothalamic vasopressin in human brain. *Brain Res* 214:349–355, 1981.
67. Schubert F, George JM, Rao MB: Vasopressin and oxytocin content of human fetal brain at different stages of gestation. *Brain Res* 213:111–117, 1981.
68. Kasting NW, Veale WL, Cooper KE: Vasopressin: A homeostatic effector in the febrile process. *Neurosci Biobehav Rev* 6:215–222, 1982.
69. Kasting NW, Veale WL, Cooper KE, et al: Effect of hemorrhage on fever: The putative role of vasopressin. *Can J Physiol Pharmacol* 59:324–328, 1982.
70. Kasting NW, Veale WL, Cooper KE, et al: Vasopressin may mediate febrile convulsions. *Brain Res* 213:327–333, 1981.
71. Berkowitz BA, Sherman S: Characterization of vasopressin analgesia. *J Pharmacol Exp Ther* 220:329–334, 1982.
72. Auerbach S, Lipton P: Vasopressin augments depolarization-induced release and synthesis of serotonin in hippocampal slices. *J Neurosci* 2:477–482, 1982.
73. Schwarzberg H, Kovacs GL, Szabo G, et al: Intraventricular administration of vasopressin and oxytocin effects the steady stable levels of serotonin, dopamine, and norepinephrine in rat brain. *Endocrinol Exp* 15:75–80, 1981.
74. Shin SH: Vasopressin has a direct effect on prolactin release in male rats. *Neuroendocrinology* 34:55–58, 1982.
75. Reppert SM, Artman HA, Swaminathan S, et al: Vasopressin exhibits a rhythmic daily pattern in cerebrospinal fluid but not in blood. *Science* 213:1256–1257, 1981.
76. Perlow MJ, Reppert SM, Artman HA, et al: Oxytocin vasopressin, and estrogen-stimulated neurophysin: Daily patterns of concentration in cerebrospinal fluid. *Science* 216:1416–1418, 1982.

77. Wang BC, Share L, Crofton JT, et al: Effect of intravenous and intracerebroventricular infusion of hypertonic solutions in plasma and cerebrospinal fluid vasopressin concentrations. *Neuroendocrinology* 34:215–221, 1982.
78. Barnard RR, Morris M: Cerebrospinal fluid vasopressin and oxytocin: Evidence for an osmotic response. *Neurosci Letters* 29:275–279, 1982.
79. Jones PM, Robinson IC: Differential clearance of neurophysin and neurohypophysial peptides from the cerebrospinal fluid in conscious guinea pigs. *Neuroendocrinology* 34:297–302, 1982.
80. Ang VT, Jenkins JS: Blood cerebrospinal fluid barrier to arginine vasopressin, desmopressin, and desglycinomide arginine-vasopressin in the dog. *J Endocrinol* 93:319–325, 1982.
81. Wang BC, Share L, Crofton JT, et al: Changes in vasopressin concentration in plasma and cerebrospinal fluid in response to hemorrhage in anesthetized dogs. *Neuroendocrinology* 33:61–66, 1981.
82. Reid AC, Morton JJ: Arginine vasopressin levels in cerebrospinal fluid in neurological disease. *J Neurol Sci* 54:295–301, 1982.
83. Hashimoto K, Ohno N, Yunoki S, et al: Characterization of corticotropin releasing factor (CRF) and arginine vasopressin in median eminence extracts on sephadex gel-filtration. *Endocrinol Jpn* 28:1–7, 1981.
84. Yasupa N, Aizawa T, Greer MA: Differential effects of dithiothreital and iodacetamide on corticotropin-releasing factor activity of bovine hypothalamic CRFs and vasopressin. *Endocrinology* 110:2074–2080, 1982.
85. Dornguist A, Carson DE, Seif SM, et al: Control of release of adrenocorticotropin and vasopressin by the supraoptic and paraventricular nuclei. *Endocrinology* 108:1420–1424, 1981.
86. Knigge KM, Joseph SA: Relationship of the central ACTH-immunoreactive opiocortin system to the supraoptic and paraventricular nuclei of the hypothalamus of the rat. *Brain Res* 239:655–658, 1982.
87. Hashimoto K, Ohno N, Aoki Y, et al: Distribution and characterization of corticotropin releasing factor and arginine vasopressin in rat hypothalamic nuclei. *Neuroendocrinology* 34:32–37, 1982.
88. Carlson DE, Dornhorst A, Seif SM, et al: Vasopressin dependent and independent control of the release of adrenocorticotropin. *Endocrinology* 110:680–682, 1981.
89. Karteszi M, Stark E, Rappay G, et al: Corticoliberin activity of rat neurohypophysis is distinct from vasopressin. *Am J Physiol* 240:689–693, 1981.
90. Buckingham JC: The influence of vasopressin on hypothalamic corticotropin releasing activity in rats with inherited diabetes insipidus. *J Physiol* (London) 312:9–16, 1981.
91. Beny J-L, Baertschi AJ: Corticotropin-releasing factors secreted by the rat median eminence in vitro in the presence or absence of ascorbic acid: Quantitative role of vasopressin and cathecholamines. *Endocrinology* 109:813–817, 1981.
92. Koob GF, Bloom FE: Behavioral effects of neuropeptides: Endorphins and vasopressin. *Ann Rev Physiol* 44:571–582, 1982.
93. De Weid D, Van Keep PA: *Hormones and the Brain*. Baltimore, University Park Press, 1980.
94. Alliot J, Alexinsky T: Effects of posttrial vasopressin injections on appetitively motivated learning in rats. *Physiol Behav* 28:525–530, 1982.
95. Judge ME, Quarterman D: Alleviation of anisomycin-induced amnesia by pre-test treatment with lysine vasopressin. *Pharmacol Biochem Behav* 16:463–466, 1982.
96. Cooper RL, McNamara MC, Thompson WG: Vasopressin and conditional flavor aversion in aged rats. *Neurobiol Aging* 1:53–57, 1980.

97. Kovacs GL, Buijs RM, Bohus B, et al: Microinjection of arginine 8-vasopressin into the dorsal hippocampus attenuates passive avoidance behavior in rats. *Physiol Behav* 28:45–48, 1982.
98. Koob GF, Le Moal M, Gaffori O, et al: Arginine vasopressin and a vasopressin antagonist peptide opposite effects on extinction of active avoidance in rats. *Regul Pep* 2:153–163, 1981.
99. Kilcoyne NN, Hoffman DL, Zimmerman EA: Immunocytochemical localization of angiotensin II and vasopressin in rat hypothalamus: Evidence for production in the same neuron. *Clin Sci* 59:57–60, 1980.
100. Vanderhaegen JJ, Lotstra F, DeMay J, et al: Immunohistochemical localization of cholecystokinin- and gastrinlike peptides in the brain and hypophysis of the rat. *Proc Natl Acad Sci USA* 77:1190–1194, 1980.
101. Tager H, Hokenboken M, Markese J, et al: Identification and localization of glucagon-related peptides in rat brain. *Proc Natl Acad Sci USA* 77:5229–6233, 1980.
102. Vale MR, Hope DB: Cyclic nucleotides and the release of vasopressin from the rat posterior pituitary gland. *J Neurochem* 39:569–573, 1982.
103. Pittman QU, Lawrence D, McLean L: Central effects of arginine vasopressin on blood pressure in rats. *Endocrinology* 110:1058–1060, 1982.
104. Liard JF, Derinz O, Tschoop M, et al: Cardiovascular effects of vasopressin infused into the vertebral circulation of conscious dogs. *Clin Sci* 61:345–347, 1981.
105. Blessing WW, Sved AF, Reis DJ: Destruction of noradrenergic neurons in rabbit brain stem elevates plasma vasopressin causing hypertension. *Science* 217:661–663, 1982.
106. Kimura T, Share L, Wang BC, et al: The role of central adrenoreceptors in the control of vasopressin release and blood pressure. *Endocrinology* 108:1829–1836, 1981.
107. Unger T, Rascher W, Schuster C, et al: *Eur J Pharmacol* 71:33–42, 1981.
108. Chevillard C, Saaverdra JM: High angiotensin-converting enzyme activity in the neurohypophysis of Brattleboro rats. *Science* 216:646–647, 1982.
109. Zerbe RL, Feuerstein G, Meyer DK, et al: Cardiovascular, sympathetic, and renin-angiotensin system responses to hemorrhage in vasopressin-deficient rats. *Endocrinology* 111:608–613, 1982.
110. Aisenbrey GA, Handelman WA, Arnold P, et al: Vascular effects of arginine vasopressin during fluid deprivation in the rat. *J Clin Invest* 67:961, 1981.
111. Andrews CE, Brenner BM: Relative contributions of arginine vasopressin and angiotensin II to maintenance of systemic arterial pressure in the anesthetized water-deprived rat. *Circ Res* 48:254, 1981.
112. Gavras H, Hatzinikolaou P, North WG, et al: Interaction of the sympathetic nervous system with vasopressin and renin in the maintenance of blood pressure. *Hypertension* 4:400–405, 1982.
113. Malayan SA, Ramsay DJ, Keil LC, et al: Effects of increases in plasma vasopressin concentration on plasma renin activity, blood pressure, heart rate, and plasma corticosteroid concentration in conscious dogs. *Endocrinology* 107:1899–1904, 1980.
114. Schwartz J. Reid IA: Effect of vasopressin blockage on blood pressure regulation during hemorrhage in conscious dogs. *Endocrinology* 109:1778–1880, 1981.
115. Young DB, McCaa RE: Lack of prolonged effect of antidiuretic hormone on the renin-aldosterone system in the dog. *Clin Exp Pharmacol Physiol* 8:267–271, 1981.
116. Imai Y, Abe K, Seino M, et al: Captopril attenuates pressor responses to norepinephrine and vasopressin through depletion of endogenous angiotensin II. *Am J Cardiol* 49:1537–1539, 1982.
117. Imai Y, Abe K, Seino M, et al: Attenuation of pressor responses to norepinephrine and pitressin and potentiation of pressor response to angiotensin II by captopril in human subjects. *Hypertension* 4:444–451, 1982.

118. Berecek KH, Murray RD, Gross F, et al: Vasopressin and vascular reactivity in the development of DOCA hypertension in rats with hereditary diabetes insipidus. *Hypertension* 4:3–12, 1982.
119. Berecek KH, Barron KW, Webb RL, et al: Vasopressin-central nervous system interactions in the development of DOCA hypertension. *Hypertension* 4:131–137, 1982.
120. Woods RL, Johnson CI: Role of vasopressin in hypertension: studies using the Brattleboro rat. *Am J Physiol* 11:727–732, 1982.
121. Matsuguchi H, Schmid PG: Acute interaction of vasopressin and neurogenic mechanisms in DOC-salt hypertension. *Am J Physiol* 242:37–43, 1982.
122. Matsuguchi H, Schmid PG: Pressor response to vasopressin and impaired baroreflex function in DOC salt hypertension. *Am J Physiol* 242:44–49, 1982.
123. Hatzinikolaou P, Gavras H, Brunner HR, et al: Role of vasopressin, catecholamines, and plasma volume in hypertonic saline-induced hypertension. *Am J Physiol* 240:827–831, 1981.
124. Morton JJ, Garcia del Rio C, Hughes MJ: Effect of acute vasopressin infusion on blood pressure and plasma angiotensin II in normotensive and DOCA salt hypertensive rats. *Clin Sci* 62:143–149, 1982.
125. Rascher W, Weidmann E, Gross F: Vasopressin in the plasma of stroke-prone spontaneously hypertensive rats. *Clin Sci* 61:295–298, 1981.
126. Lang RE, Rascher W, Unger T, et al: Reduced content of vasopressin in the brain of spontaneously hypertensive as compared to normotensive rats. *Neurosci Lett* 23:199–202, 1981.
127. Rascher W, Lang RE, Unger T, et al: Vasopressin in brain of spontaneously hypertensive rats. *Am J Physiol* 242:496–499, 1982.
128. Mohring J, Schoun J, Kintz J, et al: Decreased vasopressin control in brain stem of rats and spontaneous hypertension. *Naunyn Schmiedebergs Arch Pharmakol* 315:83–84, 1980.
129. Morris M: Neurohypophyseal response to dehydration in the spontaneously hypertensive rat. *Hypertension* 4:161–166, 1982.
130. DeLima J, Caillens H, Beaufils M, et al: Effects of furosemide-induced plasma volume reduction on plasma antidiuretic hormone in normal and hypertensive subjects. *Clin Nephrol* 15:246–251, 1981.
131. Trimarco B, Volpe M, Sacca L, et al: Inverted response of arginine vasopressin to postural change in patients with essential hypertension. *Clin Exp Pharmacol Physiol* 9:95–100, 1982.
132. Cowley AW, Cushman WC, Quillen EW, et al: Vasopressin elevation in essential hypertension and increased responsiveness to sodium intake. *Hypertension* 3:93–100, 1981.
133. Devane GW, Naden RP, Porter JC, et al: Mechanism of arginine vasopressin release in the sheep fetus. *Pediatr Res* 16:504–507, 1982.
134. Stark RI, Wardlaw SL, Daniel SS, et al: Vasopressin secretion induced by hypoxia in sheep: developmental changes and relationships to beta-endorphin release. *Am J Obstet Gynecol* 143:204–215, 1982.
135. Rose JC, Meis PJ, Morris M: Ontogeny of endocrine (ACTH, vasopressin, cortisol) response to hypotension in lamb fetuses. *Am J Physiol* 240:656–661, 1981.
136. Daniel SS, Stark RI, Hussain MK, et al: Role of vasopressin in fetal homeostasis. *Am J Physiol* 242:740–744, 1982.
137. Rose JC, Morris M, Meis PJ: Hemorrhage in newborn lambs: Effects on arterial blood pressure, ACTH, cortisol, and vasopressin. *Am J Physiol* 240:585–590, 1981.
138. Devane GW, Porter JC: An apparent stress-induced release of arginine vasopressin by human neonates. *J Clin Endocrinol Metab* 51:1412–1416, 1980.

139. Quintanilla AP: Pathophysiology of renal concentrating defects. *Ann Clin Lab Sci* 11:300–307, 1981.
140. Jamison RL, Oliver RE: Disorders of urinary concentration and dilution. *Am J Med* 72:308–322, 1982.
141. Berliner RW: Mechanisms of urine concentration. *Kidney Int* 22:202–211, 1982.
142. Bonventre JV, Lechene C: Renal medullary concentrating process is an integrative hypothesis. *Am J Physiol* 8:578–587, 1980.
143. Bonventre JV, Roman RV, Lechene C: Effect of urea concentration of pelvic fluid on renal concentrating ability. *Am J Physiol* 8:609–618, 1980.
144. Oliver RE, Roy DR, Jaminey RL: Urinary concentration in the papillary collecting duct of the rat: Role of the ureter. *J Clin Invest* 69:157–164, 1982.
145. Pennell JP, Bourgoignie JS: Water reabsorption by papillary collecting ducts in the remnant kidney. *Am J Physiol* 11:657–663, 1982.
146. Wilson DR, Sonnenberg M: Urea secretion in medullary collecting duct of the rat kidney during water and mannitol kiuresis. *Am P Physiol* 9:165–171, 1981.
147. Roman RV, Lechene C: Meclofenamate and urine concentration with and without exposure of the renal papilla. *Am J Physiol* 9:423–429, 1981.
148. Torikai S, Wang M, Klein KL, et al: Adenylate cyclase and cell cyclic AMP of rat cortical ascending limb of Henle. *Kidney Int* 20:649–654, 1981.
149. Morel F: Sites of hormone action in the mammalian nephron. *Am J Physiol* 9:159–164, 1981.
150. Hebert SC, Culpepper RM, Anoreoli TE: Sodium chloride transport in renal medullary thick ascending limb. *Am J Physiol* 10:412–431, 1981.
151. Hebert SC, Culpepper RM, Andreoli TE: ADH enhancement of transcellular sodium chloride transport: Origins at transepithelial border. *Am J Physiol* 10:432–442, 1981.
152. Hull DA, Varney DM: Effect of vasopressin on electrical potential difference and chloride transport in mouse medullary thick ascending limb of Henle's loop. *J Clin Invest* 66:792–803, 1980.
153. Imai M, Kisano E: Effects of arginine vasopressin on thin ascending limb of Henle's loop. *Am J Physiol* 12:167–172, 1982.
154. Hebert SC, Culpepper RM, Andreoli TE: Modulation of ADH effect by peribular osmolality. *Am J Physiol* 10:443–451, 1981.
155. Lestunzo LS, Windhagen EE: Effects of PTH, ADH and cyclic AMP on distal tubular calcium and sodium reabsorption. *Am J Physiol* 8:478–485, 1980.
156. Yanagawa N, Trizna W, Bar-Khayim Y, et al: Effect of AVP on the isolated perfused collecting duct. *Kidney Int* 19:705–709, 1981.
157. Levine SD, Kachadorian WA, Verna NC, et al: Effect of hydrazine on transport in toad urinary bladder. *Ad Physiol* 8F:31A–327, 1980.
158. Harmanci MC, Stern P, Kachadorian WA, et al: Vasopressin and collecting duct intramembranous particle clusters. *Am J Physiol* 8:F560–564, 1980.
159. Wade JB, Stetson DL, Lewis SA: ADH action: Evidence for a membrane shuttle mechanism. *Ann NY Acad Sci* 372:106–115, 1981.
160. Davis WL, Jones RG, Nagler MK, et al: Intracellular water transport in the action of ADH. *Ann NY Acad Sci* 372:118–130, 1981.
161. Kachadorian WA, Miller V, Rudich S, et al: Relation of ADH effects to altered membrane fluidity in toad urinary bladder. *Am J Physiol* 9:F63–69, 1981.
162. Levine S, Kuchadevian WA, Levin DN, et al: Effect of trifluoperozine on function and structure of toad bladder. Role of calmodulin in ADH-stimulation of water permeability. *J Clin Invest* 67:662–672, 1981.

163. Jackson BA, Edwards RM, Dousa TP: Measurements of cyclic AMP and cyclic GMP phosphoesterase activity. *Kid Int* 18:512–518, 1980.
164. Edwards RM, Jackson BA, Dousa TP: ADG sensitive cAMP system in papillary collecting ducts. *Am J Physiol* 9:311–318, 1981.
165. Johnson JP, Steele RE, Perkins FM, et al: Epithelial organization and hormone sensitivity of toad urinary bladder cells in culture. *Am J Physiol* 10:129–138, 1981.
166. Mendola SA, Thomas MW: Effect of monensin on osmotic water flow across the toad bladder and its stimulation by vasopressin and cyclic AMP. *J Memb Biol* 67:99–102, 1982.
167. Hardy MA, BiBona DR: Extracellular Ca^{2+} and the effect of antidiuretic hormone on the water permeability of the toad urinary bladder: An example of flow-induced alteration of flow. *J Memb Biol* 67:27–44, 1982.
168. Rosenbaum B, Lombardo G, DiScala VA: Effect of hydrostatic pressure on ADH induced osmotic water flow in toad bladder. *Pfluges Arch* 393:243–247, 1982.
169. Hull DA, Grantham JJ: Temperature effect on ADH response of isolated perfused rabbit collecting tubules. *Am J Physiol* 8:595–601, 1980.
170. Carvounis CP, Carvounis G, Arbbit LA: Role of the enderogenous kallikrein-kinin system in modulating vasopressin-stimulated water flow and urea permeability in the toad urinary bladder. *J Clin Invest* 67:1792–1796, 1981.
171. Orce GG, Castillo GA, Margolius HS: Inhibition of short circuit in toad urinary bladder by inhibition of glandular kallikrein. *Am J Physiol* 8:459–465, 1981.
172. Fejestoth G, Fahajszky T, Filep V: Effect of vasopressin one renal kallikrein excretion. *Am J Physiol* 8:388–392, 1980.
173. Kim JK, Jackson BA, Edwards RM, et al: Effect of potassium depletion on the vasopressin-sensitive cyclic AMP system in rat outer medullary tubules. *J Lab Clin Med* 99:29–38, 1982.
174. Rutecki GW, Cox JW, Robertson GW, et al: Urinary concentrating ability and antidiuretic hormone responsiveness in the potassium-depleted dog. *J Lab Clin Med* 100:53–60, 1982.
175. Beck N, Shaw JO: Thromboxane B_2 and prostaglandin E_2 in the potassium depleted rat kidney. *Am J Physiol* 9:151–157, 1981.
176. Nadvornikova H, Schuck D: The influence of a single dose of vasopressin analogs on human renal potassium excretion. *Int J Clin Pharmacol Ther Toxicol* 20:155–158, 1982.
177. Gordon JA, Peterson LN, Anderson RJ: Water metabolism after cisplatin in the rat. *Am J Physiol* 243:36–43, 1982.
178. Butkus DE, Jones FT: Reversal of copper-induced inhibition of vasopressin responsiveness by reducing agents. *Biochem Biophys Acta* 685:203–206, 1982.
179. Butkus DE, Schwartz, JH: Modulation of vasopressin action by reducing agents in Bufo marinus. *Am J Physiol* 243:52–61, 1982.
180. Handler JS, Preston AS: Vasopressin-illicited refractoriness of the response to vasopressin in toad urinary bladder. *Am J Physiol* 204:551–557, 1981.
181. Bengele HH, Mathias RS, Perkins JH, et al: Urinary concentrating defect in the aged rat. *Am J Physiol* 9:147–150, 1981.
182. Beck N, Yu BP: Effect of aging on urinary concentrating mechanisms and vasopressin-dependent cAMP in rats. *Am J Physiol* 12:121–125, 1982.
183. Kimura T, Share L: Characterization of the renal handling of vasopressin in the dog by stop-flow analysis. *Endocrinology* 109:2089–2094, 1981.
184. Vaziri ND, Skowsky R, Saiki J: Antidiuretic hormone in endstage renal disease. *J Dialysis* 4:73–81, 1980.

185. Vaziri ND, Skowsky R, Warner A: Effect of isoosmolar volume reduction during hemofiltration on plasma antidiuretic-hormone in patients with chronic renal failure. *Internat J Artificial Organs* 3:322–325, 1980.
186. Vaziri ND, Skowsky R, Saiki J, et al: Hemodialysis studies of antidiuretic hormone. *J Dialysis* 4:185–190, 1980.
187. Stokes JB: Integrated actions of renal medullary prostaglandins in the control of water excretion. *Am J Physiol* 240:471–480, 1981.
188. Roman RJ, Lechene C: Prostaglandin E_2 and F_{2x} reduce urea readsorption for the rat collecting duct. *Am J Physiol* 10:F53–60, 1981.
189. Kramer HJ, Glanzer K, Dusing R: Role of prostaglandins in the regulation of renal water excretion. *Kidney Int* 19:851–859, 1981.
190. Gross PA, Schrier RW, Anderson RJ: Prostaglandin and water metabolism: A review with emphasis in in vivo studies. *Kidney Int* 19:839–850, 1981.
191. Handler JS: Vasopressin-prostaglandin interactions in the regulation of epithelial cell permeability to water. *Kidney Int* 19:831–838, 1981.
192. Forrest JN, Schneider CJ, Goodman DB: Role of prostaglandin E_2 in mediating the effects of pH on the hydroosmotic response to vasopressin in the toad urinary bladder. *J Clin Invest* 69:499–506, 1982.
193. Selkurt EE: Role of the kidney and lung in the handling of prostaglandin E in hemorrhagic shock. *Adv Shock Res* 1:159–178, 1980.
194. Jones RL, Watson ML, Ungar A: A comparison of the effects of prostaglandins E_2 and I_2 on renal function and renin release in salt-loaded and salt-depleted anaesthetized dogs. *Q J Exp Physiol* 66:1–15, 1981.
195. Burch RM, Malushka PV: The role of thromboxane A_2 in the control of vasopressin-stimulated water flow in the toad urinary bladder. *Ann NY Acad Sci* 372:204–205, 1981.
196. Walker RM, Brown RJ, Stoff JS: Role of renal prostaglandins during antidiuresis and water diuresis in man. *Kidney Int* 21:365–370, 1982.
197. Dusing R, Herrman R, Glanzer K, et al: Renal prostaglandins and water balance: Studies in normal volunteer subjects and in patients with central diabetes insipidus. *Clin Sci* 61:61–67, 1981.
198. Belch JJ, Small M, McKenzie F, et al: DDAVP stimulates prostacyclin production. *Thromb Haemostasis* 47:122–123, 1982.
199. Padfield PL, Grekin RJ: The effects of indomethacin on vasopressin-induced antidiuresis in man. *Clin Sci* 61:493–495, 1981.
200. Zipser RD, Little TE, Wilson W: Dual effects of antidiuretic hormone on urinary prostaglandin excretion in man. *J Clin Endocrinol Metab* 53:522–526, 1981.
201. Covernier FC, Relling TE, Smith WC: Kinin-induced prostaglandin synthesis by renal papillary collecting tubule cells in culture. *Am J Physiol* 10:94–104, 1981.
202. Craven PA, DeRubertis FR: Effect of vasopressin and urea on calcium-calmodulin-dependent renal prostaglandin E. *Am J Physiol* 10:649–658, 1981.
203. Schlondorf D, Carvounis CO, Jacoby M, et al: Multiple sites for interaction of prostaglandin and vasopressin in toad urinary bladder. *Am J Physiol* 10:F625–631, 1981.
204. Holt WF, Lechene C: ADH-PGE_2 interactions in cortical collecting tubule I. Depression of sodium transport. *Am J Physiol* 10:F452–460, 1981.
205. Holt WF, Lechene C: ADH-PGE_2 interactions in cortical collecting tubule II. Inhibition of CA and P reabsorption. *Am J Physiol* 10:F461–467, 1981.
206. Craven PA, Studer RK, DeRobertis FR: Renal inner medullary prostaglandin synthesis. A calcium-calmodulin dependent process. *J Clin Invest* 68:722–732, 1981.
207. Okahawa T, Abe Y, Imanishi M, et al: Effect of calcium on prostaglandin E_2 release in dogs. *Am J Physiol* 10:F77–84, 1981.

208. Serros ER, Kirschenbaum MA: Prostaglandin dependent polyuria in hypercalcemia. *Am J Physiol* 10:F224–230, 1981.
209. Berl T, Ericksen AE: Calcium-prostaglandin interaction on the action of antidiuretic hormone in the dog. *Am J Physiol* 11:F313–320, 1982.
210. Berl T: Cellular calcium uptake in the action of prostaglandins on renal water excretion. *Kidney Int* 19:15–23, 1981.
211. Staff JS, Resa RM, Silva P, et al: Indomethacin impairs water diuresis in the DI rat: Prostaglandins independent of ADH. *Am J Physiol* 10:F231–237, 1981.
212. Ludeus JM, Taylor CV: Inhibition of ADH stimulated water flow by stable prostaglandin endoperoxide analogues. *Am J Physiol* 11:F119–125, 1982.
213. Whinnery MA, Shaw JO, Beck N: Thromboxane B_2 and prostaglandin E_2 in the rat kidney with inhibited ureteral obstruction. *Am J Physiol* 11:F220–225, 1982.
214. Strand JC, Edwards BS, Anderson ME et al: Effect of imidazole on renal function in unilateral ureteral-obstructed rat kidneys. *Am J Physiol* 9:F508–514, 1981.
215. Filbert VW, Schlondorff D: Altered prostaglandin synthesis by glomeruli from rats with unilateral ureteral ligation. *Am J Physiol* 10:F289–299, 1981.
216. Jonston PA, Bernard DB, Perrin NS, et al: Prostaglandins mediate the vasodilatory effect of mannitol in the hypoperfused rat kidney. *JCI* 68:127–133, 1981.
217. Wilson DR, Monrath V, Sonnenberg H: Prostaglandin synthesis inhibition during volume expansion collecting duct function. *Kidney Int* 22:1–7, 1982.
218. Skowsky WR, Swan L, Smith P: Effect of sex steroid hormones on arginine vasopressin in intact and castrated male and female rats. *Endocrinology* 104:105–108, 1979.
219. Forsling ML, Akerlund M, Stomberg P: Variations in plasma concentrations of vasopressin during the menstrual cycle. *J Endocrinol* 89:263–266, 1981.
220. Stromberg P, Forsling ML, Akerlund M: Effects of prostaglandin inhibition on vasopressin levels in women with primary dysmenorrhea. *Obstet Gynecol* 58:206–208, 1981.
221. Cavicchia JC, Rodriguez EM: The effect of copulation on the plasma antidiuretic activity of the male rat. *Int J Androl* 5:52–58, 1982.
222. Hammer M, Ladefoged J, Madsen S, et al: Calcium stimulated vasopressin secretion in uremic patients: an effect mediated via parathyroid hormone? *J Clin Endocrinol Metab* 51:1078–1084, 1980.
223. Baylis PH, Milles JJ, Wilkinson R, et al: Vasopressin function in hypercalcemia. *Clin Endocrinol* 15:343–351, 1981.
224. Szczepanska-Sapowska E, Brzezinski M: Interaction between effects of insulin and vasopressin on renal excretion of water and sodium in rats. *Horm Metab Res* 14:175–179, 1982.
225. Forrest JN, Goodman DBP: pH dependent prostaglandin E_2 production and somatostatin: Mediators of the action of vasopressin on the toad urinary bladder. *Ann NY Acad Sci* 372:180–192, 1981.
226. Linas SL, Berl T, Robertson GL, et al: Role of vasopressin in the impaired water excretion of glucocorticoid insufficiency. *Kidney Int* 18:58–67, 1980.
227. Schreir RW, Bichet DG: Osmotic and non-osmotic control of vasopressin release and the pathogenesis of impaired water excretion in adrenal, thyroid and edematous disorders. *J Lab Clin Med* 98:1–15, 1981.
228. Kaplan SL, Feigin RD: Syndromes of inappropriate secretion of antidiuretic hormone in children, in Barness LA (ed): *Adv Pediat Vol 27*, New Jersey, Year Book Medical Publishers, 1980, pp 247–274.
229. Narins RG, Jones ER, Stom MC, et al: Diagnostic strategies in disorders of fluid, electrolyte, and acid-base homeostasis. *Am J Med* 72:496–520, 1982.

230. Ducobu J, Dupont P: L'hypo-uricemie dors le syndrome de secretion inappropriee d'hormone antidiuretique. *Nouv Presse Med* 11:915–916, 1982.
231. Osterlind K, Hansen M, Dombernowsky P: Hypouricemia and inappropriate secretion of antidiuretic hormone in small cell bronchogenic carcinoma. *Acta Med Scan* 209:289–291, 1981.
232. Yamaji T, Ishibashi M, Katayama S: Nature of the immunoreactive neurophysins in ectopic vasopressin-producing rat cell carcinoma of the lung. Demonstrates of a putative common precursor to vasopressin and neurophysin. *J Clin Invest* 68:388–398, 1981.
233. Simpson CP, Aitken SE: Malignant histiocytosis associated with SIDAH and vitrial hemorrhages. *Can Med Assoc J* 127:302–303, 1982.
234. Singh W, Ramage C, Best P, et al: Nasal neuroglastoma secreting vasopressin: A case report. *Cancer* 45:961–966.
235. Ginsberg SJ, Comis RL, Miller M: The development of hyponatremia following combination chemotherapy for metastatic germ cell tumors. *Med Pediatr Oncol* 10:7–14, 1982.
236. Sato T, Uchigata Y, Uwadana N, et al: A syndrome of periodic adrenocorticotropin and vasopressin discharge. *J Clin Endocrinol Metab* 54:517–522, 1982.
237. Cooles PE, Borthwick LJ: Inappropriate antidiuretic hormone secretion in Wernicke's encephalopathy. *Postgrad Med J* 58:173–174, 1982.
238. Hochman MS, Kobetz SA, Handwerker JV: Inappropriate secretion on antidiuretic hormone associated with Guillain-Barré syndrome. *Ann Neurol* 11:322–323.
239. Husband C, Mai FM, Carruthers G: Syndrome of inappropriate secretion of antidiuretic hormone in a patient treated with haloperidol. *Can J Psychiatry* 26:196–197, 1981.
240. Farber MO, Roberts LR, Weinberger MH, et al: Abnormalities of sodium and water handling in chronic obstructive lung disease. *Arch Intern Med* 142:1326–1330, 1982.
241. Szatalowicz VL, Goldberg JP, Anderson RJ: Plasma antidiuretic hormone in acute respiratory failure. *Am J Med* 72:583–587, 1982.
242. Stern P, Larochelle FT, Little GA: Vasopressin and pneumothorax in the neonate. *Pediatr* 68:449–503, 1981.
243. Heim J, Laurent MC, Pawlotsky Y, et al: Intoxication par l'eau recidivante lors d'episodes de bronchite argue: syndrome de Schwartz-Bartler? *Sem Hop Paris* 58:1179–1180, 1982.
244. Lubitz L: Inappropriate antidiuretic hormone secretion and bronchiolitis. A case report. *Aust Paediatr J* 18:67, 1982.
245. Miller AC: Hyponatremia in legionnaires disease. *Br Med J* 284:558–559, 1982.
246. Rivers RP, Forsling ML, Oliver RP: Inappropriate secretion of antidiuretic hormone in infants with respiratory infection. *Arch Dis Child* 56:358–363, 1981.
247. Sigstrom L: The role of active sodium and potassium transport in hyponatremic states in infancy and childhood. *Acta Paediatr Scand* 70:353–359, 1982.
248. Bark H, LeRoith D, Nyska M, et al: Elevation in plasma ADH levels during PEEP ventilation in the dog: Mechanisms involved. *Am J Physiol* 2:E474–481, 1980.
249. Tarnow-Mordi WO, Shaw JC, Liu D, et al: Iatrogenic hyponatremia of the newborn due to maternal fluid overload: a prospective study. *Br Med J* 283:639–642, 1981.
250. Fisher RD, Rentschler RE, Nelson JE, et al: Elevation of plasma antidiuretic hormone associated with chemotherapy induced emesis in man. *Cancer Treat Rep* 66:25–29, 1982.
251. Ashraf N, Locksley R, Arieff AI: Thiazide-induced hyponatremia associated with death or neurologic damage in outpatients. *Am J Med* 70:1163–1168, 1981.
252. Gleadhill IC, Smith TA, Yium JJ: Hyponatremia in-patients with schizophrenia. *South Med J* 75:426–428, 1982.
253. Brent RH, Chodruff C: ECT as a possible treatment for SIADH: Case report. *J Clin Psychiatry* 43:73–74, 1982.

254. Nixon RA, Rothman JS, Chin W: Demeclocycline in the prophylaxis of self-induced water intoxication. *Am J Psychiatry* 139:828–830, 1982.

255. Decaux G, Unger J, Brimioulle S, et al: Hyponatremia in the syndrome of inappropriate secretion of antidiuretic hormone. Rapid correction with urea, sodium chloride and water restriction therapy. *JAMA* 247:471–474, 1982.

256. Weizman Z, Goitein K, Amit Y, et al: Combined treatment of severe hyponatremia due to inappropriate antidiuretic hormone secretion. *Pediatrics* 69:610–612, 1982.

257. Ayus JG, Olivero JV, Frommer JP: Rapid correction of severe hyponatremia with hypertonic saline solution. *Am J Med* 72:43–48, 1982.

258. Kleinschmidt-Demasters BK, Norenberg MD: Rapid connection of hyponatremia causes demyelination: Relation to central portine myelinolysis. *Science* 211:1068–1070, 1981.

259. Werder M, Ruppert RK, Bajc O, et al: Zentrale pontine myelinolyse and Schwartz-Bartler syndrome. *Schweiz Med Wochensch* 112:765–769, 1982.

260. Manning M, Sawyer WH: Antagonists of vasopressor and antidiuretic responses to arginine vasopressin. *Ann Int Med* 96:520–522, 1982.

261. Manning M, Lammek B, Kolodziejczyk AM, et al: Synthetic antagonists of in vivo antidiuretic and vasopressor response to arginine vasopressin. *J Med Chem* 24:701–706, 1981.

262. Sawyer WH, Pang PKT, Seto J, et al: Vasopressin analogs that antagonize antidiuretic responses by rats to the antidiuretic hormone. *Science* 212:49–51, 1982.

263. Manning M, Olma A, Klis WA, et al: Designs of more potent antagonists of the antidiuretic responses to arginine-vasopressin. *J Med Chem* 25:45–50, 1982.

264. Manning M, Lammek B, Kruszynkski M, et al: Design of potent and selective antagonists of the vasopressor responses to arginine-vasopressin. *J Med Chem* 25:408–414, 1982.

265. Manning M, Klis WA, Olma A, et al: Design of more potent and selective antagonists of the antidiuretic responses to arginine-vasopressin devoid of antidiuretic agonism. *J Med Chem* 25:414–419, 1982.

266. Linas SL, Anderson RV, Guggenheim SU, et al: Rob of vasopressin in the impaired water excretion in conscious rats with experimental cirrhosis. *Kidney Int* 20:173–180, 1981.

267. Bichet D, Szatalowicz V, Chaimovitz C, et al: Role of vasopressin in abnormal water excretion in cirrhotic patients. *Ann Int Med* 96:413–417, 1982.

268. Riegger GA, Liebau G, Kocksiek K: Antidiuretic hormone in congestive heart failure. *Am J Med* 72:49–52, 1982.

269. Riegger GA, Liebau G: The renin-angiotensin-aldosterone system, antidiuretic hormone and sympathetic nerve activity in an experimental model of congestive heart failure in the dog. *Clin Sci* 62:465–469, 1982.

270. Boer GJ, Van Rhbenen-Verberg CM, Vyling HB: Impaired brain development of the diabetes insipidus Brattleboro rat. *Brain Res* 255:557–575, 1982.

271. Durr J, Karakash C, Vallotton MB, et al: Abnormal water turnover associated with hypothalamic obesity. *Endocrinology* 108:1228–1232.

272. Grimaldi A, Attal B, Biro G, et al: Fievre an long course femme de soixante-dix ans relevant une histiocytose granulomateuse associant lesion ossluse femoro-tibiale et diabete insipide avec hypervatremie. *Sem Hop Paris* 58:554–558, 1982.

273. Schwartz AR, Leddy AL: Recognition of diabetes insipidus in postpartum hypopituitarism. *Obstet Gynecol* 59:394–398, 1982.

274. Gatell JM, Esmatjes E, Serra C, et al: Diabetes insipidus and anterior pituitary dysfunction after staphylococcal meningitis and multiple brain abcesses. *J Infect Dis* 146:102, 1982.

275. Adunsky A, Yaretsky A, Klajman A: Diabetes insipidus induced by postresuscitation hypoxia. *Harefua* 100:126–127, 1981.

276. Kelly PM: Systemic blastomycosis with diabetes insipidus. *Ann Int Med* 96:66, 1982.
277. Bartelheimer H: The syndrome of diabetes insipidus, diabetes mellitus, optic atrophy, deafness, and other abnormalities (DIDMOAD syndrome). Two affected sibs and a short review of the literature (98 cases). *Klein Wochenschr* 60:471–475, 1982.
278. Kehl O, Leller V: DIDMOAD syndrome (diabetes insipidus, diabetes mellitus, optic atrophy, deafness) mit zerebello-pontiner atrophie. *Schweiz Med Wochenschr* 112:348–352, 1982.
279. Kaplowitz PB, D'Ercole AJ, Robertson GL: Radioimmunoassay of vasopressin in familial central diabetes insipidus. *J Pediatr* 100:76–81, 1982.
280. Block LH, Furrer J, Locher RA, et al: Changes in tissue sensitivity to vasopressin in hereditary hypothalamic diabetes insipidus. *Klin Wochesscho* 59:831–836, 1981.
281. Zerbe RL, Robertson GL: A comparison of plasma vasopressin measurements with a standard indirect test in the differential diagnosis of polyuria. *N Engl J Med* 305:1539–1546, 1981.
282. Itabashi A, Katayama S, Yamaji T: Hypersensitivity to chlorobutanol in DDAVP solution. *Lancet* 1:108, 1982.
283. Laszlo FA, Czako L: 1-desamino, 4-valine, 8-D-arginine vasopressin (dVDAVP), a new synthetic vasopressin analog for treating diabetes insipidus. *Int J Clin Pharmacol Ther Toxicol* 20:39–43, 1982.
284. Moses AM, Moses LK, Notman DD, et al: Antidiuretic responses to injected desmopressin, alone and with indimethacin. *J Clin Endocrinol Metab* 52:910–913, 1981.
285. Christensen S: DDAVP treatment of lithium induced polyuria in the rat. *Scand J Clin Lab Invest* 40:151–157, 1980.
286. Aladjem M, Wohl R, Boichish H, et al: Desmopressin in nocturnal diuresis. *Arch Dis Child* 57:137–140, 1982.
287. Segni G, Salvaggio E, Parenti D, et al: Nuovo prospettiva terapeutica nell enuresi: la desmopressina (DDAVP). *Minerva Pediatr* 34:45–52, 1982.
288. Mannucci M, Remuzzi G, Pusiveri F, et al: Deamino-8-D-arginine vasopressin shortens the bleeding time in uremia. *N Engl J Med* 308:8–12, 1983.
289. Rose RM, Bierer BE, Thomas R, et al: A study of induced hyponatremia in the prevention and treatment of cycle cell crisis. *NEJM* 303:1138–1143, 1980.
290. Singer I: Lithium and the kidney. *Kidney Int* 19:374–387. 1981.
291. Battle D, Gaviria M, Grupp M, et al: Distal nephron function in patients receiving chronic lithium therapy. *Kidney Int* 21:477–485, 1982.
292. Aurell M, Svalandes C, Wallin L, et al: Renal function and biopsy findings in patients on long-term lithium treatment. *Kidney Int* 20:663–670, 1981.
293. Myers JB, Morgan TO, Carney SL, et al: Effects of lithium on the kidney. *Kidney Int* 18:601–608, 1980.
294. Safirstein R, Miller P, Dinman S, et al: Cisplatin nephrotoxicity in rats: defect in papillary hypertonicity. *Am J Physiol* 10:F175–185, 1981.
295. Ernst JA, Wynn RJ, Schreiner RL: Starvation with hypernatremic dehydration in two breast-fed infants. *J Am Diet Assoc* 79:126–130, 1981.
296. Jaffe KM, Kraemer MJ, Robinson MC: Hypernatremia in breast-fed newborns. *West J Med* 135:54–55, 1981.
297. Rowland TW, Zori RT, LaFleur WR, et al: Malnutrition and hypernatremic dehydration in breast-fed infants. *JAMA* 247:1016–1017.
298. Miller PD, Krebs RA, Nisal PJ, et al: Hypodypsia in geriatric patients. *Am J Med* 73:354–356, 1982.

Index

Abdomen:
   carcinomatosis of, 38
   episodic pain in, peritonitis and, 24
   hernia of, 29
   pain in, in eosinophilic cystitis, 257
Abortion, hypertonic sodium chloride, and hypernatremia, 538
Absorptiometry, dual photon, 419
Absorption, of drugs, 132–133
Acetaminophen, 152, 159, 170
   hyponatremia and, 525
   metabolism of, 138
   overdose, 88–89
   and vasopressin, 530
Acetate:
   dialysis:
      vs. bicarbonate dialysis, 57–58
      effect on blood pressure, 57
   in hyperosmolar solutions, 6
Acetazolamide, 159, 172, 320
   and citrate excretion, 323
Acetohexamide, 173
Acetohydroxamic acid, 262
Acetylcholine:
   effect of, on central nervous system, 489
   and vasopressin, 530
Acetylsalicyclic acid, 159
   dosage modification for, 142
Acid-base metabolism, 299–357
   aldosterone and, 355–357
   bone resorption and, 304–307
   calcium in, 299–304, 310
   effect of glucocorticoid on, 350–352
   hypercalcemia and, 307–309
   parathyroid hormone and, 307–309
   phosphate depletion and, 301
   potassium depletion and, 352–354
   PTH and, 399–402

   vitamin D and, 301
Acidosis:
   hyperchloremic, 333–336
      renal tubular acidosis in, 326
   organic anions and, 318
   lactic:
      congenital, enzyme deficiencies in, 341
      D-, 341–344
      experimental, treatment of, 336–341
      in McArdle's syndrome, 344–346
      peritoneal dialysis and, 38
   metabolic, 147
      bone disease and, 313–315
      in carcinoid syndrome, 336
      hydroxyapatite release and, 309
      hypercalcemia and, 310
      hypertonic sodium barbarbonate for, 538
      ketoacidosis, 329–336
      lithium induced, 327
      tetracyclines and, 147
   renal tubular, *see* Renal tubular acidosis
Acids, endogenous production of, 318
Acromegaly, 277
Acrylonitrile membrane, 64–65
Actin, in skeletal muscle, 427
Acute renal failure, *see* Renal failure, acute
Acyclovir, 159, 162
   for herpes simplex, 144
Adaptation, psycho-social, to dialysis, 84–86
Addison's disease, 277
Adenine arabinoside:
   and hyponatremia, 252
   and vasopressin, 530
Adenoma, parathyroid, phosphodiesterase in, 378
Adenosine triphosphatase, sodium-potassium (Na-K-ATPase), 275
Adhesin, 255

555

INDEX

Adipsia, primary, and hypernatremia, 538
Adrenal gland(s):
  adenoma of, 277
  congenital hyperplasia of, 277
Adrenergic nervous system, in essential hypertension, 267–274
Adrenocorticosteroids, metabolism of, 149
Adriamycin (doxorubicin), 159, 167, 204
Agenesis, renal, glomerulosclerosis and, 211
Albumin:
  CAPD and, 18
  immunization with, 200
  macroaggregated, 30
Albumin-antialbumin complex, 200
Albuminuria, 206
  dietary protein and, 205
Alcohol, inhibition of vasopressin by, 494
Alcoholism:
  chronic:
    myopathy of, 462
    osteoporosis and, 412
  hypophosphatemia and, 446–447, 453
Aldactone (spironolactone), 161
  serum magnesium and, 468
Aldosterone:
  adrenal adenoma and, 277
  effect of calcium on, 69
  plasma:
    age factors and, 287
    heparin administration and, 327
    hypertension and, 324
    and sulfuric acid feeding, in dog, 355–357
  and vasopressin, 530
  see also Hyperaldosteronism; Hypoaldosteronism
ALG, for immunosuppression, 116, 120
Alkaline phosphatase:
  serum, in osteopetrosis, 420
  total serum, 31
Alkalosis:
  metabolic, 348–350
    hypercalcemia and, 300
  respiratory, hypophosphatemia and, 445–446
  septicemia and, 443
Allergic rhinitis, minimal change nephrotic syndrome and, 211
Allergy, and eosinophilic cystitis, 257–258
Allograft:
  lesions in, 108
  rejection of, 111
  see also Renal transplantation
Allopurinol, 159, 165
  for hyperuricemia, 148

Alpha 1-adrenergic receptor, hypertension and, 270
Alpha agonist, centrally acting, 293
Alpha 1-antitrypsin, 237
Alpha 2-macroglobulin, 237–238
Alpha methyl norepinephrine, *vs.* guanabenz, 293
Alpha receptor, guanabenz and, 293
Alport's syndrome, 233–234
Aluminum:
  acute intoxication of, 30, 32
  serum, CAPD and, 22
  toxicity of, 71–72
  in renal osteodystrophy, 415–419
Aluminum hydroxide:
  in antacids, 448
  CAPD and, 23
Alzheimer's disease, 71
Amanita phalloides, 89
Amantadine, 159, 162
  elimination of, 144
Amicon hemofilter, 84, 191
Amikacin, 88, 91, 159, 162
  dosage modification for, 142
  overdose of, 39
  pharmacokinetics of, 27
Amiloride, 154
  serum magnesium and, 468
Amino acid(s):
  branched chain, 193
  essential:
    vs. nonessential, 183–187
    in TPN, 183–187
  free, CAPD and, 16
  loss of, in hemodialysis, 74–75
  new formulations of, 193
  parenteral infusion of, 175–176
    in acute renal failure, 177–187
Aminoglycoside(s), 28, 145, 162
  dosage modification of, 140
  drug interactions, 145
  excretion of, 138
  pharmacokinetics of, 141
  for urinary tract infections, 259
  see also Amikacin; Gentamicin; Tobramycin
Aminopyrine, overdose of, 89
Aminosyn, 183
Amitriptyline, 90, 134, 159, 170
  and hyponatremia, 52
  and vasopressin, 530
Ammonia:
  excretion of:
    in metabolic acidosis, 357
    in renal tubular acidosis, 316

metabolism of, 357–363
plasma, in pediatric patients, 187
production of, in elderly, 328
Ammoniagenesis, renal, pathways of, 358
Amoxicillin, 159, 163
dosage modification for, 142–146
for dysuria, 258
excretion of, 138
for urinary tract infections, 258
Amphojel, phosphate depletion with, 448
Amphotericin B, 159, 162
elimination of, 143
and vasopressin, 530
Ampicillin, 159
dosage modification for, 142, 146
excretion of, 138
Amylase, clearance of, 37
Amyl nitrate, 59
Amyloidosis, 114–115
and diabetes insipidus, 534
hemodialysis for, 83
nephrotic syndrome and, 209
renal, renal tubular acidosis and, 329
in renal transplants, 110
Analgesics, 88–89, 152, 170
dosage modification for, 142
Anastomosis, 81
Ancrod, defibrination with, 228
Anemia:
in hemodialysis patients, 63–64
microangiopathic hemolytic, 113
sickle cell, and diabetes insipidus, 533–534
due to zinc overload, 78
Anasthesia:
general, and hyponatremia, 525
hypertension and, 278
Angina pectoris, hemodialysis and, 61
Angiogram, coronary, 61
Angiography:
for coronary artery disease, 459
in pheochromocytoma, 286
Angiotensin II:
fluid intake and, 488
osmotic, 487–490
vasopressin secretion and, 494
Anion, and osmotic diuresis, 534
Anti-GMB disease, 201–204
Anorexia:
CAPD and, 20
dialysis and, 87
Antacid(s):
aluminum content of, 71, 449
drug absorption and, 133
drug interactions, 151

ingestion of, hypophosphatemia and, 448
magnesium content of, 71–72
phosphate-binding, 450
see also Aluminum hydroxide
Antiarrhythmic agents, 150, 168
Antiarthritic drugs, 147–148, 165
Antibody(ies):
acute renal failure and, 184
afinity of, 200
anti-DNA, 225
anti-Fx1A, 198–199, 212
anti-GBM, 109, 113–114
in rapidly progressive glomerulonephritis, 215
antiidiotypic, 125
antilaminin, 202
antireceptor, 125
cytotoxic, renal transplantation and, 108
lymphocytotoxic, 122, 124
production of, hybridoma technique of, 118
Anticoagulants, 148, 166
Anticoagulation, in hemodialysis patients, 66–67
Anticonvulsants, 88–90, 152–153, 170
Antidiabetic drugs, 154, 173
Antidiuretic hormone:
effect of PTH on, 403–404
see also Vasopressin
Antiemetic drugs, 153, 170
Antifungal agents, 143–144, 162
Antigen(s):
anti-GMB, 198
exogenous, 198–199
Fx1A, 198
GBM, 228
hepatitis B, 30
HLA-DR, type matching for, 120–122
native glomerular, 198
nonclassic GBM, 201
polysaccharide, 199
Antigen-antibody complexes, 200
Antigenemia, chronic hepatitis, 70
Antihistamines, 148–149, 166
Antihypertensive agents, 152, 168–169
Antilipemic drugs, 150–151, 169
Antilymphocyte globulin, immunosuppression and, 107–108
Antineoplastic agents, 149–150, 167
Antipruritics, 69
Antipyrine, overdose, 89
Antiseptics, in urinary drainage bags, 259–261
Antithrombin III, 237
Antithymocyte globulin, immunosuppression and, 107–108, 118

558 INDEX

Antitubercular agents, 144, 161
Antiviral agents, 144
Anxiety:
 hemodialysis and, 85
 hypertension and, 278
Aorta, elasticity of, 286–287
Arachidonic acid:
 peritoneal clearance and, 5
 platelets and, 64
Arginine vasopressin, see Vasopressin
Arrhythmia, cardiac, 468
 hypomagnesemia and, 459
Arsenic, 88
 poisoning, 91
Arteriovenous shunt, 81–82
Arthralgia, Henoch-Schönlein Syndrome and, 112
Arthritis:
 drugs for, 165
 inflammatory, NSAIDs for, 147
 rheumatoid, 230
Ascites:
 CAPD and, 38
 and cirrhosis, hypernatremia and, 538
 hemodialysis and, 38
 ultrafiltration and, 37–38
Ascorbic acid, for urine acidification, 259
Aspirin (acetylsalicyclic acid), 88–89, 152, 159, 170
Asthma:
 Minimal change nephrotic syndrome and, 211
 SIADH and, 527
Ataxia, and metabolic acidosis, 342
Atenolol, 159, 168
 dosage modification of, 139, 142, 152
ATG, for immunosuppression, 116, 120
Atherosclerosis, hypertension and, 286–287
Atropine:
 hemodialysis and, 59
 and vasopressin, 530
Autonomic nervous system, hemodialysis and, 59
Azathioprine, 159, 167
 and cyclosporin A, 120
 and donor-specific sensitization rate, 123–124
 for Goodpasture's syndrome, 230
 for immunosuppression, 115
 for lupus nephritis, 227
Azlocillin, 159, 163
 dosage modification for, 146
Azotemia:
 antihypertensive drugs and, 152

 control of, 191
 prerenal, 148
 renal tubular acidosis in, 315
 tetracyclines and, 147
 see also Renal failure, acute; Renal failure, chronic

B-cells, hyperactivity of, systemic lupus erythematosus and, 217
Bacteria, adhesion of, uropathogenecity and, 255
Bacteriuria, 252
 in pregnancy, 252
 in pyelonephritis, 261
 in urinary tract infections, 258
Barbiturates, 88–89
 and hyponatremia, 525
 in severe renal failure, 153
 and vasopressin, 530
Barium, and PTH secretion, 379
Baroreceptor:
 arterial, 271
 reduced sensitivity of, 287
Bartter's syndrome, hypovolemic hypotonic hyponatremia and, 524
"Basket weave" lesion, 233–234
Basophil:
 degranulation of, 211
 IgE and, 201
"Beer drinker's" hyponatremia, 525
Behçet's syndrome, and glomerulonephritis, 231
Benzodiazepine, 88
 elimination of, 153
Berger's nephropathy, 110, 112
 renal transplantation and, 109
Beta-adrenergic agonists, and renin release, 489
Beta-blockers, for hypertension, 289, 292
Betadine, for burn injury, and hypernatremia, 538
Beta-thromboglobulin, 238
 in hemodialysis patients, 65
Bicarbonate:
 absorption of, calcium and, 311
 excretion of, renal tubular acidosis and, 315
 plasma, bone resorption and, 308
 reabsorption of, 403–405
Bioavailability, drug, 132
Biphosphonate, mechanism of action, 424
Biopsy:
 percutaneous renal, 208

INDEX 559

rena immunofluoresence of, 200
for lupus nephritis, 223
Bladder, urinary:
  carcinoma of
    cyclophosphamide induced, 227
    transitional cell, 256–257
  distention of, hypertension and, 278
  emptying of, urinary tract infection and, 255
  eosinophilic cystitis of, 257
  infection of, 261
  neurogenic, urinary tract infections and, 259
  parasitic infection of, 258
Blastomycosis, and diabetes insipidus, 533
Bleomycin, 159, 167
  excretion of, 149
  hyponatremia and, 527
Blood:
  pH of, and distal acidification, 320
  transfusions of, 107, 117
  histocompatibility and, 120–126
  HLA and, 122
  immunogenicity of, 123
Blood-brain barrier, 489
Blood pressure:
  acetate and, 57
  diastolic, norepinephrine and, 271
  effect of captopril on, 61
  fluid intake and, 489
  and rate of ultrafiltration, 76
  smoking and, 291
  see also Hypertension
Blood urea nitrogen:
  in acute renal failure, 177, 185, 188–189
  hemodialysis and, 77–78
  IPD and, 33
Blood vessels, magnesium and, 461–462
Bone(s):
  biopsy of, 407
  disease:
    calcium and, 405–425
    chronic metabolic acidosis and, 313–315
    hyperparathyroid, 450
    metabolic, 433–438
    metastatic, 421
    renal tubular acidosis and, 315–317
  formation features, 406
  marrow, see Bone marrow
  metabolism of PTH, 376–377
  mineralization, 406–407
  neoplasia of, histologic features of, 422
  protein, vitamin K dependent, 420–421
  resorption of, 406
    and acid-base homeostasis, 304–307
    effect of pH on, 309–310

  hypercalcemia and, 300
  trabecular, 405
Bone marrow:
  decreased function of, 63
  donor antigen from, 117
  eosinophil in, 66
  fibrosis of, 407, 419
  suppression of, 119
Bowel:
  abnormalities of, 281
  dysfunction of, 67–68
Bradycardia, beta-blockade and, 292
Bradykinin, endogenous release of, 2
Brain:
  abscess of, 527
  atrophy of, SIADH and, 527
  thrombosis of, SIADH and, 527
  tumors of, and diabetes insipidus, 533
  water in, hemodialysis and, 32
Breastfeeding, malnutrition in, and hypernatremia, 538
Bretylium, 159, 168
  in renal insufficiency, 150
Bronchial spasm, 66
Bronchiolitus, acute, SIADH and, 527
Bronchitis, acute, SIADH and, 527
Bronchorrhea, hypovolemic hypotonic hyponatremia and, 524
BUN, see Blood urea nitrogen
Bumetanide, 159, 172
Burn, injury due to:
  Betadine for, 538
  hypophosphatemia and, 443–444
Busulfan, nephrotoxicity of, 150
Butophanol, inhibition of vasopressin due to, 494

Cafe-au-lait spot, in pheochromocytoma, 279
Calciferol, 304
Calcitonin:
  1-alpha-hydroxylase activity and, 314
  blood, in burn injury, 443
  "escape" effect of, 423
  in infants, 430
  and PTH secretion, 380
Calcium:
  cytosolic, 311–312, 378–379
  dietary, in primary hyperthyroidism, 392
  gastrointestinal absorption of, 300
  in heart muscle, 388
  intracellular, urinary acidification and, 313
  intravenous infusion of, in acid-base homeostasis, 310

Calcium (*Continued*)
  regulation of parathyroid hormone, 374
  regulation of PTH secretion, 377–380
  serum:
    IPD and, 31, 33
    phosphate therapy and, 392
    and urinary acidification, 299–304
    see also Hypercalcemia; Hypocalcemia; Hypocalciuria
Calcium blocking drugs, 169
"Calcium clamp," 380
Calcium ion influx inhibitor, in hypertension, 290
Calcium phosphate, on bone surfaces, 424
Calculi, urinary, infection and, 262
Calmodulin:
  calcium binding by, 463
  and PTH secretion, 378–379
Calories, supplementary, in hypercatabolism, 190–191
Camphor, 88
Candida parapsilosis, 26
CAPD, *see* Dialysis, continuous ambulatory peritoneal
CAPD (continuous ambulatory peritoneal dialysis) program, 9–15
Captopril, 61, 159, 168
  dosage modification of, 142, 152
Carbachol:
  intracellular pH and, 313
  urinary acidification and, 312
  and vasopressin, 530
Carbamazepine, 88, 159, 170
  and hyponatremia, 525
  and vasopressin, 494, 530
Carbenicillin, 159, 163
  dosage modification of, 142, 146
  excretion of, 138
Carbohydrates, metabolism of:
  defects in, 154
  glucose intolerance and, 154
  hemodialysis and, 84
  phosphate depletion and, 453–455
Carbon tetrachloride, peritoneal clearance of, 39
Carcinoid syndrome, metabolic acidosis in, 336
Carcinoma:
  bladder, transitional cell, 256–257
  parathyroid, 393–394
  renal cell, 256
    SIADH and, 526
  testicular, 149–150
  thyroid, 280
    medullary, 280–281

Carcinomatosis, of abdomen, 38
Cardiac output:
  hemodialysis and, 58
  hypertension and, 270, 286
Cardiomyopathy, uremic hyperparathyroidism and, 61
Cardiovascular disease:
  hypertension and, 290
  lupus nephritis and, 226
Cardiovascular drugs, 150–152, 168–169
Cardiovascular system:
  effects of vasopressin on, 503–508
  magnesium and, 458–460
Carnitine:
  deficiency, in hemodialysis patients, 86–87
  serum, CAPD and, 21, 33
  see also D,L carnitine
Carotid artery, ligation of, and diabetes insipidus, 533
Catabolism:
  in acute renal failure, 175
  Albumin for, 185
Cataract, steroid induced, 116
Catecholamine(s):
  alpha-adrenergic, 380
  beta-adrenergic, and PTH secretion, 380
  dopaminergic, and PTH secretion, 380
  metabolic pathways of, 268
  plasma:
    hemodialysis patients, 59–60
    plasma renin activity and, 277
  in uremia, 189
Catheter(s):
  blood vessel destruction and, 36
  curled, 36
  dislodgment of, 36
  peritoneal, 34
  removal of, 23
  straight, 36
  subclavian, 82
  and temporary blood access, 36
  Tenckhoff, 17, 36
  urethral, 263
Catheterization:
  indwelling, management of, 261–262
  subclavian, 82
  and urinary tract infection, 259–261
Cavernous sinus thrombosis, SIADH and, 527
CCPD, *see* Dialysis, continuous cycling peritoneal
Cefaclor, 159, 162
Cefadroxil, 159, 162
  dosage modification for, 142, 146
  for urinary tract infections, 258

INDEX **561**

Cefamandole, 159, 162
  dosage modification for, 146
  excretion of, 138
Cefazolin, 159, 163
  dosage modification for, 142, 146
  excretion of, 138
Cefonicid, 159, 163
Cefoperazone, 159, 163
Cefotaxime, 159, 163
Cefoxitin, 159, 163
  dosage modification for, 142, 146
  excretion of, 138
Cefuroxime, pharmacokinetics of, 27
Centozolone:
  and hyponatremia, 525
  and vasopressin, 530
Central nervous system:
  acetylcholine effect on, 489
  disorders of, SIADH and, 527
  drugs, 152–154, 170–171
  effect of PTH on, 386–387
  effects of vasopressin on, 500–503
  lupus and, 226
Cephalexin, 159, 163
  dosage modification for, 146
  excretion of, 138
Cephaloridine, 159, 163
Cephalosporins, 145–146, 162–163
  excretion of, 138
  for urinary tract infections, 258
Cephalothin, 159, 163
  excretion of, 138
Cephapirin, 159, 163
  pharmacokinetics of, 26–27
Cephradine, 159, 163
  dosage modification for, 142, 146
  excretion of, 138
Cerebrospinal fluid:
  homovanillic acid in, 528
  sodium concentrations in, 489
Charcoal:
  hemoperfusion, 89–90
  oral, 69
Chemiluminescence, of blood leukocytes, 25
Chemotherapy, intraperitoneal, 40
Chest pain, prostacyclin and, 67
Child(ren):
  Henoch-Schönlein Syndrome in, 112
  hypertension in, 253
  hypophosphatemia in, 455
  membranoproliferative glomerulonephritis in, 111
  nephrocalcinosis in, 323
  nephrotic syndrome in, 237

  peritoneal dialysis in, 36–37
  peritonitis in, 237
  SLE in, 227
Chlamydia trachomatis, 252
  in acute urethral syndrome, 258
Chloral hydrate, 88, 90, 159, 171
  elimination of, 153
Chlorambucil, for MCNS, 216
Chloramphenicol, 159, 164
  elimination of, 147
  metabolism of, 138
Chlordecone, 88
  poisoning, 92
Chlordiazepoxide, 159, 170
  elimination of, 153
Chlorhexidine, for urinary tract infections, 260
Chlorides, and osmotic diuresis, 534
Chlorophenoxyisobutyric acid, 150
Chlorpheniramine, 148, 159, 166
Chlorpromazine, 159, 170
Chlorpropamide, 173
  and hyponatremia, 525
  and vasopressin, 494, 530
Chlorthalidone, 159, 172
  for hypertension, 289
  and hyponatremia, 525
  and vasopressin, 530
Cholelithiasis
  clofibrate induced, 151
  in pheochromocytoma, 278
Cholesterol, serum:
  CAPD and, 15–16
  in hemodialysis patients, 72
  steroid therapy and, 116
Cholestyramine:
  binding of chlordecone, 92
  drug interaction, 151
  and osmotic diuresis, 534
Chromaffin cell, of adrenal medulla, 268
Chromatography, high pressure liquid, for phosphate analysis, 441–442
Chronic dialysis, mentally retarded and, 40
Chronic inflammatory disease, amyloidosis and, 114
Chronic obstructive pulmonary disease, 412
Chronic renal failure, *see* Renal failure, chronic
Cimetidine, 149, 159, 166
  drug interactions, 149
  effect on PTH secretion, 383
  excretion of, 138
  ketoconazole interaction, 143–144
  metabolism of, 149
  for uremic hyperparathyroidism, 61

Cirrhosis:
  with ascites, 525
    hypernatremia and, 538
  biliary, 411
  Laennec's, 411
  renal toxicity in, 148
  vasopressin secretion in, 532
  water immersion for, 239
Cisplatin, 159, 167
  excretion of, 149
  and hyponatremia, 527
Citrate:
  excretion of, acetazolamide and, 323
  tissue, metabolic acidosis and, 323
Clindamycin, 159, 164
  elimination of, 147
Clofibrate, 159, 169
  elimination of, 150
  and hyponatremia, 525
  and vasopressin, 494, 530
Clomiphene, 68
Clomipramine, and vasopressin, 530
Clonazepam, 159, 170
Clonidine, 159, 168
  vs. guanabenz, 293
  for hypertension, 289
  norepinephrine and, 272
  and vasopressin, 530
Cloxacillin, 159, 163
  excretion of, 138
Coagulation, in hemodialysis patients, 66–67
Coccidioidomycosis, systemic infection with, 70–71
Codeine, 152
Colchicine, 159, 165
  and acid-base homeostasis, 306
  and bone resorption, 307
  and diabetes insipidus, 534
  and vasopressin, 530
Colestipol, drug interaction, 151
Colistimethate, 159, 164
Colitis:
  due to CAPD, 29–30
  ischemic, 29
Collaborative Transplant Study, 121–122
Colon:
  carcinoma of, SIADH and, 526
  perforation of, 29, 67–68
Coma:
  acute hepatic, 38
  diabetic, 448
  drug induced, 87, 89, 176
  nonketotic:

hyperglycemic hyperosmolar, and osmotic diuresis, 534
    hyperosmolar, 448
  water deprivation in, hypernatremia and, 538
Concanavalin-A, T-cells and, 208
Congestive heart failure:
  hypomagnesemia in, 468
  and hyponatremia, 525
    with pneumonia, 530
  vasopressin secretion in, 532
Connective tissue disease, mixed, 230
Constipation:
  catecholamine levels and, 278–279
  in hemodialysis patients, 68
  peritonitis and, 23
Continuous cycling peritoneal dialysis
  vs. CAPD, 35
  ultrafiltration rates, 35
Coronary artery:
  lesions, 61
  magnesium in, 459
Coronary heart disease, angiography for, 459
Corticosteroids, for immunosuppression, 115
Cortisol:
  circulating, in uremia, 189
  effect of calcium on, 69
  mineralocorticoid synthesis and, 326
  and PTH secretion, 380
Cotrimoxazole, for vesicoureteric reflux, 253
Craniopharyngioma, and diabetes insipidus, 533
Creatinine:
  clearance, 7, 34
  serum:
    CAPD and, 21
    cyclosporin A and, 120
    erythrocyte deformability and, 64
    glomerulonephritis and, 214
    IPD and, 33
Cryoglobulinemia, essential mixed, 231
Cushing's syndrome, 277
  diagnosis of, 412
  iatrogenic, 115
  mineralocorticoid excess and, 534
  PTH levels in, 384
Cyclic AMP-adenylate cyclase system, 378
Cyclophosphamide, 159, 167
  for bacteriuria, 261
  dosage modification for, 142, 150
  for Goodpasture's syndrome, 230
  and hyponatremia, 525
  for lupus nephritis, 227
  for MCNS, 216

stimulation of vasopressin, 494, 530
for Wegener's granulomatosis, 231
Cyclopropane, and vasopressin release, 530
Cyclosporin A:
  for immunosuppression, 118–120
  for renal transplantation, 118
  and serum creatinine, 120
Cyst, cerebroventricular, and diabetes insipidus, 533
Cysteine, 318
  and vasopressin, 530
Cystic fibrosis, SIADH and, 527
Cystitis:
  acute, urine in, 256
  bacteriuria in, 258
  eosinophilic, 257–258
    clinical features of, 257
Cystogram, micturating, 253
Cystography, in urinary tract infections, 256
Cystoscopy:
  in bladder carcinoma, 257
  in urinary tract infections, 256
Cytochrome aa3, and lactic acidosis, 341
Cytochrome b, and lactic acidosis, 341
Cytosine arabinose, 167
Cytosine arabinoside, 159
Cytosol:
  calcium concentration in, 311–312
  norepinephrine in, 269

Dapsone, 159
Deafness:
  familial nephritis and, 234
  nerve, 233
    and diabetes insipidus, 533
Dehydration:
  extracellular fluid in, 487
  induced drinking, 487
Demeclocycline, 159, 164
  vasopressin and, 529
Dementia, dialysis, 71
Demethylchlortetracycline, and vasopressin, 530
Depression, symptoms of, 85
Dermatitis:
  bullous, 69
  seborrheic, 538
Desferrioxamine, 64
Desipramine, 159, 170
  and hyponatremia, 525
  and vasopressin, 530
Dexamethasone, 350

decreased absorption of, 68
Dextrose:
  in hyperosmolar solutions, 6
  hypertonic, 175, 178
Diabetes:
  alloxan, 464
  drugs for, 154, 173
  end-stage renal disease and, 13
  hemodialysis and, 85–86
  insulin dependent, 432
  ketoacidosis in, 329–332, 448
  osteoporosis and, 412
  vitamin D in, 432–433
  see also Diabetes insipidus; Diabetes mellitus
Diabetes insipidus:
  central, causes of, 533
  control of, 532–535
  nephrogenic, 537
    causes of, 534
Diabetes mellitus:
  CAPD and, 18–21
  hypomagnesemia in, 461
  hypovolemic hypotonic hyponatremia and, 524
  insulin-dependent, 70
  lactic acidosis and, 337
  magnesium metabolism in, 464–465
  parenteral phosphate for, 448
  uncontrolled, and osmotic diuresis, 534
Dialysate:
  acetate in, 58
    vs. bicarbonate dialysate, 75
  alkaline, 38
  base, 75–77
  bicarbonate, 34
    vs. acetate dialysate, 75
  blood in, 32
  flow rate of, 34
  hypertonic sodium chloride, and hypernatremia, 538
  osmolarity of, hypotension and, 57
  sodium concentration of, 58–59
  sodium nitroprusside and, 38
Dialysis:
  acetate, 75–76
    vs. bicarbonate, 57–58
    see also Hemodialysis
  adaptation to, 84–86
  bicarbonate, 57–58, 76
  for drug and poison overdose, 87–92
  drug dosage modification during, 141–142
  drug metabolism and, 135–136

Dialysis (*Continued*):
　hypophosphatemia during, 450
　for schizophrenia, 83
　solutions for, vasodilatory components of, 6
Dialyzer, reuse of, 80
Diaphragm:
　fluid leakage from, 30
　Starling's law and, 31
Diarrhea:
　infantile, and hypernatremia, 538
　osmotic, 538
Diastolic hypertension, *see* Hypertension, diastolic
Diatrizoate, and vasopressin, 530
Diazepam, 159, 171
　elimination of, 153
Diazoxide, 159, 168
　dosage modification for, 142
Dichloroacetate, and blood lactate, 338
Dicloxacillin, 159, 163
Diet, *see* Nutrition
Di-2-ethylhexyl phthalate, toxicity of, 79
Diflunisal, 159, 165
Digitalis, 88, 91, 151
　toxicity of, hypomagnesemia and, 468
Digitoxin, 159, 169
　elimination of, 151
　metabolism of, 138
Digoxin, 159, 169
　clearance of, 22
　elimination of, 151
　excretion of, 138
　pharmacokinetics of, 141
3,4-Dihydroxyphenylethylamine, 268
　inhibition of vasopressin, 494
Diltiazem, 150, 159, 169
　for hypertension, 290
Dimethychlortetracycline, and diabetes insipidus, 534
Dimitrophenol, and vasopressin, 530
Diphenhydramine, 148, 159, 166
Diphenylhydantoin, and vasopressin, 530
Diphosphonate:
　and acid-base homeostasis, 306
　and bone resorption, 307
　mechanism of action, 424
Dipyridamole, for glomerulonephritis, 216
Disinfectant, glutaraldehyde-based, 79
Disopyramide, 91, 159, 168
　dosage modification for, 142
　excretion of, 138
　in renal insufficiency, 150
Distribution, apparent volume of, 134

Disulfonic stilbene, and urinary acidification, 322
Diuresis:
　glucocorticoid insufficiency and, 523
　osmotic:
　　causes of, 534
　　urea and, 530
Diuretic(s), 154, 172
　for hypertension, 291
　induced hypomagnesemia, 462
　induced magnesium deficiency, 468–469
　loop, 154, 468
　magnesium-sparing, 468
　and osmotic diuresis, 534
　potassium-sparing, 154
Divalent cation, 133
DL carnitine, for plasma lipids, 87
D-mannose, 255
DNA-anti DNA complexes, SLE and, 219
Dopadecarboxylase, 268
Dopamine, 268
　antagonist, 153
　for renal damage, 143
　and vasopressin, 530
Dopamine-beta-hydroxylase, 268
Doxorubicin, 159
　proteinuria and, 204
Doxycycline, 159, 164
　metabolism of, 138
Drainage bag, urinary, antiseptic agents in, 259–261
Drowning, salt water, and hypernatremia, 538
Drug(s):
　absorption of, 131–133
　antagonism, 144
　biotransformation of, 132
　concentration in plasma, 133–134
　distribution, 131, 133–136
　dosage, 135
　　during dialysis, 141–142
　　modification of, 138–139
　dosing nomogram, 139–142
　elimination of, 136–138
　excretion of, 131
　first-pass effect of, 133
　formulation of, 132–133
　immunosuppressive, 149–150
　interaction, 133
　metabolism, 131
　overdose, therapy for, 87–92
　synergism, 143
　vasopressin secretion and, 494
　see also specific drugs and classifications

Duodenum, carcinoma of, SIADH and, 526
Dwarfism, pituitary, 277
Dysarthria, and metabolic acidosis, 342
Dyspnea, in hypertensive heart disease, 278
Dystrophy, muscular, phosphorus metabolism in, 441
Dysuria, 252
 in eosinophilic cystitis, 257
 therapy for, 258

Ebstein-Barr Virus, 118
Edema, IPD and, 33
Electrocardiogram:
 abnormalities of, magnesium depletion and, 471
 changes in, hemodialysis and, 61
Electroshock therapy, and hyponatremia, 529
Embden-Meyerhof pathway, enzyme deficiencies in, 340
Emesis, vasopressin secretion and, 494
Emetic, saline, and hypernatremia, 538
Encephalitis:
 and diabetes insipidus, 533
 SIADH and, 527
Encephalopathy:
 dialysis, aluminum toxicity and, 71
 Wernicke's, 527–528
Endocrine system:
 abnormalities of, nephrotic syndrome, 236–237
 in hemodialysis patients, 68–69
Endocytosis, epithelial cell, 201
End-stage renal disease:
 diabetes and, 13
 hemodialysis and, 13
 IPD for, 40
 patient survival and, 13–14, 86
 transplantation in, 107
 trimethoprim for, 146
End-stage renal failure, familial nephritis and, 233
Enema, hypertonic, and osmotic diuresis, 534
Enzyme, microsomal, 149
Eosinophilia:
 hemodialysis and, 66
 peripheral, 257–258
Eosinophils:
 in chronic renal failure patients, 66
 in peritonitis, 24
Epilepsy, SIADH and, 527
Epinephrine, 268
 hemodialysis and, 60

sodium ingestion and, 272
Epsilon aminocaproic acid, clearance of, 28
Erythrocyte(s):
 agglutination of, 255
 deformability of, 64
 intracellular sodium levels of, 275
 sedimentation rate, SLE and, 219
Erythromycin, 159, 164
 elimination of, 147
 for fistula infection, 71
Erythropoiesis, chloramphenicol and, 147
Erythropoietin, serum level of, 64
 CAPD and, 21
Escherichia coli, 237, 255
ESRD, *see* End-stage renal disease
Estrogen, sodium retention and, 521
Ethacrynic acid, 159, 172
 toxicity of, 154
 and vasopressin, 530
Ethambutol, 159, 162
 dosage modification for, 142
 elimination of, 144
Ethanol, and vasopressin, 530
Ethchlorvynol, 159, 171
 elimination of, 153
Ether, and vasopressin release, 530
Ethosuximide, 159, 170
Ethylchlorovynol, 88
Ethylene glycol, 88, 91
 poisoning, 39
European Working Party on High Blood Pressure in the Elderly, 289
Ewing's sarcoma, vasopressin and, 526
Exercise, hypertension and, 278

Familial nephritis, 233
Fanconi syndrome, 317
 amyloidosis and, 329
Fasting, effect of, on magnesium metabolism, 465–468
Fatty acid(s):
 L-carnitine and, 86
 oxidation of, phosphate depletion and, 455
Fenoprofen, 147, 159, 165
 induced nephrotic syndrome, 209
 toxicity of, 148
Fetus:
 vasopressin secretion in, 508–509
 vitamin D in, 429–431
 see also Neonate(s)
Fibrin, deposition of, 67

Fibrinolysis, inhibition of, 40
  hemodialysis, 40
Fibrinopeptide A, plasma concentration of, 67
Fibrosis, bone marrow, 407
Filtration, glomerular, 136–137
"First-pass effect," of drug, 133
Fistula:
  arteriovenous, 81
  infection, 71
Flucytosine, 26, 159, 162
  dosage modification for, 142
  elimination of, 143
Fludrocortisone, potassium excretion and, 324
Fluorosis, trabecular bone features of, 409
5-Fluorouracil, 159, 167
Fluphenazine, and vasopressin, 530
Flurazepam, 160, 171
  elimination of, 153
Fluroacetic acid, and vasopressin, 530
Focal sclerosising glomerulonephritis, 111–112
Folate, serum, 30
  chronic peritoneal dialysis and, 32
Follicle stimulating hormone, hemodialysis
  and, 68
Folliculitis, perforating, 70
Food:
  inorganic cations in, 318
  vitamin D in, 438
Formaldehyde, in formalin-sterilized dialyzers,
  79
Framingham Study, 286, 290
Freckling, axillary, in pheochromocytoma, 279
Frequency-dysuria syndrome, treatment of,
  258–259
Frequency syndrome, 252
Fructose biphosphatase, and lactic acidosis,
  341
Fungus, drugs against, 162
Furosemide, 160, 172
  vs. ethacrynic acid, 154
  and SIADH, 530
  stimulation of vasopressin, 494
  and urinary acidification, 322
  and vasopressin, 530
F-wave conduction, in hemodialysis patients,
  62–63

Ganglioneuromatosis, diffuse intestinal, 281
Gap junction, and bone cell activities, 421
Gardnerella vaginalis, 252
Gastroenteritis, eosinophilic, 258
Gastrointestinal tract:
  abnormalities of, 281
  disorders of, in hemodialysis patients, 67–68

Gastroparesis, 20
GBM (glomerular basement membrane):
  immune deposits in, 198–201
  injury to, 202
Gelusil, phosphate depletion with, 448
Gentamicin, 28, 160, 162
  dosage modification of, 140, 142
  nephrotoxicity of, 145
  peritoneal clearance of, 39
  pharmacokinetics of, 27
  and vasopressin, 530
Giant cell reaction, foreign body, 79
Gingiva:
  hypertrophy of, 119
  lesions of, Wegener's granulomatosis and,
    231
Glomerular filtration:
  drug clearance by, 136–137
  rate of:
    diuretics and, 154
    PTH and, 402–403
    steroid therapy and, 228
Glomerulonephritis:
  advanced sclerosing, 222
  amyloidosis and, 114
  Behçet's syndrome and, 231
  Berger's syndrome and, 112
  circulating monocytes and, 203
  crescentric, 114, 215, 230
  diffuse, 222
  focal, 222
    sclerosing, 111–112
  Goodpasture's syndrome and, 229
  hypocomplementemia and, 232
  idiopathic, 114
  immunopathogenesis of, 197–198, 203
  membranoproliferative, 110–111, 215
  membranous, 108
  mesangial proliferative, 208
  neutrophils and, 203
  poststreptococcal, 214–215
  rapidly progressive, 215
  recurrent, 109, 235
    incidence of, 236
  rejection, 109, 235
  renal transplantation and, 108–109, 114,
    234–235
  sclerotic, 222
  segmental, 222
  systemic lupus erythematosus and, 217–230
  vesicoureteric reflux, 254
  see also Glomerulopathy(ies); Nephrotic
    syndrome; Nephritis; Nephropathy
Glomerulopathy(ies):

familial, 234
membranous, 198, 212, 222
mesangial, 222
primary, therapy for, 215–216
in systemic lupus erythematosus, 109
transplant, 235
Glomerulosclerosis:
dietary protein and, 205
focal, 110–112, 220
segmental, 211
GBM injury and, 202
progressive, 205–206
Glomerulus:
basement membrane of (GBM)
immune deposits in, 198–201
injury to, 202
hypercellularity of, monocytes and, 203
hyperfiltration of, 197
IgA deposition in, 212
injury to:
B-cell mediated immunity in, 204
mediators of, 202, 204
serum sickness and, 199
lesions of, renal allografts and, 234
mesangial deposits in, 223
permselectivity of, 211
subepithelial deposits in, in lupus nephritis, 226
thrombosis of, 225, 228
Glucagon:
circulating, in uremia, 189
and PTH secretion, 380
Glucocorticoid:
deficiency of, hyponatremia and, 525
and vasopressin, 530
vitamin D and, 433
water metabolism and, 522–523
Glucose:
absorption of, peritonitis and, 41
blood, insulin and, 154
concentration of, in peritoneal cavity, 2
hypertonic, 177–181
intolerance, hypertension and, 291
synthesis of:
in acute uremia, 189
amino acids and, 188
Glucose-6-phosphatase, and lactic acidosis, 341
Glucuronide, 150
"Glutaminase I," 357
Glutathione, and vasopressin, 530
Glutethimide, 160, 171
elimination of, 153
Glyceride, and vasopressin, 530
Glycine, and vasopressin, 530

Glycogen pathways, phosphate depletion and, 454
Glycolipids, globoseries, 255
Glycolysis, phosphofructokinase and, 337
Glycoprotein, noncollagenous, nephritogenic antigens and, 228
Glycosides, cardiac, 151–152, 169
Glycosuria, phosphate depletion and, 329
Goodpasture's syndrome, 113–114, 228–230
familial nephritis and, 234
renal transplantation and, 110
Gout, NSAIDs for, 147
Graft:
bovine, 80
cadaveric, 235
protective immunologic mechanism, 125
rejection of, 108
transplant, 14
see also Renal transplantation
Granulocyte, pulmonary sequestration of, 66
Granulomatosis, Wegener's, 230
Griseofulvin, 160, 162
elimination of, 143
and vasopressin, 530
Group therapy, 86
Growth, vitamin D and, 429–431
Growth hormone, and PTH secretion, 380
Guanabenz, for hypertension, 293
Guanethidine, 160, 168
dosage modification for, 152
Gullain-Barré syndrome, SAIDH and, 527–528

Haemophilus influenzae, 252
Haemophilus parainfluenzae, 252
Haloperidol, 160, 171
and hyponatremia, 525
and SIADH, 528
and vasopressin, 530
Halothane, and vasopressin release, 530
Headache, prostacyclin and, 67
Heart:
contractility of, 60
effect of PTH on, 387–388
function of:
effect of hemodialysis on, 60–61
magnesium and, 458–459
multifocal premature ventricular contractions of, hydrochlorothiazide and, 292
phosphorylase activity in, 454
response to catecholamines, 452
see also related entries
Heart failure, renal toxicity in, 148
Heart rate, hemodialysis and, 59

568 INDEX

Heat stroke:
  classic, 346, 348
  cutaneous water loss in, 538
  exertional, 348
    lactic acidosis and, 346
  and hypernatremia, 538
Hematocrit:
  CAPD and, 21, 33
  in hemodialysis patients, 63–64
Hematoma, subdural, 527
Hematopoietic system, effect of PTH on, 387
Hematuria:
  benign familial, 233
  Berger's syndrome and, 112
  and eosinophilic cystitis, 257
  in familial nephritis, 233
  glomerular, 207
  glomerulonephritis and, 111, 214
  microscopic, 109
Hemiacidrin, for struvite stones, 263
Hemodialysis, 36
  aluminum toxicity and, 72
  amino acid loss during, 191
  anticoagulation and, 66–67
  autonomic nervous system and, 59
  vs. CAPD, 13
  cardiovascular response to, 57–60
  catecholamine metabolism in, 61
  chronic, glycosylated hemoglobin and, 40
  coagulation and, 66–67
  complications of, 78–80
  cost of, 15
  cutaneous manifestations and, 69–70
  dialysis encephalopathy and, 71
  endocrinology and, 68–69
  gastrointestinal disorders and, 67–68
  glucose-free, 40
  hematology and, 63–66
  home, failure of, 85
  hyperlipidemia and, 72–73
  infections and, 70–71
  for nonrenal disease, 82–83
  nutrition and, 73–75
  osteomalacia and, 71–72
  plasma lecithin cholesterol acetotransferase and, 40
  and pregnancy, 82
  vascular access, 80–82
Hemofilter, Amicon, 84, 191
Hemofiltration:
  continuous arteriovenous, 191
  vs. hemodialysis, 83–84
  for iron overload, 64

Hemoglobin:
  CAPD and, 18
  glycosylated, chronic hemodialysis and, 40
Hemolytic-uremic syndrome, 110, 113, 232–233
  glomerular fibrin deposition in, 233
  vs. thrombotic thrombocytopenic purpura, 232
Hemoperfusion:
  amberlite, 89
  charcoal, for acetaminophen overdose, 89
  for drug and poison overdose, 87–92
  vs. hemodialysis, 87
  resin, 90
Hemorrhage:
  and extracellular fluid, 487
  gastrointestinal, TPN for, 178
  in hemodialysis patients, 67
  intestinal, 68
  intraalveolar, Goodpasture's syndrome and, 113
  lung, Goodpasture's syndrome and, 229–230
  mediastinal, 67
  subarachnoid, 527
Henle's loop, ammonia in, 361
Henoch-Schönlein Syndrome, 110, 230
  IgA nephropathy and, 214
Heparin, 160, 166
  chronic therapy, osteoporosis and, 412
  degradation of, 67
  elimination of, 148
  hypoaldosteronism due to, 326–327
  sensitivity, 66–67
Hepatitis B, vaccine for, 70
Herbicide, 91
Hernia:
  abdominal, 29
  CAPD and, 29–30
  inguinal, 37
  of Morgagni, 29
  obturator, 29
  Richters, 29
  umbilical, 37
Herpes simplex, acyclovir for, 144
Hexadimethrine, 204
Heymann nephritis, 198, 201, 212
Histadine, 178
Histamine(s):
  endogenous release of, 2
  and PTH secretion, 380
  and vasopressin, 530
Histiocytosis, malignant, 527
Histocompatibility, and blood transfusions, 120–126

Histocompatibility complex, 110
Histocytosis, granulomatous, 533
Histocytosis X, and diabetes insipidus, 533
HLA (human leukocyte antigen) renal transplantation and, 108–110
HLA-BW35:
  Berger's syndrome and, 112
  glomerulonephritis and, 109
HLA-DR, type matching for, 120–122
HLA-DR2, and anti-GBM nephritis, 230
HLA-DRW6, graft rejection and, 122–123
Hodgkin's disease, SIADH and, 526
Hodgkin's lymphoma, SIADH and, 526
Homocystinuria, osteoporosis and, 411
Homovanillic acid, 270
  in cerebrospinal fluid, 528
Hormone(s):
  growth, 277
  sex steroid, 521
Hospitalization, duration of, 10
Host defense, 255–256
H1-receptor antagonist, 148
H2-receptor antagonist, 149
H reflex, in hemodialysis patients, 62
Human chorionic gonadotropin, hemodialysis and, 68
Human leukocyte antigen, 108–110
Hydralazine, 160, 168
  dosage modification for, 152
  in hypertension, 290
Hydrocarbon, exposure to, and Goodpasture's syndrome, 230
Hydrocele, 29–30
Hydrocephalus, and diabetes insipidus, 533
Hydrochlorothiazide, 160, 172
  for hypertension, 289, 292
Hydrothorax, 30
Hydroxyapatite, release of, metabolic acidosis and, 309
18-Hydroxycorticosterone, 326
4-Hydroxy-3-methoxyphenylglycol, 269
Hydroxyproline:
  excretion of, 432
  urinary, in osteopetrosis, 420
Hydroxy urea, 262
Hydroxyzine, 148, 160, 166
Hyperaldosteronism:
  heparin-induced, 326–327
  primary, mineralocorticoid excess and, 534
Hyperalimentation:
  intravenous, and osmotic diuresis, 534
  and magnesium metabolism, 465–468
Hyperammonemia, transient, in neonates, 36
Hypercalcemia:
  and acid-base homeostasis, 307–309
  bone resorption and, 300, 309
  CAPD for, 39
  and diabetes insipidus, 534
  diagnosis of, 385–386
  endogenous, 301
    metabolic alkalosis and, 310
  exogenous, 301
    metabolic acidosis and, 310
  familial hypocalciuric, 383
  metabolic acidosis and, 310
  parathyroid hormone and, 307
  and vasopressin-resistant polyuremia, 521
  and vasopressin, 530
  vitamin D in, 303
Hypercalciuria:
  renal, diagnosis of, 411
  sodium loading and, 439
  vitamin D in, 303
Hypercapnia, 303
Hypercarbonatemia, parathyroid hormone and, 307
Hypercatabolism:
  in acute renal failure, 176, 192
  amino acid therapy for, 186
  nutritional management of, 192–193
Hypercellularity, mesangial, 209–211
Hypercholesterolemia, hypertension and, 291
Hypercortisolism, 419
Hyperfiltration, compensatory, 205
Hypergammaglobulineamia, idiopathic, renal tubular acidosis in, 326
Hyperglycemia:
  and hyperinsulinemia, 453
  hypertonic hyponatremia and, 524
Hyperinsulinemia, and hyperglycemia, 453
Hyperkalemia:
  amino acid therapy for, 178
  distal acidification and, 352–355
  diuretics and, 154
  NSAIDs and, 148
  potassium supplements and, 292
  in renal tubular acidosis, 316
Hyperlipidemia, 30
  CAPD and, 32
  carnitine deficiency and, 86
  in hemodialysis patients, 72–73
  nephrotic syndrome and, 236
Hyperlipoproteinemia, in nephrotic syndrome, 238
Hypermagnesemia:
  in diabetes mellitus, 465
  and vasopressin, 530

Hypernatremia, 537–538
  nonpolyuric, causes of, 538
Hyperosmolar solution, 6
Hyperparathyroidism:
  hypercalcemic, renal transplantation and, 419
  metabolic alkalosis and, 301
  metabolic bone disease and, 74
  in pheochromocytoma, 280
  primary, 385
    diagnosis of, 391
    dietary calcium for, 392
    normocalcemic, 392
    oral phosphate therapy for, 392
    subtle, 392
    trabecular bone features of, 408
  secondary, 388
  uremic, 61
Hyperphosphatemia:
  amino acid therapy for, 178
  hypercalcemia and, 432
  metabolic alkalosis in, 308
  parathyroid hormone and, 307
Hyperphosphaturia, vitamin D in, 303
Hypertension:
  angina pectoris and, 61
  captopril for, 61
  in children, 253
  definition of, 286
  diastolic, 286, 288–289
  drug therapy for, 168–169, 290–293
  in elderly, 285–290
  essential:
    diuretics for, 292
    hypomagnesemia in, 461
  glomerular, 205
  glomerulonephritis and, 111, 214
  glucose intolerance and, 291
  hypercholesterolemia and, 291
  kidney function and, 113
  labile, 271
  malignant, 225
  mild, 290–291
  obesity and, 274–277, 288
  paroxysmal, 278
  pheochromocytomas and, 278–279
  plasma aldosterone and, 324
  pseudo-, 287
  race factors and, 286
  renal artery stenosis and, 206
  renal toxicity and, 148
  renin-angiotension system in, 277
  renovascular, 277
  smoking and, 291
  sodium ingestion and, 272–274
  spontaneous, 461
  due to steroids, 116
  sustained, 278
  sympathetic nervous system in, 270–271
  systolic, 286
Hypertension Detection and Follow-Up Program Study, 289, 291
Hyperthyroidism:
  renal tubular acidosis in, 326
  vitamin D and, 431–432
    metabolites in, 419–420
Hypertonic solution, 178
Hypertrichosis, 119
Hypertriglyceridemia
  CAPD and, 22
  in hemodialysis patients, 72
  isotonic hyponatremia and, 524
Hyperuricemia, in renal failure, 148
Hyperventilation, hypophosphatemia and, 445–446
Hypnotics, 153–154, 171
Hypoalbuminemia, protein synthesis and, 238
Hypoaldosteronism, hypovolemic hypotonic hyponatremia and, 524
Hypocalcemia:
  and hypocalciuria, 382
  hypomagnesemia and, 462
  and hypophosphatemia, 382
  metabolic alkalosis and, 301
Hypocaloric diet, 277
Hypocomplementemia, 111
  vasculitis and, 232
Hypocomplementemic vasculitis-urticaria syndrome, 232
Hypoglycemic agents, 154
Hypokalemia, 291–292
  cardiac complications of, 289
  and diabetes insipidus, 534
  diagnosis of, 349
  hypomagnesemia and, 462
  and vasopressin, 530
Hypomagnesemia:
  in diabetes mellitus, 461
  diagnosis of, 469–471
  in digitalis toxicity, 468
  in hypertension, 461
  and hypokalemia, 462
  in myocardial infarction, 459–460
  therapy for, 469–471
Hyponatremia:
  dilutional, 191
  drug induced, 529
  hypertonic, 523

hypervolemic hypotonic, causes of, 525
hypokalemia and, 529
hypotonic, 523
    SIADH, 523–528
    isotonic, 524
    mannitol intoxication and, 91
    in neonates, 528
    normovolemic hypotonic, causes of, 525
    pseudo-, 524
    SIADH and, 523, 526
    therapy for, 529–532
    thiazide-induced, 39
Hypoosmolality, SIADH and, 526
Hypoparathyroidism:
    metabolic alkalosis and, 301
    pseudo-, 419
    vitamin D for, 439
Hypophosphatasia:
    adult form, 411
    vitamin D and, 437
Hypophosphatemia, 442
    acute, 453
    in alcoholic patients, 446–447
    with antacid ingestion, 448
    burn injury and, 443–444
    chronic, 453
    in diabetics, 448–449
    parathyroidectomy and, 449–450
    parathyroid hormone and, 314
    postsurgical, 442–443
    posttransplantation, 444–445
    of respiratory alkalosis, 445–446
    therapy for, 455–457
Hypopituitarism, hyponatremia and, 525
Hypoplastic corpus callosum, SAIDH and, 527
Hypoproteinemia, clofibrate and, 150
Hypotension:
    acute renal failure and, 183–184
    dialysis induced, 57–58
    drug overdose and, 87
    in hypophosphatemia, 452
    orthostatic, 59, 279, 289
    prostacyclin and, 67
    risk factors for, 57
    vasopressor agents for, 191
Hypothermia:
    accidental, peritoneal dialysis for, 39–40
    drug induced, 87
Hypothyroidism:
    hyponatremia and, 525
    in nephrotic syndrome, 238
Hypouricemia, uric acid excretion in, 524
Hypovolemia, thirst and, 489
Hypoxemia, arterial, 64

Hypoxia:
    tissue, lactic acidosis and, 337
    vasopressin secretion and, 494
Hypoxic "brain death," and diabetes insipidus, 533

[125]I-fibrinogen, fibrin deposition and, 67
[131]I-metaiodobenzylguanidine, 285
Ibuprofen, 147, 160, 165
Idiopathic membranous nephropathy, 112–113
Idiopathic nephrosis, in children, 237
IgA nephropathy, 109, 212–214
    and Henoch-Schönlein Syndrome, 112
Ileus, severe adynamic, 68
Imipramine, 134, 160, 171
Immune complex:
    circulating, 200–201, 213
    deposition of, 201
    glomerular, 213
    formation of, 198–201
Immunoglobulin:
    A (IgA):
        complement fixing, 212–213
        deposition in GBM, 199
        nephropathy, 109
        C3, in glomerular basement membrane, 108–109
    E (IgE):
        dependent platelet activating factor, 201
        peritonitis and, 24
    G (IgG):
        in glomerular basement membrane, 108–109
        in Goodpasture's syndrome, 229
        SLE and, 218
        in Henoch-Schönlein syndrome, 112
    M (IgM), in glomerular basement membrane, 108–109
        anti-GBM, 202
        deposition of, 200
        hepatitis B, 70
Immunoreactivity, leucine-enkephalinlike, 495
Immunosuppression:
    discontinuation of, in renal transplant, 115–118
    for membranoproliferative glomerulonephritis, 111
    for pyelonephritis, 261
    in renal transplantation, 107
    therapy, 115–118
Immunosuppressive agents, 149–150, 167
Indomethacin, 147, 160, 165

Indomethacin, (Continued):
  and hyponatremia, 525
  and vasopressin, 530
Infant(s):
  calcitonin in, 430
  chronic peritoneum dialysis in, 36
  diarrhea in, and hypernatremia, 538
  formulas, 438
  magnesium requirements in, 465
  vitamin D and, 429–431
  see also Neonate(s)
Infection(s):
  as hemodialysis complications, 70–71
  IPD and, 33
  nephrotic syndrome and, 236
  skin, 144
  urinary tract, see Urinary tract, infection of
Infection stone, 262–263
  management of, 262
Insomnia, and metabolic acidosis, 342
Insulin, 154
  administration of, in diabetics, 19–20
  and CAPD, 154
  clearance of, 8
  intraperitoneal, 21
  resistance to, in uremia, 189
  vitamin D and, 432–433
  withdrawal, hypophosphatemia and, 448
Interleukin-1, protein degradation and, 190
Intermittent Peritoneal Dialysis, 32–34
International Study of Kidney Disease in Children, 209
Intestine(s):
  diffuse ganglioneuromatosis of, 281
  hemorrhage of, 68
  magnesium absorption of, 465
Intoxication, organic mercury, 91
Intravenous fluid, high sodium content in, and osmotic diuresis, 534
Iolbutamide, and vasopressin, 530
Ionophore A 23187:
  intracellular calcium and, 312
  intracellular pH and, 313
  osteoclast formation and, 423
IPD, see Dialysis, intermittent peritoneal
Iron:
  absorption of, 41
  deficiency of, 63
Irradiation, cell proliferation and, 423
Irritability, and metabolic acidosis, 342
Isoniazid, 160, 162
  elimination of, 144
  excretion of, 138
  for tuberculosis, 438

Isophosphamide, and vasopressin, 530
Isoproterenol, 134
  derivatives of, 292
  stimulation of vasopressin, 494
  and vasopressin release, 530
Isotonic solution, 6
Isoxazolyl, derivatives of, 146

Joint National Committee on Detection, Evaluation, and Treatment of High Blood Pressure, 290

Kaliuresis, water immersion and, 239
Kanamycin, 160, 162
  dosage modification for, 142
Ketoacidosis, 329–336
  diabetic, 329–330, 448
Ketoconazole, 160, 162
  elimination of, 143–144
Kidney:
  acid secretion by, 300
    dietary intake and, 317–322
  acidification by:
    in elderly, 328
    hypercalcemia and, 310–311
  clearance of drugs, 136
  cyctic disease of, 64
  drug excretion by, 133
  effects of vasopression on, 511–516
  failure of, drug metabolism and, 135
  function of, effect of PTH on, 389–390
  medulla, hypertonicity of, 255
  noninflammatory lesions of, 225
  parenchyma of, computed tomography of, 257
  pelvicalyceal calcifications of, 322
  polycystic, 85
  PTH metabolism by, 376
  sodium excretion by, dopamine regulation of, 277
  transplantation, in CAPD patients, 9
  see also Renal
Klinefelter's syndrome, diagnosis of, 411
Krebs cycle, enzyme deficiencies in, 340

Lactate:
  absorption in peritoneal cavity, 7
  clearance of, 38
  in isotonic solutions, 6
  in peritoneum membrane, 7
Lactation:

magnesium requirements during, 465
vitamin D deficiency and, 420
Lactic acidosis, *see* Acidosis, lactic
Lactobacillus, 252
Lactobacillus acidophillus, 342
Lactose, intolerance, hypernatremia and, 538
Lactulose, and hypernatremia, 538
Laennec's cirrhosis, diagnosis of, 411
Lanthanum, and PTH secretion, 379
Lanthanum chloride, calcium uptake and, 312
L-carnitine, 21, 33, 86–87
L-dihydroxy-phenylalanine, 268
L-dopa (L-dihydroxy-phenylalanine), 134, 268
Lecithin-cholesterol acyltransferase, 40
Legionella pneumophila, 71, 252
Leukemia:
    and diabetes insipidus, 533
    Fanconi syndrome in, 329
    SIADH and, 526
Leukocyte(s):
    polymorphonuclear, 255
    suppression of, 25–26
Leukocyte pyrogen, protein degradation and, 190
Leukocytosis, steroid induced, 115
Leukocyturia, in Wegener's granulomatosis, 231
Leutenizing hormone, hemodialysis and, 68
Libido, zinc therapy for, 68
Lidocaine, 134, 150, 160, 168
    clearance of, 149
Lincomycin, 160, 164
    elimination of, 147
Lipase, clearance of, 37
Lipid(s):
    infusions of, for renal failure, 190–191
    liver synthesis of, 238
    metabolism of, effect of PTH on, 398–399
    plasma, DL carnitine for, 87
Lipoprotein(s):
    high density, 238
        L-carnitine and, 86
    plasma, in nephrotic syndrome, 238
    pre-beta, L-carnitine and, 86
    serum, CAPD and, 15–16
Lithium, 88, 90
    dosage modification for, 142
    induced nephrotic syndrome, 209
    intoxication:
        CAPD for, 39
        and diabetes insipidus, 534
    and PTH secretion, 379
    renal acidification and, 327–328
    vasopressin and, 529–530

Lithium carbonate, 153, 160, 171
    excretion of, 138
Liver:
    acute coma of, 38
    blood flow in, cimetidine and, 149
    cirrhosis of, 425
    disease:
        alcoholic, 213
        lactic acidosis and, 337
    drug biotransformation in, 132
    drug clearance by, 136
    hypertrophy of, 238
    metabolism of, in acute renal failure, 187–190
    PTH metabolism by, 374–376
Looser's zones, 316
Lorazepam, elimination of, 153
L-tyrosine, 268
Lues granuloma, and diabetes insipidus, 533
Lung(s):
    abscess of, SIADH and, 526
    carcinoma of, SIADH and, 526
    complications of, 30
    disease of, vasopressin secretion and, 528
    drug clearance in, 136
    fibrosis, paraquat poisoning and, 91–92
    hemorrhage of:
        Goodpasture's syndrome and, 229–230
        smoking and, 230
    obstructive disease of, 289
    pathologic changes of, in hemodialysis patients, 62
    recurrent infection of, hypophosphatemia and, 453
Lupus erythematosus:
    crescent formation in, 114
    renal toxicity in, 148
    systemic:
        membrane attack complex in, 202
        renal transplantation and, 109
Lupus nephritis, 205
    monocytes in, 221
    renal biopsy for, 208
    SLE and, 225
    subepithelial deposits in, 226
    WHO classification of, 221–222
Lymphocyte(s):
    B, 65
    in hemodialysis patients, 65
    immunoreactive, 125
    mitogen stimulated, 213
    T, 65
Lymphoma, cyclosporin A induced, 118, 120
Lymphopenia, T-cell regulation and, 218

Maalox, phosphate depletion with, 448
Magnesium:
  cellular, measurements of, 457–458
  daily nutritional requirements for, 466
  deficiency:
    treatment of, 467, 469–471
  depletion of, diagnosis of, 469–471
  intestinal absorption of, 465
  intracellular, cellular function and, 469
  membrane stabilizing effect of, 458
  metabolism of:
    in diabetes mellitus, 464–465
    diuretics and, 468–469
  and PTH secretion, 379
  urinary excretion of, 465
  see also Hypermagnesemia;
    Hypomagnesemia
Magnesium hydroxide, in antacids, 448
Malabsorption syndrome, hypomagnesemia in, 462
Malic acid, and renal tubular acidosis, 317
Malnutrition:
  in acute renal failure, 175, 192
  in breastfeeding, and hypernatremia, 538
  and diabetes insipidus, 534
  IPD and, 33
  protein-calorie, in hemodialysis patients, 73–74
Manganese, and PTH secretion, 379
Manic depression, lithium for, 153
Mannitol, 88, 91
  intoxication, 39
  and osmotic diuresis, 534
Maple syrup urine disease, 36
Maprotiline, 88, 90
Marfan's syndrome, osteoporosis and, 411
Margarine, vitamin D in, 438
Mastocytosis, systemic, osteoporosis and, 412
McArdle's syndrome, lactic acidosis in, 344–346
MCNS (minimal change nephrotic syndrome), 209–211
  steroids for, 215–216
Meclofenamate, 160, 165
Medial nerve, peripheral entrapment of, 63
Mediterranean fever, familial:
  amyloidosis and, 114
  hemodialysis for, 83
Mefenamic acid, 160, 165
Megacolon, 281
Membrane:
  acrylonitrile, 64, 65
  cellulose acetate, 64
  cuprophane, 64, 65
  lysosomal, 79
  permeable polysulfone, 191
  polyacrylonitrile, 65,73, 83
  regenerated cellulose, 64, 65
Membrane attack complex, 202
Membrane integrity, phosphate depletion in, 454
Membrane permeability, CAPD and, 21
Membranoproliferative glomerulonephritis, 110–111, 215
Membranous glomerulopathy, 212
Meningitis:
  and diabetes insipidus, 533
  SIADH and, 527
Menopause, osteoporosis and, 407
Menstruation, retrograde, 32
Meperidine, 134, 160, 170
  chronic use of, 152
Meprobamate, 88, 160, 171
  dosage modification for, 142, 154
  elimination of, 153
Mercuric chloride, acute renal failure due to, 181–182
Mercury (organic), 88
Mesangial cell, HLA BW35 and, 110
Mesangial IgA nephropathy, 109–112, 213
Mesangial proliferative glomerulonephritis, 208
Mesothelium:
  absorption of, 2
  cellular degeneration of, 4
  edema of, 4
  intercellular gaps of, 2
  loss of microvillae in, 7
  permeability of, 2
Metabolic acidosis, see Acidosis, metabolic
Metanephrine, 269
Metastatic bone disease, 421
Metformin, 339
Methadone, 152, 160, 170
Methanol, 88, 91
  poisoning by, metabolic acidosis and, 348
Methaqualone, 88, 90, 160, 171
  elimination of, 1534
Methenamine, 160
  for urinary tract infections, 147
Methenamine hippurate, 259–260
Methenamine mandalate, 259–260
Methicillin, 160, 163
  excretion of, 138
Methionine, 318
  plasma, in pediatric patients, 187
Methoclopramide, 160, 170
Metholazone, 172

INDEX 575

Methotrexate, 160, 167
  dosage modification for, 142, 150
  excretion of, 138, 149
Methoxyfluorane
  and diabetes insipidus, 534
  and vasopressin, 530
Methoxytryramine, 270
Methsuximide, 88, 90
Methyldopa, 160, 168
  excretion of, 138
  vs. guanabenz, 293
  for hypertension, 289, 292
Methylprednisolone, 117
  for glomerulonephritis, 216
  for immunosuppression, 115
  for lupus nephritis, 227–228
Metoclopramide, 153
Metolazone, 160
Metoprolol, 134, 160, 168
Metronidazole, 160, 164
Mezlocillin, 160, 163
  dosage modification for, 146
Miconazole, 26, 162
  absorption of, 144
Microangiopathy, thrombotic, 225
Micrococcus, 252
Microscopy:
  immunoelectron, 228
  immunofluoresence, 209
  light, for lupus nephritis, 221
  phase contrast, 207
Micturition, hypertension and, 278
Middle molecule:
  PTH and, 391
  toxicity of, 77–78
  in uremia, 391
  uremic sickness and, 33
Milk:
  breast, vitamin D in, 430
  commercial, 430
  vitamin D in, 438
    compounds in, 426–429
Mineral, metabolism of, during pregnancy, 420
Mineralcorticoid:
  excess of, 534
  synthesis of, 326
Mineralization, tetracycline analysis of, 406–407
Minimal change nephrotic syndrome, 209–211
  steroids for, 215–216
Minocycline, 160, 164
Minoxidil, 160, 168
Mithramycin, nephrotoxicity of, 150

Mitochondria, oxidative phosphorylation in, 441
Molecule, middle, toxicity of, 77–78
Monoclonal hybridoma antithymocyte globulin, 118
Monocyte(s):
  glomerular hypercellularity and, 203
  glomerulonephritis and, 203
  in lupus nephritis, 221
Morphine, 134, 152, 160, 170
  and hyponatremia, 525
Morquio's syndrome, osteoporosis and, 411
Moxalactain, 163
Moxalactam, 160
  dosage modification for, 142, 146
Mucopolysaccharide, polysulfonated, 326
Mucosa, gastrointestinal, drug diffusion through, 133
Multiple myeloma, *see* Myeloma, multiple
Multiple sclerosis, SAIDH and, 527
Muscle(s):
  intracellular pH of, 306
  pain in, phosphorus depletion and, 452–453
  respiratory, effect of hypophosphatemia on, 453
  skeletal, *see* Skeletal muscle
Muscular dystrophy:
  phosphorus metabolism in, 441
  role of PTH in, 389
Mushrooms, 88
  toxic, 91
Myalgias, T-cell regulation and, 218
Myambutol, 159
Mycobacterium chelonei, 25
Mycobacterium tuberculosis, 25
Mycoses, systemic, 143
Myelinolysis, central pontine, and hyponatremia, 530
Myeloma:
  amyloidosis and, 114
  multiple:
    and diabetes insipidus, 534
    diagnosis of, 411
    renal tubular acidosis in, 325–326
Mylanta, phosphate depletion with, 448
Myocardial infarction, magnesium depletion in, 459–460
Myocarditis, catecholamine, 278
Myocardium:
  calcium content of, 388
  effect of phosphate depletion on, 450–452
Myopathy:
  chronic alcoholism, 462

NMR for, 441
in renal disease, 150
Myosin, calcium binding by, 463

N-acetylprocainamide, elimination of, 150
Nadolol, 160, 168
  dosage modification for, 142, 152
Nafcillin, 160, 163
  pharmacokinetics of, 26–27
Nalidixic acid, 160, 164
  for urinary tract infections, 147, 260
Naproxen, 147, 160, 165
Nasopharynx, carcinoma of, SIADH and, 526
National CAPD (continuous ambulatory peritoneal dialysis) Registry, 9
National Institutes of Health, 9, 40
Natriuresis, water immersion and, 239
Nausea:
  CAPD and, 20
  dialysis and, 87
  hemodialysis and, 78
  prostacyclin and, 67
  vasopressin secretion and, 494
N-desmethylmethsuximide, charcoal hemoperfusion of, 90
Necrosis:
  acute papillary, 148
  acute tubular, 176
  aseptic, 116
Neitilmicin, 28
  pharmacokinetics of, 27
Neomycin, drug interaction with, 151
Neonate(s):
  hyponatremia in, 528
  transient hyperammonemia in, 36
  vasopressin secretion in, 508–509
  see also Infant(s)
Neoplasia, multiple endocrine, 281
Nephramine, 186
Nephrectomy:
  and acid load, 306
  glomerulosclerosis and, 211
  for stones, 262
Nephritis:
  anti-GBM, 114, 202, 228–230
  antibodies mediating, 201
  diffuse proliferative, 225
  familial, 233
    "basket-weave," 233
  Goodpasture's syndrome and, 113
  Heymann, 198, 201
    membranous glomerulopathy and, 212
  interstitial, and diabetes insipidus, 534

lupus, 205
  and diabetes insipidus, 534
  mesangial, 220
  nephrotoxic serum, 206
  "non-Goodpasture's anti-GBM," 114
  rapidly progressing, 110
  serum sickness, 199, 201
  SLE, 219
Nephrocalcinosis:
  in children, 323
  and citrate excretion, 322–324
  medullary calcium in, 313
  in renal tubular acidosis, 315, 316, 322–324
Nephrolithiasis, 316
  in renal tubular acidosis, 321–322
Nephrons, mass of, glomerulosclerosis and, 211
Nephropathy:
  Berger's, 110, 112
  diabetic, hypotension and, 57
  experimental membranous, 198
  idiopathic membranous, 110, 112–113
  IgA, 109, 199, 200, 212–214
  membranous, 113, 208, 235
    nephrotic syndrome and, 209
  mesangial, 112
  and Schönlein-Henoch syndrome, 112
Nephrostomy, percutaneous, 263
Nephrotic syndrome, 112
  biopsy for, 208
  in children, 237
  complications of, 236–239
  congenital, 238–239
  doxorubicin and, 204
  drug induced, 209
  effect of PTH on, 389–390
  glomerulonephritis and, 214
  hormone binding proteins in, 238
  and hyponatremia, 525
  immunological alterations in, 208–209
  minimal change, 209–211
    steroids for, 215–216
  proteinuria and, 235–236
  refractory, 239
  steroid resistant, 237
  urinary loss in, 425
  see also Glomerulonephritis; Glomerulopathy(ies)
Nephrotoxicity:
  aminoglycoside induced, 145
  of cyclosporin A, 119
  synergistic, 143
Nervous system:
  adrenergic, in essential hypertension, 267–274

INDEX   577

autonomic, hemodialysis and, 59
central, *see* Central nervous system
peripheral, effect of PTH on, 386–387
sympathetic, *see* Sympathetic nervous system
N-ethylmaleimide, and vasopressin, 530
Neuroblastoma:
  nasal, SIADH and, 527
  vasopressin and, 526
Neurofibromatosis, in pheochromocytoma, 279–280
Neuroma, multiple mucosal, 281
Neuron, sympathetic, depolarization of, 269
Neuropathy:
  autonomic, CAPD and, 20
  peripheral, in hemodialysis patients, 62–63, 87
Neurotensin, and vasopressin, 530
Neurotransmitters, biosynthesis of, 268–269
Neutrophil(s):
  chemotaxis, 219
  degranulation of, 66
  glomerulonephritis and, 203
Nicotine, stimulation of vasopressin by, 494, 530
Nifedipine, 150, 160, 169
  in hypertension, 290
Nitrates, organic, 134
Nitrofurantoin, 160, 164
  for urinary tract infections, 147, 259–260
  for vesicoureteric reflux, 253
Nitrogen balance:
  in acute renal failure, 185
  amino acid therapy and, 178–181, 184
  in hemodialysis patients, 74
  protein, 187
Nitrogen mustard, for lupus nephritis, 227
Nitroprusside, urea clearances and, 6
Nitrosamine, in deionized water, 79
Nitrosoureas, nephrotoxicity of, 150
Nitrous oxide, and vasopressin, 530
Nomogram:
  dosing, 139–142
  of plasma clearance, 137
Nonrenal clearance, 136
Nonsteroidal antiinflammatory drugs, 147–148
Norepinephrine, 268
  age factors and, 287
  distribution of, 60
  hemodialysis and, 60
  in hypertension, 270–271
  hypotension and, 59–60
  inhibition of vasopressin, 494
  metabolic clearance rate, 60

obesity and, 276
production rate, 60
sodium ingestion and, 272–273
and vasopressin, 530
Normetanephrine, 269
Normovolemia, SIADH and, 526
Nortriptyline, 90, 160, 171
Norwegian study, 291
NSAID (nonsteroidal antiinflammatory drugs), 147–148
Nuclear magnetic resonance spectroscopy, 344–347
  phosphorus-31, 441–442
Nutrition:
  CAPD and, 15–17
  for hypercatabolism, 192–193
  hypertension and, 275
  magnesium metabolism and, 465–468
  parenteral, in acute renal failure, 175–192

Oat cell carcinoma, SIADH and, 526
Obesity:
  and hypertension, 274–277, 287
  hypothalmic, and diabetes insipidus, 533
Obstructive lung disease, beta blockers and, 289
Obturator hernia, 29–30
Oligodendrocyte, central pontine myelinolysis and, 530–531
Oliguria:
  in acute renal failure, 180
  NSAIDs and, 148
Oophorectomy, diagnosis of, 412
Opiate alkaloid, stimulation of vasopressin, 494
Opioid peptides, 530
  vasopressin secretion and, 495–497
Opthalmoplegia, NMR for, 441
Organic acid, secretion of, 37
Organic anions, ingestion of, 318
Organic mercury, intoxication, 91
Organic nitrate, 134
Organ of Zuckerkandl, pheochromocytoma in, 280
Organophosphorous, 88
Organ, recipient of, 14
Orthostatic hypotension, 59, 289
  pheochromocytoma and, 279
Osmolarity, vasopressin secretion and, 494
Osmoreceptor(s):
  cerebral, 487
  damage to, and primary adipsia, 538
  fluid intake and, 488

578 INDEX

Osmoregulation, high reset of, and hypernatremia, 538
Osmotic angiotensin II, 487
Osteoblast, 421
  effect of PTH on, 394
Osteoclast:
  effect of PTH on, 394
  in Paget's disease, 422
Osteodensitometry, 31
Osteodystrophy:
  and peritoneal dialysis, 31
  renal, 31
    aluminum and, 415–419
Osteofibrosis, 71
Osteogenesis imperfecta tarda, 411
Osteomalacia:
  aluminum toxicity and, 71–72
  in children, 315
  chronic metabolic acidosis in, 314
  renal tubular acidosis and, 315
  trabecular bone features of, 408
  vitamin D and, 434–436
Osteopenia, in renal tubular acidosis, 316
Osteopetrosis:
  in children, 420
  trabecular bone features of, 409
Osteoporosis:
  bone volume decrease in, 405
  diagnosis of, 410
  idiopathic, 411
  juvenile, 411
  postmenopausal, 407, 411
  secondary, 411
  senile, 411
  trabecular bone features of, 408
  vitamin D and, 437–438
Osteosclerosis, radiologic, 415
Ototoxicity, aminoglycoside induced, 145
Ovalain, and vasopressin, 530
Oxacillin, 160, 163
Oxalosis, and diabetes insipidus, 534
Oxazepam, 160
  elimination of, 153
Oxilorphan, inhibition of vasopressin, 494
Oxlinic acid, for urinary tract infections, 260
Oxypurinol, elimination of, 148
Oxytetracycline, 160, 164
Oxytocin:
  and hyponatremia, 525
  and vasopressin, 530

Paget's disease, 422
  trabecular bone features of, 409

Pain, vasopressin secretion and, 494
Palpitation, pheochromocytoma and, 278
Pancreas, carcinoma of, SIADH and, 526
Pancreatitis:
  acute, 37
    hypocalcemia and, 382
    and PTH secretion, 382–383
  hemorrhagic, 37
  peritoneal dialysis and, 37
Pancytopenia, 80
Papaverine, and lactic acidosis, 346
Parachlorophenylalanine, for diarrhea, 336
Paraproteinemia, isotonic hyponatremia and, 524
Paraquat, 88–89
Parathyroidectomy:
  for acute uremia, 386
  cardiac lesions and, 388
  in chronic renal failure, hypophosphatemia and, 449–450
Parathyroid gland:
  adenoma of, 378
  carcinoma of, 393–394
  secretory proteins of, 373–374
Parathyroid hormone:
  and acid-base homeostasis, 307–309
  anabolic effects of, 395–396
  bioassay eff, 384–385
  biosynthesis of, 371, 373
  bone resorption and, 305
  calcium regulation of, 374
  CAPD and, 21, 22
  catabolic effects of, 396
  cellular degradation of, 379
  cellular transport of, 372–373
  and euglucocerticord. 384
  metabolism of:
    bone, 376–377
    kidney, 376
    liver, 374–376
    peripheral, 372
  and plasma calcium, 300
  secretion of:
    calcium regulation of, 377–380
    humoral factors and, 380
    in vivo regulation of, 380–381
  toxicity of, 386
  in uremia, 189
  variations in, in hyperparathyroidism, 392–393
  vascular effects of, 397–398
  water metabolism and, 521–522
Parathyroid secretory protein, 373–374

INDEX

Parenteral nutrition, in acute renal failure, 175–192
Paroxysmal hypertension, 278
Parvalbumin, calcium binding by, 463
Pelvic inflammatory disease, *Chlamydia trachomatis* and, 252
Penicillin, 146, 163
   excretion of, 138
Penicillin G, 26, 160, 163
   dosage modification for, 142
   excretion of, 138
   pharmacokinetics of, 26–27
Pentazocine, 152, 160, 170
Pentobarbital, 160, 171
Pentolinium:
   norepinephrine and, 272
   in pheochromocytoma, 283–284
Penylbutazone, 160
Peptides, proteolytic activity of, 190
Perforating granuloma annulare, vitamin D and, 439–440
Pericarditis:
   dialysis for, 40
   IPD and, 33
   relapsing, 87
Peripheral nervous system, effect of PTH on, 386–387
Peripheral neuropathy, hemoperfusion for, 62–63, 87
Peripheral vascular disease:
   CAPD and, 32
   pindolol for, 292
Peritoneography, of catheter placement, 37
Peritoneal dialysis:
   chronic peritoneal, in infants, 36
   continuous ambulatory peritoneal, 1
     acute aluminum intoxication and, 32
     albumin and, 18
     aluminum hydroxide and, 23
     ascites and, 38
     calcium balance and, 15
     vs. CCPD, 35
     cost of, 15
     dextrose and, 16
     diabetics and, 16, 18
     in end-stage renal disease, 9
     free amino acid and, 16
     grafts and, 17
     hemoglobin and, 18, 21
     high density lipoprotein cholesterol and, 16
     hypertriglyceridemia and, 22
     insulin administration and, 19
     magnesium balance and, 15
     nitrogen balance and, 15, 17
     nondiabetics and, 16, 18
     nutrition and, 15–17
     parathyroid hormone and, 21
     phosphorus balance and, 15
     plasma lipid and, 16
     potassium and, 15–18
     serum cholesterol and, 15
     serum creatinine and, 21
     serum lipoprotein cholesterol and, 16
     serum phosphate and, 31
     serum triglyceride and, 15, 18, 21, 32
     sexual activity and, 20
     tyrosine-phenylalanine ratio and, 15
     very low density lipoprotein-cholesterol and, 15
     very low density lipoprotein-triglyceride and, 15, 16
   continuous cycling peritoneal, 1, 34–36
   creatinine clearance of, 7
   glucose absorption from, 3
   intermittent peritoneal, 1, 18, 22, 32–34
     vs. CAPD, 33
     chronic, 33
   for accidental hypothermia, 39–40
   in children, 36
   iron absorption and, 41
   maple syrup urine disease and, 36
   osmotic agents in, 4
   osteodystrophy and, 31
   for psoriasis, 83
   theophylline clearance of, 7
Peritoneum:
   clearance of, 6
   microcirculation of, 2, 41
   net sieving coefficients of, 5
   transport in, 7–9
   ultrafiltration by, 1–5
   ultrastructural analysis of, 4
Peritonitis:
   acute, in rats, 3
   asymptomatic, 24
   CAPD and, 22–24, 23
   in children, 237
   fungal, 26
   glucose absorption and, 2
   in hemodialysis patients, 68
   infectious, 23
   in rats, 3
   nonbacterial, 24–25
   organisms causing, 25
   pneumococcal, 237
   protein loss and, 2
   starch, 24

ultrafiltration and, 2
Pesticides, 91
Phagocytosis:
  of blood leukocytes, 25
  of staphylococcus, 256
  of yeast, 256
Phenacetin:
  neuropathy, and diabetes insipidus, 534
  and vasopressin, 530
Phenformin:
  and hyponatremia, 525
  and lactic acidosis, 337, 340
  and vasopressin, 530
Phenobarbital, 160, 171
  digitoxin interaction, 152
  dosage modification for, 142, 154
  elimination of, 153
Phenolsulfotransferase, 269
Phenothiazine(s):
  elimination of, 153
  and vasopressin, 530
Phenylalanine, in acute uremia, 189
Phenylbutazone, 88, 147, 165
  digitoxin interaction, 152
  overdose, 89
Phenylephrine, 59
4-Phenylethanulamine-N-methyltransferase, 268
Phenytoin, 88, 90, 160, 170
  cimetidine interaction, 149
  digitoxin interaction, 152
  metabolism of, 138
  pharmacokinetics of, 135
Pheochromocytoma, 277–286
  diagnosis of, 282–286
  etiology of, 279–281
Phosphate(s):
  depletion of, 303
    antacid ingestion and, 448
    metabolic consequences of, 450–455
  deprivation of, in acute acid load, 305
  homeostasis, PTH in, 402
  mobilization of, from bone, 449
  oral, for hyperparathyroidism, 392
  parenteral administration of, 457
  for diabetes mellitus, 448
Phosphate-dependent glutaminase, 357
Phosphate-independent glutaminase, 357
Phosphaturia, vitamin D in, 303
Phosphoenolpyruvate carboxykinase, 341
Phosphofructokinase, 337
Phospholipid(s):
  metabolism of:

  effect of PTH on, 398–399
  phosphate depletion and, 455
  renal, 14 C-labeled choline in, 182
Phosphorus:
  depletion of, biochemical consequences of, 456
  metabolism of, disorders of, 440–442
  -31 nuclear magnetic resonance, 441–442
  in urine, 448
  see also Hypophosphatemia
Phosphorylase kinase, in hypercatabolic renal failure, 189
Pindolol, 160, 169
  for hypertension, 292
Pine oil, 88
Piperacillin, 160, 163
  dosage modification for, 142, 146
Piroxicam, 147, 160, 165
Pituitary dwarfism, 277
Pituitary gland:
  postpartum necrosis of, 533
  surgery to, and diabetes insipidus, 533
Pituitary-ovarian function, 68
Plasma clearance, 136–138, 139
Plasmapheresis:
  for anti-GBM antibodies, 230
  clearance of quinine, 39
  for glomerulonephritis, 216
  for Goodpasture's syndrome, 230
  for lupus nephritis, 228
Platelet(s):
  aggregation, 65, 238
  concentration of, in pheochromocytoma, 285
  effect of PTH on, 388–389
  factor IV, 65
  in hemodialysis patients, 64–65
  IgE activation of, 201
Plethysmography, body, 30
Pleura, effusion of, 30
Pneumonia:
  in congestive heart failure, and hypernatremia, 538
  SIADH and, 526
  TPN for, 178
Pneumothorax, acute, SIADH and, 527
Poisoning:
  ethylene glycol, 39
  metal, 91
  methanol, 348
  mushroom, 91
  self-, 90
  solvent, 91

therapy for, 87–92
uremic, 63
Polyanion, in peritoneal dialysis, 4
Polyarteritis nodosa, 230
   SIADH and, 527
Polycation, circulating, in proteinuria, 204
Polycystic kidney disease, 85
Polylysine, 204
Polyneuropathy, 147
Polysaccharide dextran, 199
Polyuria in acute renal failure, 180
   differential diagnosis of, 535–536
   vasopressin-resistant, hypercalcemia and, 521
Polyuria, vasopressin-resistant, 515
Porphyria, acute intermittent, 527
Porphyria cutanea tarda, 69
Porphyrin, plasma level of, 69
Postmenopause, osteoporosis and, 407
Poststreptococcal glomerulonephritis, 214–215
Potassium:
   dietary, depletion of, 352–354
   excretion of, fludrocortisone and, 324
   plasma, hydrochlorothiazide and, 292
   serum:
      amino acids and, 178
      CAPD and, 16, 33
   supplements, and digitalis therapy, 292
Potency, sexual, zinc therapy for, 68
Povidone iodine, for urinary tract infections, 261
Prazosin, 160, 169
Prednisolone, for immunosuppression, 115
Prednisone:
   for Goodpasture's syndrome, 230
   for immunosuppression, 115
Pregnancy:
   hemodialysis and, 82
   mineral metabolism during, 420
   normovolemic hypotonic hyponatremia and, 525
   PTH during, 420
   SLE and, 227
Primidone, 160, 170
Probenecid, 148, 160, 165
Procainamide, 160, 168
   excretion of, 138
   pharmacokinetics of, 141
   in renal insufficiency, 150
Progressive systemic sclerosis, 113
Prolactin, and PTH secretion, 380
Proliferative lupus nephritis, 221
   monocytes in, 221

Proparathyroid hormone, 371
Propoxyphene, 134, 160, 170
   chronic use of, 152
   intoxication, and diabetes insipidus, 534
   and vasopressin, 530
Propranolol, 134, 160, 169
   for hypertension, 292
   metabolism of, 138
Prostacyclin, 65
   as anticoagulant, 67
Prostaglandin:
   endogenous release of, 2
   formation of, 64
   inhibition of, 147
   and PTH secretion, 380
   regulation of vasopressin, 516–521
Prostaglandin E:
   antiinflammatory effect of, 206–207
   and glomerulonephritis, 207
   and vasopressin release, 530
Prostaglandin E2, protein degradation and, 190
Prostaglandin I2, as anticoagulant, 67
Prostate, carcinoma of, SIADH and, 526
Prostatitis, 258
Protamine, 204
   and mesothelial permeability, 6
   and peritoneal permeability, 7
Proteases, circulating, 192
Protein(s):
   binding of, 137
   catabolism, 176
   degradation:
      in nonuremic postoperative patients, 193
      pharmacological therapy for, 192
   degradation of, 185, 188
   depletion of, and diabetes insipidus, 534
   dietary:
      albuminuria and, 205
      glomerular sclerosis and, 205
   magnesium binding to, 458
   metabolism, tetracyclines and, 147
   plasma, drug binding to, 134–135
   secretory, of parathyroid gland, 373–374
   synthesis, hypoalbuminemia and, 238
   tube feeding of, and osmotic diuresis, 534
   vitamin D binding, 425–426
Proteinuria:
   antilaminin and, 202
   circulating polycations in, 204
   and eosinophilic cystitis, 257
   in familial nephritis, 233
   glomerulonephritis and, 214

glomerulosclerosis and, 111, 211
light-chain, 329
mechanisms of, 204–205
methylprednisolone and, 228
in Wegener's granulomatosis, 231
Proximal convoluted tubule, acidification in, 313
Pruritis, 66
in hemodialysis patients, 69
Pruvate dehydrogenase complex, enzyme deficiencies in, 340
Pseudofracture, 316
Pseudohypertension, 287
Pseudohyponatremia, isotonic hyponatremia and, 524
Pseudohypoparathyroidism, 419
vitamin D for, 439
Pseudomonas repacia, 25
Psoriasis:
hemodialysis for, 82
peritoneal dialysis for, 7, 38–39
Psychogenic polydipsia, hyponatremia and, 525
Psychosis(es):
acute, SIADH and, 527
exacerbated, hyponatremia and, 525
Psychotherapeutic drugs, 170–171
in hyponatremia, 529
PTH, *see* Parathyroid hormone
Puberty, vitamin D and, 431
Purine nucleotide cycle, 359
Puromycin aminonucleoside, proteinuria and, 204
Purpura:
Henoch-Schönlein, IgA nephropathy and, 214
nonthrombocytopenic, 112
thrombotic thrombocytopenic, 232
Pyelography, intravenous, 253
in urinary tract infections, 256
Pyelolithotomy, for stones, 262
Pyelonephritis, 251
chronic, 252
immunosuppression for, 261
Pyrasolone, overdose, 89
Pyruvate carboxylase, and lactic acidosis, 341
Pyruvate dehydrogenase, 338
Pyuria, and eosinophilic cystitis, 257

Quinidine, 88, 150, 161, 168
clearance of, 22
digoxin interaction with, 151
and intracellular calcium, 312
metabolism of, 138
Quinine, 88, 90
peritoneal dialysis of, 39

Radiation, ultraviolet, vitamin D and, 438
Radioimmunoassay, 64
of PTH, 384
Rapidly progressive glomerulonephritis, 215
Rapidly progressive nephritis, 114
Raynaud's phenomenon
pindolol for, 292
T-cell regulation and, 218
Rectum, bleeding from, 29
Rehabilitation, 84–86
Rejection, of transplant:
immunosuppression for, 115–118
management of, 107
"Rejection glomerulonephritis," 109, 235
Renal artery stenosis, 206
acute, and diabetes insipidus, 534
Renal cell carcinoma, 256
Renal clearance, 136–137
Renal disease, progression of, 205–206
Renal failure:
acute, 37
amino acid therapy for, 179
due to antibiotics, 184
due to glomerulonephritis, 176
in hemolytic uremic syndrome, 133
due to hypotension, 184, 186
liver metabolism in, 187–190
muscle metabolism in, 187–190
NSAIDs and, 148
parenteral nutrition for, 175–192
pregnancy and, 82
due to radio contrast material, 184
due to rhabdomyolysis, 184
due to sepsis, 184
survival rates from, 178
chronic:
amino acid infusion for, 177
CAPD for, 434
hemodialysis, 83
and osmotic diuresis, 534
PTH in, 402
vitamin D and, 433–434
IgA nephropathy and, 214
permanent, Wegener's granulomatosis and, 231
pharmacology of drugs in, 131–154
progressive, glomerulosclerosis and, 211
see also Uremia; Uremic syndrome

INDEX **583**

Renal tubular acidosis:
  and bone disease, 315–317
  citrate excretion and, 322–324
  diagnosis of, 411
  distal, 316
    in systemic disease, 325–326
  hyperkalemic, 316, 324–325
  hypovolemic hypotonic hyponatremia
    and, 524
  idiopathic distal, 323
  nephrocalcinosis in, 322–324
  proximal, 316
Renal tubular cell, regeneration of, 181
Renal tubular transport, of bicarbonate,
    effect of PTH on, 403
Renal vein, thrombosis of, nephrotic syndrome
    and, 238
Renin:
  effect of calcium on, 69
  plasma:
    age factors and, 287
    obesity and, 276
    water immersion and, 239
Reserpine, 161, 169
Respiratory failure, acute, SIADH and, 527
Respiratory function, CAPD and, 30–31
Respiratory muscle, effect of
    hypophosphatemia on, 453
Reticuloendothelial system, immune complex
    removal by, 201
Retinopathy, chronic hypertensive, 278
Rhabdomyolysis:
  acute, hypocalcemia and, 383
  acute renal failure and, 184
  drug-induced coma and, 176
Rheumatoid arthritis, with vasculitis, 230
Rheumatoid factor:
  glomerular disease and, 231
  IgM deposits and, 231
Rhinitis, allergic, MCNS and, 211
Rickets:
Richter's hernia, 29–30
Rickets:
  in renal tubular acidosis, 316–317
  vitamin D for, 439
Ricter's hernia, 29–30
Rifampicin, for tuberculosis, 438
Rifampin, 161, 162
  elimination of, 144
Rocky Mountain spotted fever, SAIDH and,
    527

Salicylate(s), 147

overdose, 89
Saralasin, reduced renal damage with, 143
Sarcoid granuloma, and diabetes insipidus,
    533–534
Sarcoidosis, membranous glomerulopathy
    and, 212
Schizophrenia, dialysis for, 83
Scintigram, of pheochromocytoma, 285
Scleroderma, 113
  and renal transplants, 110
Sclerosis:
  of peritoneum, 26
  progressive systemic, 113
Secobarbital, 161, 171
Sedatives, 88–90, 153–154, 171
Sepsis, acute renal failure and, 176, 183–184
Septicemia, respiratory alkalosis and, 443
Septooptic dysplasia, and diabetes insipidus,
    533
Serotonin:
  antagonists, 336
  intraplatelet, 389
Serum sickness nephritis, 199, 201
Sex hormones, steroid, and water balance, 521
Sexual intercourse, urinary tract infections and,
    259
Sheehan syndrome, and diabetes insipidus, 533
SIADH (syndrome of inappropriate ADH
    secretion), 523–528
Sicca syndrome, T-cell regulation and, 218
Sickle cell anemia, and diabetes insipidus,
    533–534
Silicon, intoxication, 79–80
Similac, 430
Sipple's syndrome, 280
Sisomicin, 28
  pharmacokinetics of, 27
Sjögren's syndrome, and diabetes insipidus,
    534
Skeletal muscle:
  effect of phosphorus depletion on,
    452–453
  effect of PTH on, 388
  magnesium and, 462–464
Skeleton:
  coupling factor in, 425
  effects of PTH on, 394–396
Skin, water loss by, 538
SLE, *see* Systemic lupus erythematosus
Smoking, cigarette:
  hypertension and, 291
  lung hemorrhage and, 230
Sodium:
  body, hypernatremia and, 537–538

584 INDEX

excretion of:
  clonidine and, 290
  dopamine regulation of, 277
ingestion of, and hypertension, 272–274
loading, hypercalciuria and, 439
mucosal, 312
and osmotic diuresis, 534
retention of, estrogen and, 521
serosal, 312
see also Hyponatremia; Hypernatremia
Sodium bicarbonate, hypertonic, for postcardiac arrest, 538
Sodium-calcium exchange system, 312
Sodium chloride:
  in hyperosmolar solutions, 6
  hypertonic, in renal failure, 538
Sodium docuste, peritoneal clearance and, 6
Sodium nitroprusside, 38
Sodium phosphate, hypertonic, and hypernatremia, 538
Sodium valproate, 170
Somatostatin:
  and PTH secretion, 380
  and vasopressin, 530
Spectroscopy, nuclear magnetic resonance, 344–347
Spermatogenesis, zinc therapy for, 68
Sphymomanometry, 287
Spinal cord, injury to, urinary tract infections and, 259
Spirography, 30
Spironolactone, 154, 161, 172
Splenectomy, transplantation and, 108
Splenomegaly, 80
Staphlococci, coagulase negative, 251
Staphylococcus aureus, 24, 25
Staphylococcus epidermidis, 251
Staphylococcus saprophyticus, 251–252
Status asthmaticus, SIADH and, 527
Steroid(s):
  for Berger's syndrome, 112
  for idiopathic membranous glomerulopathy, 216
  for immunosuppression, 115
  for lupus nephritis, 227
  for MCNS, 215–216
Stomach, drug absorption in, 133
"Strawberry gums," 231
Streptococcus bovis, 342
Streptococcus pneumoniae, 237
Streptomycin, 161, 162
  dosage modification for, 142
Streptozotocin, nephrotoxicity of, 150

Stroke, hypertension and, 286
Strontium, and PTH secretion, 379
Struvite stone, 263
Subarachnoid hemorrhage, SIADH and, 527
Substance P, and vasopressin, 530
Sucrose, in hyperosmolar solutions, 6
Sulfafurazole, for vesicoureteric reflux, 253
Sulfamethoxazole, 161, 163
  dosage modification for, 142
  for dysuria, 258
  elimination of, 146
Sulfasalazine, drug interaction, 151
Sulfasoxazole, for urinary tract infections, 258
Sulfinpyrazone, 148, 161
Sulfisoxazole, 163
  elimination of, 146
Sulfisoxole, 161
Sulfonamide, 146, 163
Sulfuric acid, in dog, and aldosterone, 355–357
Sulindac, 147, 161, 165
Sural nerve, sensory potential of, peripheral neuropathy and, 62
Surgery, patient in, hypophosphatemia of, 442–443
Sweating:
  electrolyte loss by, 489
  excessive, hypovolemic hypotonic hyponatremia and, 524
  pheochromocytoma and, 278
Sympathetic nervous system:
  hemodialysis and, 59
  and hypertension, 270
Syndrome of Inappropriate ADH Secretion (SIADH), 523–528
Systemic lupus erythematosus:
  crescent formation in, 114
  and glomerulonephritis, 217–220
  membrane attack complex in, 202
  renal manifestations of, 217–230
  renal transplantation and, 109
Systemic vascular resistance, effect of acetate on, 57
Systemic vasculitis, 230–233
Systolic hypertension, 286

Tachycardia:
  hydrochlorothiazide induced, 292
  pheochromocytoma and, 279
T-cell:
  regulation, systemic lupus erythematosus and, 218

INDEX

sensitization, 208
Telangiectasias, multiple gastric, 68
Terbutaline, 134
Testes, carcinoma of, 149–150
Testosterone, serum, and plasma zinc, 68
Tetracycline, 146, 161, 164
    calcium chelates, 406–407
    for chlamydial infection, 259
    contraindications for, 146
    excretion of, 138
Thallium, 88
    poisoning, 91
Theophylline, 88, 90–91
    cimetidine interaction, 149
    clearance of, 7
    metabolism of, 138
    and vasopressin, 530
Therapy, group, 86
Thiazides, and vasopressin, 530
Thioglycolate, and vasopressin, 530
Thiopental, and vasopressin, 530
Thioridazine:
    and hyponatremia, 525
    and vasopressin, 530
Thiothixene, and vasopressin, 530
Thirst, 487–491
    and metabolic acidosis, 342
    stimulators of, 489
Thoracolumbar system, 268
Thrombin:
    clotting time of, 66–67
    inhibitors of, 237
Thrombocytopenia:
    hemolytic uremic syndrome and, 113
    T-cell regulation and, 218
Thrombosis:
    cavernous sinus, 527
    glomerular, 225
    nephrotic syndrome and, 236–237
    renal vein, 238
Thrombotic diathesis, in nephrotic syndrome, 238
Thymoma, SIADH and, 526
Thyrocalcitonin, 306
Thyroid:
    carcinoma of, in pheochromocytoma, 280
    medullary, carcinoma of, 281, 432
    vitamin D in, 431–432
Thyroid hormone, deficiency, urinary dilution and, 523
Thyroid stimulating hormone, in congenital nephrotic syndrome, 238
Thyrotoxicosis, diagnosis of, 412

Thyroxine:
    in congenital nephrotic syndrome, 238
    in hemodialysis patients, 69
    in nephrotic syndrome, 238
Ticarcillin, 161, 163
    dosage modification of, 142, 146
    excretion of, 138
    pharmacokinetics of, 26–27
Timolol, 161, 169
Tinnitus, diuretic induced, 154
T lymphocyte, fenoprofen and, 209
Tobramycin, 162
    dosage modification for, 142
    pharmacokinetics of, 28
Tobramycin sulfate, 161
Tolazamide, 173
Tolbutamide, 161, 173
    elimination of, 154
    and hyponatremia, 525
Tolmetin, 161, 165
    nephrotic syndrome due to, 209
Tomography, computed
    of peritoneum, 38
    of pheochromocytoma, 285
    in pyelonephritis, 257
    of trabecular bone mass, 415
"Total body clearance," 136
Toxin, removal of, 88
Toxocara cati, 258
TPN (total parenteral nutrition), in acute renal failure, 175–192
Tracheotomy, in congestive heart failure, and hypernatremia, 538
Tranquilizers, 88–90
Transferrin, in hemodialysis patients, 73
Transfusion, exchange, and hypernatremia, 538
Transplantation, in CAPD patients, 17–18
Transplantation:
    renal:
        in CAPD patients, 17–18
        and diabetes insipidus, 534
        glomerular lesions in, 234–235
        glomerulonephritis in, 108–110, 235
        history of, 107
        and HLA mismatches, 119
        hypercalcemic hyperparathyroidism and, 419
        hypophosphatemia in, 444–445
        immunosuppression, 107–108
        and osmotic diuresis, 534
        rejection of, 109, 115–118
        in siblings, 124

Transplant glomerulonephritis, 109
Tranylcypromine:
  and hyponatremia, 525
  and vasopressin, 530
Trauma:
  colorie supplementation for, 190
  head, and diabetes insipidus, 533
  peripheral amino acid release and, 190
  SIADH and, 527
Tremor, cyclosporin A and, 119
Triamterene, 154, 161, 289
  serum magnesium and, 468
Tricyclic agent, elimination of, 153
Tricyclic amine, 88, 90
Trifluoperazine, and vasopressin, 530
Triglyceride(s), serum:
  CAPD and, 15
  carnitine and, 86
  in hemodialysis patients, 72
  and plasma immunoreactive insulin, 73
  steroid therapy and, 116
Triiodothyronine:
  in hemodialysis patients, 69
  in nephrotic syndrome, 238
  serum, vitamin D and, 431
  and vasopressin, 530
Trimethoprim, 161, 164
  dosage modification for, 142
  elimination of, 146
Trimethoprim-sulfamethoxazole
  for dysuria, 258
  pharmacokinetics of, 27
  for urinary tract infection, 258
Troponin, calcium binding by, 463
Tryosine-hydroxylase, 268
Tuberculoma, vasopressin and, 526
Tuberculosis:
  and diabetes insipidus, 533
  drugs for, 144
  increased incidence of, in hemodialysis patients, 70–71
  PTH in, 438–439
  SIADH and, 526
  vitamin D in, 438
Tubular necrosis, acute, and diabetes insipidus, 534
Tubular transport, drug clearance by, 136–137
Tubule:
  distal convoluted, acidification in, 318
  proximal convoluted, acidification in, 313
Tumor(s):
  bone, hypercalcemia and, 421
  giant cell, malignant, 422

  medullary thyroid, 281
  metastatic
    and diabetes insipidus, 533
    SIADH and, 527
  primary, SIADH and, 527
  renin-secreting, 277
Turner's syndrome, diagnosis of, 412
Tyrosine-phenylalanine ratio, CAPD and, 15

Ulnar nerve, peripheral entrapment of, 63
Ultrafiltration:
  ascites and, 37–38
  blood pressure and, 76
  of peritoneum, 1–5
  for psoriasis, 82–83
  rate of, 57, 84
Ultraviolet, radiation, 69
Urea:
  clearance of, 8
  nitrogen:
    in acute renal failure, 177, 185, 188–189
    hemodialysis and, 77–78
    IFD and, 33
  production of, 147
Ureaplasma urealyticum, 252
Urease inhibitor, 262
Uremia:
  acute, electrocardiogram abnormalities and, 386
  control of, in animals, 8
  essential amino acids in, 177
  glucose interance in, 154
  iron absorption in, 41
  PTH in, 389
    immunoreactivity of, 390–391
  symptoms of, 33
  see also Renal failure
Uremic bone disease, trabecular bone features of, 409
Uremic poisoning, 63
Uremic syndrome:
  PTH and, 386
Ureter, carcinoma of, vasopressin and, 526
Urethra:
  dilatation of, 259
  diverticular, 256
  shortness of, 255
Urethral syndrome, 252
  acute, treatment of, 258–259
Urethritis, nonspecific, in men, 252
Urethrotomy, internal, 259

Uric acid, nephropathy, and diabetes insipidus, 534
Urinary acidification, *see* Urine, acidification of
Urinary bladder, *see* Bladder, urinary
Urinary drainage bag, antiseptic agents in, 259–261
Urinary tract:
  bleeding of, 207
  infection of:
    acute nonobstructive, 257
    catheter associated, 261
    in children, 253
    diagnosis of, 256–258
    host parasite interaction and, 255–256
    microorganisms in, 251–252
    recurrent, 259
    therapy for, 258–261
  irritability of, 257
  obstruction of, and osmotic diuresis, 534
Urine:
  acidification of, 259
    in elderly, 328
    glucocorticoids and, 351
    hypercalcemia and, 310–311
  analysis of, for proteinuria, 235–236
  concentration of, 509–511
  dilution of, 509–511
    glucocorticoids and, 522
    thyroid hormone and, 523
  drugs in, 136–137
  metabolites of, in pheochromocytoma, 282
  midstream, bacteria in, 256
  opsonic effect of, in acute cystitis, 256
Urography, excretory, in urinary tract infections, 256
Uropathogenecity, bacterial adhesion and, 255
Uropathy, obstructive, 150
Urticaria, hypocomplementemia and, 232
Urticaria pigmentosa, osteoporosis and, 412

Valproic acid, 161
Valsalva maneuver, 59
Vancomycin, 28, 161, 164
  excretion of, 138, 147
  pharmacokinetics of, 27, 28
Vanillylmandelic acid, 269
Vascular disease, peripheral
  CAPD and, 32
  pindolol for, 292
Vascular resistance, systemic, effect of acetate on, 57

Vascular tone, magnesium and, 461
Vasculitis, systemic, 230–233
Vasoconstriction, neurogenic, sodium ingestion and, 274
Vasodilator, for hypertension, 290
Vasopressin:
  antidiuretic response to, 511
  calcium-dependent-secretion, 495
  in cirrhosis, 532
  in congestive heart failure, 532
  drug regulation of, 494
  hyponatremia and, 525
  inhibition of, 530
  nonosmotic mediation of, 497–500
  osmotic mediation of, 497–500
  peripheral action of, drugs facilitating, 530
  release of, drugs stimulating, 530
  secretion of:
    hemodynamic mechanisms of, 490
    neurophysiology of, 492–495
    thirst and, 489
  structure of, 531
  synthesis of, 491–492
  therapy, 536–537
  volume mediation of, 497–500
Vasopressinoid acid, and vasopressin, 530
Verapamil, 150, 161, 169
  for hypertension, 290
  for peripheral vasodilation, 462
Vesicoureteric reflux, 252
  in children, 253
  grades of, 254
Vesicoureteric valve, urinary tract infection and, 255
Vibrio alginalyticus, 25
Vinblastine:
  and hyponatremia, 527
  and vasopressin, 530
Vincristine:
  and hyponatremia, 525
  stimulation of vasopressin, 494
  vasopressin and, 530
Viomycin sulfate, 161
Virus:
  drugs against, 162
  Ebstein-Barr, 118
Vitamin A, in hemodialysis patients, 75
Vitamin B6, deficiency, in chronic renal failure, 75
Vitamin D:
  and acid-base homeostasis, 300–304
  binding proteins, 425–426
  compounds in milk, 426–429

deficiency:
  distal acidification and, 301, 303
  osteoporosis and, 412
 excess, metabolic alkalosis and, 301, 303
 Fifth International Workshop on, 440
 glucocorticoid and, 433
 in nephrotic syndrome, 239
 and perforating granuloma annulare, 439–440
 for rickets, 439
 and PTH secretion, 380
 seasonal variation in, 438
 in tuberculosis, 438
Vitamin K, bone protein and, 420–421
Vomiting:
 CAPD and, 20
 IPD and, 33

Warfarin, 161, 166
 cimetidine interaction with, 149
 elimination of, 148
Wasting, in acute renal failure, 192
Water:
 deprivation of, hypernatremia and, 538
 excretion of:
  in diabetes insipidus, 523
  glucocorticoids and, 522
 metabolism of, 487–538
  glucocorticoids and, 522–523
  parathyroid hormone and, 521–522
  thyroid hormone and, 523
Water balance, hormone regulation of, 521
Water immersion, for nephrotic syndrome, 239
Water transport, effect of PTS on, 403–404
Wegener's granulomatosis, 230
 and diabetes insipidus, 533
 immune complexes in, 231
Werner's syndrome, 411
Wernicke's encephalopathy, SAID and, 527–528
White blood cell(s):
 effect of PTH on, 388–389
 in hemodialysis patients, 65–66
Wilson's disease, dialysis for, 39
World Health Organization, classification of lupus nephritis, 221–224

Xanthine oxidase, inhibition of, 148

Zinc, and serum testosterone, 68
Zomepirac, 161, 165
Zuckerkandl, organ of, pheochromocytoma in, 280